Neurodevelopmental Disabilities

Dilip R. Patel · Donald E. Greydanus ·
Hatim A. Omar · Joav Merrick
Editors

Neurodevelopmental Disabilities

Clinical Care for Children and Young Adults

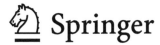 Springer

Editors

Dilip R. Patel
Department of Pediatrics and Human
 Development
Kalamazoo Center for Medical Studies
Michigan State University College
 of Human Medicine
Kalamazoo, MI 49008-1284
USA
patel@kcms.msu.edu

Hatim A. Omar
Adolescent Medicine and Young Parent
 Programs, Kentucky Clinic
Department of Pediatrics
Kentucky Children's Hospital
University of Kentucky College
 of Medicine
Lexington, KY, USA
haomar2@uky.edu

Donald E. Greydanus
Department of Pediatrics and Human
 Development
Kalamazoo Center for Medical Studies
Michigan State University College
 of Human Medicine
Kalamazoo, MI 49008-1284
USA
greydanus@kcms.msu.edu

Joav Merrick
National Institute of Child Health and
 Human Development, Health Services
 Office of the Medical Director, Division
 for Mental Retardation
Ministry of Social Affairs and Social
 Services
POBox 1260, IL-91012 Jerusalem
Israel

Kentucky Children's Hospital
University of Kentucky
Lexington, KY, USA
jmerrick@zahav.net.il

ISBN 978-94-007-0626-2   e-ISBN 978-94-007-0627-9
DOI 10.1007/978-94-007-0627-9
Springer Dordrecht Heidelberg London New York

Library of Congress Control Number: 2011922661

Printed on acid-free paper

Springer is part of Springer Science+Business Media (www.springer.com)

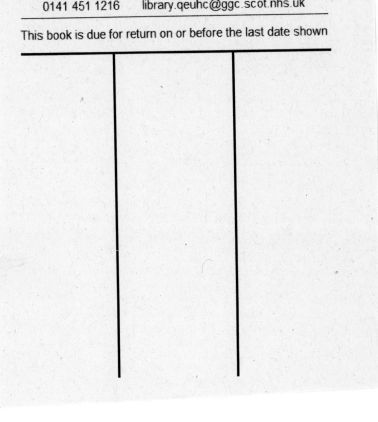

Foreword

I am very pleased to write the foreword to this book. There are a number of other related books on the subject, most notably *Developmental–Behavioral Pediatrics* now in its 4th edition [1] *Capute and Accardo's Neurodevelopmental Disabilities in Infancy and Childhood* now in its 3rd edition [2] and Rubin and Crocker's *Medical Care for Children and Adults with Developmental Disabilities* now in its 2nd edition [3], which plumb the depths of what we know about child development, developmental delays, differences and disabilities, and health care. Yet, there is always something we do not know, always something new to understand, to comprehend, and process. The fact that within the past 50 years we have seen the field of developmental pediatrics arise from relative obscurity to legitimacy in the formation of the specialties of developmental behavioral pediatrics and neurodevelopmental pediatrics within the universe of pediatrics in the United States is a testament to the realization and appreciation of the importance of promoting child health and development in our world today.

Furthermore, we have seen, in the past 50 years, the greater appreciation and respect for individuals with developmental disabilities. The dark and ugly era influenced by the pseudo-science of eugenics and the systematic marginalization and rejection of individuals with developmental disabilities by a society, which created places far from the active centers of family, community and society, morphed into overcrowded, unsanitary, and unconscionable institutions. These institutions were opened to public view in the 1960s and 1970s in the United States, as well as in the United Kingdom and Europe, then subsequently, with the Glasnost of the early 1990s, the opening of the Soviet institutions. In the past five decades we have seen deinstitutionalization, community integration, self-determination, and affirmation of the rights of individuals with intellectual and developmental disabilities in so many ways. We have witnessed laws that have assured the promotion of early intervention for infants from birth to 3 years of age, the education for all "handicapped children," employment and living opportunities for adults, the recognition of self-determination as a right, and the capstone, Americans with Disabilities Act that serves to open all of society to all people with disabilities.

The pioneering efforts that arose after the horrors of the prequel and sequel of the Second World War have promoted, through the United Nations, Human Rights for all citizens, particularly those most vulnerable – in this context, individuals with disabilities and the children of the world. Whereas in the dark ages of the first half of the twentieth century, individuals who were different were ostracized and excluded from society resulting in disruption and destruction of the values upon which our lives depend, the second half of the twentieth century has seen inclusion of individuals who are different with a spirit of acceptance, acknowledgment, and appreciation of differences between people.

In our own time we have witnessed advances in knowledge and understanding of child development, we have developed strategies and programs to improve the health and well-being of children with developmental disabilities and their families in the communities in which they live, and, in the process, we have enriched all of society. This has connected us in a myriad of ways that affirm our values of respect and personal dignity for all and for the recognition that we are all imbued with the spirit of life, that we are all interdependent upon one another, and that the ultimate measure of an individual or a society is in how the most vulnerable members of society are treated.

One of the important landmarks mentioned in the chapter on health care in this book is the turning point in the 1960s in the United States. This was initiated not originally by the then president John F. Kennedy but by his mother, Rose Kennedy, who pressed upon him and advocated for the need to address the plight of individuals with – what was then called – mental retardation. The formation and formulation of the University Affiliated Facilities, Mental Retardation Research Centers, and of the National Institute of Child Health and Development created for us – now 50 years later – the research underpinnings of what we have learned about children and adults with intellectual and developmental disabilities and the training of professionals in the interdisciplinary clinical practice of providing the necessary services in early identification, early intervention, and comprehensive care – not to mention strategies for prevention and health promotion at primary, secondary, and tertiary levels, education and social opportunities. These institutions reflect the pillars of health and well-being for our society, research, clinical practice, public health policies, and, most important of all, advocacy.

It is with this background that we now can look at this book *Neurodevelopmental Disabilities: Clinical Care for Children and Young Adults* edited by Patel, Greydanus, Omar, and Merrick. This book is by no means a repetition or a replay of the classic texts mentioned above but serves to supplement and complement existing texts by bringing an up-to-date, well-researched set of thoughtfully considered chapters to provide a readily readable and accessible way to consider the current world of child development. It offers pediatricians and other providers of child health and developmental services a way in which to confront the common reality of differences, delays, and disabilities for children and their families in the long term and in the big picture. As they point out and elaborate, it is not only important to understand the fundamentals of child development and to identify and evaluate children who are developing differently also necessary to know and understand how to make diagnoses, develop treatment plans, and communicate with families and other members of society in order to assure the optimal outcome for the child, the family, the community, and ultimately for society.

Specifically the chapters are oriented in *Google Map* kind of way – looking from the big picture to the small details, from child development in general to many specific genetic and acquired conditions in particular. Each chapter is well researched and well presented to give the reader a good grasp of the subject and a good set of references to explore in greater depth if desired. Apart from the standard set of necessary chapters in such a textbook, they have enriched the table of contents with an examination of families – parents, siblings, and other caregivers – and, in particular, the situation of the child who is adopted. I am also pleased to see the consideration given to sexuality, pain, the child with a chronic illness, and the sensitive subject of end of life and palliative care.

Although the focus of the book is on the developmental, learning, and behavioral aspects of neurodevelopmental disabilities, they do touch on the medical care of children from the clinical practice to the public health perspective. Furthermore, they tackle the challenge that all pediatricians confront, and more so to the families, when the children reach adolescence and adulthood, and they graduate from school, need to have an adult oriented physician, leave home, find a job, and begin to live as independently as possible.

Thus, I commend the editors and authors for a well-constructed and well-written book, and I recommend this book as an extremely useful and valuable text for the medical student, the resident, and for the practicing pediatrician as well as for other professionals who provide care for children.

Personally, for me it is gratifying to seeing the fruits of all the work that has gone before being translated into the promotion of good health and development for all children with freedom from unnecessary pain and suffering. But we cannot rest here, we must move forward to increase our knowledge and ability to make this a reality for all children at a global level.

Atlanta, GA   I. Leslie Rubin, MD

References

1. Carey WB, Crocker AC, Elias ER, Feldman HM, Coleman WI, editors. Developmental–behavioral pediatrics. 4th ed. Philadelphia, PA: WB Saunders; 2009.
2. Accardo PJ, editor. Capute and Accardo's neurodevelopmental disabilities in infancy and childhood. 3rd ed. Baltimore, MD: Paul H Brookes; 2008.
3. Rubin IL, Crocker AC, editors. Medical care for children and adults with developmental disabilities. 2nd ed. Baltimore, MD: Paul H Brookes; 2006.

Contents

Contributors

Erin Tentis Berglund, PhD Gillette Children's Specialty Healthcare, St Paul, MN, USA, ETBerglund@gillettechildrens.com

Katherine Bergwerk, MD Private Prictice, Nof Ayalon, IL-99785 Israel, bergwerk@bezeqint.net

Lynn M. Breau, PhD, RPsych School of Nursing and Departments of Psychology and Pediatrics, Dalhousie University, Halifax, Nova Scotia, Canada, B3H 3J5; Pediatric Complex Pain Team, IWK Health Centre, Halifax, Nova Scotia, Canada, lbreau@dal.ca

Bantu Chhangani, MD Sleep Medicine, Saint Mary's Neuroscience Program, Grand Rapids, MI, USA, bantuchhangani@yahoo.com

Teresa Crumpton, AuD Department of Speech Pathology and Audiology, Western Michigan University, Kalamazoo, MI 49008-5355, USA, teresa.crumpton@wmich.edu

Gary Diamond, MD, FAAP, FAACPDM Department of Pediatrics, Sackler School of Medicine, Tel Aviv University, Tel Aviv, Israel; Institute of Child Development and Neurology, Schneider Children's Medical Center of Israel, Clalit Health Services, 49202 Petah-Tiqva, Israel; Department of Pediatrics, Albert Einstein College of Medicine, Rose F Kennedy Center, Center for the Evaluation and Rehabilitation of Children, Bronx, NY, USA, diamondg@clalit.org.il

Nancy N. Dodge, MD, FAAP Michigan State University, Lansing, MI, USA; Neurodevelopmental Pediatrics, Helen DeVos Children's Hospital, Grand Rapids, MI 49503, USA, nancy.dodge@devoschildrens.org

Ilan Feldberg, MD, DMD, MHA Health Services, Division for Mental Retardation, Ministry of Social Affairs, National Institute of Child Health and Human Development, IL-91012 Jerusalem, Israel, feldberg5@walla.com

Donald E. Greydanus, MD, Dr HC (ATHENS) Department of Pediatrics and Human Development, Kalamazoo Center for Medical Studies, Michigan State

University College of Human Medicine, Kalamazoo, MI 49008-1284, USA,
greydanus@kcms.msu.edu

Robin Joseph, MA School of Psychology, Walden University, Minneapolis, MN,
USA, rjoseph@waldenu.edu

Manmohan K. Kamboj, MD Associate Professor, Section of Endocrinology,
Metabolism and Diabetes, Nationwide Children's Hospital, Columbus, OH 43205,
USA, Manmohan.Kamboj@Nationwidechildrens.org

Isack Kandel, MA, PhD Office of the Medical Director, Health Services,
Division for Mental Retardation, Ministry of Social Affairs, National Institute of
Child Health and Human Development, IL-91012 Jerusalem, Israel,
kandel.isack@gmail.com

Bharti Katbamna, PhD Department of Speech Pathology and Audiology,
Western Michigan University, Kalamazoo, MI 49008-5355, USA,
bharti.katbamna@wmich.edu

Jeffrey L. Koh, MD, MBA Department of Anesthesiology and Perioperative
Medicine, Doernbecher Children's Hospital, Oregon Health and Science
University, Portland, OR, USA; Department of Pediatrics, Doernbecher Children's
Hospital, Oregon Health and Science University, Portland, OR, USA,
kohj@ohsu.edu

Margo Adams Larsen, PhD Family Institute, PC, Grand Forks, ND 58201,
USA, dr.adamslarsen@gmail.com

Meir Lotan, MScPT, PhD Department of Physical Therapy, Ariel University
Center of Samaria, IL-40700 Ariel, Israel; Ariel and Israeli Rett Syndrome
Association, National Evaluation Team, National Rett Syndrome Clinic, Chaim
Sheba Medical Center, Ramat-Gan, Israel, ml_pt_rs@netvision.net.il

Joav Merrick, MD, MMedSci, DMSc National Institute of Child Health and
Human Development, Health Services, Office of the Medical Director, Division for
Mental Retardation, Ministry of Social Affairs and Social Services, POBox 1260,
IL-91012 Jerusalem, Israel; Kentucky Children's Hospital, University of Kentucky,
Lexington, KY, USA, jmerrick@zahav.net.il

Mohammed Morad, MD Office of the Medical Director, Health Services,
Division for Mental Retardation, Ministry of Social Affairs, National Institute of
Child Health and Human Development, IL-91012 Jerusalem, Israel; Kentucky
Children's Hospital, University of Kentucky, Lexington, KY, USA; Department of
Family Medicine, Faculty of Health Sciences, Ben Gurion University of the Negev,
Beer-Sheva, Israel; Clalit Health Services, Beer-Sheva, Israel, morad@bgu.ac.il

Ahsan Nazeer, MD Department of Psychiatry, Kalamazoo Center for Medical
Studies, Michigan State University, Kalamazoo, MI 49048, USA,
nazeer@kcms.msu.edu

Nickola Wolf Nelson, PhD, CCC-SLP Department of Speech Pathology and Audiology, PhD Program in Interdisciplinary Health Sciences, Western Michigan University, Kalamazoo, MI 49008-5355, USA, nickola.nelson@wmich.edu

Hatim A. Omar, MD Adolescent Medicine and Young Parent Programs, Kentucky Clinic, Department of Pediatrics, Kentucky Children's Hospital, University of Kentucky College of Medicine, Lexington, KY, USA, haomar2@uky.edu

Dilip R. Patel, MD, MD, FAAP, FSAM, FAACPDM, FACSM Department of Pediatrics and Human Development, Kalamazoo Center for Medical Studies, Michigan State University College of Human Medicine, Kalamazoo, MI 49008-1284, USA, patel@kcms.msu.edu

Helen D. Pratt, PhD Behavioral Developmental Pediatrics, Pediatrics Program, Department of Pediatrics and Human Development, Kalamazoo Center for Medical Studies, Michigan State University College of Human Medicine, Kalamazoo, MI 49008-1284, USA, pratt@kcms.msu.edu

Yehuda Senecky, MD Institute of Child Development and Neurology, Schneider Children's Medical Center of Israel, Clalit Health Services, 49202 Petah-Tiqva, Israel, SENEKIMI@ZAHAV.NET.IL

Regan E. Settles, MS Department of Psychology, University of Kentucky, Lexington, KY, 40506-0044, USA, regan.settles@uky.edu

Helen M. Sharp, PhD Department of Speech Pathology and Audiology, Western Michigan University, Kalamazoo, MI 49008, USA, helen.sharp@wmich.edu

Rachel F. Steffens, MS Department of Psychology, University of Kentucky, Lexington, KY, 40506-0044, USA, rachel.steffens@uky.edu

Stephen M. Tasko, PhD Department of Speech Pathology and Audiology, Western Michigan University, Kalamazoo, MI 49008, USA, stephen.tasko@wmich.edu

Helga V. Toriello, PhD Department of Pediatrics and Human Development, Michigan State University College of Human Medicine, East Lansing, MI, USA; Director of Genetics, Spectrum Health, Grand Rapids, MI 49503, USA, helga.toriello@spectrum-health.org

John A. Yozwiak, PhD Division of Adolescent Medicine, Department of Pediatrics, Kentucky Clinic, University of Kentucky College of Medicine, Lexington, KY 40536-0284, USA, jayozw00@uky.edu

About the Editors

Donald E. Greydanus, MD, FAAP, FSAM, FIAP (H), is professor of pediatrics and human development at Michigan State University College of Human Medicine (East Lansing, Michigan, USA) and director of the Pediatrics Residency Program at Michigan State University/Kalamazoo Center for Medical Studies (Kalamazoo, Michigan, USA). Received the 1995 American Academy of Pediatrics' Adele D. Hofmann Award for "Distinguished Contributions in Adolescent Health", the 2000 Mayo Clinic Pediatrics Honored Alumnus Award for "National Contributions to the field of Pediatrics," and the 2003 William B. Weil, Jr., M.D. Endowed Distinguished Pediatric Faculty Award from Michigan State University College of Medicine for "National & International Recognition as well as Exemplary Scholarship in Pediatrics." Received the 2004 Charles R. Drew School of Medicine (Los Angeles, CA) Stellar Award for "Contributions to Pediatric Resident Education" and awarded an honorary membership in the Indian Academy of Pediatrics – an honor granted to only a few pediatricians outside of India. Was the 2007 visiting professor of pediatrics at Athens University, Athens, Greece, and received the Michigan State University College of Human Medicine Outstanding Community Faculty Award in 2008. Past chair of the National Conference and Exhibition Planning Group (Committee on Scientific Meetings) of the American Academy of Pediatrics and member of the Pediatric Academic Societies' (SPR/PAS) Planning Committee (1998 to present). Member of the Appeals Committee for the Pediatrics' Residency Review Committee (RRC) of the Accreditation Council for Graduate Medical Education (Chicago, IL) in both adolescent medicine and general pediatrics. Numerous publications in adolescent health and lectureships in many countries on adolescent health. E-mail: Greydanus@kcms.msu.edu

Joav Merrick, MD, MMedSci, DMSc, is professor of pediatrics, child health, and human development affiliated with Kentucky Children's Hospital, University of Kentucky, Lexington, United States, and the Zusman Child Development Center, Division of Pediatrics, Soroka University Medical Center, Ben Gurion University, Beer-Sheva, Israel, the medical director of the Health Services, Division for Mental Retardation, Ministry of Social Affairs, Jerusalem, the founder and director of the

National Institute of Child Health and Human Development. Numerous publications in the field of pediatrics, child health, and human development, rehabilitation, intellectual disability, disability, health, welfare, abuse, advocacy, quality of life, and prevention. Received the Peter Sabroe Child Award for outstanding work on behalf of Danish Children in 1985 and the International LEGO-Prize ("The Children's Nobel Prize") for an extraordinary contribution toward improvement in child welfare and well-being in 1987. E-mail: jmerrick@internet-zahav.net.

Hatim A. Omar, MD, FAAP, professor of pediatrics and obstetrics and gynecology and director of the Section of Adolescent Medicine, Department of Pediatrics, University of Kentucky, Lexington. Dr. Omar has completed residency training in obstetrics and gynecology as well as pediatrics. He has also completed fellowships in vascular physiology and adolescent medicine. He is the recipient of the Commonwealth of Kentucky Governor's Award for community service and volunteerism. He is the recipient of the Commonwealth of Kentucky Governer's Award for community service and volunteerism in 2000, KY Teen Pregnancy Coalition Award for outstanding service 2002, awards for suicide prevention from the Ohio Valley Society for Adolescent Medicine and Kentucky Pediatric Society in 2005 and 2007, Sexual Abuse Awareness Month Award for his work with sexual abuse victims from the KY association of sexual assault professionals in 2007, Special Achievement Award from the American Academy of Pediatrics 2007 and the Founders of Adolescent Medicine Award from the AAP in 2007. He is well known internationally with numerous publications in child health, pediatrics, adolescent medicine, pediatric, and adolescent gynecology. E-mail: haomar2@uky.edu

Dilip R. Patel, MD, MD, FAAP, FSAM, FAACPDM, FACSM, is professor in the Department of Pediatrics and Human Development at the Michigan State University College of Human Medicine, East Lansing, Michigan, USA. He is a full-time teaching faculty member in the Pediatric Residency Program at the Michigan State University Kalamazoo Center for Medical Studies, Kalamazoo, Michigan, USA. Dr. Patel has subspecialty training and interests in neurodevelopmental disabilities, developmental–behavioral pediatrics, adolescent medicine, and sports medicine. He has published numerous papers on a wide-ranging topics in these areas and has edited several special symposia and books. E-mail: patel@kcms.msu.edu

Chapter 1
Neurodevelopmental Disabilities: Introduction and Epidemiology

Dilip R. Patel and Joav Merrick

Abstract Developmental disabilities or neurodevelopmental disabilities (include intellectual disability) are a diverse group of chronic disorders that begin at any-time during the development process (including conception, birth, and growth) up to 22 years of age and last throughout an individual's lifetime. Major disabilities include intellectual disability, learning disabilities, communication disorders, autism spectrum disorders, cerebral palsy, and neural tube defects. This chapter provides an introduction and reviews epidemiology of major disabilities.

Introduction

Developmental disabilities or neurodevelopmental disabilities (include intellectual disability) are a diverse group of chronic disorders (see Table 1.1) that begin at any-time during the development process (including conception, birth, and growth) up to 22 years of age and last throughout an individual's lifetime [1]. The underlying basis for these disorders lies in fundamental deficits in the developing brain due to genetic, prenatal, perinatal, metabolic, and other factors [2]. Developmental disabilities affect 17% of individuals younger than 18 years of age in the United States [1]. Prevention along with early recognition and intervention is critically important to mitigate the enormous personal and socioeconomic impact of these disorders.

The World Health Organization has developed the International Classification of Functioning, Disability, and Health (ICF), which consists of three key components – body function and structure, activity, and participation – that provides a framework for delineating disabilities (see Table 1.2) [2, 3]. The three key components of functioning and disability are inter-related and may interact with the health condition (e.g., disorder or disease) and personal and environmental factors.

D.R. Patel (✉)
Department of Pediatrics and Human Development, Kalamazoo Center for Medical Studies, Michigan State University College of Human Medicine, Kalamazoo, MI 49008-1284, USA
e-mail: patel@kcms.msu.edu

D.R. Patel et al. (eds.), *Neurodevelopmental Disabilities*,
DOI 10.1007/978-94-007-0627-9_1, © Springer Science+Business Media B.V. 2011

1

Table 1.1 Major categories of developmental disabilities

Intellectual disability
Learning disabilities
Communication disorders
Autism spectrum disorders
Neurobehavioral disorders
Neurogenetic disorders
Neurometabolic disorders
Neuromuscular disorders
Cerebral palsy
Other neuromotor disorders
Sensory impairments
Disabilities associated with chronic diseases
Traumatic brain injuries
Spinal cord injuries

Table 1.2 World Health Organization International Classification of Functioning, Disability, and Health

Normal function	Lack of normal function
Body function: the physiological functions of the body	Impairment: problems in the body function as a significant deviation or loss
Body structures: anatomic parts of the body	Impairments: problems in structure as a significant deviation or loss
Activity: the execution of a task or action by an individual	Activity limitation: difficulties an individual may have in executing activities
Participation: involvement in a life situation	Participation restrictions: problems an individual may have in involvement in life situation
Functioning: a global term used to encompass body functions, body structures, activities, and participation	Disability: a global term used to encompass problems with body functions, body structures, activity limitations, and participation restrictions

http://www.who.int/classifications/icf/en/

   In the United States, according to the Individuals with Disability Education Improvement Act (2004) the term child with a disability means a child with intellectual disability, hearing impairments (including deafness), speech or language impairments, visual impairments (including blindness), serious emotional disturbance, orthopedic impairments, autism, traumatic brain injury, other health impairments, or specific learning disabilities [4]. A child with disability as defined by the IDEA needs special education and related services, as may be required to assist a child with a disability to benefit from special education, and includes the early identification and assessment of disabling conditions in children.

   The term infant or toddler with a disability means an individual under 3 years of age who needs early intervention services because she/he is experiencing developmental delays, as measured by appropriate diagnostic instruments and procedures in one or more of the areas of cognitive development, physical development, communication development, social or emotional development, and adaptive development or has a diagnosed physical or mental condition that has a high probability of resulting in developmental delay.

According to the Americans with Disabilities Act (ADA) the term "disability" means, with respect to an individual, a physical or mental impairment that substantially limits one or more major life activities of such individual, a record of such an impairment, or being regarded as having such an impairment [5]. Major life activities include, but are not limited to, caring for oneself, performing manual tasks, seeing, hearing, eating, sleeping, walking, standing, lifting, bending, speaking, breathing, learning, reading, concentrating, thinking, communicating, and working. A major life activity also includes the operation of a major bodily function, including, but not limited to, functions of the immune system, normal cell growth, digestive, bowel, bladder, neurological, brain, respiratory, circulatory, endocrine, and reproductive functions.

Intellectual Disability

According to the American Association of Intellectual and Developmental Disabilities (AAIDD), intellectual disability "is a disability characterized by significant limitations both in intellectual functioning and in adaptive behavior as expressed in conceptual, social, and practical adaptive skills" [6, 7]. The assessment of intellectual functioning and adaptive behavior must take into consideration the expectations based on individual's age and culture [8]. The influence on cognitive assessment of sensory, motor, communication, or behavioral factors should also be appropriately considered in administration of assessment instruments and interpretation of their results [8].

In the United States a widely used definition is the one from the IDEA that defines intellectual disability as "significantly sub-average general intellectual functioning, existing concurrently with deficits in adaptive behavior and manifested during the developmental period that adversely affects a child's educational performance" [4]. According to the *Diagnostic and Statistical Manual of Mental Disorders*, 4th edition, text revision (DSM-IV-TR), intellectual disability (or mental retardation) is defined as an intelligence quotient (IQ) of approximately 70 or below on an individually administered standardized test of intelligence concurrent with deficits in adaptive functioning in two of the following areas: communication, self-care, home living, social or interpersonal skills, use of community resources, self-direction, functional academic skills, work, leisure, health, and safety. All definitions stipulate that the onset of disability must occur before the age of 18 years [9–11].

The severity of intellectual disability can be categorized based on a combination of level of intellectual functioning, adaptive functioning, and intensity of supports needed [8, 9, 12]. When the level of intellectual functioning cannot be reliably assessed, but there is a high level of confidence based on clinical judgment, a diagnosis of intellectual disability can be made without specifying the severity of intellectual functioning [7, 8].

The reported prevalence of intellectual disability reflects consideration of the definition used, method of ascertainment of the data, and the characteristics of the population studied [13, 14]. Based on the typical bell-shaped distribution of intelligence in the general population and 2 standard deviations below the mean as a cutoff point, approximately 2.5% of the population is expected to have intellectual disability. Most epidemiological studies consider those with an IQ score of 50 or less as having severe and those above 50 as having mild intellectual disability [10–15]. Eighty-five percent of individuals with intellectual disability have mild intellectual disability [9–12]. The prevalence of severe intellectual disability has remained the same over several decades at 0.3–0.5% of the population in the United States [12]. Based on the United States National Center for Health Statistics 1997–2003 National Health Interview Survey, the prevalence of intellectual disability among children aged 5–17 years is estimated to be 7.5 per 1,000 [12]. Intellectual disability is reported to be twice as common in males as in females. The recurrence risk of intellectual disability in families with one previous child with severe intellectual disability is reported to be between 3 and 9% [8, 11, 12].

Mild intellectual disability is associated predominantly with environmental risk factors, and a specific etiology can be identified in less than half of the affected individuals [12–14]. On the other hand, underlying biological or neurological etiology can be identified in more than two-thirds of affected individuals who have severe disability [8, 11, 13]. The most common identified conditions in children with severe intellectual disability include chromosomal disorders, genetic syndromes, congenital brain malformations, neurodegenerative diseases, congenital infections, inborn errors of metabolism, and birth injury [12–14].

Learning Disabilities

The term learning disability describes difficulties in specific areas of learning that have a direct relation to academic performance. The terms learning disabilities (LDs) and learning disorders are often used interchangeably in the literature. The main types of learning disabilities are reading disability (dyslexia), mathematics disability (dyscalculia), disorder of written expression (dysgraphia), and non-verbal learning disability (NVLD) [16, 17]. The failure to achieve academically in children who have LDs occurs in the presence of age-appropriate teaching and learning experiences and is not the result of cognitive deficits or sociocultural factors [16, 17]. Early identification is crucial to prevent academic failure, behavioral disturbances, low self-esteem, early school dropout, and lifelong implications for academic success, occupation, socioeconomic well–being, and consequently health.

A child is considered to have a specific learning disability if the child does not achieve adequately for the child's age or to meet grade-level educational standards in one or more of the specific areas, when provided with learning experiences and instruction appropriate for the child's age or state-approved grade-level standards [4].

To ensure that underachievement in a child suspected of having a specific learning disability is not due to the lack of appropriate instruction in reading or math, the following must be taken into consideration, as part of the evaluation: data that demonstrate that prior to, or as a part of, the referral process, the child was provided appropriate instruction in regular education settings, delivered by qualified personnel, and data-based documentation of repeated assessments of achievement at reasonable intervals, reflecting formal assessment of student progress during instruction, which was provided to the child's parents [4]. The public agency must promptly request parental consent to evaluate the child to determine if the child needs special education and related services.

Specific LD is diagnosed when the child or adolescent's scores on an individually administered standardized achievement test (in reading, mathematics, or written expression) are substantially below that expected based on his/her age, level of education, and IQ. Because LDs can occur at all levels of IQ the definitional concept of discrepancy between ability and achievement is an area of controversy and debate in the LD literature [4, 16, 17].

Specific reading disability is fairly common, with up to 17.5% of children being affected [18, 19]. Dyslexia is highly comorbid with other developmental problems, including impairments in language, motor skills, and behavioral control [20]. Reading disability is also a contributor to juvenile delinquency and leads to higher rates of recidivism [21]. Dyslexia is identified in 80% of children who have LDs.

Specific mathematics disorder (also known as dyscalculia) is also fairly common, seen in 3–6% of school-age children [22–24]. It is more common in girls than in boys, possibly related to environmental, rather than biological, factors. The presence of dyscalculia should prompt physicians to look for medical and psychiatric syndromes, given that mathematics disorder is present at higher-than-average rates in conditions such as epilepsy and fragile X syndrome [22–26].

Of all the LDs, the disorder of written language (also called written language disorder or WLD) is the least researched [27, 28]. However, a study from Minnesota found that, by age 19 years, 6.9–14.7% of the subjects met criteria for WLD, which is about as common as reading disorder [27]. Boys with WLD outnumbered girls 2–3:1, and 25% of all subjects had WLD without a comorbid reading disorder.

Communication Disorders

Language is a system of symbolic knowledge represented in the brain used for meaningful communication. The English language has 44 phonemes. A phoneme is a unit of sound in speech. A morpheme (word) refers to the smallest meaningful unit of language. Speech is the production of sounds of words. Communication disorders are common in school-age children identified in 12–14% of students. In school-age children the prevalence of expressive language disorder is reported to be 3–7% and mixed receptive–expressive disorder to be 3–5% [9]. The reported prevalence of phonologic disorder is 2% by 6–7 years of age and 0.5% by 17 years of age and that for stuttering ranges 0.8–1.0% in adolescents [9].

Autism Spectrum Disorders

Autism spectrum disorders (ASDs) are a group of developmental disabilities characterized by significant deficits in social, communication, and behavioral domains [29, 30]. Autistic disorder, Asperger syndrome, and pervasive developmental disorder not otherwise specified (PDD NOS) are the three ASDs. Persons who have autistic disorder have significant language delays, social and communication challenges, and unusual behaviors and interests [30]. A significant percentage of them also have intellectual disability. Persons who have Asperger syndrome manifest deficits in social domain and have unusual behaviors and interest; however, they typically do not have deficits in language or intellectual ability. Persons with pervasive developmental disorder, not otherwise specified, have some features of autistic disorder and some features of Asperger syndrome, but do not meet all the criteria for either disorder [30].

Centers for Disease Control and Prevention reports that the overall prevalence of ASDs in the United States is 9.0 per 1,000 population in children aged 8 years [29]. The average prevalence of ASDs is four times higher in males than in females [30]. The risk for a second child having an ASD, when an older sibling has ASD, is 5–6% [29, 30]. In the United States, the average prevalence of ASDs identified among children aged 8 years has increased by 57% from 2002 to 2006.42 The prevalence of ASDs has increased 10-fold over the past 50 years [29, 30]. Although various reasons have been postulated for the increased prevalence, the exact reasons have not been clearly elucidated [3–32].

Of the estimated 4 million children born in the United States each year approximately 27,000 will eventually be diagnosed with ASD [30]. Assuming a constant prevalence rate over the past 20 years, approximately 600,000 persons between the ages of 0 and 21 have an ASD [30–33]. The prevalence rate of ASD in Asia and Europe is reported to be between 0.6 and 1% [30–33].

There is high covariance between the ASDs and IDs, as between 50 and 70% of individuals with ASDs will have some type of ID; conversely, as many as 40% of those with IDs will have an ASD [34]. In children with IDs, the most reliable prevalence rate of comorbid pervasive developmental disorders (PDDs) is 16.7%, which was derived using DSM-IV-TR criteria [9, 35]. The ASD-ID combination tends to increase the severity of both disorders, leading to more subjective distress, less functional ability, and greater need for community services.

No cause is found in most cases of ASDs [36, 37]. There are some genetic syndromes, both common (e.g., Down syndrome and fragile X syndrome) and rare (e.g., adenylosuccinate lyase deficiency), that are associated with higher-than-expected rates of autism [38]. It is unclear if there is something inherent in those syndromes that predisposes to the development of autistic features or whether the risk is secondary to the intellectual impairment that is commonly seen in many genetic disorders.

Cerebral Palsy

According to American Academy of Cerebral Palsy and Developmental Medicine, cerebral palsy (CP) describes a group of permanent disorders of development of movement and posture, causing activity limitation, that are attributed to nonprogressive disturbances that occurred in the developing fetal or infant brain [39, 40]. The motor disorders of CP are often accompanied by disturbances of sensation, perception, cognition, communication, and behavior, by epilepsy, and by secondary musculoskeletal problems. CP is classified as spastic (hemiplegia, diplegia, quadriplegia), dyskinetic (choreoathetoid, dystonia), hypotonic, or mixed [39–41].

The worldwide incidence of CP is estimated to be 2–3 per 1,000 live births [39, 42–44]. Each year about 10,000 babies born in the United States develop CP [45]. Because initial symptoms and signs suggestive of CP may resolve during first few years of life, the prevalence of CP is generally higher in infancy. Despite a tremendous improvement in obstetric and neonatal care, the overall prevalence of CP has remained the same since the 1950s [40, 41]. This trend is partly explained by the fact that most low birth weight and premature babies now survive. Although prematurity and low birth weight are significant risk factors for developing CP, multiple other risk factors have been identified [39–46].

Myelomeningocele

Neural tube defects (NTDs) result from failure of the neurulation that is failure of the closure of the neural tube during development of central nervous system as expected between the third and fourth week of in utero development [47, 48]. Although any segment of spinal level can be affected, 75% of cases involve the lumbosacral level [49]. Myelomeningocele is the most severe type of NTD in which there is a defect in the vertebral column through which the meninges and the spinal cord protrude at the level of the defect [48].

The prevalence of NTDs varies in different regions of the world [49]. In the United States, the incidence of NTDs is 1 in 4,000 live births [47, 49]. In Wales and Ireland, the prevalence is three to four times higher, whereas in Africa it is much lower [49]. The variability in prevalence rates of NTDs in different regions of the world is believed to be due to a combination of genetic and environmental factors. Lumbar myelomeningocele, which is three to seven times more common in females than in males, accounts for most cases of myelomeningocele [47–49].

A significant decrease (50%) in the prevalence of NTDs has been reported over the past four decades [49]. Some of the reasons believed to have contributed to the decrease in prevalence of NTDs include routine and widespread supplementation with folic acid, prenatal diagnosis and subsequent decision to terminate pregnancy by some couples, and improved nutrition as well as general health of women [47, 49].

Dual Diagnosis

The reported prevalence rates of psychiatric disorders in persons who have developmental disabilities have been quite inconsistent, depending on the studies' choice of variables, such as subject age (child, adolescent, adult, or elderly), setting (clinical or community), location (family home, residential care, or state hospital), degree of intellectual impairment (mild, moderate, or severe), developmental diagnosis (specific developmental syndrome vs. nonspecific etiology), psychiatric diagnosis (specific disorders vs. grouped as "mental illness"), and evaluation method (chart review, survey, or clinical interview). Another important challenge to the accurate measurement of psychopathology in the developmental disabilities is the difficulty in differentiating psychiatric symptoms from the clinical features associated with some of the developmental disabilities themselves [50–55]. Taking these technical issues into consideration, the rates of some behavioral and emotional disorders do appear to be higher in the persons who have developmental disabilities than they are in comparison groups ranging from 20 to 50% [51–55].

Hearing Loss

Sounds can be described in terms of their frequency (or pitch) and intensity (or loudness). Frequency is measured in hertz (Hz). A person, who has hearing within the normal range, can hear sounds that have frequencies between 20 and 20,000 Hz, with the most important sounds in daily activities in the 250–6,000 Hz range. Speech includes a mix of low- and high-frequency sounds. Vowel sounds like "u" have low frequencies (250–1,000 Hz) and are usually easier to hear. Consonants like "s," "h," and "f" have higher frequencies (1,500–6,000 Hz) and are harder to hear. Consonants convey most of the meaning of what we say. Someone who cannot hear high-frequency sounds will have a hard time understanding speech. Intensity, or loudness, is measured in decibels (dB). A person with hearing within the normal range can hear sounds ranging from 0 to 140 dB. A whisper is around 30 dB. Conversations are usually 45–50 dB. Sounds that are louder than 90 dB can be uncomfortable to hear. A loud rock concert might be as loud as 110 dB. Sounds that are 120 dB or louder can be painful and can result in temporary or permanent hearing loss.

Impairments in hearing can happen in either frequency or intensity, or both. Hearing loss severity is based on how well a person can hear the frequencies or intensities most often associated with speech. Severity can be described as mild, moderate, severe, or profound. The term "deaf" is sometimes used to describe someone who has an approximately 90 dB or greater hearing loss or who cannot use hearing to process speech and language information, even with the use of hearing aids. The term "hard of hearing" is sometimes used to describe people who have a less severe hearing loss than deafness.

Hearing loss can affect one or both ears and can be conductive, sensorineural, mixed, or central. Approximately 30% of children who are deaf or hard of hearing also have one or more other developmental disabilities, such as intellectual disabilities, cerebral palsy, vision impairment, or epilepsy. Hearing loss can affect a child's ability to learn both to speak and to understand spoken language. This is especially true if the child is born with a hearing loss or loses his/her hearing before 2 years of age. People with hearing loss may communicate using speech (sometimes called oral communication), sign language (sometimes called manual communication), or a combination of both. Oral communication focuses on speech, listening with hearing aids, and sometimes lip reading. Manual communication includes sign language.

Vision Impairment

The incidence, prevalence, and causes of childhood vision impairment vary widely in different parts of the world depending on the available health resources, general nutritional status and well-being, socioeconomic status, screening, and preventive practices. Vision impairment means that a person's eyesight cannot be corrected to a "normal" level. Vision impairment may be caused by a loss of visual acuity, where the eye does not see objects as clearly as usual. It may also be caused by a loss of visual field, where the eye cannot see as wide an area as usual without moving the eyes or turning the head. There are different ways of describing how severe a person's vision loss is. The World Health Organization defines "low vision" as visual acuity between 20/70 and 20/400, with the best possible correction, or a visual field of 20° or less. "Blindness" is defined as a visual acuity worse than 20/400, with the best possible correction, or a visual field of 10° or less. Someone with a visual acuity of 20/70 can see at 20 ft what someone with normal sight can see at 70 ft. Someone with a visual acuity of 20/400 can see at 20 ft what someone with normal sight can see at 400 ft. A normal visual field is about 160–170° horizontally. Vision impairment severity may be categorized differently for certain purposes. In the United States, for example, the term "legal blindness" indicates that a person is eligible for certain education or federal programs. Legal blindness is defined as a visual acuity of 20/200 or worse, with the best possible correction, or a visual field of 20° or less.

Visual acuity alone cannot tell you how much a person's life will be affected by their vision loss. It is important to also assess how well a person uses the vision they have. Two people may have the same visual acuity, but one may be able to use his/her vision better to do everyday tasks. Most people who are "blind" have at least some usable vision that can help them move around in their environment and do things in their daily lives. A person's functional vision can be evaluated by observing them in different settings to see how they use their vision. A functional vision evaluation can answer questions such as these: can the person scan a room to find someone or something? What lighting is best for the person to do different tasks? How does the person use his/her vision to move around in a room or outside?

Vision impairment changes how a child understands and functions in the world. Impaired vision can affect a child's cognitive, emotional, neurological, and physical development by possibly limiting the range of experiences and the kinds of information a child is exposed to. Nearly two-thirds of children with vision impairment also have one or more other developmental disabilities, such as mental retardation, cerebral palsy, hearing loss, or epilepsy. Children with more severe vision impairment are more likely to have additional disabilities than are children with milder vision impairment.

Conclusions

Developmental disabilities or neurodevelopmental disabilities (include intellectual disability) are a diverse group of chronic disorders that begin at anytime during the development process (including conception, birth, and growth) up to 22 years of age and last throughout an individual's lifetime. The World Health Organization has developed the International Classification of Functioning, Disability, and Health (ICF), which consists of three key components – body function and structure, activity, and participation – that provides a framework for delineating disabilities. The three key components of functioning and disability are inter-related and may interact with the health condition (e.g., disorder or disease) and personal and environmental factors. The reported prevalence of intellectual disability reflects consideration of the definition used, method of ascertainment of the data, and the characteristics of the population studied. Based on the typical bell-shaped distribution of intelligence in the general population and 2 standard deviations below the mean as a cutoff point, approximately 2.5% of the population is expected to have intellectual disability. Specific reading disability is fairly common, with up to 17.5% of children being affected. Centers for Disease Control and Prevention reports that the overall prevalence of ASDs in the United States is 9.0 per 1,000 population in children aged 8 years. The worldwide incidence of CP is estimated to be 2–3 per 1,000 live births. The prevalence of NTDs varies in different regions of the world. In the United States, the incidence of NTDs is 1 in 4,000 live births. The prevalence and causes of vision impairment vary in different parts of the world depending on multiple factors.

Acknowledgments This chapter is adapted with permission from authors' previous works [56, 57]. The sections on hearing loss and vision impairment are adapted from (public domain) United States Centers for Disease Control, http://www.cdc.gov/ncbddd/dd/ddhi.htm and http://www.cdc.gov/ncbddd/kids/vision.html, accessed July 12, 2010.

References

1. Accardo PJ, editor. Cupute and Accardo's neurodevelopmental disabilities in infancy and childhood. 3rd ed. Vol 1 and 2. Baltimore, MD: Paul Brookes; 2008.
2. World Health Organization. The international classification of functioning, Disability, and Health. Geneva: WHO; 2001.
3. Cieza A, Stucki G. The international classification of functioning Disability and Health: its development process and content validity. Eur J Phys Rehabil Med. 2008;44: 303–13.
4. The Individuals with Disabilities Education Improvement Act of 2004. 20 USC 1400 HR 1350 PL 108–446. http://idea.ed.gove accessed 1/27/2010.
5. The American with Disabilities Act. http://www.ada.gov accessed 1/27/2010.
6. What we mean by disability. http://www.socialsecurity.gov accessed 12/17/2009.
7. American Association of Intellectual and Developmental Disabilities. Intellectual disability: definition, classification, and systems of supports. 11th ed. Washington, DC: American Association of Intellectual and Developmental Disabilities; 2010.
8. Luckasson R, Borthwick-Duffy S, Buntix WHE, et al. Mental retardation: definition, classification, and system of supports. 10th ed. Washington, DC: Am Assoc Ment Retardation; 2002.
9. American Psychiatric Association. Diagnostic and statistical manual of mental disorders. 4th ed. Text Revision. Washington, DC: American Psychiatric Association; 2000. pp. 39–84.
10. Walker WO, Johnson CP. Mental retardation: overview and diagnosis. Pediatr Rev. 2006;27(6):204–12.
11. Shapiro BK, Batshaw M. Mental retardation (intellectual disability). In: Kliegman RM, Behrman RE, Jenson HB, Stanton BF, editors. Nelson Textbook of Pediatrics. 18th ed. Philadelphia, PA: Elsevier Saunders; 2007. pp. 191–6.
12. Intellectual disability. http://www.cdc.gov/ncbddd/dd/mr3.htm accessed 12/15/2009.
13. McDermott S, Durkin MS, Schupf N, Stein ZA. Epidemiology and etiology of mental retardation. In: Jacobson JW, Mulick JA, Rojahn J, editors. Handbook of intellectual and developmental disabilities. New York, NY: Springer; 2007. pp. 3–40.
14. Yeargin-Allsopp M, Murphy CC, Cordero JF, Decouflé P, Hollowell JG. Reported biomedical causes and associated medical conditions for mental retardation among 10-year-old children, metropolitan Atlanta, 1985 to 1987. Dev Med Child Neurol. 1997;39:142–9.
15. Curry CJ, Stevenson RE, Anghton D, et al. Evaluation of mental retardation: recommendations of a consensus conference. Am J Med Genet. 1997;72:468–77.
16. Lagae L. Learning disabilities: definitions, epidemiology, diagnosis, and intervention strategies. Pediatr Clin North Am. 2008;55(6):1259–68.
17. Shapiro B, Church RP, Lewis MEB. Specific learning disabilities. In: Batshaw ML, Pellegrino L, Roizen NJ, editors. Children with Developmental Disabilities. 6th ed. Baltimore, MD: Paul H Brookes; 2007. pp. 367–86.
18. Shaywitz BA, Shaywitz SE. Dyslexia. Continuum. 2001;17–36.
19. Shaywitz SE, Shaywitz BA. Dyslexia (specific reading disability). Biol Psychiatry. 2005;57:1301–9.
20. Grizzle KL. Developmental dyslexia. Pediatr Clin North Am. 2007;54:507–23.
21. Shelley-Tremblay J, O'Brien N, Langhinrichsen-Rohling J. Reading disability in adjudicated youth: prevalence rates, current models, traditional and innovative treatments. Aggress Violent Behav. 2007;12:376–92.
22. Shalev RS. Dyscalculia. Continuum. 2001;60–73.
23. Shalev RS, Gross-Tsur V. Developmental dyscalculia. Pediatr Neurol. 2001;24:334–42.
24. Butterworth B. The development of arithmetical abilities. J Child Psychol Psychiatr. 2005;46:3–18.
25. Shalev RS, Manor O, Gross-Tsur V. Developmental dyscalculia: a prospective six-year follow-up. Dev Med Child Neurol. 2005;47:121–5.

26. Shalev RS, Auerbach J, Manor O, Gross-Tsur V. Developmental dyscalculia: prevalence and prognosis. Eur Child Adolesc Psychiatry. 2000;9:58–64.
27. Katusic SK, Colligan RC, Weaver AL, Barbaresi WJ. The forgotten learning disability: epidemiology of written-language disorder in a population-based birth cohort (1976–1982), Rochester, Minnesota. Pediatrics. 2009;123:1306–13.
28. Deuel RK. Dysgraphia. Continuum. 2001;7:37–59.
29. Centers for Disease Control and Prevention. Prevalence of autism spectrum disorders – autism and developmental disabilities monitoring network, United States, 2006. MMWR. 2009; 58(SS 10):1–24.
30. Autism spectrum disorders. http://www.cdc.gov/ncbddd/autism accessed 12/15/2009.
31. Rapin I, Tuchman RF. Autism: definition, neurobiology, screening, diagnosis. Pediatr Clin North Am. 2008;55(5):1129–46.
32. Wing L, Potter D. The epidemiology of autism spectrum disorders: is the prevalence rising? MRDDRR. 2002;8(3):151–61.
33. Hughes JR. A review of recent reports on autism: 1000 studies published in 2007. Epilepsy Behav. 2008;13:425–37.
34. Matson JL, Shoemaker M. Intellectual disability and its relationship to autism spectrum disorders. Res Dev Disabil. 2009;30:1107–14.
35. de Bildt A, Sytema S, Kraijer D, Minderaa R. Prevalence of pervasive developmental disorders in children and adolescents with mental retardation. J Child Psychol Psychiatry. 2005;46: 275–86.
36. Folstein SE. The clinical spectrum of autism. Clin Neurosci Res. 2006;6:113–7.
37. Battaglia A, Carey JC. Etiologic yield of autistic spectrum disorders: a prospective study. Am J Med Genet Part C. 2006;142C:3–7.
38. Cohen D, Pichard N, Tordjman S, Baumann C, Burglen L, Excoffier E, et al. Specific genetic disorders and autism: clinical contribution towards their identification. J Autism Dev Dis. 2005;35:103–16.
39. Cerebral palsy. http://www.cdc.gov/ncbddd/dd/cp3 accessed 12/15/2009.
40. Paneth N. Establishing the diagnosis of cerebral palsy. Clin Obstetr and Gynecol. 2008;51(4):742–8.
41. Horstmann HM, Bleck EE. Orthopaedic Management in Cerebral Palsy. 2nd ed. London: Mac Keith Press; 2007. pp. 1–46.
42. O'Shea TM. Cerebral palsy in very preterm infants: new epidemiological insights. Ment Retard Dev Disabl Res Rev. 2002;8(3):135–45.
43. Nelson KB. The epidemiology of cerebral palsy in term infants. Ment Retard Dev Disabl Res Rev. 2002;8(3):146–50.
44. Murphy N, Such-Neibar T. Cerebral palsy diagnosis and management: the state of the art. Curr Probl Pediatr Adolsc. 2003;33(5):141–76.
45. Ashwal S, Russman BS, Blasco PA, Miller G, Sandler A, Shevell M, Stevenson R. Academy of neurology practice parameter: diagnostic assessment of the child with cerebral palsy. Neurology. 2004;62:851–63.
46. Dodge N. Cerebral palsy: medical aspects. Pediatr Clin North Am. 2008;55(5):1189–208.
47. Mitchell LE, Adzick NS, Melchionne J, Pasquariello PA, Sutton LN, Whitehead AS. Spina bifida. Lancet. 2004;364:1885.
48. Dias MS, Partington M. Embryology of myelomeningocele and anencephaly. Neurosurg Focus. 2004;16(2):1–16.
49. Liptak GS. Neural tube defects. In: Batshaw ML, Pellegrino L, Roizen NJ, editors. Children with Developmental Disabilities. 6th ed. Baltimore, MD: Paul H Brookes; 2007. pp. 419–38.
50. Kerker BD, Owens PL, Zigler E, Horwitz SM. Mental health disorders among individuals with mental retardation: challenges to accurate prevalence estimates. Pub Health Rep. 2004;119:409–17.
51. Emerson E. Prevalence of psychiatric disorders in children and adolescents with and without intellectual disability. J Intellect Disabil Res. 2003;47:51–58.

52. Morgan VA, Leonard H, Bourke J, Jablensky A. Intellectual disability co-occurring with schizophrenia and other psychiatric illness: population-based study. Br J Psychiatry. 2008;193:364–72.
53. Simonoff E, Pickles A, Charman T, Chandler S, Loucas T, Baird G. Psychiatric disorders in children with autism spectrum disorders: prevalence, comorbidity, and associated factors in a population-derived sample. J Am Acad Child Adolesc Psychiatry. 2008;47:921–9.
54. Hurtig T, Kuusikko S, Mattila M-L, Haapsamo H, Ebeling H, Jussila K, et al. Multi-informant reports of psychiatric symptoms among high-functioning adolescents with Asperger syndrome or autism. Autism. 2009;13:583–98.
55. Hofvander B, Delorme R, Chaste P, Nydén A, Wentz E, Ståhlberg O, et al. Psychiatric and psychosocial problems in adults with normal-intelligence autism spectrum disorders. BMC Psychiatry. 2009;9:35.
56. Patel DR, Merrick J. Intellectual disability. In: Greydanus DE, Patel DR, Pratt HD, Calles J Jr, editors. Behavioral pediatrics. 3rd ed. New York, NY: Nova Science; 2009. pp. 39–50
57. Patel DR, Greydanus DE, Calles J Jr, Pratt HD. Developmental disabilities across the life span. Dis Mon. 2010;56(6):299–398.

Chapter 2
Basic Concepts of Developmental Diagnosis

Dilip R. Patel

Abstract Development generally follows four domains, namely motor, speech and language, social–emotional, and cognitive. Development is considered typical when it is progressing as expected. The predominant signs and symptoms of atypical development vary depending on the age of the infant or the child. For example, a delay in achieving motor milestones as expected is generally recognized early in infancy, atypical language development is more often recognized in early childhood, and academic difficulties are recognized in late childhood and adolescence. This chapter reviews the basic concepts and definitions applied in the study of developmental problems, the main features of common conditions considered in the differential diagnoses of developmental disorders, and describes signs that should prompt further developmental evaluation.

Introduction

Development generally follows four domains and has a typical progression when it is proceeding as expected: (1) motor development consists of fine motor and gross motor domains; (2) speech and language development has both receptive and expressive domains; (3) social–emotional development is a reflection of or a combination of development in other domains that includes fine motor adaptive abilities, overall communication abilities, and cognitive abilities; and (4) cognitive development generally refers to visual–perceptual, visual–motor, and problem-solving skills and abilities [1–6]. Language development is a good indicator of overall cognitive development [2].

The typical development is based on certain key principles [1–5, 7, 8]: (1) gross motor development progresses in a cephalo-caudal sequence whereas fine motor

D.R. Patel (✉)
Department of Pediatrics and Human Development, Kalamazoo Center for Medical Studies, Michigan State University College of Human Medicine, Kalamazoo, MI 49008-1284, USA
e-mail: patel@kcms.msu.edu

D.R. Patel et al. (eds.), *Neurodevelopmental Disabilities*,
DOI 10.1007/978-94-007-0627-9_2, © Springer Science+Business Media B.V. 2011

Table 2.1 Developmental surveillance, screening, and evaluation

Process	Goal	Definition
Surveillance	Identify children who *may have* developmental problems	Gathering and synthesizing information about developmental progress of the child based on history, observations by parents or other caretakers and health-care practitioners, and during periodic visits on a longitudinal and continuous basis over time
Screening	Identify children *at risk* of a developmental disorder	The administration of a brief standardized screening test
Evaluation	Identify a *specific developmental disorder* and its etiology if known	A diagnostic process that may involve appropriate laboratory, genetic, or metabolic testing; neuroimaging studies and psychological testing as well as specialist consultations

development progresses from midline to lateral; (2) the primitive reflex patterns have to be lost or integrated into evolving complex motor patterns for later (sequential) voluntary motor development to proceed; (3) all children do not attain developmental milestones at the same rate or at the same time; there is a range of normal variation of typical development; (4) not all typically developing children progress at the same rate in all developmental domains; however, the sequence of typical development is the same in all children; and (5) development progresses from generalized and reflexive responses to more specific and purposeful responses. These key concepts are useful when applied in developmental screening, surveillance, and evaluation (see Table 2.1) [5].

Definitions

Global developmental delay generally refers to a significant developmental delay in two or more developmental domains in children less than 5 years of age and is not necessarily based on measured intelligence quotient (IQ) because it is difficult to measure IQ reliably before 5 or 6 years of age [2, 5, 7, 8]. Developmental quotient (DQ) is a measure of rate of developmental progression in a given developmental domain. It is calculated as follows: developmental quotient (DQ) = [developmental age (DA)/chronologic age (CA)] × 100 [2]. A significant delay in development is a DQ that is equal to or less than 70 in a given domain. Atypical development can be described as a delay, deviation, dissociation, or regression (see Table 2.2) [2–5].

IQ generally can be measured in children 6 years of age, and it is a measure of cognition or intelligence [2, 5, 8, 9]. It is calculated as follows: intelligence quotient (IQ) = [mental age (MA)/chronologic age (CA)] × 100. Standardized tests of intelligence, individually administered, measure IQ. Intellectual disability is defined as significantly subaverage intellectual functioning (IQ of 70 or less with a standard

Table 2.2 Characterization of atypical development

Atypical development	Definition
Delay	Significantly delayed attainment of milestones or skills in one or more domains, but in a correct sequence, compared to that of typically developing children
Deviation	Attainment of developmental skills in a given domain that is out of sequence, for example, when an infant rolls from supine to prone before prone to supine
Dissociation	Attainment of developmental skills at significantly different rates between two or more domains of development. For example, when there is delayed motor development relative to other domains in cerebral palsy
Regression	Loss of previously acquired developmental milestones or skills or failure to acquire new skills

error of measurement of 5 on an individually administered standardized intelligence test) with limitations in adaptive behavior as expressed in conceptual, social, and practical adaptive skills [10–15].

Clinical Features

Infants

Predominant Delay in Motor Milestones

Generally, in infants, delayed or atypical motor development manifests earlier than other domains of development. Because there is a range of periods during which infants attain typical milestones, the most common cause of apparent motor delay is a normal variation or maturational lag [2, 4]. The most significant cause of motor delay in infancy is cerebral palsy which consists of motor delay, abnormal tone, and posture [2, 3, 7, 8, 16, 17].

Clinical presentation and features of infants and children with cerebral palsy may vary depending on its type and severity [16, 17]. A child over 2 months of age with cerebral palsy may have poor head control, stiff legs, and scissoring. A child over 6 months of age may still not have head control, may not sit unsupported, and might preferentially use only one extremity. A child over 10 months of age might crawl by pushing off with one hand and leg while dragging the opposite hand and leg and may not sit without support. A child over 12 months of age might not be crawling and may not stand with support. A child over 24 months of age may not be yet walking or able to push a toy with wheels.

Other causes of predominant motor delay include traumatic insults to the central nervous system damage (kernicterus, birth injury, stroke, metabolic insults, and congenital infections); spinal cord disorders (myelomeningocele, Werdnig–Hoffmann disease); myopathies; muscular dystrophies; and benign congenital hypotonia [4, 7, 8, 11, 12].

Atypical Development Affecting Social, Cognitive, and Language Milestones

A full evaluation for autism, significant cognitive delay, or language impairment is mandatory in infants with the following: no babbling, pointing, or other gestures by 12 months of age, no single words by 16 months, no two word spontaneous phrases by 24 months of age, and any loss of previously acquired language or social skills [5–8]. A deficiency in joint attention, that is, the ability to attend both an object and a person at the same time (e.g., when the infant or child points to or shows an object to her mother and simultaneously looks at her), is often an early sign in infants and toddlers with autism [6].

Other conditions to consider in infants with predominant language, cognitive, and social delays include hearing impairment, severe cognitive deficits, genetic disorders, inborn errors of metabolism including hypothyroidism, and severe nutritional or environmental deprivation.

Developmental regression may occur in autism between 18 and 24 months [4]. Some of the less common conditions associated with progressive encephalopathy with onset before age 2 years include metabolic conditions such as disorders of amino acid metabolism, lysosomal storage disease, hypothyroidism, mitochondrial diseases, tuberous sclerosis, Lesch–Nyhan syndrome, Rett syndrome, Canavan disease, and Pelizaeus–Merzbacher disease [4].

Children

Atypical Language Development

Speech and language problems may present as any number of symptoms including poor intelligibility (normal 25% by age 2, 50% by age 2, 75% by age 3, and 100% by age 4), persistent baby talk, mispronunciations of words, or lack of spontaneous speech [18–24]. Speech is the production of sounds for words, prosody is the pattern of rhythm, stress, and intonation of the speech, and language is a system of symbolic knowledge represented in the brain used for meaningful communication [18–20]. The English language has 44 phonemes. A phoneme is a unit of sound in speech. Airflow obstruction accompanies the production of consonant sounds, whereas it does not in the case of vowel sounds. A morpheme (word) refers to the smallest meaningful unit of language. The basic components of the language appear in Table 2.3 [18–24].

Main causes of atypical development in preschool-age children are autism spectrum disorders, intellectual disability, and developmental language disorders [3, 5–8, 12, 14]. Children with autism have qualitative impairment in communication skills, qualitative impairment in social relatedness, and a range of atypical stereotypical behaviors [6, 26]. Their motor development is normal. Autism spectrum disorders typically are recognized by age 3 years, some as early as 18 months or earlier [6]. Parents usually first notice unusual behaviors and language difficulties in the child. They may describe the child as not socially responsive to others or who may intensely focus on one item for a long period of time. The child may

Table 2.3 Basic components of language

Structure or form of language	Phonology	Sound system of the language that is made of phonemes. Use of phonemes and conventions for their combinations
	Grammar	Morphology: rules or conventions for constructing meaningful words, e.g., adding -s/-es to a word to indicate plural (duck/ducks)
		Syntax: rules or conventions for constructing meaningful phrases or sentences and their relationship, e.g., word order "Daddy go there." But "There Daddy go" is not typical English structure
Content of language	Lexicon	Vocabulary
	Semantics	Relationship among words. Symbols representing universal concepts. Meaning of words (e.g., in relation to objects, agents, an action, states, attributes, or locations). Meaning and relationship of abstract concepts (e.g., idioms and proverbs)
Use of language	Pragmatics	Rules or conventions for use of language in a socially and culturally appropriate manner and in the appropriate context, e.g., turn taking, eye contact, maintaining a topic in conversation

demonstrate withdrawn, aggressive, or self-abusive behavior, may have poor eye contact, become attached to a particular toy, and excessively line up toys or other objects [27]. A child with autism spectrum disorder may not play pretend games, want others to leave him alone, have trouble understanding other people's feelings, and demonstrate echolalia [6, 27, 32]. Asperger syndrome demonstrates normal cognitive and language abilities and predominant deficits in social development [23–35].

Children with intellectual disability have predominant deficits in cognitive and language abilities. Their social development is consistent with their mental age, and they have no motor deficits. Some of the signs of intellectual disability that the parent may observe include – that the child is late to sit, crawl, or walk; learn to talk; have trouble speaking; find it hard to remember things; have trouble understanding social roles; have trouble seeing the results of their actions; or have trouble solving problems [12–14]. There is no identifiable specific cause in most children with mild intellectual disabilities. The likelihood of identifying a specific etiology increases as the severity of intellectual disability increases. Some of the known causes of intellectual disability include fragile X syndrome, fetal alcohol syndrome, other genetic syndromes, lead toxicity, iron deficiency, brain malformations or dysgenesis, and tuberous sclerosis [9, 11–15]. Fragile X syndrome is the most common inherited form of intellectual disability [14].

Children with developmental language disorders have predominant deficits in various aspects of language development, while their social, motor, and cognitive development is normal [18–20, 24]. Differential diagnosis of speech and language delay or disorders includes speech and voice disorders, hearing impairment, developmental language disorders, intellectual disability, autism spectrum disorders, maturational language delay, and lack of environmental stimulation for language learning and literacy. A bilingual home environment is not a cause for language delay.

The various subtypes of developmental language disorders have been described that are based on particular aspects of the language that is affected [18–24]. Expressive language disorders predominantly affect speech production. In verbal dyspraxia (also called developmental apraxia of speech), the child will have difficulty in planning, sequencing, and executing voluntary speech sounds [24]. The speech is disfluent, unintelligible, and significantly delayed with inconsistent articulation errors. Speech programming deficit disorder is characterized by fluent, unintelligible, jargon and is considered by most speech–language pathologists to be similar to verbal dyspraxia and both largely to be speech production problems [20, 24].

Mixed receptive–expressive language disorders are characterized by deficits in both comprehension and expression of speech [19, 20]. Verbal auditory agnosia or word deafness is characterized by profound impairment in comprehension of spoken words [18–20, 24]. Children are mostly non-verbal or have very limited verbal expression. This is a rare condition in children. In phonologic or syntactic deficit disorder, the comprehension or the ability to recognize phonological rules receptively is mostly preserved or is relatively better (in most children) than expression [19, 20, 24]. It is characterized by significant omissions, distortions, and substitutions of words, and the speech is telegraphic, with limited vocabulary and grammatical errors. The child tends to use short sentences and has difficulty in repetition of words or sentences [18].

Higher order processing disorders of language are more complex disorders. Lexical deficit disorder or lexical–syntactic deficit is characterized by severe deficits in word finding and paraphrasing, jargon, and pseudo-stuttering [19, 20, 24]. There is significant deficiency in understanding of connected speech, impoverished syntax, and syntactic distortions. Spontaneous language is relatively better than language on demand. The child may respond to simple commands, and his/her ability to decode wh-questions is limited. Semantic–pragmatic deficit disorder is characterized by poor discourse of connected speech, though the child may apparently be talkative [20]. The phonology and syntax (often simplified syntax) are preserved. Other characteristics of this disorder include atypical choices of words, word-finding deficits, significant deficits in comprehension and verbal reasoning, and tangential and stereotyped speech often with echolalia [20, 24]. Children manifest deficiencies in conversational skills characterized by speaking aloud to no one in particular, poor maintenance of the topic, and responding inaccurately or out of context to commands and questions. This is a rare condition in children.

Developmental speech disorders are described in Table 2.4 [19]. Selective mutism is failure to speak in specific social situations, such as in school, whereas the child is able to speak in other situations such as at home. Twenty to 30% of children with selective mutism have associated articulation problems and language delays. Some children may use gestures to communicate in specific situations. Child may manifest shyness, clinging, temper tantrums, or oppositional behaviors.

Table 2.4 Developmental speech disorders

Disorder	Description
Speech sound disorder	Also described as functional articulation disorder or phonological disorder. Characterized by errors in articulation and speech sounds, consistent substitution of simple sounds for complex sounds or single consonants for blended consonants, dropped consonants, and errors within words. Problem may not be recognized until preschool
Stuttering	Disturbed speech fluency with atypical rate and rhythm and repetitions of sounds, syllables, words, and phrases generally accompanied by evidence of stress or physical tension. There may be sound prolongations, interjections, pauses within words, and blocking of words. Typical onset between 2 and 7 years with peak at age 5 years
Resonance disorders	Can be either hypernasal or hyponasal voice due to anatomical factors. Hypernasality may be due to dysfunction of the velopharyngeal mechanism, seen, for example, in cleft palate. Hyponasality is seen, for example, in nasal congestion, upper respiratory infections, nasal anomalies, and hypertrophied adenoids
Dysarthria	Due to dysfunction of the neuromuscular or motor mechanism for speech production (e.g., cerebral palsy). Characterized mainly by inconsistent misarticulations of speech sounds and words, poor intelligibility, and slow speech
Verbal dyspraxia and speech programming disorder	Both terms describe similar types of largely speech production problems. These disorders may significantly influence expressive language as well

Regression of Previously Acquired Skills or Failure to Acquire Expected New Skills

Main causes of developmental regression include autistic regression, Rett syndrome, childhood disintegrative disorder, and Landau–Kleffner syndrome [4, 18]. Rett syndrome demonstrates loss of developmental milestones after a period of normal development, autistic behaviors, characteristic abnormal wringing hand movements, and a deceleration in head circumference [4]. Following early regression there is some recovery, but then stagnation and late motor deterioration ensue. Some of the other features in children with Rett syndrome include hyperventilation, breath holding, air swallowing, bruxism, gait dyspraxia, neurogenic scoliosis, autonomic dysfunction, inappropriate laughing and screaming spells, and intense eye communication.

Childhood disintegrative disorder (CDD) is a rare condition characterized by loss of previously acquired motor, language, and social skills [4]. It has very high male predominance, and the typical onset is between 3 and 4 years of age. The much later onset of loss of skills after a period of normal development differentiates it from Rett disorder. Children with CDD have very low IQ and often develop seizures. These children also lose bowel and bladder control.

Landau–Kleffner syndrome (LKS) typically occurs between ages 3 and 8 years [4]. After the first 3 years of normal development the child loses language skills.

Non-verbal cognitive abilities and social skills are not affected. Abnormal pattern of sleep EEG and seizures, especially during night, are characteristic of LKS.

Less common causes of progressive encephalopathy with developmental regression with onset after 2 years of age include genetic/metabolic lysosomal storage disease; disorders of gray matter such as ceroid lipofuscinosis and mitochondrial disorders; white matter diseases such as adrenoleukodystrophy, Alexander disease, acquired human immunodeficiency syndrome encephalopathy, and post-infectious subacute sclerosing panencephalitis [4].

Early Learning Difficulties and Behavioral Symptoms

Early (about third-grade) academic or learning difficulties can present as poor grades, delay in completing assignments, inattention, delay in learning new skills, and difficulties in comprehending or reading [36, 37]. These children may also be shy and withdrawn and have behavioral problems at school. Differential diagnosis should include attention-deficit/hyperactivity disorder, sensory impairments, specific learning disability, developmental coordination disorder, and intellectual disability or borderline intellectual functioning [36].

Vision and hearing impairment may be associated with other developmental disabilities. A child with visual impairment might close or cover one eye; squint the eyes or frown; complaint that things are blurry or hard to see; have trouble reading or doing other close-up work or hold objects close to eyes; blink more than usual or seem cranky when doing close-up work such as looking at a book. A child with complete or partial hearing impairment might not turn to the source of a sound from birth to 3 or 4 months of age; may not say single words, such as "dada" or "mama" by 1 year of age; and turn head when he/she sees you but not if you only call out his/her name. This often is mistaken for not paying attention or just ignoring.

Developmental coordination disorder affects school-age children and persists into adolescent years. Difficulties in motor coordination will cause substantial impairment in academic function or activities of daily living. Earliest manifestations may include difficulty in sucking and swallowing, drooling during infancy, speech difficulties, and delayed motor milestones during early childhood. Parents may observe that the child has difficulties with many of the fine motor tasks such as using scissors, tying shoe laces, or buttoning or unbuttoning. They also may drop objects, have poor handwriting, or will frequently bump into furniture or other people. Differential diagnosis in these children include attention-deficit hyperactivity disorder (ADHD), visual impairment, and intellectual disability.

Adolescents

Academic Difficulties

Developmental learning disabilities or disorders are the main consideration in older children and adolescents with difficulties with school work [36–51]. In addition to specific signs associated with learning disorders, these children may present with behavioral problems. The differential diagnoses should also include anxiety disorders, attention-deficit hyperactivity disorder (ADHD), pervasive developmental disorders, and disruptive behavior disorders. In adolescents also consider substance abuse and depressive disorders.

Developmental learning disorder is diagnosed when the child's or adolescent's scores on an individually administered standardized achievement test (in reading, mathematics, or written expression) are substantially below that expected based on his/her age, education, and level of intelligence (on individually administered standardized tests) [36, 37]. Reading disorder may not be apparent until fourth grade, especially if mild and in children with high IQ [38–41]. Some of the clinical features of reading disorder include delayed language, problems with rhyming words or words that sound alike, difficulty in learning letters of the alphabet, spelling errors, difficulty in reading (decoding) unfamiliar or nonsense words or single words, and slow reading [38–41].

Children with mathematics disorder will demonstrate problems with skills in arithmetic by the end of second or third grade [42–48]. Some of the features include difficulties understanding or naming mathematical terms, operations, or concepts; difficulties decoding or recognizing mathematical symbols or signs; difficulties copying numbers or figures, following sequences of mathematical steps, counting, or multiplication tables [42–48]. Disorder of written expression is apparent by the end of the fifth grade and manifests problems with writing skills, which include grammatical errors, punctuation errors, poor paragraph organization, spelling errors, and very poor handwriting [47, 48]. Non-verbal learning disability demonstrates difficulties with problem-solving, visual–spatial, and visual–perceptual deficits, while the language-based skills and intelligence are normal [47].

Diagnosis

A detailed prenatal, birth, perinatal, neonatal, and developmental history is the most essential aspect in the diagnostic evaluation of children with atypical development. Certain elements of physical examination deserve particular emphasis. In infants, examination should focus on neurological and developmental assessment. The examination should document serial measurements of height, weight, and head circumference on appropriate graphs. Also a meticulous search of dysmorphic features or congenital anomalies should be an integral component of the examination. In addition, in adolescents the examination should include assessment of Tanner stage and mental status examination.

Any parental concern about development, hearing, or vision is an indication for further evaluation of developmental or sensory problems. Hearing evaluation is mandatory in all children with symptoms or signs of developmental disorder. Current guidelines recommend universal hearing screening by 1 month of age with subsequent diagnostic audiological testing completed by 3 months of age.

Table 2.5 Examples of developmental screening instruments

Category of screening	Examples of screening instruments
General development	Ages and Stages Questionnaires
	Battelle Developmental Inventory Screening Tool, 2nd edition
	Bayley Infant Neurodevelopmental Screen
	Brigance Screens-II
	Child Development Inventory
	Child Development Review – Parent Questionnaire
	Denver-II Developmental Screening Test
	Infant Development Inventory
	Parents' Evaluation of Developmental Status
Gross motor	Early Motor Pattern Profile
	Motor Quotient
Language and cognitive	Capute Scales
	Communication and Symbolic Behavioral Scales Developmental Profile: Infant, Toddler Checklist
	Early Language Milestone Scale-2

For those infants identified having hearing impairment treatment intervention should start by age 6 months. Hearing screening is also part of periodic health maintenance examinations. Vision screening should be part of periodic health maintenance examinations in all children.

Developmental screening with appropriate standardized screening instrument (see Table 2.5) is part of the periodic health maintenance examinations in the primary care setting at 9, 12, and 30 months of age [5]. If there is no periodic health maintenance exam at 30 months, then perform it at 24 months of age [5]. Similarly screening for autism with standardized autism screening tools (Modified CHAT is the most widely used screening tool) should be routine at the 18- and 24-month visit [6]. If office screening yields suspicion for a developmental disorder, a more formal and advanced testing is necessary. Clinical psychologists with special expertise

Table 2.6 Suggested consultations and collaborations for evaluation and management

Problem	Suggested consultation
All children with significant developmental delay, with a DQ of 70 or less, should have formal psychological testing	Formal psychological testing and evaluation by clinical psychologist
Developmental regression	Child neurologist, clinical geneticist, metabolic disease specialist
Disorders of speech and language	Speech–language pathologist
Symptoms and signs suggestive of autism spectrum disorders	Neurodevelopmental specialists, other clinical specialists with expertise in autism
Additional consultations based on history, signs and symptoms, and initial psychological and laboratory testing	Child neurologist, neurodevelopmental disabilities physician, endocrinologist, genetics, and other specialists

in the diagnostic testing of children with developmental disorders should perform diagnostic psychological testing.

Consider neuroimaging, electroencephalography, tests for genetic disorders, and specific laboratory tests for metabolic disorders based on history, examination, and consultation with appropriate medical specialists [5, 6, 8, 9, 52] (Table 2.6).

Conclusions

Developmental progression is generally described in four main domains, namely motor, speech–language, social–emotional, and cognitive. The predominant presentations of atypical progression of development vary depending on the age of the infant or the child. Developmental quotient is used as a measure of developmental progression in a given developmental domain, whereas intelligent quotient is used to describe the level of cognition or intelligence. Atypical development can be described as delay, deviation, dissociation, or regression. A thorough history and examination are the cornerstones of developmental diagnosis. Early recognition of atypical developmental progression is essential, because early interventions have been shown to be more effective than late interventions in general. Comprehensive guidelines have been published recently by the American Academy of Pediatrics and the American Academy of Neurology for developmental screening and evaluation.

Acknowledgment This chapter is modified and adapted from author's previous work [53].

References

1. Pellegrino L. Patterns in development and disability. In: Batshaw ML, Pellegrino L, Roizen NJ, editors. Children with developmental disabilities. 6th ed. Baltimore: Paul H Brookes; 2007. pp. 217–28.
2. Accardo PJ, Accardo JA, Capute AJ. A neurodevelopmental perspective on the continuum of developmental disabilities. In: Accardo PJ, editor. Capute and Accardo's neurodevelopmental disabilities in infancy and childhood. 3rd ed. Baltimore: Paul H Brookes; 2008. pp. 3–26.
3. Illingworth RS. The development of the infant and young child: Normal and abnormal. 7th ed. London: Churchill Livingstone; 1980. pp. 53–72.
4. Fenichel GM. Psychomotor retardation and regression. In: Fenichel GM, editor. Clinical pediatric neurology. 5th ed. Philadelphia: Elsevier; 2006. pp. 117–48.
5. American Academy of Pediatrics. Identifying infants and young children with developmental disorders in the medical home: an algorithm for developmental surveillance and screening. Pediatrics 2006;118 (1):405–20.
6. Johnson CP, Myers SM. Council on children with disabilities. Identification and evaluation of children with autism spectrum disorders. Pediatrics. 2007;120 (5):1183–215.
7. Shevell MI. Global developmental delay. Pediatr Clin North Am. 2008;55 (5):1071–84.
8. Shevell MI, Ashwal S, Donley D, et al. Practice parameter: evaluation of the child with global developmental delay. Neurology. 2003;60:367–79.
9. Moeschler JB, Shevell MI. Committee on Genetics. Clinical genetic evaluation of the child with mental retardation or developmental delays. Pediatrics. 2006;117:2304–16.
10. American Association of Intellectual and Developmental Disabilities. Intellectual Disability: Definition, Classification, and Systems of Supports. 11th ed. Washington, DC: American Association of Intellectual and Developmental Disabilities; 2010.

11. Luckasson R, Borthwick-Duffy S, Buntix WHE, et al. Mental retardation: definition, classification, and system of supports. 10th ed. Washington, DC: Am Assoc Ment Retard; 2002.
12. Walker WO, Johnson CP. Mental retardation: overview and diagnosis. Pediatr Rev. 2006;27 6:204–12.
13. Shapiro BK, Batshaw M. Mental retardation (intellectual disability). In: Kliegman RM, Behrman RE, Jenson HB, Stanton BF, editors. Nelson textbook of pediatrics. 18th ed. Philadelphia: Elsevier Saunders; 2007. pp. 191–6.
14. Intellectual disability. http://www.cdc.gov/ncbddd/dd/mr3.htm. Accessed 15 Dec 2009.
15. VanKarnebeck CDH, Janswiejer MCE, Leenders AGE, et al. Diagnostic investigation in individuals with mental retardation: a systematic literature review of their usefulness. Eur J Human Genet. 2005;13:2–65.
16. Cerebral palsy. http://www.cdc.gov/ncbddd/dd/cp3 (2009). Accessed 15 Dec 2009.
17. Paneth N. Establishing the diagnosis of cerebral palsy. Clin Obstetr Gynecol. 2008;51 4: 742–8.
18. Stuart S. Communication disorders. In: Batshaw ML, Pellegrino L, Roizen NJ, editors. Children with developmental disabilities. 6th ed. Baltimore: Paul H Brookes; 2007. pp. 313–24.
19. Sharp HM, Hillenbrand K. Speech and language development and disorders in children. Pediatr Clin North Am. 2008;55 (5):1159–74.
20. Simms MD. Language disorders in children: classification and clinical syndromes. Pediatr Clin North Am. 2007;54:437–67.
21. McLeod S, McKinnon DH. Prevalence of communication disorders compared with other learning needs in 14,500 primary and secondary school students. Int J Lang Commun Disord. 2007;42 Suppl 1:37–59.
22. Lindsay G, Dockrell JE, Strand S. Longitudinal patterns of behaviour problems in children with specific speech and language difficulties: child and contextual factors. Br J Educ Psychol. 2007;77:811–28.
23. Mawhood L, Howlin P, Rutter M. Autism and developmental receptive language disorder – a follow-up comparison in early adult life. I: cognitive and language outcomes. J Child Psychol Psychiatry. 2000;41:547–59.
24. Nelson NW. Language and literacy disorders: infancy through adolescence. Boston: Allyn Bacon Pearson Imprint; 2010.
25. Centers for Disease Control and Prevention. Prevalence of autism spectrum disorders. Autism and developmental disabilities monitoring network, United States, 2006. MMWR. 2009;58 SS 10:1–24.
26. Autism spectrum disorders. http://www.cdc.gov/ncbddd/autism (2009). Accessed 15 Dec 2009.
27. Rapin I, Tuchman RF. Autism: definition, neurobiology, screening, diagnosis. Pediatr Clin North Am. 2008;55 (5):1129–46.
28. Wing L, Potter D. The epidemiology of autism spectrum disorders: is the prevalence rising? MRDDRR. 2002;8 (3):151–61.
29. Hughes JR. A review of recent reports on autism: 1000 studies published in 2007. Epilepsy Behav. 2008;13:425–37.
30. Matson JL, Shoemaker M. Intellectual disability and its relationship to autism spectrum disorders. Res Dev Disabil. 2009;30:1107–14.
31. de Bildt A, Sytema S, Kraijer D, Minderaa R. Prevalence of pervasive developmental disorders in children and adolescents with mental retardation. J Child Psychol Psychiatry. 2005;46: 275–86.
32. Folstein SE. The clinical spectrum of autism. Clin Neurosci Res. 2006;6:113–17.
33. Battaglia A, Carey JC. Etiologic yield of autistic spectrum disorders: a prospective study. Am J Med Genet Part C. 2006;142C:3–7.
34. Cohen D, Pichard N, Tordjman S, Baumann C, Burglen L, Excoffier E, et al. Specific genetic disorders and autism: clinical contribution towards their identification. J Autism Dev Dis. 2005;35:103–16.

35. Myers SM, Johnson CP. Council on children with disabilities. Management of children with autism spectrum disorders. Pediatrics. 2007;120 (5):1162–82.
36. Lagae L. Learning disabilities: definitions, epidemiology, diagnosis, and intervention strategies. Pediatr Clin North Am. 2008;55 (6):1259–68.
37. Shapiro B, Church RP, Lewis MEB. Specific learning disabilities. In: Batshaw ML, Pellegrino L, Roizen NJ, editors. Children with developmental disabilities. 6th ed. Baltimore: Paul H Brookes; 2007. pp. 367–86.
38. Shaywitz BA, Shaywitz SE. Dyslexia. Continuum. 2001;17–36.
39. Shaywitz SE, Shaywitz BA. Dyslexia (specific reading disability). Biol Psychiatry. 2005;57:1301–9.
40. Grizzle KL. Developmental dyslexia. Pediatr Clin North Am. 2007;54:507–23.
41. Shelley-Tremblay J, O'Brien N, Langhinrichsen-Rohling J. Reading disability in adjudicated youth: prevalence rates, current models, traditional and innovative treatments. Aggress Violent Behav. 2007;12:376–92.
42. Shalev RS. Dyscalculia. Continuum. 2001;8:60–73.
43. Shalev RS, Gross-Tsur V. Developmental dyscalculia. Pediatr Neurol. 2001;24:334–42.
44. Butterworth B. The development of arithmetical abilities. J Child Psychol Psychiatr. 2005;46:3–18.
45. Shalev RS, Manor O, Gross-Tsur V. Developmental dyscalculia: a prospective six-year follow-up. Dev Med Child Neurol. 2005;47:121–5.
46. Shalev RS, Auerbach J, Manor O, Gross-Tsur V. Developmental dyscalculia: prevalence and prognosis. Eur Child Adolesc Psychiatry. 2000;9:58–64.
47. Katusic SK, Colligan RC, Weaver AL, Barbaresi WJ. The forgotten learning disability: epidemiology of written-language disorder in a population-based birth cohort (1976–1982), Rochester, Minnesota. Pediatrics. 2009;123:1306–13.
48. Deuel RK. Dysgraphia. Continuum. 2001;7:37–59.
49. Rosenberger PB. Management of learning disabilities. Continuum. 2001;125–30.
50. Goldston DB, Walsh A, Arnold EM, Reboussin B, Daniel SS, Erkanli A, et al. Reading problems, psychiatric disorders, and functional impairment from mid- to late adolescence. J Am Acad Child Adolesc Psychiatry. 2007;46:25–32.
51. Feldman E, Levin BE, Lubs H, Rabin M, Lubs ML, Jallad B, et al. Adult familial dyslexia: a retrospective developmental and psychosocial profile. J Neuropsychiatry Clin Neurosci. 1993;5:195–99.
52. Ashwal S, Russman BS, Blasco BS, Miller PA, Sandler G, Shevell A, Stevenson M, American R. Academy of Neurology practice parameter: diagnostic assessment of the child with cerebral palsy. Neurology. 2004;62:851–63.
53. Patel DR. Principles of developmental diagnosis. In: Greydanus DE, Feinberg A, Patel DR, Homnick D, editors. The pediatric diagnostic examination. New York, NY: McGraw Hill Medical; 2008. pp. 629–44.

Chapter 3
Psychological Assessment and Testing

Margo Adams Larsen, Erin Tentis Berglund, Robin Joseph,
and Helen D. Pratt

Abstract Assessment of patients diagnosed with developmental disabilities requires the clinician to understand that presenting problems are the culmination of a complex array of contributing factors. Development is influenced by biological, neurological, cognitive, and psychosocial factors, as well as their contributions to the functioning of the patient. Neurodevelopmental challenges specifically impact the growth and maturation of the nervous system and these interactions within an individual. Psychological assessment can often assist the medical provider through a more comprehensive investigation of these various factors. In particular, assessments focused on neuropsychological functioning in children with neurodevelopmental disorders can assist care providers in understanding how the individual patient's functioning is impacted and can provide suggestions on how the environment must be adapted to allow the patient to navigate the maturation process with obstacles minimized and function maximized.

Introduction

In this growing age of managed care and required medical referrals, it is increasingly likely that children and adolescents will present to primary care settings with concerns related to developmental delay in one or more of their developmental domains (see Table 3.1) as well as general medical issues that may have implications for adaptive functioning. While schools must provide assessment of youth with neurodevelopmental disabilities (as early as age 3 years), the schools have strict guidelines for implementing an Individual Education Plan (IEP). The process usually cannot be completed in a timely manner or the school is unable to provide the

M.A. Larsen (✉)
Family Institute, PC, Grand Forks, ND 58201, USA
e-mail: dr.adamslarsen@gmail.com

D.R. Patel et al. (eds.), *Neurodevelopmental Disabilities*,
DOI 10.1007/978-94-007-0627-9_3, © Springer Science+Business Media B.V. 2011

Table 3.1 Domains of function that impact psychological development

Motor	*Language*
Fine motor	Receptive language
Gross motor coordination	Expressive language
Control of large and small muscles (smoothness rate, rhythm, sequence, symmetry, left–right differences)	Written language
Postural control	Comprehension of language nuances (syntax, semantics, learning new words, social language, conversation skills)
Balance	*Auditory*
Motor planning	Hearing (ability to understand language and coordinate that information with other events and actions in the environment and within one's self)
Agility/flexibility	
Strength	*Perceptual motor*
Endurance	Eye–hand coordination
Visual	Visual–spatial (discriminating shapes, position, relative size, foreground, background relationships, form, constancy, speed in relation to self, others, and objects)
Discrimination	
Acuity	Trajectory judgment
Tracking	Temporal sequencing
Attention	Awareness of sequential ordering
Extraocular muscle control (resting balance, control of movement, visual motor coordination)	Awareness of time and sequence
	Judging velocity of moving objects
Cognitive	Body position sense
Attention	Proprioceptive and kinesthetic sense (body image, body awareness, strength, awareness of body in space, awareness of strength, touch)
Mental processing speed (alertness)	
Memory	*Social/emotional*
Thinking (knowledge of specifics, comprehension, application, analysis, synthesis, evaluation, decision making, problem solving, and the ability simultaneously to monitor multiple events and people	Regulation and modulation of emotions
	Ability to establish new friendships
	Ability to maintain peer and family relationships
	Integrative/adaptive
	Everyday functioning related to communication, daily living skills, social skills, and community living

Reprinted with permission from [1, 2]

type of assessment required (i.e., intellectual, neurodevelopmental, neuropsychological, behavioral, and psychosocial) to address the medical referral question. Youth identified early in life with developmental risks or concerns are often referred to early intervention programs (varying in title by state) to monitor, track, and ensure engagement with appropriate services prior to the time that public educational settings would take over. It may even be the case that youth across the age span with various medical conditions (e.g., head injury, spina bifida, cerebral palsy, diabetes, metabolic conditions, chronic illness, physical disabilities, and brain tumors) are often referred for psychological assessment via primary or specialty care, long before the academic process is involved. Youth who have non-specific delays combined with average to above average intellectual function are often able to adapt to their environments well enough to mitigate significant maturational, academic, social, or emotional deficits until they reach situations that require higher order functioning (e.g., fourth grade academic demands, entering middle school or high school). In order to better understand the concept of assessment, a discussion related to "normal" neurodevelopment or "normal" development will be helpful.

Neurodevelopment in a broad sense refers to the growth and maturation of the nervous system, as well as sensory and perceptual abilities of the child [1, 3–9]. Normal growth and development is characterized by individual variations in the rate of progression and achievement of milestones and the sequential nature of this progression. Although largely determined by genetic factors, environmental factors (such as opportunity, nutrition, and social context) also play a significant role in overall development of a child or adolescent [10]. Capute noted that motor milestones are mostly influenced by maturation of the neurological system; on the other hand, social and adaptive skills are influenced largely by environmental factors, such as social expectations, education, and training [3]. The term neurodevelopment encompasses various domains which can be broadly categorized as physical or somatic, neurological, sensory-perceptual, cognitive, and psychosocial or emotional [10].

Disability or Delay

Historically, psychologists test children who present with symptoms of developmental disabilities to determine their cognitive strengths and weaknesses to assist with the development of interventional programming. The World Health Organization in 2002 recommended that the focus should be on what individuals can do in a standard environment (capacity) and in their usual environment (performance) [11]. The word function includes body functions, activities, and participation, while disability is used as an umbrella term for impairments, activity limitations, and participation restrictions. Environmental factors include all factors that interact with all functions. The deficit model of disability is obsolete; a functional model is the current approach to viewing disability [12]. Terminology used to describe individuals with impairments has shifted from reification (i.e., the disabled person or the person with disabilities) to a description of ability versus inability. Assessment is used to identify the relative extent or magnitude of strengths and weaknesses, thereby identifying areas of impairment. Medical diagnosis (and to a large degree, educational diagnosis) focuses specifically on the extent or magnitude of impairment. Four classifications are noted: (a) body functions (parts of the body affected); (b) body structure (the nature of the change in the respective body structure); (c) activity and participation (capacities and limitations); and (d) environmental factors (accommodations or barriers) [11].

Children with known neurodevelopmental deficits are likely to present with an array of functional challenges affecting motor and sensory domains. These challenges may also translate into difficulties with the neurotransmission of information within the brain, typically referred to as "processing" difficulties. Finally, the practical application of these skills (adaptive and otherwise) also may display difficulties. Comprehensive assessment that reviews all aspects of the child's functioning is therefore essential to best capture the totality of the implications of neurodevelopmental deficits for a specific individual. By assessing, documenting, and describing the normative and qualitative functioning in various neurocognitive domains, care providers will be best equipped to focus on accommodations or treatments that will most effectively limit the impact of the neurodevelopmental challenge.

The procedures of psychological assessment are defined based upon the presenting symptoms related to developmental delays, questions or concerns to be addressed based on the referral source, and any further concerns or questions raised by family or other care/educational providers. The assessment may simply document the current developmental functioning or it may be comprehensive to address multiple questions as well as provide data to support and identify services needed to accommodate, ameliorate, or eliminate obstacles in a variety of life settings (e.g., academics, social, home); to develop appropriate treatment planning and execute accordingly; and to guide program placement.

Collecting Background Information

Assessments most often begin with the psychologist collecting background information. Obtaining a thorough history would include acquiring information related to development (e.g., gross motor, fine motor, speech, and self-help milestones), specific behavioral concerns and history of behavioral problems (e.g., duration, intensity, onset, and changes), medical history (e.g., prenatal, birth, medical, and psychiatric information), family history (e.g., family demographics, dynamics, and family medical/genetic factors), academic history (e.g., grades completed, need for, and type of, special education), psychosocial history (e.g., social, emotional, and behavioral information), and use of available resources (e.g., speech therapy, counseling, support groups), as well as any additional information deemed important by the psychologist. Assessment requires collecting information from a comprehensive set of records including school, medical, and other service/caregiver domains. Teacher evaluations, school observations, and team conversations should augment the school records that could include special education evaluation reports, report cards, IEP documentation or 504 Accommodation documentation, and notation of any behavioral difficulties such as truancy and suspensions. This data collected from the interview and collaborative resources assists the clinician in developing a comprehensive understanding of the child, in terms of family-based strengths and weaknesses as well as school-based strengths and weaknesses, to add to the information gathered through standardized test data. The culmination of this assessment is a report that documents the background information, observational data collected, results of the standardized assessments conducted, applicable diagnosis, and specific recommendations that address the referral questions.

Observational Data Collection

Behavior can be influenced by the environment through antecedent and consequential events, as well as be reflexive to physiological circumstances. When either reflexes or antecedents and consequences are structured in a way that adversely impacts others much of the time and to a moderate to strong degree, the humans exhibiting them are typically referred for evaluation and assessment. Behavioral observation allows for the clinician to examine specific actions directed at particular symptoms or behaviors that are problematic for an individual or others with whom the individual must interact. Behaviors theoretically serve four major functions: (1) to obtain attention, (2) to escape unpleasant experiences, (3) to receive something tangible (object), and (4) internal satisfaction (covert stimulation). Behavioral observation makes it possible for the clinician to define a target behavior so that it is clear what response or behavior is of concern and allows for the identification of appropriate and effective interventions across a variety of functional domains, such that both strengths and weaknesses can be best assessed.

Testing Circumstances

A psychological assessment requires many variables be controlled to allow for the best assessment possible and increase the likelihood of a valid outcome. Specifically, evaluators must be trained and fully prepared in administering the procedures for the assessment, commonly referred to as a protocol. To be well prepared, the evaluator may need to memorize the entire protocol, ready various forms and materials that will be utilized, and be very familiar with the assessment procedures that are being applied. The testing conditions are also important. Most administration manuals specify how the materials should be presented, such as in a well-lit, low-noise workspace with a table and chair of appropriate height to provide a comfortable atmosphere for the assessment. Any deviations from these standardized procedures should be noted in the testing report and should be considered by the report writer when interpreting the findings. For example, a child with cerebral palsy who is seen in a wheelchair with a tray may not utilize a table for testing; this should be noted in the report. When assessing children and adolescents with neurodevelopmental disabilities, it is often imperative to adapt some aspect of the testing protocol to the particular patient. For example, written tasks may be omitted for youth with significant fine motor struggles; they may be allowed to respond aloud instead. Any adaptation should be noted as well. Evaluator error is always possible and should also be noted in the report if it occurred. Another aspect to the assessment is how the assessment is introduced to the examinee and how the examinee responds to the evaluator (rapport). Obviously, an assessment with an examinee who understands the reasons for the evaluation and who has a good working relationship with the evaluator is likely to result in more accurate estimates of functioning.

From the perspective of the child, anxiety related to the testing situation or to assessments in general may impact performance. As most psychological testing is done without parents present in the room, preparation for this situation is well advised as some children, particularly those who are young or shy, may experience initial discomfort separating from their parents. Generally, careful explanation regarding the current assessment will help alleviate worries and enhance performance. In situ assessment related to state of functioning (anxious versus relaxed) and prompted coping skills are often useful in reducing anxiety during psychological assessment. However, as with other test circumstances, these should be documented in the report. For an individual who has recently (within the past year) been evaluated, re-testing may demonstrate improved performance due to learning and recollection of the test, resulting in a more elevated performance than would be truly representative of the individual's daily functioning. Patients who are sophisticated testers (e.g., are knowledgeable about testing or have taken test-taking courses) are likely to perform better than would be expected based on testing skills as opposed to their daily functioning skills in the domain being assessed. Psychological measures can be very sensitive and often can influence an individual's learning, such that re-testing utilizing the same measure and materials within too close temporal proximity can confound the results and overestimate functioning for the examinee.

Testing Conditions

Testing Environment

Traditionally, psychological testing focuses on examining the patient while employing carefully constructed models of administration and using strict guidelines for the actions of the psychologist during the administration. However, infants, children, and adolescents with developmental disabilities require assessments that may not be originally considered by many psychologists. Such alterations may involve the use of standardized tests not normally included in a "full battery." For example, children and adolescents with language-based impairments may provide a better picture of their functional abilities if the testing included an emphasis on non-verbal instruments. Similarly, youth with motor impairments such as cerebral palsy are often better assessed if measures do not require hand–eye coordination to perform at optimal level. Likewise, youth who have known visual impairments would be better evaluated using measures that do not require sight or permit alternative forms of recognition. The focus of evaluation of youth who present with functional impairments should be on identifying obstacles to their successful progression through the maturation process (from birth to adulthood). There are times in the assessment of neurodevelopmental disabilities where standardized assessment procedures are completely useless, for example, the scenario of a quadriplegic patient who is non-verbal and who has been determined to only have self-regulated control of eye gaze/blinking. This individual will not be able to validly complete a typical intellectual assessment, and the examiner must be creative in their chosen assessment procedures to address referral questions to document intellectual capacity. For example, a very basic applied behavioral assessment could be chosen to quantify the responses to behavioral demands such as eye blink, gazing, and visual picture identification.

Appropriate Time Between Testing Referrals

In general, unless a head injury or memory problem is apparent, a good guideline for reassessment is at least 1 year for psychological and neuropsychological assessments; however, assessment of mood, attention, or psychosocial aspects may be more frequent. Neurodevelopmental assessments may occur much more frequently, especially between birth and 3 years, as treatment outcomes are often measured by their direct impact on growth related to developmental markers. Evaluators may choose to utilize comparative measures or alternative forms rather than repeating the same measure as well. Evaluator compliance with administration standards reduces the differences between examinees. However, the impact of the examinee on the assessment situation is often described in the behavioral observations section of the report, where characteristics thought to impact the test results are described (e.g., disruptive behavior throughout the assessment; wore glasses; required encouragement and motivation).

Daily functioning and adaptive skills are very important variables to consider in the assessment procedures. Behavior does not occur in a vacuum of unrelated materials. Antecedents (what came 3–5 seconds before), behavior (what the patient does), consequences (what came 3–5 seconds after the behavior), development (adaptive functioning the patient typically displays), as well as environment (what the patient's surroundings are) are essential to better understanding the patient's experiences and lead to more comprehensive diagnostic patterns and pictures.

Ethical Concerns and Cautions

The American Psychological Association (APA) Code of Ethics outlines a "standard of care" for all practicing, licensed psychologists [13]. Within this code are specific guidelines related to assessment and test results (Section 9 and 4). An examiner must consider in his or her report all variables that might explain the findings, such as culture and educational exposure. As well, psychologists are to ensure the security of assessments, provide reports and full explanations of the assessment results to patients or their representative (e.g., parents), and provide raw data to appropriately informed requesting parties.

Confidentiality and sharing of test results are also guided by the APA Ethics Code (Sections 9 and 4). Psychologists have the utmost responsibility to maintain an individual's confidentiality and to ensure that no harm may come as a result of releasing their private information (e.g., test reports, raw scores). Reports are only released when the appropriate release forms are signed and are likely to only be released to professionals who will have an understanding and background in reviewing the report without disposition. Reports are generally not released to families unless a disposition meeting has been scheduled to fully review the results and findings. HIPAA regulations have added further regulatory intervention with regard to the sharing of protected health information and patient records, and aside from the "standard of care" or ethical guidelines that are set out for the psychological profession, there are state and federal laws that require the confidentiality and security of medical/psychological records. With this said, obtaining a release at the time a referral is made will assist all parties in the assessment and disposition process.

Psychological Report

A very brief review of principle and statistical concepts related to psychological assessment is warranted for a better understanding of the discussion of various assessments to follow. The reader may wish to refer to Fig. 3.1 to identify the concepts discussed. A psychological test is a measure that has been empirically derived to assess the differences between one individual's performances compared to that of many other similar individuals or between an individual's performance compared across situations. A psychological test generally has a standardized method of administration, requirements of training for those administering and interpreting the test, and direct implications for the examinee's psychological, educational, or career-orientated functioning. Thus, Anastasi defined a psychological test as "an objective and standardized measure of a sample of behavior" [14]. Psychological assessments are used to predict how well an individual may perform given a certain set of circumstances and in turn to predict or generalize to daily life (current and future) functioning for the examinee. By definition, psychological tests have been standardized, meaning their validity (what they are measuring), reliability (consistency in measurement), method (manualized documentation so each administration is identical), and use (qualification of administrator) have rigorously been scrutinized prior to publication. The Mental Measurements Yearbook (MMY) provides information regarding publisher, purpose of the assessment, and published reviews, on nearly every English-published psychological assessment [15]. As well, the Standards for Educational and Psychological Testing provides information regarding the requirements for assessments to be considered empirically valid.

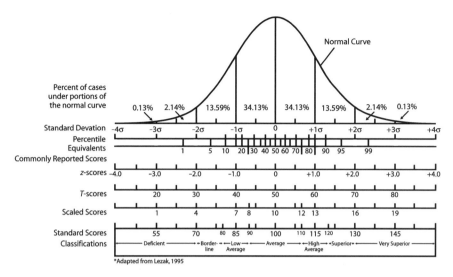

Fig. 3.1 Distribution of Standard Scores (adapted from Lezak, 1995)

Psychological tests are "controlled" for the purposes of protection of the public, to increase validity and reliability, as well as to protect copyright and "trade secrets" [16].

Norms

Norms broadly refer to the performance of the standardization sample on the same assessment. These may be broken down and presented in age-based groups, grade-based groups, gender-based groups, or some combination thereof. Norms are commonly used as a method of comparing the examinee's performance and functionality to that of the standardization group.

Statistical Concepts and the Bell Curve

The basis of most psychological assessments is a normal distribution or the use of corrected statistical analyses to allow for extrapolation to the normal curve distribution of scores. This is also referred to as the Bell Curve and represents the population frequency and distribution of scores for IQ, achievement, and functioning in a variety of domains (see Fig. 3.1).

All normal curve distributions have the following characteristics: 68.7% of the population falls between 1 standard deviation above and below the mean; 95.4% of the population falls between 2 standard deviation above and below the mean; and 99.7% of the population falls between 3 standard deviation above and below the mean. Standard deviation (SD) is a statistical measure of variability, while the mean (M) is a statistical measure of the average score. In considering deficits, generally 1.5 SD below the mean or greater (e.g., 2 SD below, 3 SD below) is a cut-off point representing significant deviations from expected or typical performance and reflective of a need for intervention. In contrast, an individual scoring at least 1.5 SD above the mean is thought to be gifted. The normal curve allows not only estimates of deviation based on where performance falls under the curve but also translation of these data points into a variety of more frequently used, user-friendly "scores."

Percentiles

Percentiles are generally understandable and comparable by parents and non-professionals; however, it is important to understand that percentile units are not standard or equal. Thus, at the middle of the distribution, small differences in standard scores translate into great differences in percentiles, and at the extremes of a distribution, large differences in standard scores are required to have much difference in percentiles. Percentiles are utilized in providing relative position of an examinee's performance based on the normative sample.

Standard Scores

Standard scores are utilized more frequently as the method of summarizing or reporting an examinee's performance. Standard scores represent performance as a product of deviation from the mean based in standard deviation units and can be translated into scores based upon the normative sample. Generally, in most psychometric assessments, standard scores have a mean of 100 and a standard deviation of 15. For example, Wechsler IQ scores are reported as standard scores, such that a child who has an IQ value of 70 would fall 2 standard deviation below the mean and be classified with deficient intellectual abilities. On the Wechsler series assessments, as well as other tests, a scaled score is often used to describe performance on a subtest. Scaled scores are a form of standard score in which the mean is 10 and the standard deviation is 3. A child is classified in the Very Superior range on Block Design from the WISC-IV by earning a subtest score of 18.

Other versions of comparative scores also exist. For example, another expression of the standard score is a T-score, for which the mean is 50 and the standard deviation is 10 points; a T-score of 45 falls in the normal range (i.e., within 1 SD below or above the mean of the normative sample). Yet another translation of standard scores is z-score (refer to Fig. 3.1), which is a product of the following calculation: obtained performance minus the mean of the normative sample, divided by the standard deviation of the normative sample. For z-scores, the comparative mean is expected to be 0 and the standard deviation is known to be 1. Thus, a student who has a z-score of –2 in preferred hand dexterity is performing 2 SD below the normative mean, and performance would be classified as deficient.

Confidence Intervals

Confidence intervals are another method of providing information regarding a person's performance. In fact, this is commonly provided to demonstrate the non-static nature of assessment scores. Test reliability and error contribute to obtain performance scores considered estimates of the individual's true performance. Confidence intervals provide a range within which the true score is likely to fall, given a statistical confidence value (usually 90 or 95%). Thus, a Wechsler IQ Index score may be 90, but have a confidence interval range from 85 to 95.

A Word of Warning About Grade Equivalence

It is important to understand the concept of grade equivalence, particularly in achievement or academic testing. Grade equivalence refers to the examinee's performance on the test and the grade level of others who performed similarly. Grade equivalence does not relate to the grade level of achieved performance on the test. For example, an individual in 5th grade who obtained a standard score of 85 may have a grade equivalence of grade 4 on the assessment. This means that the level of performance for the individual was able to be achieved by all children in a 4th grade sample who took the same measure. It does not mean that the score of 85 was at a 4th grade work level. Grade equivalence is not a good basis for comparison as the concept is often misunderstood; in addition, grade equivalence does not take into account differences in instruction or inequality in grade units and may have cast implications when utilized improperly.

Neuropsychological Testing and Psychological Testing

A neuropsychological evaluation seeks to utilize various psychological assessment measures along with behavioral observations and assessments to understand how the structures in any given brain are functioning. Specifically, neuropsychologists utilize various assessment procedures to better understand the implications of problematic brain functioning or structure (i.e., hemorrhage, arteriovenous malformations, cerebral palsy, seizure, TBI, toxin exposure, etc.). Thus, psychological assessment serves as a basis for more advanced interpretations and recommendations. For example, a right-handed 8-year-old presents for neuropsychological assessment. Comprehensive psychological assessment of various measures is completed, and the findings suggest that the psychologist may report the child has strong verbal skills and very weak non-verbal skills. Further neuropsychologically driven assessment may also review poor visual–motor integration skills, fine motor or sensory delays, and extremely strong verbal memory skills. The neuropsychologist may report the child's performance was consistent with a non-verbal learning disability and implicate the left hemisphere substriatal pathway. Thus, a more brain/behavior detailed impression would be expected.

Psychometric Testing Measures

A variety of standardized assessment measures have been developed to assess constructs of intellectual functioning, academic achievement, developmental progress, memory, and cognitive capacities. A brief description of areas of assessment is provided and commonly used measures are reviewed. The information provided is not meant to be an endorsement of the tool, nor is the list exhaustive; however, most of the measures described are generally considered to be reliable, valid assessment tools when utilized by a licensed, trained professional. In the following pages, the reader will find an overview of several common psychological assessment tools, reviewed in categories relating to the psychological functions they are designed to assess.

Cognitive Assessment

Cognitive assessment tools (see Table 3.2) estimate an individual's global cognitive functioning. These have typically been referred to as "IQ tests." However, testing theory and psychological assessment are now more sophisticated and "IQ tests" are comprised of multiple tasks or batteries. These batteries are able to assess multiple domains of cognitive functioning such as language skills, non-verbal performance abilities, mental agility, and memory.

Measures like the Wechsler Intelligence Scales include standard scores for the various domains of functioning, and a score that provides an overall functioning estimate, or Full Scale Intellectual Quotient. In years gone by this Full Scale value was considered the intellectual quotient. Theories now put much less emphasis on this single number and focus more on functioning in the various assessed domains.

Verbal or Language Skills

Verbal skills are also evaluated (see Table 3.3). These are the language skills thought to represent the functioning of the most dominant brain hemisphere in lateralized individuals. Assessment tools for this domain typically involve auditory or visual instructions and language-based assessment strategies and focus on assessing receptive language, expressive language, and verbal memory functions if a comprehensive evaluation is conducted.

Non-verbal or Performance Skills

Non-verbal or performance skills (see Table 3.4) are another domain area of psychological testing. Non-verbal skills are thought to represent the functioning of the non-dominant hemisphere in lateralized individuals. Assessment tools for this functioning domain include batteries that involve no language-based instructions (e.g.,

Table 3.2 Cognitive assessment measures

Wechsler Preschool and Primary Scale of Intelligence – 3rd edition (WPPSI-III) (Wechsler; Psychological Corporation)	2 years, 6 months–7 years, 3 months	14 subtests; yields Full Scale, verbal and performance IQ scores
Wechsler Intelligence Scale for Children – 4th edition (WISC-IV) (Wechsler; Psychological Corporation)	6 years–16 years, 11 months	15 subtests; yields Full Scale IQ, verbal comprehension, perceptual reasoning, working memory, and processing speed indices
Wechsler Adult Intelligence Scale – 3rd edition (WAIS-III) (Wechsler; Psychological Corporation)	16 years–adulthood	14 subtests; yield Full Scale IQ, verbal comprehension, perceptual organization, working memory, and processing speed indices
Wechsler Abbreviated Scales of Intelligence (WASI) (Wechsler; Psychological Corporation)	6 years–adulthood	4 subtests; brief IQ screener; yields Full Scale, Verbal, and Performance IQ estimates
Mullen Scales of Early Learning (Mullen) (Mullen; AGS Publishing)	Birth–68 months	5 subtests; yields gross motor, visual reception, fine motor, receptive language, and expressive language scores
Stanford-Binet – 5th edition (SB-V) (Roid; Riverside Publishing)	2 years–adulthood	10 subtests; yields Full Scale, verbal, and non-verbal IQ scores as well as four index scores
Kaufman Brief Intelligence Test – 2nd edition (KBIT-2)	4–90 years	Verbal and non-verbal domain scores based on three subtests: Verbal knowledge and riddles and matrices

Table 3.3 Verbal language assessment measures

Peabody Picture Vocabulary Test – 3rd edition (PPVT-III) (Dunn and Dunn; American Guidance Services, Inc.)	2 years, 6 months–90+	Assesses English receptive vocabulary skills
Expressive Vocabulary Test (EVT) (Williams; American Guidance Services, Inc.)	2 years, 6 months–90+	Assesses English expressive vocabulary skills
Boston Naming Test – II (Goodglass and Kaplan; Pro-Ed, Inc.)	5 years–adult	Assesses expressive language skills and provides measures to evaluate assistance of phonological and multiple choice cues

mimed), tasks that involve language instructions but no verbal responses (e.g., creating a block design to match a visual stimuli; copying a complex diagram), or tasks that utilize visual-based stimuli requiring a language-based response (e.g., determine a visual matched pair and state the letter of the matched stimuli). Memory functions can be assessed in non-verbal domains as well.

Table 3.4 Non-verbal or performance assessment measures

Universal Test of Nonverbal Intelligence (UNIT) (Bracken and McCallum; Riverside Publishing Company)	5 years–17 years, 11 months	Six subtests; no verbalizations required; yields Full Scale IQ, memory, reasoning, symbolic, and non-symbolic quotients
Comprehensive Test of Nonverbal Intelligence (CTONI) (Hammill, Pearson, Wiederholt; Pro-Ed, Inc.)	6–89 years	Six subtests; yields non-verbal IQ, picture non-verbal IQ, and geometric non-verbal IQ indices
Ravens Standard Progressive Matrices (Ravens; Harcourt Assessment, Inc.)	Child–adult norms	Assesses reasoning through pictures
Benton Judgment of Line Orientation (Benton; Psychological Assessment Resources, Inc.)	Child–adult norms	Measures visuospatial judgment
Leiter International Performance Scale Revised (Leiter-R; Stoelting Company)	2–20 years	Completely non-verbal assessment tool administered in mime
Wechsler Nonverbal Scales of Ability (WNV) (PsychCorp; Harcourt Assessment, Inc.)	2 years–21 years, 11 months	Four subtests; yields a Full Scale IQ score; utilizes a variety of non-verbal responses (pointing, puzzles, writing symbols)

Executive Functioning

Executive functioning (see Table 3.5) is another domain particularly of interest in individuals with attention and behavior regulation problems. The frontal lobe is thought to be involved heavily in organization, planning, and regulation of various behaviors and is highly taxed on tasks that assess executive skills. These assessment tools emphasize attention, organization, short-term memory, mental shifting, and sustained mental focus. These tasks challenge the workings of the frontal lobe and are typically found in neuropsychological assessments and assessments for attention-based disorders.

Memory Functions

Memory functions (see Table 3.6) can be assessed in a variety of ways. Recall memory can involve free or cued/prompted responses, while recognition memory involves providing a verbal or visual stimuli and asking if it was one learned/seen before. In addition, memory can be assessed as a function of time. Immediate recall is assessed after a brief delay, such as 10 s exposure to the stimuli and 5 s delay before recall. Delayed recall is assessed after a much longer delay, typically 30 min, and may occur after single review of materials or multiple repetitions of the target materials. These methods of memory assessment help determine aspects of memory that may be stronger or weaker comparatively. Some assessment tools will also add

Table 3.5 Assessment of executive function measures

Measure	Age range	Description
Behavior Rating Inventory of Executive Function (BRIEF) (Gioia et al.; Psychological Assessment Resources, Inc.)	5–18 years	Parent-, teacher-, and self (teenagers)-report forms; assesses seven areas of executive functioning, as well as three broad scores: behavioral regulation index, metacognition index, and global executive composite
Conners Continuous Performance Task – 2nd edition (CPT-II) (Conners; Multi-Health Systems, Inc.)	Pre-school–kindergarten (Kiddie CPT); 6 years–adulthood (CPT-II)	20-min computer test to assess attention; tracks omission errors, commission errors, response times, and latency in responding
Test of Variables in Attention (TOVA) (Leark et al.; Universal Attention Disorders, Inc.)	6–19 years	25-min computer test to assess attention; yields omission errors, commission errors, response time, and variability in response time; two versions available – visual and auditory
Wisconsin Card Sorting Test (WCST) (Heaton et al.; Psychological Assessment Resources, Inc.)	6 years, 6 months–adulthood	Assesses abstract reasoning/problem solving; yields information regarding errors, ability to learn abstractly, perseveration, and ability to shift and maintain set
Children's Categories Test (CCT) (Boll; Psychological Corporation)	Level I: 5–8 years Level II: 9–16 years	Non-verbal assessment of abstract reasoning
Tower of London (Culbertson and Zillmer; Psychological Assessment Resources, Inc.)	7 years–adult	Assesses visual problem solving skills including planning and organizing
Trail Making Test (Reitan; Reitan Neuropsychological Laboratory, Inc.)	5 years–adult	Assesses mental fluency as well as ability to shift set
Test of Everyday Attention for Children (TEA-Ch) (Manly et al.; Pearson Assessment)	6–16 years	Assesses various aspects of attention yet minimizes the need for other skills (e.g., language, dexterity); examines selective attention, sustained attention, and attentional control/switching

Table 3.6 Memory assessment measures

Children's Memory Scale (CMS) (Cohen; Psychological Corporation)	5–16 years	Yields immediate and delayed scores for both verbal memory and visual memory, general memory, delayed recognition, learning, and attention/concentration
Wide Range Assessment of Memory and Learning – 2nd edition (WRAML2) (Sheslow and Adams; Jastak Associates, Inc.)	5 years–adulthood	Six core and four optional subtests; yields verbal and visual memory as well as attention/concentration scores; also has four recognition memory and three delayed recall subtests
Wechsler Memory Scale – 3rd edition (WMS-III) (Wechsler; Psychological Corporation)	16 years–adulthood	Six core and five optional subtests; yields three domain scores: immediate memory, general memory (delayed), and working memory
Rey Complex Figure Task (Meyers and Meyers; Psychological Assessment Resources, Inc.)	6 years–adulthood	Assesses visuospatial construction and visual memory; yields scores for copy, short-term recall, long-term recall, and recognition
California Verbal Learning Test – Children's Version (CVLT-C);	CVLT-C: 5–16 years	All similar measures assessing ability to recall unrelated information in the form of word lists; generally yield scores related to learning ability, immediate recall, delayed recall, and recognition
California Verbal Learning Test – 2nd edition (CVLT—II) (Dellis et al.; Psychological Corporation)	CVLT-II: 16 years–adulthood	
Rey Auditory Verbal Learning Task (RAVLT) (Schmidt; Western Psychological Services)	RAVLT: 7 years–adulthood	

an element to purposefully assess impeded memory such as a distracter list. Both verbal and non-verbal (i.e., visual) memory can be assessed.

Neuropsychological Measures

Specialized neuropsychological measures (see Table 3.7) are utilized to assess the function of particular brain systems and are typically conducted by assessing a function using two or more methods or tasks. In addition, sensory functioning is typically assessed using neuropsychological tools that focus on one or more of the five sensory areas (i.e., visual, auditory, olfaction, gustatory, sensorimotor) and their integration and processing within the brain's neurocircuitry. For example, auditory and visual processing may be emphasized for individuals thought to have attentional disorders as these areas are fundamental to the comprehension and execution of instructions. Individuals with traumatic brain injury may require

Table 3.7 Examples of neuropsychological assessment batteries

NEPSY-II (Korkman, Kirk, & Kemp; NCS Pearson, Inc.)	3–16 years, 11 months	Assesses domains of neurocognitive functioning, including attention and executive functioning, language, memory and learning, sensorimotor, social perception, and visuospatial processing
Halstead-Reitan Neuropsychological Test Battery (HRNB; Reitan Neuropsychological Laboratories)	5 years–adulthood	Assesses memory, abstract reasoning, language, sensory/motor, and perception domains
Luria-Nebraska Neuropsychological Battery (LNNB; Golden, Purisch, & Hammeke; Western Psychological Services)	15 years–adult	Assesses various areas within motor, sensory, language, memory, and reasoning domains
Luria-Nebraska Neuropsychological Battery for Children (LNNB-C; Golden; Western Psychological Services)	8–12 years	Assesses various areas within motor, sensory, language, memory, and reasoning domains

evaluation of all sensory areas to determine the nature and severity of injury or recovery. Oftentimes, a neuropsychological evaluation relies on a combination of tools assessing a variety of domains (e.g., cognitive, verbal, non-verbal, executive function, academic), as described throughout this section. Additionally, neuropsychologists may use all or part of specifically designed neuropsychological batteries, such as the NEPSY-Second Edition, the Halstead-Reitan Battery, or the Luria-Nebraska Neuropsychological Battery.

Academic or Achievement Assessments

Academic assessments (see Table 3.8) examine achievement skills in the areas of reading, writing/spelling, and arithmetic, including basic knowledge (e.g., math facts or word reading), problem solving and higher order skill sets (e.g., essay writing), and the comprehension of these concepts. In addition, as grade levels increase, assessment tools are available for specific subject areas such as science, social studies, and geography. Brief measures as well as multi-concept measures are available. For individuals in high school, this assessment area may also include career and vocational interest and skills.

Developmental or Adaptive Assessments

Developmental assessments (see Table 3.9) are utilized to estimate an individual's functioning compared to developmental constructs, concepts, and criterion. While

Table 3.8 Achievement assessment measures

Wide Range Achievement Test – 4th edition (WRAT-4) (Wilkinson; Wide Range, Inc.)	5 years–adulthood	Four subtests: sentence comprehension, word reading, spelling, and math computation
Bracken Basic Concepts Scale – Revised (BBCS-R) (Bracken; Psychological Corporation)	2 years, 6 months–8 years	Assesses knowledge of basic concepts learned during preschool and early elementary; 11 skills assessed
Wechsler Individual Achievement Test – 3rd edition (WIAT-III) (Wechsler; Psychological Corporation)	4–85 years	Nine subtests; yields composite scores for reading, mathematics, written language, and oral language
Woodcock-Johnson – III (WJ-III) (Woodcock et al.; Riverside Publishing)	2 years–adulthood	12 standard and 10 supplemental subtests; yields scores for reading, oral language, mathematics, written language, and academic knowledge

Table 3.9 Developmental assessment measures

Bayley Scales of Infant Development – 3rd edition (Bayley) (Bayley; Psychological Corporation)	1–42 months	Direct examination of the child; assesses mental, motor, and behavioral skills; cognitive, language, personal/social, and fine/gross motor skills also assessed
Vineland Adaptive Behavior Scales (Vineland); and Vineland Adaptive Behavior Scales – 2nd edition (VABS-II) (Sparrow et al.; American Guidance Services, Inc.)	Birth–adulthood	Parent questionnaire or interview; yields general adaptive composite score and communication, daily living skills, socialization, and motor skills domain scores
Development Profile – 3 (DP-3) (Alpern et al.; Western Psychological Services)	Birth–155 months	Parent interview; also involves observation; assesses physical, adaptive, social-emotional, cognitive, and communication skills
Adaptive Behavior Assessment System – 2nd edition (ABAS-II) (Harrison and Oakland; Harcourt Assessment, Inc.)	Birth–adulthood	Parent questionnaire or interview; separate forms for various age brackets; yields general adaptive composite score as well as conceptual, social, and practical domains; separate form for teachers
Ages and Stages Questionnaire (Squires et al.; Brookes Publishing Company)	4–60 months	Parent report form; used to screen/monitor five areas of development: communication, gross motor, fine motor, problem solving, and personal-social skills; available in English, Spanish, French, and Korean
Denver Developmental 2nd edition (Denver II) (Denver Developmental Materials, Inc.)	Birth–6 years	Parent report form; screens a child's adaptive functioning compared to normal developmental expectations; English and Spanish versions

likely most familiar to the medical provider for infants through preschool age, these tools have become increasingly utilized in the comprehensive assessment of children with any type of developmental impairment such as Asperger's syndrome, autistic disorder, or neurologically involved children. Age estimates are often used as comparative methods.

Behavioral Symptom Assessment

Behavioral symptoms (see Table 3.10) and behavioral functioning are assessed through interview, observation, behavioral assessment techniques, and various standardized measures to augment the behavioral assessment procedures previously described. Comprehensive approaches would be recommended for children with behavioral problems in conjunction with behavioral assessment and the planning of behavioral programming.

Emotional Functioning Assessment

Emotional functioning (see Table 3.11) is typically assessed through multiple methods, including self-report, parent/teacher report, and interview. There also are very specific tools utilized for specific symptom areas that are helpful when considering the diagnosis of anxiety disorders, obsessive compulsive disorders, depression, social skill deficits, and self-concept concerns.

Personality Assessment

For the older adolescent, assessments of behavioral characteristics that may represent an emerging personality style (see Table 3.12) are available. It should be noted that behavioral theory would suggest caution in the assessment of "personality" in individuals below the age of 18 years.

The Psychological Assessment Report

In general, when psychological assessment has been conducted, a report should be generated. The report should include a review of the referral concerns, historical information for the child, a list of psychometric assessment tools used, current functioning status, behavioral observations, and specific scores related to any standardized assessment procedures conducted (this may be in a brief or comprehensive format). The report should provide a review of the individual's performance. There should be a dialogue discussing the impression of the findings related to the referral question, providing a diagnosis when appropriate. Psychological diagnoses are made based on the most current Diagnostic and Statistical Manual of Mental Disorders (DSM) which is published by the American

Table 3.10 Behavioral self-report/other report measures

Measure	Age	Description
Child Behavior Checklist (CBCL) (Achenbach and Rescorla; Department of Psychiatry, University of Vermont)	18 months–18 years	Yields scores for 14 subscales as well as internalizing, externalizing, and total problems; corresponds to the youth self-report (ages 11–18) and teacher report form
Conners' Rating Scales – Revised (CRS-R) (Conners; Multi-Health System Inc.)	3–17 years	Parent-, self (ages 12–17)-, and teacher report forms; yields seven subscales and seven index scores; emphasis on symptoms of ADHD
ADHD Rating Scales – IV (DuPaul et al.; Guilford Press)	5–18 years	Separate parent and teacher report forms; yields three scores: inattention, hyperactivity/impulsivity, and total score
Vanderbilt ADHD Diagnostic Rating Scale (Woraich et al.; J Abnorm Child Psychol)	6–12 years	Parent and teacher report forms; free to download; based on DSM-IV criteria for ADHD, ODD, and CD
Asperger Syndrome Diagnostic Scale (ASDS) (Myles et al.; Pro-Ed, Inc.)	5–18 years	Parent, teacher, and professional questionnaire forms; yields diagnostic indicator and functioning in cognitive, maladaptive, language, social, and sensorimotor areas
Childhood Autism Rating Scale – 2nd edition (CARS) (Schopler et al.; Western Psychological Services)	2 years and older	Standard and high functioning versions of rating booklets, as well as parent/caregiver questionnaire; yields diagnostic indicator score based on 15 areas of functioning
Gilliam Asperger's Disorder Scale (GADS) (Gilliam; PRO-ED, Inc.)	3–22 years	Questionnaire completed by parent, teacher, or professional; assesses four scales: social interaction, restricted patterns of behavior, cognitive patterns, and pragmatic skills; yields a diagnostic indicator score
Gilliam Autism Rating Scale – 2nd edition (GARS) (Gilliam; PRO-ED, Inc.)	3–22 years	Screening instrument completed by parents and teachers; includes three subscales: stereotyped behaviors, communication, and social interaction; yields a diagnostic indicator score, the autism index

Table 3.11 Emotional assessment measures

Piers-Harris Children's Self-Concept Scale – 2nd edition (Piers and Herzberg; Western Psychological Services)	7–18 years	Self-report form; yields six subscale scores and total score
Children's Depression Inventory (CDI) (Kovacs; Multi-Health Systems, Inc.)	7–17 years	27-item self-report form; yields five subscale and total depression scores
Suicide Ideation Questionnaire (SIQ) (Reynolds; Psychological Assessment Resources)	Adolescents, grades 7–12	Separate forms for junior high and high schools; screening tool for suicidal ideation
Revised Children's Manifest Anxiety Scale – 2nd edition (RCMAS) (Reynolds and Richmond; Western Psychological Services)	6–19 years	49-item self-report form; yields total anxiety score as well as three subscales; also has a defensiveness scale
State-Trait Anxiety Inventory for Children (STAIC) (Spielberger; Mindgarden, Inc.)	Grades 4–6	Self-report measure; 20 items assess state (fluctuating) anxiety and 20 items assess trait (consistent) anxiety
Roberts Apperception Test for Children – 2nd edition (RATC) (McArthur and Roberts; Western Psychological Resources)	6–18 years	Requires youth to create stories describing stimuli on cards presented to them; yields scores in several domains, including available resources, problem Identification, resolution, emotion, outcome, and unusual or atypical response
Social Skills Rating Scale (SSRS) (Greshem and Elliot; American Guidance Services)	3–18 years	Parent-, teacher-, and self-report forms; assesses three areas of social skills: social skill, problem behaviors, and academic competence

Psychiatric Association. The current edition at the time of this publication is the DSM-IV:TR [17]. Diagnoses are made using a five-axis system:

- Axis I: Transient Disorders (e.g., anxiety disorder, major depression)
- Axis II: Life-Long Disorders (e.g., mental retardation, personality disorders)
- Axis III: Medical Disorders that relate (e.g., diabetes, visual processing disorder)
- Axis IV: Areas of Functional Impact (e.g., family, school, development, health)
- Axis V: Global Assessment of Functioning (i.e., number 0–100 subjectively describing functioning level)

More than one diagnoses may be listed under a given axis. A diagnosis is required for billing and reimbursement purposes (now mandated to be an ICD diagnosis), as well as qualification for certain resources such as case management (state and federally funded programs) and school accommodations (medical and psychological diagnoses are often "translated" into educational diagnoses or categories for service provision). Once a diagnosis is identified, recommendations typically will follow.

Table 3.12 Character assessment measures

Children's Personality Questionnaire (IPAT)	8–12 years	Self-report objective measure; assesses several personality dimensions including shyness, assertiveness, and emotional stability
Louisville Behavior Checklist (Miller; Western Psychological Services)	4–17 years	Parent report objective measure
Minnesota Multiphasic Personality Inventory – Adolescent (MMPI-A) (Butcher et al.; National Computing Services, Inc.)	12–18 years	Self-report objective measure; 478 items; yields scores related to response style/validity, drug/alcohol use, and psychopathology
Millon Adolescent Clinical Inventory (MACI) (Millon; National Computing Services)	13–19 years	Self-report objective measure; 160 items; yields scores related to personality patterns, clinical syndromes, and response style/validity
Rorschach Inkblot Test (Exner; John Wiley and Sons)	5 years–adulthood	Projective measure; requires the individual to identify and describe perceptions on a stimulus card
Thematic Apperception Test (TAT) (Murray; Harvard University Press)	4 years–adulthood	Projective measure; requires the individual to create a story about a picture on a stimulus card; administered twice, on consecutive days

Recommendations

Recommendations in the report should reflect or respond to the initial consultation or referral questions and may provide comprehensive management ideas for school, home, and professional treatment providers. Recommendations may include suggestions for referrals for further evaluation, therapeutic issues, behavioral interventions, and/or academic accommodations; specific ideas, recommendations, and suggestions for intervention; and/or resources for education and additional information may also be included.

Referrals

Following psychological or neuropsychological assessment there may be further aspects of the child's functioning that are of concern. For example, these assessments may have highlighted questions about audiological or visual functioning, fine or gross motor functioning, or social communication skills, resulting in further referrals to specialty providers to specifically assess these functional areas. At times, these areas need to be evaluated prior to a psychological diagnosis being made. For example, finger agnosia, gait instability, and verbal memory problems may warrant referral to a pediatric neurologist prior to a psychological or educational diagnosis being made, which might erroneously identify attention deficit disorder versus a seizure disorder. All psychological assessment assumes medical diagnoses are not responsible for impairments in performance, and thus, testing that highlights areas of significant weakness may simply have been overlooked prior to referral. Common referrals are to certified audiologists, vision specialists, occupational therapists, physical therapists, speech and language pathologists, neurologists, and, when complex neurochemical issues are potentially involved, pediatric psychiatrists. As some managed care companies do not reimburse for assessing learning disabilities, a recommendation for academic evaluation through the school district to assess for the presence and nature of a learning disability may be made. Additionally, if chemical dependency is an area of concern, a referral for a chemical dependency evaluation may be warranted. A referral to a child life specialist may occur if a child struggles during medical procedures; the child life specialist would help the child cope with the procedure through distraction tactics and education. A referral for therapeutic recreation involvement may assist families in learning about and accessing leisure activities based on their child's neurodevelopmental functioning. Most often, the psychologist would coordinate these referrals through the primary care provider.

Other Recommendations

Additional recommendations based on the psychological evaluation may be made, specifically pertaining to the home or school settings. Specific classroom accommodations may be recommended. For instance, for a child with ADHD, preferential seating may be suggested. Similarly, a child with cerebral palsy and subsequent fine motor and writing struggles may be allowed note taking assistance. A myriad of school accommodations are available; oftentimes, developing these accommodations for youth with neurodevelopmental disabilities takes both creativity and flexibility on the part of the adult.

Specific recommendations for the home may be made as well. These may pertain to ensuring sufficient adult supervision, such as for children with autistic disorder. It may be suggested that a poster of pictures of home rules, rather than a written poster, be used for children with speech and language difficulties. Utilization of a sticker chart or other forms of positive reinforcement may be suggested for all children, regardless of the presence or absence of neurodevelopmental concerns.

Regardless of the diagnosis, a psychological evaluation should provide information regarding an individual's areas of strengths and needs. Based on these results, it will be important for parents, teachers, and other care providers in the child's life to have reasonable expectations for the child. It is essential that the child, family, and care providers have education regarding the child's diagnosis at a level that is understandable to them. In addition, explanation of recommendations will help motivate those involved to fully participate in the changes suggested. In general, it is most helpful to increase the communication between home and school and between these environments and those of the treatment providers involved in the child's care.

Conclusions

Psychological assessment can often assist the medical provider's investigation of factors that impact their patient's ability to maximize function and successfully navigate the maturational process. For patients who have neurodevelopmental challenges, specialized assessment can provide very critical information to assist with the planning on interventions to ensure positive growth and development. Psychologists with specialized training in evaluating and treating children, adolescents, and young adults can be significant additions to the physician's team and improve patient outcomes.

References

1. Pratt HD, Patel DR, Greydanus DE. Sports and the neurodevelopment of the child and adolescent. In: DeLee JC, Drez DD, Miller MD, editors. Orthopaedic sports medicine. 2nd ed. Philadelphia, PA: WB Saunders; 2002. pp. 624–43.
2. Pratt, HD. Neurodevelopmental Issues in the assessment and treatment of deficits in attention, cognition, and learning during adolescence. Adolesc Med. 2002;13(3):579–598.
3. Capute AJ, Accardo PJ. A neurodevelopmental perspective on the continuum of developmental disabilities. In: Capute AJ, Accardo PJ, editors. Developmental disabilities in infancy and childhood. 2nd ed. Baltimore, MD: Paul H Brookes; 1996. pp. 1–24.
4. Caterino MC. Age differences in the performance of basketball dribbling by elementary school boys. Percept Mot Skills. 1991;73:253–4.
5. Dixon SD, Stein MT, editors. Encounters with children: pediatric behavior and development. 3rd ed. Philadelphia, PA: Mosby; 2000.
6. Dyment PG. Sports and the neurodevelopment of the child. In: Stanitski CL, DeLee JC, Drez DD, editors. Pediatric and adolescent sports medicine. Philadelphia, PA: WB Saunders; 1994. pp. 12–15.
7. Finch CF, Elliott BC, McGrath AC. Measures to prevent cricket injuries: an overview. Sports Med. 1999;28(4):263–72.
8. Lews BJ. Structuring movement experiences for pre-school children. Child Care Health Dev. 1978;4:385–95.
9. Linder MM, Townsend DJ, Jones JC, et al. Incidence of adolescent injuries in junior high-school football and its relationship to sexual maturity. Clin J Sports Med. 1995;5:167–70.
10. Patel DR, Greydanus DE, Calles JL Jr, Pratt HD. Developmental disabilities across the lifespan. Dis Mon. 2010;56(6):299–398.
11. World Health Organization. Towards a common language for functioning, disability and health: the international classification of functioning, disability and health. Geneva: WHO; 2002.
12. Bricher G. Disabled people, health professionals and the social model of disability: Can there be a research relationship? Disabil Soc. 2000;15(5):781–93.
13. Anastasi A. Psychological testing. 6th ed. New York, NY: Macmillan; 1988: p. 23.
14. American Psychological Association. American psychological association ethical principles of psychologists and code of conduct. Washington, DC: APA; 2002.
15. Spies RA, Carlson JF, Geisinger KF, editors. The eighteenth mental measurements year book. Nebraska: University Nebraska Press; 2010.
16. AERA, APA, NCME. Standards for educational and psychological testing. Hanover: Sheridan Press; 1999.
17. American Psychiatric Association. Diagnostic and statistical manual of mental disorders. 4th ed. Text revision. Arlington, VA: APA; 2000.

Chapter 4
Inborn Errors of Metabolism

Manmohan K. Kamboj

Abstract Inborn errors of metabolism (IEMs) are a set of relatively uncommon complicated medical conditions involving abnormalities in the complex biochemical and metabolic pathways of the human body system. They involve great complexity of the underlying pathophysiology, biochemical workup, and analysis and have complicated therapeutic options for management. These children are often sick with significant complications and high rates of morbidity and mortality. The understanding of these complex disorders requires special in-depth training and experience. Most primary care physicians are less familiar with these disease conditions and therefore less willing to deal with them because of the complexity involved. There are metabolic specialists available, mostly in large medical centers, with expertise to deal with these intricate complicated issues. Primary care physicians and pediatricians usually are the first point of contact for most of these newborns, children, or adolescents, however. Therefore, it is important that primary care physicians become comfortable in being able to recognize early signs and symptoms, be able to initiate appropriate diagnostic and therapeutic interventions, and be able to make appropriate referrals. This chapter summarizes the key issues basic to understanding IEMs.

Introduction

Inborn errors of metabolism (IEMs) have been known for approximately the past 100 years, with the term being first used by Sir Archibald Garrod (1857–1936) in 1902 [1]. The initial disorders described were alkaptonuria, benign pentosuria, albinism, and cystinuria at that time, to be followed by description of one of the

M.K. Kamboj (✉)
Associate Professor, Section of Endocrinology, Metabolism and Diabetes, Nationwide Children's Hospital, Columbus, OH 43205, USA
e-mail: Manmohan.Kamboj@Nationwidechildrens.org

D.R. Patel et al. (eds.), *Neurodevelopmental Disabilities*,
DOI 10.1007/978-94-007-0627-9_4, © Springer Science+Business Media B.V. 2011

major IEMs, namely phenylketonuria (PKU), by Ivar Asbjørn Følling (1888–1973) in 1934. Since that time, advances in medicine have uncovered more than 500 IEMs [2].

Definition

The term metabolism encompasses the net result of a multitude of complex biochemical processes that occur in living organisms to maintain cellular activities. These processes are organized into specific metabolic pathways with the primary function to maintain daily life activities. Each pathway depends on certain substrates and specific enzymes to ensure smooth functioning. IEMs are a group of heritable genetic disorders interfering with these metabolic pathways in different ways, leading to inadequate functioning of a particular pathway. This interference in the normal enzymatic or metabolic pathway has varying consequences, including deficiency of a particular end product or excessive accumulation of a substrate that may be toxic. Either of these two scenarios leads to significant morbidity and mortality by hampering normal functioning of a particular metabolic pathway.

Epidemiology

The incidence of IEMs is highly variable among the many specific clinical entities, ranging from 1 in 400 US African Americans for hemoglobinopathies, 1 in 4,500 for congenital hypothyroidism, 1 in 15,000 for PKU, to 1 in 100,000 for most of the fatty acid disorders (except MCAD) and organic acidemias. Incidences of some common inborn errors are listed in Table 4.1 [3]. Some of the common metabolic disorders are listed in Table 4.2 [3, 4].

Etiopathogenesis

Several patterns of inheritance are possible for the different IEMs. It is important to detail a three- to four-generation pedigree to evaluate the mode of inheritance accurately.

Autosomal recessive (AR) inheritance is the most common mode of inheritance for metabolic disorders. In this case, both the parents are heterozygous for the mutant gene; hence, they do not express the disorder, but the offspring are homozygous for that particular gene defect; hence, they express the defect and present clinically with the disorder. The family history is generally negative in the parents, but there may be a history of early neonatal deaths or a clinical disorder expressed as a concern. Consanguinity has an increased chance of expression of an AR disorder. Rarely, these mutations may occur de novo [5].

X-linked recessive inheritance may also be seen in some IEMs, in which one copy of the mutated gene on the X-chromosome is sufficient for causing the

Table 4.1 Some common disorders of inborn errors of metabolism

Disorders of carbohydrate metabolism
- Glycogen storage diseases
- Galactosemia

Disorders of amino acid metabolism (aminoacidurias)
- PKU
- Maple syrup urine disease
- Homocystinuria
- Tyrosinemia
- Nonketotic hyperglycemia

Disorders of organic acid metabolism (organic acidemias)
- Methylmalonic acidemia
- Propionic acidemia

Disorders of fatty acid oxidation
- Short-chain acyl coenzyme A (CoA) dehydrogenase (SCAD)
- Medium-chain acyl CoA dehydrogenase (MCAD)
- Long-chain acyl CoA dehydrogenase (LCAD)
- Very long-chain acyl CoA dehydrogenase (VLCAD)

Disorders of mitochondrial metabolism
- Mitochondrial myopathy, encephalopathy, lactic acidosis, and stroke-like episodes (MELAS)
- Glutaric aciduria
- Pyruvate dehydrogenase deficiency

Disorders of urea cycle
- Carbamoyl phosphate synthetase deficiency
- Ornithine transcarbamylase deficiency
- Arginosuccinate deficiency

Peroxisomal disorders
- Adrenoleukodystrophy
- Zellweger syndrome
- Chondrodysplasia punctata
- Adult Refsum disease

Disorders of the steroid pathway
- Congenital adrenal hyperplasia
- Smith–Lemli–Opitz syndrome

Disorders of lipid storage
- Tay–Sachs disease
- Gaucher's disease
- Metachromatic leukodystrophy

Disorders of purine metabolism
- Lesch–Nyhan syndrome

Transport disorders
- Cystinosis
- Hypercholesterolemia

Lysosomal disorders
- Mucopolysaccharidoses (MPS)
- MPS I (Hurler and Scheie disease)
- MPS II (Hunter disease)
- MPS III (Sanfilippo disease)
- MPS IV (Morquio disease)
- MPS VI
- MPS VII

Table 4.1 (continued)

- Glycoproteinosis
- Sphingolipidosis
- Combined defects
- I-cell disease

Disorders of metal metabolism

- Wilson disease
- Hemochromatosis
- Menkes disease

Others

- Hypothyroidism
- Hemoglobinopathies
- MELAS

Table 4.2 Incidence of some inborn errors of metabolism

Congenital hypothyroidism	1:4,500
Congenital adrenal hyperplasia	1:10,000
PKU	1:15,000
Galactosemia	1:30,000
Other aminoacidurias	1:100,000
Homocystinuria	
MSUD	
Organic acidemias	1:100,000
Fatty acid oxidation disorders	1:100,000
MCAD	1:15,000

Abbreviation: MSUD, maple syrup urine disease.

disorder. Therefore, in this mode of inheritance, the disorder is transmitted from a carrier mother to her male offspring. Also, de novo mutations are observed with a much higher incidence in this pattern of inheritance [5].

Autosomal dominant (AD) inheritance is a less common mode of inheritance for IEMs. The incidence of de novo mutations causing AD disorders is much higher than in other patterns of inheritance. AD transmission generally means that one of the parents has the disease; 50% of the progeny have the disorder, and there is an equal gender distribution [5].

A mitochondrial mode of inheritance is also seen in some IEMs. It is interesting to note that the mitochondrial DNA is always maternal in origin; therefore, a mutation in the mitochondrial DNA is inherited only from the mother. Mitochondrial DNA is prone to de novo mutations; hence, diseases transmitted in this manner may be found to be sporadic in occurrence [5].

Table 4.3 lists the modes of inheritance of some common IEMs [5].

Clinical Features

IEMs may present early in the newborn period, later on in early or late childhood, or much later in adulthood. A high index of suspicion needs to be maintained for IEMs,

Table 4.3 Modes of inheritance in some common inborn errors of metabolism

AR inheritance
- PKU
- Maple syrup urine disease
- Glycogen storage disease
- Galactosemia
- Organic acidurias
- MCAD
- Zellweger syndrome

X-linked recessive (XLR) inheritance
- Ornithine carbamylase deficiency
- Fabry disease
- Pyruvate dehydrogenase deficiency

AD inheritance
- Marfan syndrome
- Acute intermittent porphyria
- Familial hypercholesterolemia

Mitochondrial inheritance
- Kearns–Sayre syndrome
- Leigh syndrome

because the symptomatology of these disorders is often nonspecific and hence may lead to a workup for other medical conditions. The clinical presentation attributable to IEMs may be subclassified into a few broad categories.

Early-Onset Disorders

Silent Disorders

IEMs in this category do not cause life-threatening signs and symptoms in infancy but present later on in the early childhood period with mental retardation and developmental delay. This group includes PKU and congenital hypothyroidism [6].

Disorders Presenting with Acute Metabolic Encephalopathy

This group includes urea cycle disorders, organic acidemias, and aminoacidurias. These conditions may present with metabolic disturbances caused by accumulations of precursors or metabolites, which are reflected early in the newborn period with poor feeding, lethargy, persistent vomiting, seizures, hypotonia, apnea, respiratory distress, tachypnea, and tachycardia. These newborns usually end up getting a workup for sepsis with this type of presentation [6]. These features are attributed to the toxic effect of metabolites on the central nervous system, causing a picture of a metabolic encephalopathy. The biochemical features are significant for metabolic acidosis, hyperammonemia, or other metabolic abnormalities.

Disorders Presenting with Metabolic Acidosis

This group generally includes organic acidemias. These neonates exhibit severe metabolic acidosis with an increased anion gap along with elevated organic acid intermediates specific for the defect or lactate. Lactic acidosis is present in disorders of pyruvate metabolism including pyruvate dehydrogenase deficiency, defects in gluconeogenesis, pyruvate carboxylase deficiency, and mitochondrial disorders [7].

Disorders Presenting with Hyperammonemia

Many newborns with defects in the urea cycle, organic acidemias, and transient hyperammonemia of the newborn (THAN) present with metabolic encephalopathy and hyperammonemia.

Disorders Presenting Later on in Childhood

This group of IEMs includes lysosomal storage disorders, Tay–Sachs disease, Gaucher's disease, and metachromatic leukodystrophy. These disorders generally present with progressive neurologic deterioration [8].

Other clinical signs and symptoms, including generalized nonspecific manifestations; neurologic signs and symptoms; developmental disorders; dysmorphic phenotypes; and disorders in the gastrointestinal, hematologic, and dermatologic systems, are summarized in Table 4.4 [6, 7, 9]. One of the most unique and intriguing features of IEMs is the presence of specific odors in some of these metabolic disorders. Some of these are listed in Table 4.5 [7, 9–11].

Diagnosis

Clinical presentation should raise suspicion of an IEM. Details of history, including a family history of consanguinity, similar disorders in close and extended family, and any neonatal deaths, should be sought. Details of relation of symptoms to eating in terms of timing and in relation to specific type of food consumption, cyclic pattern of vomiting, lethargy, and behavioral changes should be inquired about. Signs manifested on clinical examination, including hepatosplenomegaly, skin lesions, and neurologic deficits, should guide one toward an initial laboratory workup. In children who may be critically ill, it is important to consider and then rule out options in the differential diagnosis of the specific clinical scenario. General laboratory investigations indicated are listed in Table 4.6 [6, 12]. Additional specific biochemical workup should be decided based on details of the history, clinical presentation, results of preliminary laboratory investigations, and suspicion of a specific IEM. It is preferred that extra blood and urine samples be drawn and saved for later investigations. A second tier of laboratory workup that may be indicated is listed

Table 4.4 Important clinical signs and symptoms of inborn errors of metabolism

Dysmorphism
- Peroxisomal disorders
- Zellweger syndrome
- Lysosomal storage disorders
- Mucopolysaccharidosis
- Mucolipidosis
- Gangliosidosis
- Homocystinuria
- Smith–Lemli–Opitz syndrome

Neurologic manifestations
- Seizures: seen in any IEM because of toxic metabolites
- Pyridoxine dependent
- Folinic acid dependent
- Secondary to hypoglycemia
- Peripheral neuropathy
- Mitochondrial disorders
- Lysosomal storage disorders
- Hypotonia
- Fatty acid oxidation disorders
- Peroxisomal disorders
- Urea cycle disorders
- Mitochondrial disorders
- Pompe's disease
- Glycogen storage disorders
- Myopathy
- Glycogen storage diseases
- Fatty acid oxidation disorders
- Mitochondrial disorders
- Ataxia
- Peroxisomal disorders
- Mitochondrial disorders
- Lysosomal storage disorders
- Lethargy or coma
- Aminoacidurias
- Organic acidemias
- Urea cycle disorders
- Fatty acid oxidation defects
- Mitochondrial disorders

Developmental delay
- May occur in all IEMs: rare

Gastrointestinal manifestations
- Hepatomegaly or splenomegaly
- Lysosomal storage disorders
- Glycogen storage diseases
- Jaundice or liver dysfunction
- Galactosemia
- Fatty acid oxidation disorders
- Tyrosinemia
- Peroxisomal disorders
- $\alpha1$-Antitrypsin deficiency
- Niemann–Pick disease

Table 4.4 (continued)

Cardiac manifestations
- Hypertrophic cardiomyopathy
- Glycogen storage disease: type 2
- Pompe's disease
- Mucopolysaccharidosis
- Dilated cardiomyopathy
- Fatty acid oxidation disorders
- Organic acidemias
- Mitochondrial disorders

Ophthalmologic manifestations
- Lenticular cataracts
- Galactosemia
- Mitochondrial disorders
- Corneal opacities
- Fabry disease
- Mucopolysaccharidosis
- Cystinosis
- Cherry red macular spots
- Tay–Sachs disease
- Galactosialidosis
- Niemann–Pick disease
- GM1 gangliosidosis
- Dislocated lens
- Homocystinuria
- Marfan syndrome
- Molybdenum cofactor deficiency
- Sulfite oxidase deficiency
- Retinitis pigmentosa
- Abetalipoproteinemia
- Peroxisomal disorders
- Mitochondrial disorders

Hydrops fetalis: nonimmune
- Lysosomal storage disorders
- Mitochondrial disorders
- Neonatal hemochromatosis
- Glycogen storage disease: type 4

Dermatologic manifestations
- Skin rash
- Acrodermatitis enteropathica
- Ichthyosis
- X-linked ichthyosis
- Sjögren–Larsson syndrome
- Angiokeratomas
- Fabry disease
- Lysosomal storage disorders

in Table 4.7. Special precautions may be needed in the drawing and processing of some of these samples. The samples for plasma ammonia, lactate, and pyruvate should be obtained without the use of a tourniquet and need to be transported on ice for immediate analysis in the laboratory; pyruvate samples should be collected

Table 4.5 Odors characteristic of some inborn errors of metabolism

Odor	Metabolic disorder
Fruity odor	Methylmalonic acidemia
	Propionic acidemia
Burnt sugar/maple syrup-like	Maple syrup urine disease
Mousy/musty	Phenylketonuria
Sweaty socks, cheese-like	Isovaleric acidemia
Malt-like	Methionine malabsorption
Cat urine	3-Methylcrotonic acidemia
	3-Hydroxy, 3-methyl glutaric aciduria
Fish-like	Trimethylaminuria
	Carnitine excess
Cabbage-like	Tyrosinemia

Table 4.6 Initial laboratory investigations for inborn errors of metabolism

Blood
- Complete blood cell count
- Comprehensive metabolic panel, including
  - Liver and kidney function
  - Electrolytes
  - Uric acid
  - Serum ammonia
  - Arterial blood gas

Urine
- Urinalysis
- pH
- Color
- Odor
- Specific gravity
- Ketones
- Urine-reducing substances

in perchlorate to prevent degradation [12]. Table 4.8 lists correlations with some alterations in laboratory evaluations with possible IEMs [12].

Newborn Screening

Newborn screening (NS) for genetic disorders in all newborns endeavors to make early and timely diagnosis of otherwise potentially life-threatening or debilitating inherited disorders. For a genetic disorder to be considered for NS, several criteria should be justified. These include the following: the particular genetic disorder should result in significant morbidity or mortality; should have a known mechanism of pathogenesis; should offer the potential of prevention or adequate treatment; should have an easy, inexpensive, and rapid test available for screening; should have reliable follow-up confirmatory testing available; and the cost-to-benefit ratio of

Table 4.7 Additional laboratory investigations for inborn errors of metabolism

Blood or plasma
- Quantitative amino acids
- Lactate
- Aldolase, creatine kinase
- Acylcarnitine profile
- Lipid profile

Urine
- Quantitative amino acids
- Organic acids
- Myoglobin

Imaging
- MRI: brain
- Echocardiogram

Biopsy
- Muscle biopsy
- Skin biopsy

Genetic studies
- As specifically indicated

Table 4.8 Laboratory findings in inborn errors of metabolism

Metabolic acidosis with increased anion gap	Organic acidemias
Respiratory alkalosis	Urea cycle disorders
Hyperammonemia	Urea cycle disorders
	Organic acidemias
Lactic acidosis	Mitochondrial disorders
	Glycogen storage diseases
	Disorders of
	Glyconeogenesis
	Pyruvate metabolism
	Organic acidemias
	Fatty acid oxidation disorders
	Aminoacidurias
High lactate/pyruvate ratio (normal: 10:1–20:1)	Mitochondrial disorders
	Pyruvate carboxylase deficiency
Acylcarnitine profile abnormalities	Fatty acid oxidation disorders
	Organic acidemias
Hypoglycemia	Glycogen storage disease
With ketosis	Organic acidemias
Without ketosis	Maple syrup urine disease
	Fatty acid oxidation disorders
	Disorders of ketogenesis
Quantitative amino acid profiles	Specific defects in amino acid metabolism have specific patterns
Urine organic acids	Specific defects in amino acid metabolism have specific patterns

incorporating the testing in the NS should be less than the cost of diagnosing, testing, and managing the condition otherwise [3, 13].

NS was initially stated for PKU in 1959 by Robert Guthrie (1916–1995); since then, it has expanded to include an extended list of predominantly IEMs and some hematologic and endocrine disorders [8]. Advances in biochemical testing with tandem mass spectrometry have facilitated the incorporation of many genetic disorders in the NS. Common disorders screened for are listed in Table 4.9 [3, 14, 15]. Most NS programs in the United States are state controlled and state specific, and different states include different disorders in their specific NS programs. Many other countries worldwide offer variable genetic NS programs as well. It is therefore important to remember to look into the specific screening program that a particular newborn underwent. Moreover, it is imperative to realize that a normal newborn screen does not rule out all inborn or inherited disorders. The aim of the NS is to make an early diagnosis for the conditions being screened for. There may be false-positive and false-negative results. Once positive NS is obtained for an IEM, the primary care physician or pediatrician should perform a clinical examination and make an

Table 4.9 Genetic disorders available for screening on the newborn screening programs

Amino acid disorders
- PKU
- Homocystinuria
- Tyrosinemia
- Maple syrup urine disease
- Nonketotic hyperglycinemia
- Citrullinemia
- Arginosuccinate deficiency
- Hyperornithinemia

Carbohydrate disorders
- Galactosemia

Fatty acid oxidation disorders
- SCAD
- MCAD
- LCAD
- VLCAD
- Carnitine palmityl transferase (CPT) deficiency

Organic acidemias
- Methyl malonic acidemia
- Propionic acidemia
- Isovaleric acidemia
- Glutaric acidemia
- β-Methyl crotonyl CoA carboxylase (MCC) deficiency

Other IEMs
- Biotinidase deficiency

Endocrine disorders
- Hypothyroidism
- Congenital adrenal hyperplasia

Hematologic disorders
- Various hemoglobinopathies

assessment and then seek consultation with the metabolic or genetic specialist who has expertise in the field for initiating further diagnostic testing and implementing the required therapeutic measures. These patients should be closely followed, preferably by the metabolic specialists. Early therapeutic intervention can lower morbidity and mortality significantly.

The aim of the NS is to make an early diagnosis for the previously mentioned conditions. There may be false-positive and false-negative results. Once positive NS is obtained for an IEM, the primary care physician or pediatrician should initiate dialog with the metabolic or genetic specialist who has expertise in the field for initiating further clinical examination and assessment, diagnostic testing, and implementation of the required therapeutic measures. These patients should preferably be followed closely by the metabolic specialist. With this early intervention, morbidity and mortality can be significantly lowered.

Principles of Management

General Principles of Treatment

The general measures of treatment are put into place before a definitive diagnosis of a specific IEM is made. Some of these interventions include withholding of all dietary oral intake until some specific investigations and guidelines can be established, preferably after consultation with metabolic specialists. In most cases, intravenous dextrose fluid with saline may be initiated after adequate hydration with normal saline. Acidosis may also need correction by replacement with bicarbonate [16].

Specific Therapeutic Measures

The specific therapeutic options are disease specific and are instituted once a particular IEM is diagnosed. These measures are geared toward addressing the specific concerns of the particular underlying defect. Figure 4.1 represents the underlying approaches to treatment strategies for various IEMs [8]. Table 4.10 outlines some of the specific therapeutic options available for various metabolic disorders [8].

Conclusions

The clinical outcome of children depends on multiple factors. These include severity of the underlying metabolic defect, ability to make the diagnosis early, availability of specific adequate treatment options, and appropriate institution of the therapeutic measures. Depending on all these variables, some IEMs have a relatively better prognosis than others. Many of these children are living longer, but many may be at high risk for developing progressive neurologic deficits, learning disabilities, and mental retardation. A study done to evaluate response to treatment in IEMs revealed improvement in clinical parameters in approximately half of the patients who have metabolic disorders [17].

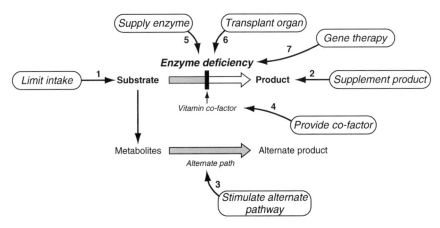

Fig. 4.1 Approaches to treatment of IEMs. Treatment can be directed at (1) limiting the intake of a potentially toxic compound, (2) supplementing the deficient product, (3) stimulating an alternate metabolic pathway, (4) providing a vitamin cofactor to activate residual enzyme activity, (5) supplying the enzyme itself, (6) transplanting a body organ containing the deficient enzyme, and (7) [7] gene therapy (with permission from Batshaw and Tuchman [8], p. 339)

Table 4.10 Examples of treatment approaches for inborn errors of metabolism

Approaches	Disorder	Specific treatment
Restrict diet	PKU	Phenylalanine restriction
	Maple syrup urine disease	Branch chain amino acid restriction
	Galactosemia	Galactose restriction
Supplement-deficient product	Congenital hypothyroidism	Synthroid
	Glycogen storage disease	Cornstarch
	Urea cycle disorders (except argininemia)	Arginine
Stimulate alternate pathway	Urea cycle disorders	Sodium phenylbutyrate
	Organic acidemias	Carnitine
	Isovaleric acidemia	Glycine
	Wilson disease	Penicillamine
Supply vitamin cofactor	Multiple carboxylase deficiency	Biotin
		Pyridoxine
	Homocystinuria	Vitamin B_{12}
	Methylmalonic acidemia	
Replace enzyme	Severe combined immunodeficiency (SCID)	PEG-ADA

Table 4.10 (continued)

Approaches	Disorder	Specific treatment
Transplant organ	Metachromatic leukodystrophy	Bone marrow
	Ornithine transcarbamylase deficiency	Liver
		Liver
	Tyrosinemia	Liver
	Glycogen storage disease	
Use gene therapy	SCID	Retrovirus gene transfer
Use other therapies or emerging technologies	Inhibit pathway: tyrosinemia	NTBC
	Use substrate deprivation: PKU	Recombinant enzyme

With permission from Batshaw and Tuchman [8, p. 340].

Acknowledgment This chapter is adapted with permission from Kamboj [18].

References

1. Garrod AE. The incidence of alkaptonuria: a study in chemical individuality. Lancet. 1902;2:1616–20.
2. Saudubray JM, Chappentier C. Clinical phenotypes: diagnosis/algorithms. In: Scriver CR, Beaudet AL, Sly WS, et al. editors. Metabolic and molecular bases of inherited disease. 8th ed. New York, NY: McGraw-Hill; 2001. pp. 1327–403.
3. Tiller GE. Inborn errors of metabolism. In: Sabella C, Cunningham RJ III, editors. Intensive review of pediatrics. 2nd ed. Philadelphia, PA: Lippincott Williams Wilkins; 2006. pp. 353–61.
4. Sutton VR Overview of the classification of inborn errors of metabolism. Up to date. www.uptodate.com(2010). Accessed 19 Mar 2010.
5. Clarke JTR. General principles. In: A clinical guide to inherited metabolic diseases. 3rd ed. New York, NY: Cambridge University Press; 2006. pp. 1–27.
6. Burton BK. Inborn errors of metabolism in infancy: a guide to diagnosis. Pediatrics. 1998;102(6):E69.
7. Sutton VR Presenting features of inborn errors of metabolism. Up to date. www.uptodate.com(2010). Accessed 19 Mar 2010.
8. Batshaw ML, Tuchman M. PKU and other inborn errors of metabolism. In: Batshaw ML, editor. Children with disabilities. 5th ed. Baltimore, MD: Paul H Brookes; 2002. pp. 333–45.
9. Ellaway CJ, Wilcken B, Christodoulou J. Neonatology for the generalist: clinical approach to inborn errors of metabolism presenting in the newborn period. J Paediatr Child Health. 2002;38:511–17.
10. Wappner RS. Biochemical diagnosis of genetic diseases. Pediatr Ann. 1993;22(5):282–92.
11. Mace JW, Goodman SI, Centerwall WR, et al. The child with an unusual odor. A clinical resume. Clin Pediatr (Phila). 1976;15(1):57–62.
12. Sutton VR Overview of the evaluation of inborn errors of metabolism. Up to date. www.uptodate.com(2010). Accessed 19 Mar 2010.
13. Sielski LA Newborn screening. Up to date. www.uptodate.com(2010). Accessed 19 Mar 2010.
14. Korson MS. Advances in newborn screening for metabolic disorders: what the pediatrician needs to know. Pediatr Ann. 2000;29(5):294–301.
15. McCandless SE. A primer on expanded newborn screening by tandem mass spectrometry. Prim Care. 2004;31(3):583–604.

16. Kwon KT, Tsai VW. Metabolic emergencies. Emerg Med Clin North Am. 2007;25(4): 1041–60.
17. Treacy E, Childs B, Scriver CR. Response to treatment in hereditary metabolic disease: 1993 survey and 10-year comparison. Am J Hum Genet. 1995;56(2):359–67.
18. Kamboj M. Clinical approach to the diagnoses of inborn errors of metabolism. Pediatr Clin North Am 2008;55(5):1113–29.

Chapter 5
Genetic Evaluation in Developmental Disabilities

Helga V. Toriello

Abstract Developmental disabilities are a relatively common reason for referral to a pediatric subspecialist. Although there are numerous reasons for the child being affected with a developmental disability, genetic causes are not an uncommon cause. A genetics evaluation can often identify this cause, and the family counseled appropriately regarding cause, prognosis, and recurrence risks. This chapter describes the various steps in the genetics evaluation process.

Introduction

Developmental disability is a common child health concern and poses a number of challenges in terms of recognition, diagnosis of the underlying condition, determination of the etiology, and understanding the natural history and prognosis. The purpose of this chapter is to provide guidance for determination of the genetic etiology of an individual's developmental delay or intellectual disability (DD/ID). This is a multi-step process and involves obtaining detailed information about family history, prenatal and postnatal medical history, and developmental history. The review of that information is followed by a detailed physical examination, ascertaining the presence of not only major anomalies but also minor anomalies. The aim of this examination is to determine whether a child is dysmorphic or not, which then helps guide the approach to testing, which is generally one of the last steps in the process.

H.V. Toriello (✉)
Department of Pediatrics and Human Development, Michigan State University College of Human Medicine, East Lansing, MI USA; Director of Genetics, Spectrum Health, Grand Rapids, MI 49503, USA
e-mail: helga.toriello@spectrum-health.org

D.R. Patel et al. (eds.), *Neurodevelopmental Disabilities*,
DOI 10.1007/978-94-007-0627-9_5, © Springer Science+Business Media B.V. 2011

Family History

When obtaining a family history, the goal should be to get information on three generations, which includes the proband (individual who brought the family to the physician's attention), the parents, siblings (full and half), aunts and uncles, grandparents, cousins, and great-grandparents. It is important to ask not only about similarly affected individuals but also about any significant medical or developmental concerns in family members. This is important because some conditions may have variable expression, and obtaining information on other possibly affected family members helps provide a more complete picture of the condition present in the family. For example, a child with a history of seizures and cognitive impairment has a father with normal cognitive development, but a number of unusual skin changes and a history of having had a cardiac rhabdomyoma as a child. That history would point toward a possible diagnosis of tuberous sclerosis in both the father and the child. In addition to medical conditions in the family, it is important to determine whether the parents are related to each other. This is useful information to have, because it then makes the chance that the child has an autosomal recessive condition much more likely.

Prenatal History

It is first important to obtain a history of previous pregnancies. For example, how many were liveborn? Were there any miscarriages, and if so, when in the pregnancy did these occur? Were there any stillbirths? Was a cause of the stillbirth(s) found? The next step is to determine the parents' ages when the proband was born. Did the mother have any prenatal testing, either serum screening or combined ultrasound and serum screening, or invasive diagnostic procedures such as chorionic villus sampling or amniocentesis? Did the mother have any infectious diseases during the pregnancy? Was there an elevation in body temperature for a period of time? Did she take any prescription or illicit drugs or did she consume alcoholic beverages?

Medical and Developmental History

Weight, height, and head circumference at birth and at the time of the evaluation are crucial to obtain. In addition, determination of whether these are consistent with parental and sibling heights and weights is important. The fact that a child is "larger" than the rest of the family may point toward an overgrowth syndrome. Document developmental milestones; if there are delays, determine if the delay is cognitive, motor, or both. Ascertain which other medical specialists a child has seen. It may be necessary to request copies of medical evaluations done by those specialists, but these could be useful in determining a diagnostic approach. Finally, determine whether hearing and vision have been evaluated and whether any deficits were identified. If the child has any major anomalies, determine what type, with the major types including

- *Malformation.* This form of anomaly is caused by abnormal development of a structure during embryogenesis and is considered to be an intrinsic defect of development. Examples of malformations include cleft lip/palate, ventricular septal defect, or polydactyly.
- *Deformation.* A deformation is the result of constraint or compression of an already formed part of the body. Deformations usually occur during the fetal period and may even occur postnatally. Examples include clubbed feet and plagiocephaly.
- *Disruption.* This is also a secondary effect on an intrinsically normal structure, but is related to an extrinsic agent causing tissue destruction or cell death. One example is amniotic bands.
- *Dysplasia.* This term applies to abnormal development of a particular tissue. For example, an ectodermal dysplasia is a condition in which ectodermally derived structures (skin, hair, teeth, and nails) are involved to some degree.

If there are multiple anomalies present, other terms are used to describe the various patterns of anomalies. These are as follows:

- *Syndrome.* A syndrome is a specific pattern of anomalies which generally have an identified cause, for example, Down syndrome and trisomy 21, Rett syndrome, and MECP2 mutation.
- *Sequence.* This term is used to describe multiple anomalies which occur in a cascading effect as the result of a primary anomaly. For example, a child with spina bifida may have hydrocephalus and clubbed feet as well, but the hydrocephalus and clubbed feet are a direct result of the primary anomaly, spina bifida.
- *Association.* This refers to the co-occurrence of several anomalies more often than expected by chance. The cause is not known. The best known association is the VACTERL association, in which the variable combination of vertebral, anal, cardiac, tracheoesophageal, renal, and limb anomalies occurs.

Physical Evaluation

Even if no major anomalies are present, a child may still have a syndrome. It is therefore important for the clinician to do a careful physical evaluation looking for minor anomalies and determining whether the child is dysmorphic or not. The first step in this process is to observe the entire child, before "picking apart" his or her appearance [1]. Does the child resemble other family members? If not, what are the key physical features that cause phenotypic differences? The second step is to then objectively document these features. Whenever possible, measurements should be done to verify subjective impressions. For example, hypertelorism (widely spaced eyes) can be verified by measuring the interpupillary distance; small hands can be verified by measuring the distance from the tip of the middle finger to the first bracelet crease on the wrist, and so on. After this physical evaluation, the physician might have a short differential diagnosis list. The next step is to then look for key physical manifestations to support or rule out the suspected diagnosis. For example, if the clinician suspects Kabuki syndrome on the basis of long palpebral fissures and lower lid ectropion, determination of the presence of fetal fingertip pads, trapezoidal philtrum, and fleshy earlobes can be done to help verify the diagnosis. This approach is particularly important in cases where no confirmatory testing is available. If a diagnosis is not readily apparent, then the detailed list of findings can lead to a search of the literature or dysmorphology databases in an attempt at achieving a list of possible diagnoses [1].

Testing

In the section above, it is noted that molecular testing can be done to confirm a diagnosis. But if no diagnosis is suspected, what laboratory tests might be useful in determining the possible etiology of the condition? There have been a number of studies investigating the utility of the various tests that are available, as well as practice parameters published by professional societies describing the benefits of various tests. This chapter is not meant to be a comprehensive review of all of these articles, but rather an attempt at synthesis of some of the important points raised by many of them.

Battaglia et al. [2] in 1999 performed a retrospective review of 120 patients (excluding those with Down syndrome) who had various investigations. Following testing, 42% of patients were diagnosed, with a chromosome anomaly found in 12%, fragile X in 3%, and a metabolic disorder in 2.5%. The authors stated that in this group, 16% had a known multiple congenital anomaly/"mental retardation" syndrome, with two of those individuals likely having been diagnosed by the use of fluorescent in situ hybridization (FISH). Other investigative procedures used were skeletal radiographs, electroencephalograms (EEG), and magnetic resonance imaging (MRI) of the head. Although a fairly high number of MRI scans were abnormal, only 7.5% were diagnostically useful. Conversely, although the EEG was abnormal in a similar number of patients (8.3%), the authors believed that these studies were diagnostically useful. In 2005, Bradinova et al. [3] summarized their findings in a similar study, with a similar number of patients ($N = 100$). Fifteen percent of their patients were diagnosed clinically, with five of those diagnoses confirmed by molecular or FISH studies. Twenty percent had a cytogenetic abnormality; however, in contrast to the study described above [2], children with Down syndrome were included in the tabulation. If these children are excluded, the proportion of those with a chromosome anomaly was 9%. Fragile X was present in 2% and a metabolic disorder found in some. It is difficult to determine how many of their patients did indeed have a metabolic disorder; the authors state that a metabolic disorder was suspected, but not proven, in 7%, which they then stated was in agreement with the published rate of 1%. EEGs and MRIs were also used to investigate this population of patients, with similar results to that of Battaglia et al. [2]. Nineteen percent of their patients had MRI abnormalities, with a diagnosis achieved in 13% of that group (or 2.5% of the total). The EEG was useful in achieving a diagnosis in 7%.

Although Rauch et al. [4] primarily focused on cytogenetic approaches to the evaluation of an individual with DD/ID, they reported an interesting observation in that in 5.6% of the mothers of males skewed X-inactivation was found. This was suggestive of an X-linked condition affecting the boy.

Recently, Engbers et al. [5] found that metabolic disorders are likely responsible for a greater number of causes than had been reported by others. In a recent study that re-evaluated children with DD/ID and previously normal metabolic studies, they found that 2.8% in this group were found to have a metabolic disorder. Reasons for increased detection included repetition of initial studies, incorporation of testing for creatine deficiency disorders, correct preservation of the fluid prior to analysis, expansion of testing to other tissues (e.g., cerebrospinal fluid), and use of loading or fasting tests.

Van Karnebeek et al. [6] reported on a systematic review of the literature in an attempt at determining a rational approach to making a diagnosis in a child with DD/ID. They also found that a dysmorphological exam was most useful in achieving a diagnosis, citing a diagnostic frequency of 62%. Among investigative techniques, there was extensive discussion regarding results of karyotyping, but with no total percentage reported (although it could be inferred from the discussion that the combination of routine karyotype with subtelomeric FISH was diagnostic in approximately 10–12% of patients). The yield of fragile X testing was low, with 2% or fewer individuals found to have fragile X. It was noted that the frequency of fragile X was higher in those with moderate to severe degrees of cognitive impairment, compared to that in a group of individuals with mild impairment. This group also found a low frequency of metabolic disorders in this group, citing a median frequency of 1%. Finally, MRI was diagnostic in very few patients in the articles reviewed by the authors, with most groups reporting diagnoses achieved with MRI between 0.9 and 3.9%. As a result of this review, the authors recommended a step-wise approach to diagnosis in children with DD/ID. This can be summarized as follows:

- Clinical history and detailed physical examination, paying attention to dysmorphic features.
- If no diagnosis is achieved, standard cytogenetic analysis, followed by FISH for subtelomeric rearrangements, if indicated (generally the combination of moderate to severe CI combined with dysmorphic features).
- Fragile X and metabolic studies have a relatively low yield, but if indications are present (e.g., positive family history for fragile X and cognitive regression or suggestive physical findings such as hepatomegaly for metabolic disorders) should have a higher yield.
- Although brain imaging often finds abnormalities, the frequency of diagnoses made with this approach is low.

Professional societies have also developed recommendations for the diagnostic approach to the child with DD/ID. The American College of Medical Genetics [7] published their recommendations in 1997, with these recommendations including a careful physical examination, including documentation of dysmorphic features as well as the behavioral phenotype; chromosome analysis, consideration of testing for fragile X, citing a 2% yield in the studies they reviewed; metabolic testing under suggestive circumstances; and intracranial imaging.

In 2005 Shevell et al. [8] published a practice parameter on behalf of the American Academy of Neurology, in which an evidence-based approach was taken to development of these guidelines. Their recommendations were as follows:

- Routine cytogenetic testing, with a yield of almost 4% in the studies reviewed by the group, is indicated. The use of subtelomeric FISH, with a yield of 6.6%, should also be considered, if a karyotype is normal.
- Testing for fragile X, with an estimated yield of 2.6%, should be considered, particularly in those with a positive family history of DD/ID.
- Metabolic testing has a low yield of 1%, and should not be done routinely. However, in certain situations (such as consanguinity, isolated population) or if clinically indicated, the yield increases to 5%.
- Neuroimaging should be considered to be part of the diagnostic process; here again, the frequency of abnormalities detected is fairly high (49–65% for MRI) although it was not stated how frequently the MRI finding was diagnostic.
- Additional studies to consider include testing for Rett syndrome in females with moderate to severe impairment (yield unknown) and EEG studies (yield ~1%).

Finally, the American Academy of Pediatrics [9] published their recommendations in 2006, which were similar to those made by other groups. This group also stressed the importance of the dysmorphologic exam, as well as the neurologic exam in the diagnostic approach. In many cases, the dysmorphologic exam was sufficient to establish the diagnosis, whereas the neurologic exam was useful in determining the need for further studies or referral to other specialists. Cytogenetic testing, including subtelomeric FISH in the case of a normal karyotype, is also recommended, with a yield of over 10% for both tests together. Fragile X testing, despite its relatively low yield of 2%, should at least be considered in the diagnostic evaluation of the child with DD/ID. Given the high sensitivity and specificity of the test, it is not unreasonable to have a fairly low threshold for offering this test, at least in cases of males with DD/ID. Metabolic studies have a similarly low yield of 1%, but here routine screening is not recommended. Instead, metabolic studies should be done on the basis of clinical findings in the patient.

It can be readily apparent that chromosome analysis with the inclusion of FISH for subtelomeric rearrangements is clearly one of the most important tests to use in the diagnostic approach. However, cytogenetic testing has recently undergone a remarkable evolution. DNA-based techniques, primarily chromosomal microarray (CMA), which determine copy number variants (CNVs) have become a recent tool for clinical use. In this process, the DNA from the patient and from a control is labeled and cohybridized to a known genomic sequence. Differences in the intensity of fluorescence between the genomes of the patient and the control indicate CNVs, many of which are pathogenic microdeletions or microduplications [10]. It should be noted here that not all CNVs are associated with disease or impairment; the estimated mean number of CNVs each person has is thought to be at least 800 [11]. Nonetheless, Rauch et al. [4], in their investigation of the diagnostic yield of various genetic tests used in the evaluation of patients with unexplained DD/ID, found that using CMA would have the highest yield of any single test (28.9%) and was thus suggested by the authors to be considered a first-tier test. More recently, Wincent et al. [12] studied 160 patients with idiopathic DD/ID and multiple congenital anomalies and found a CNV in 22.5%; 13.1% were considered causal, whereas 9.4% were of unknown significance. Among the 21 patients with a pathogenic CNV, all but four had previously had a normal karyotype.

Recently Miller et al. [13] reviewed the evidence for using CMA as the first step in the investigation of DD/ID, as well as for the investigation of multiple congenital anomalies and/or autism spectrum disorders (ASD). They recommended that CMA be used as a first-tier test for the above-listed indications, with this recommendation being based on a review of 21,698 patients. The diagnostic yield was 12.2% higher than that of a G-banded karyotype. As a result of the widespread use of this technique, a few microdeletions or microduplications have been found to be particularly common. Three of these are described below.

15q13.3 Deletion

This microdeletion is associated with mild to moderate DD/CI, seizures and/or abnormal EEG, and mildly dysmorphic facial features. These features include upslanting, widely spaced eyes, prominent philtrum, and full everted lips. The hands may also show minor anomalies, including clinodactyly or short fourth metacarpals [14].

16p11.2 Deletion

Most individuals with this relatively common microdeletion present with DD/CI and speech delay. Autism spectrum disorders are also fairly common in those with this microdeletion, having been reported in at least 20%, depending on the mode of ascertainment [15]. Most have macrocephaly, and mildly dysmorphic features have been described. These are rather variable, but can include flat facial profile, hypertelorism, and smooth philtrum. Recently, it has been reported that obesity or overweight are relatively more common in individuals with this deletion who are more than 4 years of age, becoming a constant manifestation in those in their teens or older [16].

17q21.31 Deletion

This microdeletion is thought to be one of the most common microdeletions found on microarray analysis, with an estimated population frequency as high as 1/13,000

[17]. Individuals with this deletion have mild to moderate DD/ID. Phenotypic manifestations include low birth weight, severe neonatal hypotonia, poor feeding, and a dysmorphic facial appearance, which includes a long face, blepharoptosis, so-called pear-shaped nose, broad chin, and apparently low-set ears. The facial phenotype becomes more striking over time [18]. None of these conditions had been recognized prior to the institution of microarrays in the diagnostic repertoire, and it is expected that more relatively common microdeletion or microduplication syndromes will be described over time.

However, there are some caveats regarding microarray testing. Parental testing is often, if not always, needed for interpretation of the results, particularly if the CNV is not associated with a well-known microdeletion or microduplication syndrome. Paciorkowski and Fang [10] recently proposed four levels of evidence to be used in the interpretation of CMA results. Level I evidence is stated to be a very clear genotype–phenotype correlation, in which there is a well-defined association between the syndrome and the CNV. A well-known example of this is the association of Williams syndrome with the deletion of 7q11. Level II evidence is termed possibly new genotype–phenotype correlation and applies to the situation where there is an evolving genotype–phenotype correlation. In this situation, there have been one or more reports in the literature, but there is a less consistent phenotype among the various reports. Level III evidence is called possibly new genotype–phenotype correlation and pertains to the situation where a CNV has not been reported to be a benign variant, but for which there is no information in the literature. Level IV evidence is termed uninterpretable, whereby multiple CNVs (none of which are reported as normal variants *or* associated with a disease phenotype) are found or are also found in a parent who is phenotypically unaffected. In addition, CMA cannot identify balanced chromosomal rearrangements such as translocations or inversions or differentiate free trisomies from Robertsonian translocations [4, 19]. Some aneuploidies can be missed, such as an XYY case if the wrong gender control is used [20]. Marker chromosomes may also be missed, depending on the size, marker composition, and array coverage of the specific chromosomal area [21]. Detection of mosaicism has been reported, but the accuracy of detecting low levels described by some groups has been questioned by others [19, 21]. Finally, triploidy will not be detected by some forms of microarray.

Summary

In summary, as of 2010, a reasonable genetic evaluation of a child with DD/CI should consist of the following:

- Review of family history, medical and developmental history, and thorough dysmorphology examination.
- Chromosomal microarray analysis as a first-tier test. Since a recent study noted no correlation between the detection rate and the degree of ID, there is no reason to not consider testing an individual with mild ID [12].

- Fragile X, particularly in a male.
- Consider metabolic testing, but attempt to do more of a targeted approach, as well as investigate other types of samples (e.g., cerebrospinal fluid, if clinically indicated). However, it may be reasonable to screen for creatine deficiency disorders, which are relatively common and may be treatable, and congenital disorders of glycosylation, because regression (a hallmark of metabolic disorders) is often not present [2, 22].
- Consider neuroimaging and/or EEG if indicated. As pointed out by Engbers et al. [23], an MRI was most likely to be diagnostic in cases of movement or pyramidal disorders, epilepsy, or abnormal head circumference. The authors further suggested that if other evaluations (e.g., genetic, metabolic, or cytogenetic) are uninformative, an MRI could provide useful clues to the actual diagnosis.
- If the pedigree pattern is suggestive of X-linked inheritance, consider testing the mother for skewed X inactivation or testing for mutations in X-linked genes known to be associated with DD/ID. Since approximately 15% of inherited DD/ID is caused by genes on the X chromosome, this is not unreasonable [24].

It is anticipated that within the next few years, whole genome sequencing will become an available tool for diagnosing children with DD/ID. Coupled with microarray analysis and testing for trinucleotide repeat expansion conditions (e.g., fragile X), it is anticipated that with these newer technologies, most children with DD/ID will be able to be diagnosed. This in turn will improve care and management of affected children.

References

1. Hall BD, Toriello HV. The pediatric diagnostic examination. New York, NY: McGraw-Hill; 2008.
2. Battaglia A, Bianchini E, Carey JC. Diagnostic yield of the comprehensive assessment of developmental delay/mental retardation in an Institute of child Neuropsychiatry. Am J Med Genet. 1999;82:60–66.
3. Bradinova I, Shopova S, Simeonov E. Mental retardation in childhood: clinical and diagnostic profile in 100 children. Genet Couns. 2005;16:239–48.
4. Rauch A, Hoyer J, Guth S, Zweier C, Kraus C, Becker C, Zenker M, Huffmeier U, Thiel C, Ruschendorf F, Nurnberg P, Reis A, Trautmann U. Diagnostic yield of various genetic approaches in patients with unexplained developmental delay or mental retardation. Am J Med Genet. 2006;140A:2063–74.
5. Engbers H, Berger R, van Hasselt P, de Koning T, de Sain-van der Velden MGM, Kroes HY, Visser G. Yield of additional metabolic studies in neurodevelopmental disorders. Ann Neurol. 2008;64:212–17.
6. Van Karnebeek CDM, Jansweijer MCE, Leenders AGE, Offringa M, Hennekam RCM. Diagnostic investigations in individuals with mental retardation: a systematic literature review of their usefulness. Eur J Hum Genet. 2005;13:6–25.
7. Curry CJ, Stevenson RE, Aughton D, Byrne J, Carey JC, Cassidy S, Cunniff C, Graham JM, Jones MC, Kaback MM, Moeschler J, Schaefer GB, Schwartz S, Tarleton J, Opitz J. Evaluation of mental retardation: recommendations of a consensus conference. Am J Med Genet. 1997;72:468–77.

8. Shevell M, Ashwal S, Donley D, Flint J, Gingold M, Hirtz D, Majnemer A, Noetzel M, Sheth RD. Practice parameter: evaluation of the child with global developmental delay. Neurol. 2003;60:367–80.
9. Moeschler JB, Shevell M. Committee on genetics. clinical genetic evaluation of the child with mental retardation or developmental delays. Pediatrics. 2006;117:2304–16.
10. Paciorkowski AR, Fang M. Chromosomal microarray interpretation: what is a child neurologist to do? Pediatr Neurol. 2009;41:391–8.
11. Tyson C, Harvard C, Locker R, Friedman JM, Langlois S, Lewis ME, et al. Submicroscopic deletions and duplications in individuals with intellectual disability detected by array-CGH. Am J Med Genet. 2005;139A:173–85.
12. Wincent J, Anderlid BM, Lagerberg M, Nordenskjold M, Schoumans J. High-resolution molecular karyotyping in patients with developmental delay and/or multiple congenital anomalies in a clinical setting. Clin Genet. 2010;doi:10/1111/j.1399–004.2010.01442.x.
13. Miller DT, Adam MP, Aradhya S, Biesecker LG, Brothman AR, Carter NP, et al. Consensus statement: chromosomal microarray is a first-tier clinical diagnostic test for individuals with developmental disabilities or congenital anomalies. Am J Hum Genet. 2010;86:749–64.
14. Sharp AJ, Mefford HC, Li K, Baker C, Skinner C, Stevenson RE, et al. A recurrent 15q13.3 microdeletion syndrome associated with mental retardation and seizures. Nat Genet. 2008;40:322–8.
15. Shinawi M, Liu P, Kang SH, Shen I, Belmont JW, Scott DA, et al. Recurrent reciprocal 16p11.2 rearrangements associated with global developmental delay, behavioural problems, dysmorphism, epilepsy, and abnormal head size. J Med Genet. 2010;47:332–41.
16. Walters RG, Jacquemont S, Valsesia A, deSmith AJ, Andersson D, Falchi M, et al. A new highly penetrant form of obesity due to deletions on chromosome 16p11.2. Nature. 2010;463:671–5.
17. Slavotinek AM. Novel microdeletion syndromes detected by chromosome microarrays. Hum Genet. 2008;124:1–17.
18. Tan TY, Aftimos S, Worgan L, Susman R, Wilson M, Ghedia S, et al. Phenotypic expansion and further characterisation of the 17q21.31 microdeletion syndrome. J Med Genet. 2009;46:480–9.
19. Xiang B, Li A, Valentin D, Nowak NJ, Zhao H, Li P. Analytical and clinical validity of whole-genome oligonucleotide array comparative genomic hybridization for pediatric patients with mental retardation and developmental delay. Am J Med Genet. 2008;146A:1942–54.
20. Shearer BM, Thorland EC, Gonzales PR, Ketterling RP. Evaluation of a commercially available focused array CGH platform for the detection of constitutional chromosome anomalies. Am J Med Genet. 2007;143A:2357–70.
21. Lu X, Shaw CA, Patel A, Li J, Cooper ML, Wells WR, et al. Clinical implementation of chromosomal microarray analysis: summary of 2513 postnatal cases. PLoS One. 2007;28:e327.
22. Toriello HV. Intellectual disability and genetic influences. Int J Disabil Hum Dev. 2008;7:349–54.
23. Engbers JM, Nievelstein RAJ, Gooskens RHJM, Kroes HY, van Empelen R, Braams O, et al. The clinical utility of MRI in patients with neurodevelopmental disorders of unknown origin. Eur J Neurol. 2010;17:815–22.
24. Bashiardes S, Kousoulidou L, van Bokhoven H, Ropers HH, Chelly J, Moraine C, et al. A new chromosome X exon-specific microarray platform for screening of patients with X-linked disorders. J Mol Diagn. 2009;11:562–8.

Chapter 6
Neurodevelopmental Disorders in Common Syndromes

Helga V. Toriello

Abstract Numerous genetic syndromes have had the cognitive and behavioral components of the phenotype delineated, leading to improved diagnosis of the condition, as well as to better management and interventional approaches. This article is a review of some of what is known about the neurodevelopmental aspects of some of the more common genetic syndromes.

Introduction

Although the cognitive aspects of various syndromes have been recognized for years, more recently clinical geneticists and others have come to recognize the importance of delineating the behavioral profile as well. As defined by some, the behavioral phenotype encompasses motor, cognitive, communicative, and social aspects of the specific condition under study [1]. From a diagnostic standpoint, the behavioral phenotype may be as, if not more, important than clinical features in terms of recognizing the syndrome.

Additional information that can be gained from studying cognitive and behavioral phenotypes of individuals with syndromes is that we gain an understanding of genetic influences on brain function, which can then be applied to both research and intervention [2, 3]. The following is a summary of what is known about the neurodevelopmental aspects of a number of genetic syndromes. This is not meant to be an exhaustive list but to provide insight into what we know about some of these conditions.

H.V. Toriello (✉)
Department of Pediatrics and Human Development, Michigan State University College of Human Medicine, East Lansing, MI, USA; Director of Genetics, Spectrum Health, Grand Rapids, MI 49503, USA
e-mail: helga.toriello@spectrum-health.org

D.R. Patel et al. (eds.), *Neurodevelopmental Disabilities*,
DOI 10.1007/978-94-007-0627-9_6, © Springer Science+Business Media B.V. 2011

Angelman Syndrome

Angelman syndrome (AS) is caused by the loss of maternally imprinted genetic material on chromosome 15q, in the so-called Prader–Willi/Angelman region. The phenotype of AS includes severe developmental delay/intellectual disability (DD/ID), significant speech impairment, ataxia, microcephaly, and a characteristic facial appearance (large appearing mouth, prominent chin). A unique behavioral profile is part of this phenotype and is characterized by (inappropriate) happy disposition with frequent laughter, often accompanied by hand flapping. Developmental delays are first noted during the first year; however, the unique manifestations of AS do not become apparent until the second year of life, and it can sometimes take several years before the correct diagnosis is made.

A recent review of cognitive profiles in individuals with AS reported that in a group of children with AS, intellectual disability (ID) in the severe to profound range of impairment was found, with developmental ages ranging between 3 and 17 months in this group. Results of evaluations of adaptive behavior scales found that the average adaptive behavior composite was 49, and individually correlated with the child's cognitive abilities. However, there were differences among the different adaptive behaviors that were measured, with motor skills most impaired and socialization least impaired [4]. Speech impairment is generally considered to be severe, with none or limited use of words, although receptive speech is better than expressive speech [5].

A fairly specific behavioral phenotype has been reported for AS and is included in the Consensus on Clinical Diagnosis of Angelman Syndrome [6]. Relatively consistent behaviors include frequent laughter or smiling, excitability (e.g., hand flapping), hyperactivity, tongue thrusting, drooling, fascination with water, and sleep disturbances (as evidenced by too little or disrupted sleep). Additionally reported behaviors include feeding problems, fixation on food, hyperphagia, and increased heat sensitivity. Recently, Berry et al. [7] evaluated 91 individuals with either molecularly proven or clinically suspected AS and compared their behavior to a control group of similar intellectually impaired individuals. Their goal was to confirm that the above-listed behaviors were indeed specific to AS. As compared to the control group, the authors found that poor attention span and impulsivity were less common in the AS group, whereas hyperactivity, chewing or mouthing of objects, eating nonfood items, food fads, gorging of food, fascination with water, hand flapping, and sleep disturbance were significantly more common than in the control group. Interestingly, outbursts of laughter were *not* found more often than in the control group, so these authors suggested that this and short attention span are not relatively common in AS, as is suggested by the consensus report. The laughter, which is thought to be pathognomonic, has been further studied to determine the context in which it occurs. It was initially thought to be unprovoked and to occur inappropriately; more recently it has been suggested to be related to context, although it may occur in situations that are not considered to be pleasant (e.g., having blood drawn). It may also increase during periods of anxiety; however, in general it does appear to occur more frequently in social situations and less in nonsocial situations [1].

Down Syndrome

Down syndrome (trisomy 21) is caused by an extra copy of chromosome 21. Individuals with Down syndrome (DS) all have some degree of cognitive impairment and are more likely to have cardiac anomalies, early onset Alzheimer disease, and various other health concerns. The cognitive deficits can be characterized as deficiencies in learning, memory, and language, with morphosyntax, verbal short-term memory, and explicit long-term memory usually impaired, and visuospatial short-term memory, associative learning, and implicit long-term memory usually preserved [8]. Motor delays are also common in DS, with these children acquiring motor skills more slowly than their age-matched peers. Even in their second decade of life, DS children are more likely to have specific motor impairments, including difficulty with precise limb movement (e.g., stepping over a stick on a balance beam) or with finger movements (e.g., pivoting thumb and index finger). Gross motor tasks such as push-ups are more difficult as well [9]. Recently, Fidler et al. [9] demonstrated that praxis skills (praxis is defined as the planning, execution, and sequencing of movements) were significantly impaired in children with DS as compared to matched controls with comparable intellectual disability. Since praxis is involved in many skills of everyday living, it was not surprising that a correlation between praxis skills and function on the daily living skills domain of the Vineland Adaptive Behavior Scales was found. As a result of finding a specific profile of praxis deficits, the authors recommended that this information be used for intervention planning by occupational therapists and other practitioners.

Behavioral manifestations of Down syndrome have also been well studied. Dykens et al. [10] provided a good summary of what was known up to the time of publication regarding the behavioral phenotype of individuals with Down syndrome. Children with DS are more likely to be diagnosed with attention-deficit hyperactivity disorder (ADHD), conduct disorder, or oppositional disorder than are typically developed children. The latter two conditions manifest as noncompliance, disobedience, or aggressive behavior. The aggressive behaviors were less likely to be extreme (e.g., fighting) and more likely to be low-level aggression, such as disobedience, argumentativeness, or attention demanding. Adolescents with DS have not been as well studied, but in the few studies that have evaluated behavior in this group, internalizing symptoms, such as withdrawal and depression, are more common. In addition, parents of DS adolescents often report that these individuals are less likely to be outgoing, cheerful, or affectionate, and in general are "less fun." Additionally, adults with DS exhibit less aggressive behavior than do adults with cognitive impairment in general.

Conversely, older adults have also been well characterized, given the significant frequency of dementia in this group. Indeed, although approximately 50% of adults with DS who are 50 years or older show clinical signs of dementia, most individuals who are 40 years or older have neuropathologic changes that are typical of dementia. Cognitive decline is therefore not unexpected in adults with DS. In addition to Alzheimer disease, adults with DS are more prone to depression, as evidenced by frequent withdrawal, mutism, low mood, passivity, decreased appetite, and insomnia. Some individuals with depression have experienced hallucinations. It is noteworthy that in the DS population, as opposed to in the general population, individuals exhibited behavioral and personality changes more commonly than memory problems in the preclinical stages of Alzheimer disease. However, Adams and Oliver [11] found that behavioral changes were more common in those with cognitive decline, as evidenced by a number of neuropsychological tests.

Fragile X Syndrome

Fragile X syndrome is considered to be the most common cause of inherited cognitive impairment. The cause of fragile X syndrome (FXS) is a trinucleotide (cytosine–guanine–guanine) expansion within the *FMR1* gene, thus leading to lack of production of fragile X protein, FMRP. This lack of FMRP is thought to be the basis of the cognitive and behavioral features of the FXS phenotype. The physical phenotype is fairly subtle, with males generally having a long face, large and/or protruding ears, average to large head size, and after puberty, macroorchidism. Female carriers can also have subtle facial features similar to those of males with FXS. The number of repeats considered to be in the normal range is 5–40. However, when there are 59–200 repeats, there is said to be a premutation in that gene present. Above 200 repeats, the gene is considered fully mutated, and as a result, fully methylated (shut off) and not expressed. The remaining range of repeats, 41–58, is said to be in the intermediate or gray zone [12]. Both males and females can have premutations or full mutations, with the effect determined by their genetic status. The mutation can be present in every cell or only in some cells (in which case the individual is said to be mosaic).

Males with the full mutation have been described as having a characteristic cognitive and behavioral phenotype. The cognitive phenotype is essentially deficits in executive functions. This includes deficits in processing and remembering sequential information, short-term memory deficits, visuospatial abnormalities, visual–motor coordination deficits, and pragmatic language deficits. However, strengths include vocabulary, verbal working memory, and long-term memory for meaningful and learned information [13]. Children with FXS have a slower rate of development than do their peers, so although it may appear that there is a decline in IQ over time, this is not caused by regression, but rather a divergent trajectory of development [14]. Males that have full mutations generally have an average IQ of 41, whereas males that are mosaic for the full mutation have an average IQ of 60. In some instances, males may have a full mutation which is not methylated, so their cognitive ability falls within the "normal" range.

Behaviorally, young boys with FXS show gaze aversion (considered the hallmark manifestation of FXS) [14], tactile defensiveness, sensitivity to noise and taste, perseveration in speech, or hand flapping, and other stereotypies. Adult males with FXS are more likely to exhibit autistic behavior, as well as to be more shy, socially withdrawn, and less energetic than are comparably cognitively impaired males. However, both males (and females) with fragile X can also exhibit hyperactivity, impulsivity, tantrums, aggression, destructiveness, and self-injurious behavior [15]. Interestingly, the degree of aggression has been found to correlate with a polymorphism (benign variant) of a serotonin transporter, 5-HTTLPR, with homozygotes for one form of polymorphism being more aggressive and destructive than homozygotes for the other form [16]. Males with premutations have not been as well studied, although the studies that have been done have found that these males are more likely to have alcohol dependence, obsessive–compulsive disorders, learning disability, and executive function deficits. However, the IQ of these individuals was not significantly different from that of controls [17].

Females with the full mutation can have significant cognitive impairment, but this is related to the pattern of X inactivation (remember, in females, one of the X chromosomes becomes inactivated during embryogenesis). At least half of the women with a full mutation have an IQ in the borderline or mildly cognitively impaired range. Furthermore, women with a full mutation whose cognition falls within the normal range are still more likely to have executive function deficits and some behavioral differences. These include greater deficits in socialization, and being rated as withdrawn or depressed more often than controls [18]. Females with a premutation do not have any discernible executive function problems; however, there is some evidence that these women are more likely to have social phobia, panic disorder and/or agoraphobia, and anxiety disorders [19]. It should not be surprising that women with a full mutation also exhibit impaired social interaction, as well as impulsivity, shyness, moodiness, and inattention [15].

Klinefelter (XXY) Syndrome

Klinefelter syndrome (KS) is caused by the presence of an extra X chromosome in a male. Males with KS have the combination of testicular failure, tall stature for the family, and a relatively characteristic cognitive and behavioral profile. Cognitively, boys with KS tend to be in the normal range, but IQ scores tend to be less than those of their siblings or control males. The literature reports that most males with KS have lower verbal IQ than performance IQ, although the degree of difference can vary across the lifespan; in addition, some studies have found the reverse in that performance IQ is lower than verbal IQ [20]. In addition, a recent study found that the lower full-scale IQ is attributable to deficits in both verbal and nonverbal cognitive abilities. For example, Bruining et al. [21] recently described 51 boys with Klinefelter syndrome and found that the total IQ was 80; the mean performance IQ was 86, whereas the mean verbal IQ was 78.

It is not surprising therefore that language and speech impairments are also common, and are present at all ages. Speech and language delays, as evidenced by delays in early expressive language and speech milestones, are noted in most males with KS. In the early school years, problems with reading, spelling, and writing (but not arithmetic skills) are common. In addition, these boys have difficulties with articulation, word finding, and phonemic processing. During the second decade, impaired reading, spelling, and arithmetic are prevalent, with most of these boys receiving special education. In early adulthood, these gaps widen, with KS males being several grade levels below age-matched controls [22]. In addition, boys with KS also have a higher frequency of motor problems, as demonstrated by decreased strength, running speed, and agility [23].

It has been known for some time that attention deficit is more common in these boys. Recently, however, in the group of 51 boys with Klinefelter syndrome mentioned above, Bruining et al. [21] found that 63% had ADHD, whereas 27% had autism spectrum disorders. Bishop et al. [24] also found an increased frequency of ASD in a smaller group of 19 boys with KS, with 11% of their sample being affected. They emphasized that not only should there be awareness of the high frequency of psychopathology in these boys but also in any boy who is exhibiting behavioral problems, especially in conjunction with a nonverbal learning disability, a karyotype should be done. In addition, Boks et al. [25] found that among a group of 31 adult males with KS, 10 (32%) had a psychiatric disorder, including two with a psychotic disorder (schizophrenia and delusional disorder).

Perhaps the most comprehensive review of the behavioral characteristics of KS males was provided by Visootsak and Graham [26]. They summarized findings of other studies, which in general had found that males with KS were friendly, kind, and helpful, although could also be timid, immature, and reserved. One study had found that during childhood, being shy, quiet, and underactive was not uncommon. Most disliked rough games and cried easily when bullied by other children. Older males with KS described themselves as more sensitive, apprehensive, and insecure than were their peers. However, as Visootsak and Graham [26] point out, many of these studies were done on males who were not receiving testosterone replacement therapy. This treatment has been shown to increase self-esteem and a feeling of well-being in this group of males. In addition, males diagnosed prenatally or at birth had fewer behavioral problems as compared to males who were diagnosed postnatally, likely because of anticipatory guidance in the former group.

Visootsak and Graham [26] also reviewed cognitive and social function of males with variant forms of KS. In those with a 48, XXYY karyotype, the full-scale IQ is lower, with a range of 70–80. The verbal IQ is significantly lower than the performance IQ, with a 13-point difference between the averages of the two. In addition, the verbal IQ has been found to decrease with age, with the performance IQ remaining the same. As in the XXY group, language-based learning disabilities are common. These boys are also described as shy and reserved, although they can also have ADHD, impulsivity, aggression, and mood instability. More specific information was provided by a large study of 95 males with XXYY, in which Tartaglia et al. [27] found that 72% had ADHD, 28% had autism spectrum disorder, and 47% had a mood disorder.

Males with a 48, XXXY karyotype have a lower total IQ than do XXY males, with language being more severely impaired in the former group. As a group, they are described as being immature, passive, and subject to temper tantrums and outbursts; however, they are less likely to have internalizing and externalizing maladaptive behavior.

Neurofibromatosis

Neurofibromatosis (NF) is an autosomal dominant disorder with several manifestations and wide variability in expression. The most common features of NF include multiple café au lait macules, freckling, neurofibromas, optic nerve gliomas, and Lisch nodules of the iris. Both cognitive and behavioral functions are impaired in many individuals with this condition. In general, 6–7% of children with NF fall in the cognitively impaired range (IQ < 70). Children whose IQ is in the normal range are still found to function at a lower level than are their siblings, with over 60% having an IQ 10 or more points lower than that of their siblings. Visuospatial deficits are more common than language deficits and more severe than IQ would predict (whereas language skills were no more deficient than IQ would predict). In addition, fine motor skills and motor speed are reduced in NF children as compared to their unaffected siblings [28].

In general, children with NF have a significantly increased risk for social and emotional problems. Dilts et al. [29] had proposed that the behavioral phenotype for NF includes social and attention problems, deficits in motor development and visual–motor integration, and a greater frequency of internalizing as compared to externalizing problems. Specifically, Noll et al. [30] found that the social problems could be characterized as being more sensitive and isolated, with fewer friends and reciprocated friendships. Attention problems were generally not accompanied by hyperactivity, and the frequency of ADHD comorbid conditions, oppositional defiant disorder and conduct disorder, was not increased in children with NF.

Noonan Syndrome

Noonan syndrome (NS) is an autosomal dominant condition characterized by a characteristic facial phenotype, short stature, and pulmonic stenosis. The facial phenotype changes with age but in general consists of hypertelorism, ptosis, and prominent nasolabial folds [31]. Few studies have investigated cognitive and behavioral functions; however, the studies that have been done have found deficits in both. Lee et al. [32] investigated a cohort of 48 children with NS and found that the full-scale IQ was 84, with a slightly higher performance score than verbal score. Wingbermuhle et al. [33] elaborated on the cognitive findings in NS and pointed out that language skills in children with NS tend to develop slower, with articulation disorders common. In addition, motor delays and clumsiness are commonly reported, with almost half of the children with NS receiving a diagnosis of developmental coordination disorder. These motor skills will often improve with time, however.

In addition, children with NS have been noted to have an increased frequency of behavioral problems, with social problems (characterized by immaturity, lack of interaction with peers, and diminished insight into social situations), stubbornness, restlessness, impulsivity, and mood problems commonly mentioned [33]. The personality of the individual with NS is rarely described, but Collins and Turner [34] noted that the child with NS is generally confident, happy, and talkative, whereas the adult is likely to be friendly and agreeable.

Prader–Willi Syndrome

Prader–Willi syndrome (PWS) is a genetic condition caused by the lack of expression of paternally derived genes on chromosome 15q11–13, in the Prader–Willi/Angelman region. The two main subtypes of PWS are deletion of the paternally derived chromosome 15 and uniparental disomy of the maternally derived chromosome 15. The phenotype of PWS consists of short stature, hypogonadism, infantile hypotonia, childhood-onset hyperphagia, and obesity. Cognitive impairment is virtually always present, as are characteristic behavioral abnormalities.

In general, the degree of cognitive impairment is in the borderline to mild/moderate range. Copet et al. [35] evaluated 85 adults with PWS and found that the average full-scale IQ was 52, with verbal and performance IQs in the same range (VIQ = 53, PIQ = 52.5). The PIQ was significantly better in the deletion group than in the nondeletion group (although in the deletion group PIQ = VIQ), whereas the VIQ was significantly greater than the PIQ in the nondeletion group (VIQ > PIQ). Similarities and differences were found between the two groups in terms of subtests. In both groups, vocabulary subtest was identified as a strength, whereas digit span, digit symbol, and digit symbol coding were found to be weaknesses. The deletion subgroup had specific weaknesses in the comprehension and picture completion subtests, and relative strengths in object assembly (with this identified strength likely correlating to the jigsaw puzzle ability noted in individuals with PWS). The nondeletion group had weakness in the picture arrangement subtest, whereas it had strengths in the information and similarity verbal subtests. These findings are highly suggestive of distinct cognitive profiles in individuals with PWS being dependent on genotype. Further evidence for distinctive genetic differences comes from the study by Whittington et al. [36], in which individuals with the two subtypes of PWS were compared to their unaffected sibs. Whereas the correlation of between those with nondeletion PWS and their siblings was 0.5, the correlation between those with deletion PWS and their siblings was –0.07.

PWS is also associated with a specific behavioral phenotype, which consists of excessive interest in food, skin picking, difficulty with changes in routine, temper tantrums, obsessive and compulsive behaviors, and mood fluctuations. The skin picking has been further characterized as squeezing, scratching, biting, rubbing, pricking, cutting, or digging at the skin; this is found in 95% of those with PWS [37]. The obsessive and compulsive behaviors are not those that are seen in obsessive–compulsive disorder (e.g., checking and cleaning) but rather more like ritualistic behaviors such as hoarding and insistence on routines. The repetitive behaviors seen in PWS have been compared to those seen in autism spectrum disorders, with the nondeletion group identified as especially at increased risk for autistic symptoms. Even here, however, there are subtle differences in the types of ritualistic behaviors in the PWS group and the ASD group in that those with PWS were more likely to collect and store objects, whereas those with ASD were more likely to line up objects [38]. In addition, those in the nondeletion group are also more likely to have psychosis (as many as 28% in some studies) and sleep disorders, whereas those with deletions are more likely to have skin picking, mood lability, food stealing, withdrawal, sulking, nail biting, hoarding, and overeating [39].

It has been shown that these behaviors increase with age, peaking in early adulthood. However, adults with PWS have reduced rates of maladaptive and compulsive behavior, similar to the rates in young children with PWS and markedly lower than the rates in adolescents and young adults with PWS. This is in contrast to the situation in those with cognitive impairment in general, whereby increases in psychiatric problems are found with increasing age [40].

Rett Syndrome

Rett syndrome (RS) is an X-linked dominant neurodevelopmental disorder in females characterized by initially normal development, with subsequent regression with loss of skills between the ages of 6 and 18 months. The main manifestations include acquired microcephaly, loss of purposeful hand movements, and loss of communication and motor skills. The cognitive level in girls with RS has been estimated to be at a level of 8 months or less [41]. However, adaptive behavior skills are slightly higher, with communication at a mean of 11 months, daily living skills at a mean of 14 months, and socialization at a mean of 10 months. This suggests that despite the severe degree of cognitive impairment, girls with RS are able to have some interaction with people and to learn some simple self-help skills. However, Demeter [42] has suggested that using an alternative approach to cognitive assessment might yield a better understanding of what girls with RS can achieve.

A lengthy list of behaviors has also been generated for RS. These behaviors have been assigned to various domains, with these domains (and examples) including general mood (screaming spells, inconsolable crying, abrupt mood swings, and unexplained irritability); breathing problems (breath holding, swallowing air); hand behaviors (lack of purposeful grasp, difficulty stopping repetitive hand movements); repetitive facial movements (grimacing, tongue movements); body rocking and expressionless face; nighttime behaviors (spells of screaming or laughter during the night); fear/anxiety (apparent panic, holding parts of the body rigidly); walking, standing (walks with a stiff-legged gait, leans on objects when standing); other (appears isolated, hand wounds from repetitive hand movements).

The cause of Rett syndrome is a mutation in the *MECP2* gene, which encodes methyl-CpG-binding protein 2. A recent study has shown differences in the behavioral phenotype based on the genotype. For example, those with the R294X mutation were more likely to have mood difficulties, body rocking, and nighttime behaviors, and less likely to have hand behaviors or repetitive facial movements. Conversely, those with the T158M mutation were less likely to have mood disturbances and were more likely to have hand behaviors [43].

Smith-Magenis Syndrome

Smith-Magenis syndrome (SMS) is a genetic disorder caused by microdeletion of chromosome 17p11.2 or mutation of the *RAI1* gene. The cardinal manifestations include both physical and behavioral characteristics, with the physical manifestations including midface hypoplasia, upslanting palpebral fissures, broad nasal bridge, and tented upper lip with a prominent philtrum. Most children with SMS have cognitive impairment, with that impairment becoming more apparent with age. In a recent study of young children (age 3 years or less), Wolters et al. [44] found that the mean developmental index on the Bayley Scales was 66.6. However, in this group of 11 children, two fell within the lower limits of normal (85–115). Both receptive and expressive language were delayed, with expressive more delayed than receptive. Gross motor milestones were mildly to moderately delayed, for example, independent walking was achieved at approximately 20 months. Oral–motor dysfunction is also common in these children.

Overall, the Vineland Adaptive Behavior Scales score was in the mildly delayed range (average score 76.3). However, one of the domains, the socialization score, was within the normal range, whereas the other three (daily living, communication, and motor skills) were depressed. In this small sample of 11 young children, none were found to have evidence of autistic behavior.

As children with SMS age, cognitive impairment becomes more apparent, as do the hallmark behavioral abnormalities. Among 29 children with SMS, Udwin et al. [45] found that the FSIQ was between 41 and 60 in 22, and 40 or below in seven. The mean FSIQ was 53.9. There was no significant difference between verbal and performance IQs. Adults with SMS had comparable findings, although the range of IQs in this group was <40–68, with the mean FSIQ 55.8.

In both groups, areas of strength were long-term memory, computational skills, and perceptual skills, whereas areas of weakness were visuomotor coordination, sequencing, and response speed. In terms of adaptive behavior, the domains of daily living skills and motor skills were relative weaknesses, whereas the domains of communication and socialization were relative strengths [46]. This correlates with the finding that among adults, dependence on caretakers was greater than would be expected by the cognitive level, and it was suggested that the behavioral disturbances in these individuals affected their ability to develop independence skills [45].

The behavioral disturbances include impulsivity, aggression, tantrums, attention seeking, sleep disturbances, stereotypies, and self-injurious behavior. The latter two are especially striking and may be fairly specific to SMS. The stereotypies include the so-called spasmodic upper body squeeze, which is a form of self-hugging when the individual is happy or excited. The second stereotypy is the licking of the finger followed by the flipping of the page of a book (the so-called lick and flip) seen in a significant proportion of individuals with SMS. The self-injurious behavior is unusual in that in addition to skin picking, head banging, and hand or wrist biting which can be seen as a manifestation in other syndromes [47], individuals with SMS are prone to pulling out their fingernails or toenails, or to inserting objects into body orifices such as the ears, nose, rectum, or vagina [47, 48]. Sleep disturbance is another distinctive manifestation of SMS and generally manifests as an apparent perturbation of circadian rhythm. Individuals with SMS generally have frequent and prolonged nighttime arousal, early awakening, and daytime sleepiness. REM sleep is said to be reduced as well.

A specific personality type has also been described, with individuals with SMS described as generally being friendly and outgoing but prone to excessive aggression and temper tantrums. Repetitive questioning has also been noted, as has a preference for adult contact [49].

Sotos Syndrome

Sotos syndrome (SS) is a genetic condition associated with pre- or postnatal-onset overgrowth, generally affecting head circumference, weight, and length. The face is said to be mildly dysmorphic and includes tall, prominent forehead, downslanting palpebral fissures, and prominent jaw (more apparent with age). Cognitive abilities can range between normal cognitive achievement and moderate cognitive impairment. Most with SS will have learning disabilities, even if cognitive function is in the normal range. Language impairments are not uncommon, and numeracy impairment is also reported to be common. Behavioral aspects of SS include deficits in social functioning or autistic features. Additional behavioral concerns that are more common in SS individuals include hyperactivity, temper tantrums, sleep problems (typically early morning awakening), emotional immaturity, and anxiety [50, 51].

Tuberous Sclerosis

Tuberous sclerosis (TS) is an autosomal dominant genetic disorder that affects a number of organ systems, including the brain, eye, skin, kidneys, and heart. To date, two genes, *TSC1* and *TSC2*, have been identified as causative of this condition. Cognitive impairment has been known to be a component manifestation for a long time; more recently, however, the behavioral aspects of this condition have been elucidated. Although most individuals with TS have an IQ that is within the normal range, another 30% fall within the severely to profoundly impaired range (IQ < 21). The impairment, when present, is generally apparent by 1 year of age, with no evidence of "catch-up" by 30 months of age. Even if cognitive impairment is not present, language delay is common. Both children and adults with TS and normal intelligence can have deficits in attentional skills and executive function, as well as memory dysfunction [52]. Social and communication deficits, as well as motor deficits, have also been noted in some individuals with normal cognitive function.

Several behavioral manifestations have been described and include both autism spectrum disorders, ADHD and related conditions, aggression, emotional lability, anxiety and sleep disorders, and temper tantrums. Some of these behaviors are age specific. For example, developmental disorders, social impairment, and disruptive behaviors are more common in childhood and adolescence, whereas adults show more anxiety and depressed symptoms, alcoholism, and obsessive–compulsive disorders [51, 53]. Individuals with cognitive impairment are also more likely to exhibit autism spectrum disorders or disruptive behaviors. A recent study of self-injurious behavior (SIB) in 257 individuals with the diagnosis of TS found that 10% of these individuals exhibited SIB [54]. Positive correlations with the presence of SIB included a history of seizures, autism, and location of cerebral tubers. A second study investigated the genotype–phenotype correlations comparing those with a *TSC1* mutation to those with a *TSC2* mutation. In the past, it had been suggested that those with a *TSC2* mutation are more often cognitively impaired than are those with a *TSC1* mutation. However, this study found that there is sufficient overlap between those with a *TSC1* mutation and those with a *TSC2* mutation to not be useful in predicting the onset of seizures or the degree of cognitive impairment solely on the basis of the gene that is mutated [55]. That being said, there is reasonably good evidence that one particular mutation in the *TSC2* gene, the R905Q mutation, is associated with an unusually mild condition, with hypomelanotic macules and focal seizures that either remit spontaneously or are easily controlled with medication. In addition, individuals who have the TSC clinical diagnosis, but no identified mutation, are more likely to have milder brain features than are those with either a TSC1 or a TSC2 mutation [55].

Turner Syndrome

Turner syndrome is a chromosomal condition in which a female is missing all or part of one of her X chromosomes. When all or one of the Xs is missing, the karyotype is written as 45, X. However, in some individuals, a deletion of part of one of the Xs can be sufficient to cause the Turner syndrome phenotype. In general, females with Turner syndrome have short stature, coarctation of the aorta, a specific cognitive profile, and an increased risk of impaired psychosocial skills. Rovet [56] has reviewed neurocognitive deficits in Turner syndrome in relationship to neuronal and hormonal influences. These deficits (and examples of effects) include spatial ability (puzzle assembly, directional sense); visualization (visual imagery, part–whole perception); visuomotor (design copying, visual sequencing); memory (visual memory, short-term recall); attention (inhibitory control, auditory attention); executive function (planning, fluent production); and language (verbal fluency, articulation). However, not all aspects of memory, attention, executive function, or language are affected, with spared areas including verbal and rote memory; sustained attention and focusing; set shifting; and expressive and receptive language, respectively. Overall, females with Turner syndrome are two to fourfold more likely than non-Turner females to have some sort of cognitive difficulty.

Females with Turner syndrome are also more likely to have various psychological problems, although the incidence of severe psychopathology is not significantly elevated. Among psychological problems that have been identified, social relationships seem to be the area that is most consistently identified as a problem area. Burnett et al. [57] recently reviewed the literature on social cognition in Turner syndrome and noted that females with Turner syndrome tend to have fewer friends, to participate in fewer social activities, to have greater attentional and social difficulties, and to withdraw from social interactions more often than do control females.

Velocardiofacial Syndrome

Velocardiofacial syndrome (VCFS) is caused by a deletion of part of the long arm of chromosome 22, in the q11 region. Cardinal manifestations include effects on the face (narrow palpebral fissures, long, wide nose, small chin), palate (velopharyngeal insufficiency, cleft or highly arched palate) and heart (congenital cardiac defects, particularly those that are considered conotruncal). Mild cognitive impairment is an extremely common manifestation of this condition, as are some characteristic behavioral manifestations.

De Smedt et al. [58] recently reported on the results of cognitive testing on a large sample of children ($N = 103$) with VCFS. The average IQ was 73, with a range of 50–109. In general, the VIQ was greater than the PIQ, although there were exceptions. It is noteworthy that the FSIQ in familial cases (i.e., inherited from a parent) was significantly lower, with an average of 65. However, the number of children in this group was small ($N = 11$). Oskarsdottir et al. [59] also evaluated cognitive function, obtained similar results for FSIQ and a higher VIQ than PIQ. However, they also evaluated other functions, with the following results. Early development was delayed in most, with unusual forms of crawling (e.g., shuffling in a sitting position), late walking, delayed attainment of bladder control, and inability to ride a bicycle by age 7 years. Not all of the children with delayed attainment of motor skills had cognitive impairment, so this did not correlate with IQ. Executive function was also impaired in many. In general, evidence for a nonverbal learning disability was found in these children. However, delayed speech and language development were also common, being described as one of the most consistent findings in children with VCFS. Children with VCFS are essentially nonverbal through 30 months but show improvement between the ages of 3 and 4 years [60]. As a result of these findings, it is obvious that children with VCFS should have a multi-disciplinary approach so that each child can be provided with adequate treatment and support.

Kiley-Brabeck and Sobin [61] also found greater executive dysfunction in these children and correlated this deficit to poor social skills. Compared to their nonaffected siblings, children with VCFS had significantly lower social skills. Specific deficits in the areas of cooperation, assertion, and responsibility were found, whereas self-control skills did not differ from those of their control siblings. This led to the authors suggesting that in a child with VCFS and poor social skills, executive dysfunction be sought; conversely, in a child with VCFS and executive dysfunction, social skills should be evaluated.

In addition to learning and social problems, almost half of the individuals with VCFS have an autism spectrum disorder (ASD), ADHD, or both. Within the ASD spectrum, autism was relatively rare, with most children having what the authors called an autistic-like condition. In their study group, 20% of individuals with VCFS had ADHD only, 15% had ASD only, and 10% had a combination of ADHD and ASD. In addition, a few adults had other psychiatric diagnoses, including depression, anxiety disorder, or psychotic symptoms, as evidenced by delusions or hallucinations.

Antshel et al. [62] compared ADHD in children with VCFS to idiopathic ADHD and found some notable differences between the two groups. In general, children with VCFS were more likely to have the inattentive type of ADHD. Niklasson et al. [63] also evaluated children with VCFS for the presence of ADHD (with or without comorbid ASD) and found that it was present in over half of the children studied. In general, among the 13 children with ADHD, 10 had the inattentive form, whereas 3 had the combined form.

Williams Syndrome

Williams syndrome is a genetic condition caused by deletion of a small segment of the long arm of chromosome seven, in the region designated as 7q11.23. Individuals with Williams syndrome have a characteristic facial appearance (including periorbital puffiness, full cheeks and lips, wide mouth with widely spaced teeth, and a long smooth philtrum), supravalvular aortic stenosis, transient hypercalcemia, and short stature. Individuals with Williams syndrome (WS) also have cognitive impairment as well as a specific behavioral phenotype. Cognitive impairment is present in almost all individuals with WS, with the degree of impairment ranging from borderline to moderate (although the rare individual with no cognitive impairment or severe cognitive impairment exists) [64]. Although language skills are said to be a strength of those with WS, delayed language development is common, with many, if not most, children producing their first words at 3 years of age. However, by school age, language is relatively preserved in relation to general intelligence, although exceptional linguistic ability is not thought to occur [65]; indeed, within this category, pragmatic abilities are more limited than expected for the child's developmental level. Nonetheless, individuals with WS do have a relative strength in concrete vocabulary and grammatical ability [64]. Weaknesses identified in individuals with WS include the above-mentioned pragmatics, as well as relational/conceptual vocabulary. Additionally, those with WS show strengths in concrete nonverbal reasoning and verbal short-term memory, and severe deficits in visuospatial construction. Therefore, it is important to realize that individuals with WS do not have strong language skills across the board, but rather a composite of strengths and weaknesses within this domain.

Those with WS are also said to have good social skills, and in some of the early papers, the children were described as having a "cocktail party manner." A strength in social skills is supported by the findings of Mervis and John [64], who found that on the Scales of Independent Behavior, performance on the Social Interaction and Communication Skills scale was significantly better than on the remaining scales (motor skills, personal living skills, and community living skills). Personality-wise, children with WS are more likely to be gregarious, people-oriented, visible, tense, and sensitive than are others with ID [66]. In addition, children with WS are more likely to have attention problems; one study even found that all children scored in the clinical range for ADHD [67].

In addition, individuals with WS commonly have an anxiety disorder (including specific phobia, generalized anxiety disorder, and separation anxiety), oppositional or conduct disorder, and low motivation [64]. In terms of phobias, a striking number of fears are seen in those with WS, including earthquakes, thunderstorms, carnival rides, and being teased to name a few of the over 50 different fears that had been identified in these individuals [68].

Finally, mention should be made of the third reported strength of WS individuals (speech and social ability being the other two, discussed above), that being music ability. Dykens et al. [68] reported that individuals with WS are more likely to play an instrument, take music lessons, and be rated as more skilled in playing. Among those that did participate, levels of anxiety or fears were lower than those in the comparison groups of children with Prader–Willi syndrome and Down syndrome.

Conclusions

Many, if not most, syndromes have complex phenotypes that include physical features, cognitive deficits, and/or behavioral manifestations. In order to maximize the potential in any child with a syndrome, medical, educational, and behavioral needs must all be met. In addition, scientists can learn by studying these syndromes and their cognitive and behavioral phenotypes to better understand how the brain functions.

References

1. Pelc K, Cheron G, Dan B. Behavior and neuropsychiatric manifestations in Angelman syndrome. Neuropsych Dis Treat. 2008;4:577–84.
2. Reiss AL. Childhood developmental disorders: an academic and clinical convergence point for psychiatry, neurology, psychology and pediatrics. J Child Psychol Psychiatr. 2009;50:87–98.
3. Fisch GS, Carpenter N, Howard-Peebles PN, Holden JJA, Tarleton J, Simensen R, Nance W. Studies of age-correlated features of cognitive-behavioral development in children and adolescents with genetic disorders. Am J Med Genet. 2007;1434A:2478–89.
4. Peters SU, Goddard-Finegold J, Beaudet AL, Madduri N, Turcich M, Bacino CA. Cognitive and adaptive behavior profiles of children with Angelman syndrome. Am J Med Genet. 2004;128A:110–13.
5. Williams CA, Dagli AI, Driscoll DJ. Angelman syndrome. In: Pagon RA, Bird TC, Dolan CR, Stephens K, editors. GeneReviews [Internet]. Seattle, WA: Univ Washington; 2008.
6. Williams CA, Beaudet AL, Clayton-Smith J, Knoll JH, Kyllerman M, Laan LA, et al. Angelman syndrome 2005: updated consensus for diagnostic criteria. Am J Med Genet. 2006;140A:413–18.
7. Berry RJ, Leitner RP, Clarke AR, Einfeld SL. Behavioral aspects of Angelman syndrome: a case control study. Am J Med Genet. 2005;132A:8–12.

8. Lott IT, Dierssen M. Cognitive deficits and associated neurological complications in individuals with Down's syndrome. Lancet Neurol. 2010;9:623–33.
9. Fidler DJ, Hepburn SL, Mankin G, Rogers SJ. Praxis skills in young children with Down syndrome, other developmental disabilities, and typically developing children. Am J Occ Ther. 2005;59:129–38.
10. Dykens EM. Psychiatric and behavioral disorders in persons with Down syndrome. MRDD Res Rev. 2007;13:272–8.
11. Adams D, Oliver C. The relationship between acquired impairments of executive function and behavior change in adults with Down syndrome. J Intellect Disabil Res. 2010;54:393–405.
12. Saul RA, Tarleton JC. FMR1-related disorders. In: Pagon RA, Bird TC, Dolan CR, Stephens K, editors. GeneReviews [Internet]. Seattle, WA: Univ Washington; 2010.
13. Cornish K, Kogan C, Turk J, Manly T, James N, Mills A, Dalton A. The emerging fragile X permutation phenotype: evidence from the domain of social cognition. Brain Cogn. 2005;57:53–60.
14. Lightbody AA, Reiss AL. Gene, brain, and behavior relationships in fragile X syndrome: evidence from neuroimaging studies. Devel Disabil Res Rev. 2009;15:343–52.
15. Tsouris JA, Brown WT. Neuropsychiatric symptoms of fragile X syndrome. CNS Drugs. 2004;18:687–703.
16. Hessl D, Tassone F, Cordeiro L, Koldewyn K, McCormick C, Green C, et al. Brief report: aggression and stereotypic behavior in males with fragile X syndrome – moderating secondary genes in a "single gene" disorder. J Autism Dev Disord. 2007;38:184–9.
17. Moore CJ, Daly EM, Schmitz N, Tassone F, Tysoe C, Hagerman RJ, et al. A neuropsychological investigation of male premutations carriers of fragile X syndrome. Neuropsychologia. 2004;42:1934–47.
18. Freund LS, Reiss AL, Abrams MT. Psychiatric disorders associated with fragile X in the young female. Pediatrics. 1993;91:321–9.
19. Bourgeois J, Coffey S, Rivera SM, Hessl D, Gane LW, Tassone F, et al. Fragile X premutation disorders – expanding the psychiatric perspective. J Clin Psychiatr. 2009;70:852–62.
20. Boone KB, Swerdloff RS, Miller BL, Geschwind DH, Razani J, Lee A, et al. Neuropsychological profiles of adults with Klinefelter syndrome. J Int Neuropsychol Soc. 2001;7:446–56.
21. Bruining H, Swaab H, Kas M, van Engeland H. Psychiatric characteristics in a self-selected sample of boys with Klinefelter syndrome. Pediatrics. 2009;123:e865–70.
22. Gerschwind DH, Boone KB, Miller BL, Swerdloff RS. Neurobehavioral phenotype of Klinefelter syndrome. MRDD Res Rev. 2000;6:107–16.
23. Ross JL, Roeltgen DP, Stefanatos G, Benecke R, Zeger MPD, Kushner H, et al. Cognitive and motor development during childhood in boys with Klinefelter syndrome. Am J Med Genet. 2007;146A:708–19.
24. Bishop DVM, Jacobs PA, Lachlan K, Wellesley D, Barnicoat A, Boyd PA, et al. Autism, language and communication in children with sex chromosome trisomies. Arch Dis Child. 2010 July 23 (epub ahead of print).
25. Boks MPM, de Vette MHT, Sommer IE, van Rijn S, Giltay JC, Swaab H, Kahn RS. Psychiatric morbidity and X-chromosomal origin in a Klinefelter sample. Schizophren Res. 2007;93: 399–402.
26. Visootsak J, Graham JM Jr. Social function in multiple X and Y chromosome disorders: XXY, XYY, XXYY, XXX. Dev Disabil Res Rev. 2009;15:328–32.
27. Tartaglia N, Davis S, Hench A, Nimishakavi S, Beauregard R, Reynolds A, et al. A new look at XXYY syndrome: medical and psychological features. Am J Med Genet. 2008;146A: 1509–22.
28. Hyman SL, Shores A, North KN. The nature and frequency of cognitive deficits in children with neurofibromatosis type 1. Neurol. 2005;65:1037–44.
29. Dilts CV, Carey JC, Kircher JC, Hoffman RO, Creel D, Ward K, et al. Children and adolescents with neurofibromatosis 1: a behavioral phenotype. Devel Behav Pediatr. 1996;17:229–39.

30. Noll RB, Reiter-Purtill J, Moore BD, Schorry EK, Lovell AM, Vannatta K, Gerhardt CA. Social, emotional, and behavioral functioning of children with NF1. Am J Med Genet. 2007;143A:2261–73.
31. Van der Burgt I. Noonan syndrome. Orphanet J Rare Dis. 2007 doi: 10.1186/1750–1172–2–4.
32. Lee DA, Portnoy S, Hill P, Patton MA. Psychological profile of children with Noonan syndrome. Dev Med Child Neurol. 2005;47:35–38.
33. Wingbermuhle E, Egger J, van der Burgt I, Verhoeven W. Neuropsychological and behavioral aspects of Noonan syndrome. Horm Res. 2009;72 suppl:15–23.
34. Collins E, Turner G. The Noonan syndrome: a review of the clinical and genetic features of 27 cases. J Pediatr. 1973;83:941–50.
35. Copet P, Jauregi J, Laurier V, Ehlinger V, Arnaud C, Cobo A-M, et al. Cognitive profile in a large French cohort of adults with Prader–Willi syndrome: differences between genotypes. J Intellect Disabil Res. 2010;54:204–15.
36. Whittington J, Holland A, Webb T. Relationship between the IQ of people with Prader–Willi syndrome and that of their siblings: evidence for imprinted gene effects. J Intellect Disabil Res. 2009;53:411–18.
37. Morgan JR, Storch EA, Woods DW, Bodzin D, Lewin AB, Murphy TK. A preliminary analysis of the phenomenology of skin-picking in Prader–Willi syndrome. Child Psychiatr Hum Dev. 2010;41:448–63.
38. Greaves N, Prince E, Evans DW, Charman T. Repetitive and ritualistic behaviour in children with Prader–Willi syndrome and children with autism. J Intellect Disabil Res. 2006;50: 92–100.
39. Ho AY, Dimitropoulos A. Clinical management of behavioral characteristics of Prader–Willi syndrome. Neuropsych Dis Treat. 2010;6:107–18.
40. Dykens EM. Maladaptive and compulsive behavior in Prader–Willi syndrome: new insights from older adults. Am J Ment Retard. 2004;109:142–53.
41. Perry A, Sarlo-McGarvey N, Haddad C. Brief report: cognitive and adaptive functioning in 28 girls with Rett syndrome. J Autism Dev Disord. 1991;21:551–6.
42. Demeter K. Assessing the developmental level in Rett syndrome: an alternative approach? Eur Child Adolesc Psychiatr. 2000;9:227–33.
43. Robertson L, Hall SE, Jacoby P, Ellaway C, de Klerk N, Leonard H. The association between behavior and genotype in Rett syndrome using the Australian Rett syndrome database. Am J Med Genet. 2006;141B:177–83.
44. Wolters PL, Gropman AL, Martin SC, Smith MR, Hildenbrand HL, Brewer CC, Smith ACM. Neurodevelopment of children under 3 years of age with Smith-Magenis syndrome. Pediatr Neurol. 2009;41:250–8.
45. Udwin O, Webber C, Horn I. Abilities and attainment in Smith-Magenis syndrome. Dev Med Child Neurol. 2001;43:823–8.
46. Madduri N, Peters SU, Voigt RG, Llorente AM, Lupski JR, Potocki L. Cognitive and adaptive behavior profiles in Smith-Magenis syndrome. J Dev Behav Pediatr. 2006;27:188–92.
47. Shelley BP, Robertson MM. The neuropsychiatry and multisystem features of the Smith-Magenis syndrome: a review. J Neuropsychiatr Clin Neurosci. 2005;17:91–97.
48. Dykens EM, Smith ACM. Distinctiveness and correlates of maladaptive behaviour in children and adolescents with Smith-Magenis syndrome. J Intellect Disabil Res. 1998;42:481–9.
49. Taylor L, Oliver C. The behavioural phenotype of Smith-Magenis syndrome: evidence for a gene–environment interaction. J Intellect Disabil Res. 2008;52:830–41.
50. Mouridsen SE, Hansen MB. Neuropsychiatric aspects of Sotos syndrome. A review and two case illustrations. Eur Child Adolesc Psychiatr. 2002;11:43–48.
51. Sarimski K. Behavioural and emotional characteristics in children with Sotos syndrome and learning disabilities. Dev Med Child Neurol. 2003;45:172–8.
52. De Vries P, Humphrey A, McCartney D, Prather P, Bolton P, Hunt A. Consensus clinical guidelines for the assessment of cognitive and behavioural problems in tuberous sclerosis. Eur Child Adolesc Psychiatr. 2005;14:183–90.

53. Kopp CM, Muzykewicz DA, Staley BA, Thiele EA, Pulsifer MB. Behavior problems in children with tuberous sclerosis complex and parental stress. Epilepsy Behav. 2008;13: 505–10.
54. Staley BA, Montenegro MA, Major P, Muzykewicz DA, Halpern EF, Kopp CMC, et al. Self-injurious behavior and tuberous sclerosis complex: frequency and possible associations in a population of 257 patients. Epilepsy Behav. 2008;13:650–3.
55. Napolioni V, Moavero R, Curatolo P. Recent advances in neurobiology of tuberous sclerosis complex. Brain Dev. 2009;31:104–13.
56. Rovet J. Turner syndrome: a review of genetic and hormonal influences on neuropsychological functioning. Child Neuropsychol. 2004;10:262–79.
57. Burnett AC, Reutens DC, Wood AG. Social cognition in Turner syndrome. J Clin Neurosci. 2010;17:283–6.
58. De Smedt B, Devriendt K, Fryns JP, Vogels A, Gewillig M, Swillen A. Intellectual abilities in a large sample of children with velo-cardio-facial syndrome: an update. J Intellect Disabil Res. 2007;51:666–70.
59. Oskarsdottir S, Belfrage M, Sandstedt E, Viggedal G, Uvebrant P. Disabilities and cognition in children and adolescents with 22q11 deletion syndrome. Dev Med Child Neurol. 2005;47:177–84.
60. Murphy KC. The behavioural phenotype in velo-cardio-facial syndrome. J Intellect Disabil Res. 2004;48:524–30.
61. Kiley-Brabeck K, Sobin C. Social skills and executive function deficits in children with 22q11 deletion syndrome. Appl Neuropsychol. 2006;13:258–68.
62. Antshel KM, Faraone SV, Fremont W, Monuteaux MC, Kates WR, Doyle A, et al. Comparing ADHD in velocardiofacial syndrome to idiopathic ADHD. J Atten Disord. 2007;11 1:64–73.
63. Niklasson L, Rasmussen P, Oskarsdottir S, Gillberg C. Autism, ADHD, mental retardation and behavior problems in 100 individuals with 22q11 deletion syndrome. Res Dev Disabil. 2009;30:763–73.
64. Mervis CB, John AE. Cognitive and behavioral characteristics of children with Williams syndrome. Am J Med Genet. 2010;154C:229–48.
65. Cassasco X, Castillo S, Aravena T, Rothhammer P, Aboitiz F. Williams syndrome: pediatric, neurologic, and cognitive development. Pediatr Neurol. 2005;32:166–72.
66. Klein-Tasman BP, Mervis CV. Distinctive personality characteristics of 8-, 9-, and 10-year olds with Williams syndrome. Dev Neuropsychol. 2003;23:269–90.
67. Rhodes SM, Riby DM, Park J, Fraser E, Campbell LE. Executive neuropsychological functioning in individuals with Williams syndrome. Neuropsychologia. 2010;48:1216–26.
68. Dykens EM, Rosner BA, Ly T, Sagun J. Music and anxiety in Williams syndrome: a harmonious or discordant relationship? Am J Ment Retard. 2005;5:346–58.

Chapter 7
Autism Spectrum Disorders

Ahsan Nazeer

Abstract Autism spectrum disorders are becoming more recognized in the general population. With increased awareness, primary care physicians are diagnosing these disorders at an earlier age. The following is a brief review of the proposed diagnostic changes in DSM-V, and recommendations for making a diagnosis and for treatment planning.

Introduction

Autism is a neuro-developmental disorder that despite having a history of spanning well over 100 years has only recently gained widespread recognition. The history of autism is not linear and marred with misconceptions on one side and scientific breakthroughs on the other. In 1943, Leo Kanner (1894–1981), an Austrian–American psychiatrist, identified a cluster of symptoms in 11 children (eight boys and three girls) that he later identified as "autism." He recounted 11 case studies in his seminal paper "Autistic Disturbances of Affective Contact" in which he described these children as having "autistic aloneness" [1]. He described these children to be born without the ability to make social relationships and identified some characteristic features including limited ability to develop relationships, language delays, aloofness, lack of imagination, and persistence on sameness. One year later, in 1944, Vienna-born physician Hans Asperger (1906–1980) identified a similar symptom cluster during his work with 200 families and interestingly identified that cluster as "autistic psychopathy." He occasionally called these children "little professors" and found them to have little empathy and inability to form relationships [2]. Unfortunately, Asperger's work remained un-noticed until 1980 when

A. Nazeer (✉)
Department of Psychiatry, Kalamazoo Center for Medical Studies, Michigan State University, Kalamazoo, MI 49048, USA
e-mail: nazeer@kcms.msu.edu

D.R. Patel et al. (eds.), *Neurodevelopmental Disabilities*,
DOI 10.1007/978-94-007-0627-9_7, © Springer Science+Business Media B.V. 2011

Lorna Wing (1928–), a British psychiatrist, translated his work into English and published "Asperger's Syndrome: A Clinical Account" in 1981 [3]. The years following the initial identification of autistic disorder were a period of significant diagnostic uncertainties, with some clinicians using autistic criteria too broadly and some too narrowly. As the term "autism" was borrowed from Eugen Bleuler (1857–1939), who, in 1911, used it to identify schizophrenic psychopathology, for some, autism remained synonymous with childhood schizophrenia.

Finally, in 1978, Sir Michael Rutter (1933–) [4] identified four core symptom clusters of autistic disorder: social impairment, language disturbances, insistence on sameness, and onset before 30 months of age. These criteria, with modifications and changes, were later incorporated into the Diagnostic and Statistical Manual of Mental Disorders (DSM-III) systems of classification [5].

Definition

Autism spectrum disorders (ASDs) are characterized by impairment in social interactions, language deficits, and ritualistic and repetitive behaviors with onset prior to 3 years of age.

The DSM system of classification has adapted to ongoing research and better understanding of the psychopathology of autistic disorders. DSM-IV TR (text revision) identifies five disorders under the broader category of autism spectrum disorder that includes autistic disorder, Asperger's disorder, childhood disintegrative disorder, Rett's disorder, and pervasive developmental disorder NOS (not otherwise specified). DSM-V that is scheduled for publication in 2013 [6] has proposed the following changes in the autism spectrum disorder category:

1. Rett's disorder will be excluded from DSM-V.
2. Childhood disintegrative disorder, Asperger's disorder, and pervasive developmental disorder-not otherwise specified will be merged into a single diagnosis of autistic disorder.
3. Diagnostic criteria for autistic disorder will be changed as below:

   a. The domains of social interaction and communication will be merged into social/communication deficits and restricted interests will be renamed fixed interests/repetitive behaviors.
   b. In the social/communication domain, DSM-V will require all of the following criteria to be met: deficits in non-verbal and verbal communication, lack of social reciprocity, and lack of peer relationships.
   c. In the fixed interests/repetitive behavior domain, DSM-V will require any two of the following three criteria to be met: stereotypic behaviors or unusual sensory symptoms, adherence to routines, and restricted interests.

With emerging knowledge, there continues to be a possibility of further changes in the proposed DSM-V criteria until its publication in 2013. By that time, it is advisable for clinicians to continue using the following DSM-IV-TR criteria [7] to diagnose and document autism spectrum disorders.

Autistic Disorder

In order to qualify for a diagnosis of autistic disorder, DSM-IV-TR requires impairment in social interactions (lack of social reciprocity, impairment in eye contact, failure to develop peer relationships), impairment in communication (delay in language acquisition, impairment in ability to initiate or sustain conversation, repetitive use of language), and stereotypic pattern of behavior (restricted pattern of interest, inflexible routines, and repetitive motor mannerisms), all with onset prior to 3 years of age.

Asperger's Disorder

Asperger's disorder is a part of autism spectrum disorder in which impairment in social interactions and stereotypic patterns of behavior are present with normal intelligence and relatively normal language development. Individuals with Asperger's disorder do not have any clinically significant delays in language or cognitive development.

Childhood Disintegrative Disorder (CDD)

CDD, also called Heller's syndrome, is a relatively rare disorder that presents with features of normal development until 2 years of age and then loss of social, intellectual, and language skills by 3–4 years of age (by 10 years of age as per DSM-IV-TR).

Rett's Syndrome

Rett's disorder presents with normal development until at least 6 months of age followed by deceleration in head growth, loss of social skills, mental retardation and characteristic hand-wringing movements. DSM-V is proposing to exclude this disorder from DSM system as autistic symptoms are present for only a minimal period of time through the total course of this disorder.

Pervasive Developmental Disorder-Not Otherwise Specified (PDD-NOS)

DSM-IV-TR reserves this category for individuals who present with impairment in social interactions, communication skills, or stereotypic behaviors but do not meet the full diagnostic criteria of autistic disorder, Asperger's disorder, childhood disintegrative disorder, and Rett's disorder.

Epidemiology

With the changes in diagnostic criteria over the last 10–15 years, recent reports have suggested that the prevalence of autistic disorders is on the rise. Fombonne [8] in his review of 43 studies, published since 1966, identified the median prevalence for the autistic disorders to be 60–70/10,000. In the United States, the Center for Disease Control and Prevention's Autism and Developmental Disabilities Monitoring Network [9] has reported an average prevalence of 1 in 110 children. No precise explanation of the recent rise in the prevalence is known but theories range from more awareness in medical and general populations to the broadening of diagnostic criteria. The mean male–to-female ratio among studies is 4:1. This difference in sex ratio diminishes in children with moderate to severe mental retardation with a male-to-female ratio of 2:1.

At this time there are no clear theories of etiology of autism spectrum disorders. Higher rates of seizures and mental retardation among these individuals point toward biological factors. The following is a brief summary of the etiological factors playing a role in the development of these disorders.

Genetic Factors

Current research suggests autistic disorders to be neuropsychiatric in origin with a high level of inheritance. Twin studies in autism have established the notion that identical twins are highly concordant for the development of autistic disorders [10]. Autistic children also have increased number of family members with autism or autistic traits. Studies have also shown increased prevalence of other psychiatric disorders, including depression and anxiety, in immediate family members. These findings suggest the possible interactions of more than one gene in the causation of these disorders.

Numerous techniques have been used to identify potential genetic loci for autistic disorders. Linkage and association studies have identified certain chromosomes and genes of interest including chromosomes 2, 5, 7, 11, 16, 17, and 18. Two chromosomes 15q11–q13 and 22q11.2 have shown particular promise in this regard. Gene deletions on both of these chromosomes present with specific phenotypes. Deletion on chromosome15q presents with Prader–Willi/Angelman syndrome, while the deletion on chromosome 22q presents with velo-cardio-facial (VCFS) syndrome. Maternal 15q11–13 duplications are one of the most commonly observed phenomena and can be found in 1–3% of autistic patients [11]. Researchers have also found increased prevalence of autistic disorders in patients with neurogenetic syndromes including fragile X, tuberous sclerosis, and Turner's syndrome. Fragile X is the most common genetic cause of mental retardation and autism in males. One-third of autistic children have fragile X syndrome, whereas only 12% of children with fragile X syndrome are autistic.

Tuberous sclerosis (TSC) presents with mental retardation, hamartomatous lesions, seizures, and adenoma sebaceum. Wood's lamp examination is used to examine the "ash leaf" macules.

Rett's syndrome is an X-linked disorder with incidence of 1 in 15,000 females. Mutations in MECP2 were identified in 1999 and later studies found 70–80% of the patients with Rett's syndrome to have mutations in this gene. Individuals with Rett's syndrome present with microcephaly, hand-wringing movements, and autistic features.

Environmental Factors

While genetic factors have clearly been implicated in the causation of autism, the role of environmental factors is still an area of ongoing debate. Thimerosal, a mercury-containing preservative that was used in vaccines to prevent fungal and bacterial contamination, has been implicated as causing autism. Multiple European and Canadian cohort studies have not supported this association, and studies have found that the incidence of autism spectrum disorders continued to increase after discontinuation of thimerosal in vaccines. In a meta-analysis performed by the Institute of Medicine, more than 200 studies on thimerosal and autism were reviewed, but no association was found.

Other environmental factors [12] of interest include prenatal exposure to thalidomide (in the first trimester), valproic acid, rubella infection, and misoprostol.

Clinical Features

The clinical presentation of autism spectrum disorders is heterogeneous and depends upon the age of the patient, severity of symptoms, and associated comorbidities. Despite this variability in presentation, identification of core symptoms as described by DSM continues to be the mainstay of the diagnosis. The following is a brief description of the core symptoms of autism.

Impairment in social skills: Lack of social reciprocity is one of the hallmark features of autism spectrum disorders. This impairment is evident from early infancy; parents usually report their child as "aloof" who does not like to be cuddled or touched. They usually do not imitate the actions of parents, such as clapping hands, saying "bye bye," or playing social games like peek-a-boo. Infants as young as 6 months of age tend to avoid social stimuli and prefer non-social interactions. They tend to show more interest in stationary inanimate objects. Because their attachment with parental figures is impaired, they do not develop stranger anxiety.

A recent study [13] has found nine features that predict the future development of autism and distinguish between ASD and other developmental disorders.

Authors have noted that repetitive movements of objects (e.g., lining up objects, collecting objects) were better able to distinguish between ASD and developmental disorder during early ages than were repetitive movements of the body or social communication problems.

Researchers at CDC and the Interdisciplinary Council on Developmental and Learning Disorders [14] have emphasized the following warning signs in children at risk of developing autism spectrum disorders:

- Failure to respond to sounds during the first 2 months of life
- Failure to initiate reciprocal behavior with parents by 4 months
- Failure to start or initiate interactions with parents at 9 months of age
- Using parents' body parts as an extension of their own body, for example, using their hands to pick up toys

"Impaired joint attention" is another cardinal feature of autism. Joint attention is the phenomenon in which the child attends to the same object in the environment that his parents are attending to. A normal child then shifts his/her gaze from the object to the parent and back to the object and then communicates with gestures and limited verbal skills. This is usually considered a pre-verbal phase of development and is important for language, communication, and social development at 9 months of age.

Impairment in communication: Speech and language development starts earlier in infancy. The first 2–3 years represent the steepest part of the learning curve and neurodevelopment for a child as it develops comprehensive speech and language abilities. Normally, children start babbling randomly around 3–4 months of age and start imitating parent's speech by 10–12 months. By 12 months most children can say 1–2 words and increase their vocabulary to 5–20 words by 18 months of age. Any lag in the above-mentioned sequence constitutes language delays. DSM-IV defines language delays as the "inability to speak a single word by 2 years and communicative phrases by 3 years of age." It should be noted that infants and toddlers with intact cognition and hearing learn receptive language, learn to express patterns of intonation and rhythm and body language, and can be taught to express needs and desires using sign language at an earlier age than when communication by speech begins. Parents also usually learn to interpret their child's babblings sooner than do strangers.

Speech and language abnormalities in autism are dependent upon the severity of the disorder. Deficits range from limited to no speech and language abilities in severely autistic children to minimal abnormalities in articulation and pragmatics (social use of language) in individuals with a mild form of autism. Children who can speak may have deviant language development with pronoun reversal, echolalia, and pedantic speech being some of the examples of this deviance. Others have difficulties with pragmatics or the correct social use of language. They also have difficulty in initiating and sustaining conversations. The quality of their speech is monotonous and sometimes chanting in nature. Because of the concrete nature of their speech and thought process, they have difficulty in understanding proverbs and metaphors which results in a speech that is factual and is limited to the content of the matter.

Ritualistic interests and activities: "Restricted interests" constitute an important feature of autistic disorders. Around 2–5 years of age, children start engaging themselves in some form of ritualistic behavior, but in most of the instances, these are neither fixed nor intense. Autistic children on the other hand engage themselves in behaviors that are intense in nature. They are time consuming and persist for extended periods of time. Some of these behaviors include opening and closing a door multiple times, spinning toys, touching different objects, and watching ceiling fan spinning. Children may have finer and more sophisticated interests including preoccupations with computers, dinosaurs, trains, and Roman mythologies. They spend extensive amounts of time gathering information about their topics of interest. These children usually enjoy these activities, like to talk about them, and feel motivated to continue pursuing these interests. This is in contrast to obsessions of sufferers of obsessive compulsive disorder (OCD) in which individuals complete a ritualistic act in order to avoid or suppress unwanted intrusive thoughts and feelings. Some autistic individuals develop compulsions during the course of their illness for which a specialty referral is usually warranted to differentiate these symptoms from other ritualistic behaviors.

Diagnosis

Early identification and intervention is the key for better long-term outcomes in these children. Several organizations [15–17] including the American Academy of Pediatrics (AAP) and the American Medical Association (AMA) have provided practice parameters and guidelines to assist primary care physicians with this task. For a detailed discussion, the reader is referred to the above-mentioned guidelines.

Broadly, assessment of autistic disorders includes multiple components done by multidisciplinary teams. Some of the components of a thorough assessment are as follows:

Clinical and Developmental History

Core symptoms of autism are easier to elicit in school age children than in infants or preschool children. Studies have found impairments in verbal and non-verbal behaviors along with impairments in symbolic play to be the key features aiding in early diagnosis. Table 7.1 summarizes the observable symptoms and historical information from the core domains that can be elicited in the initial evaluation.

Medical Assessment

Medical examination is meant to rule out any associated medical or genetic disorder that could contribute to the overall psychopathology. Table 7.2 summarizes the important components of medical history and physical examination.

Table 7.1 Psychiatric history and mental status examination

A. Social interactions:
Able to relate with others
Ability to reciprocate affection and love by others
Number of friends and quality of friendships
Eye contact
Ability to understand other's emotions and feelings
Lack of socially appropriate facial expressions

B. Communication:
History of language delays
Ability to communicate with others (because of social ostracism or peer
    rejection, children with autism may not feel the need for interactions with
    others)
Ability to comprehend speech
Difficulties with articulation and pronunciation
Immature use of grammar
Lack of empathy
Problems in social use of language
Echolalia
Pronoun reversals
Pedantic speech (speech that is focused on details, long-winded, one sided and
    in which the individual keeps on talking about his favorite topic irrespective
    of the discussion at hand)

C. Restricted interests and repetitive behaviors:
Hand flapping
Head banging
Rocking
Preoccupation with parts of objects
Restricted interests that are abnormal in frequency and intensity (e.g., a 4-year
    old getting interested in the mechanical functioning of railroad steam
    engines)

Laboratory Tests

History and physical examination help guide clinicians toward specific tests with
the highest yield. Overall, the following tests should be considered: audiology and
vision testing, complete blood count, basic metabolic panel, urine analysis, fasting
lipid and glucose levels, EKG, EEG, chromosomal analysis for karyotyping and
fragile X, and imaging studies including brain MRI, if indicated.

Autism Rating Scales

Numerous rating scales are available to assist in the diagnosis. Table 7.3 summarizes
some commonly used scales.

Clinicians can also consider referring the patient for further specialized testing.
Table 7.4 summarizes some of the assessments that can be ordered.

Table 7.2 Medical history and physical examination

A. Medical history:
Detailed prenatal, birth, and post-natal history of any medical complications
Use of medications during first trimester
Family history of autism, schizophrenia
History of genetic transmission of diseases among family members
History of ear infections
History of generalized viral illness or streptococcal throat infection (for PANDAS)
Chronic gastrointestinal problems (some studies have pointed toward an association between chronic GI infections and development of autism)
Vaccination history and response to vaccinations
Response to pain
History of seizures

B. Physical examination:
Height, weight, and vital signs
Wood's lamp examination for tuberous sclerosis
Crude tests like clapping to test the hearing
Visual acuity
Head circumference (increased head circumference is a nonspecific symptom but was initially pointed out by Kanner and later by others)
Detailed neurological examination to review any localized deficits
Soft neurological signs including fine and gross motor impairment (e.g., clumsiness, which some authors have suggested to be a symptom of Asperger's disorder)

Table 7.3 Autism rating scales

Checklist for Autism in Toddlers (CHAT)	Quick ≤ 5 min screen for children between 18 and 24 months of age. Suitable for primary care offices. Sensitivity ranges from 0.18 to 0.40
Childhood Autism Rating Scale (CARS)	Observer rated 15-item questionnaire for children older than 2 years of age. Sensitivity ranges from 0.92 to 0.98 with a specificity of 0.85
Autism Behavior Checklist (ABC)	57-item questionnaire for children 18 months of age or above. Completed by the parents and carries a sensitivity of 0.38–0.58 with a specificity of 0.76–0.97
Social Communication Questionnaire (SCQ)	40-item questionnaire that is based on the Autism Diagnostic Interview-Revised and is used for children older than 4 years. Cutoff scores of >14 carry a positive predictive value of greater than 90%. Carries a sensitivity of 0.85–0.96 and a specificity of 0.80

Treatment

Behavioral and educational treatments are the mainstay of the management of autistic disorders. Psychopharmacology is important to treat the behavioral problems and comorbid psychiatric disorders.

Despite the fact that DSM-V has simplified the diagnosis, inherent variability and population differences make it necessary to create individual plans for affected individuals. Following is a brief description of some therapeutic modalities.

Table 7.4 Other tests that can be considered

Speech and language testing	Speech and language pathologists screen, diagnose, and treat the speech impairment associated with autistic disorders. They evaluate mechanics of speech, including the syntax (language form), pragmatics (social use of language), and semantics (content of speech). Strengths and weaknesses are noted and a comprehensive plan for speech therapy is complied
Neuropsychological assessment (NPT)	NPT is the mainstay of the assessment of children with autism spectrum disorders. NPT helps identify cognitive and neuropsychiatric deficiencies including impairment in executive functioning, sensorimotor issues, verbal and non-verbal intelligence, and visual–spatial skills. Areas of strength and weakness are delineated to help with the development of a sound educational plan
Educational assessment	Educational assessment usually takes place in the schools. Emphasis is placed on assessing the child's abilities in arithmetic, reading, and writing
Occupational assessment	Occupational assessment is focused on identifying the child's strengths and skills in different domains including self-care, play, and safety. Sensory integration problems are noted and appropriate treatments are instituted

Psycho-educational Interventions

There are three models of psychoeducational interventions:

1. *Treatment and Education of Autistic and Communication Handicapped Children (TEACCH)*: TEACCH is probably the most well-known educational program for children with autism. It was founded by Eric Schopler at the University of North Carolina and is widely used all over the world. This program uses the concept of "culture of autism" that consists of the understandings that autistic children have preference for visual presentation of material, have difficulty with social aspects of communications, tend to prefer a structured routine, have preferred activities, and have problems with attention. This program addresses cognition, communication, perception, and motor skills. This program can be instituted in different settings including self-contained classrooms and at home with the help of therapists, while parents are encouraged to be co-therapists.
2. *The Denver model*: Based on the Piaget's theory of cognitive development, it was first introduced by Sally Rogers at the University of Colorado. This model uses the play-based approach and similar to the TEACCH model builds upon the pre-existing skills of the autistic children. Communication and social skills are the main focus of this model and play is used to gradually develop these skills. Supporting data for these early interventions (children less than 30 months) are still scant and major randomized, controlled trials are still lacking.
3. *Applied behavioral analysis (ABA)*: ABA is considered to have the most established evidence base among the three psycho-educational approaches. Numerous

studies have shown efficacy in improving language, cognitive, and adaptive functioning. The underlying assumption of this strategy is that autistic children have difficulty in learning from their environment. Based upon learning theory, ABA helps the child learn, maintain, and utilize appropriate behaviors in different settings. It provides tools that focus on simple instructions and reinforcements. In ABA, first a maladaptive behavior is identified. Then, a detailed analysis is conducted of the precedents of the behavior, the behavior itself, and its natural consequences. These elements are then targeted and modified to alter the behavior. In ABA, the individual's behaviors are influenced by rewards and negative behaviors are ignored or changed systematically. Later the rewards are removed to promote self-sustenance of the desired behaviors. The rewards/reinforces are then reused to teach a new behavior to the individual.

Miscellaneous Interventions

1. *Social skills training*: Social skills training is mostly provided in school in 30-min-long, twice weekly sessions that include role playing, modeling, and coaching. Children are taught the basic underpinnings of social functioning including proper eye contact, postures, gestures, and rules of engagement in reciprocal conversations.
2. *Occupational therapy*: Occupational therapy focuses on sensory and motor coordination difficulties that autistic individuals present. Therapists encourage the child to participate in games to improve motor coordination.
3. *Support groups*: Family support groups provide a venue to share information, instill hope, assist with advocacy, support problem solving, and improve the parents' psychological well-being. Autism support groups are available in many larger communities and also via the Internet. Some of them include Autism Speaks, Autism Society of America (ASA), Asperger Syndrome and High Functioning Autism Association (AHA), and National Association of Autism (NAA).
4. *Vocational training and rehabilitation*: Vocational rehabilitation programs provide services for autistic and other individuals with disabilities to help them maintain an independent or semi-independent life. Counselors help with finding a job that is appropriate for the individual's interest and capabilities; they also help with placement. They also provide continued support and crisis management to help continue the employment.

Pharmacological Interventions

Autism is associated with numerous psychiatric comorbidities including attention deficit hyperactivity disorder (ADHD), conduct disorder, anxiety and mood disorders, and in rare cases psychosis [18]. These comorbid disorders usually respond well to psychopharmacological management. The following is a brief summary of symptom-focused treatments.

Aggression: Aggression including irritability, impulsivity, and self-injurious behavior is one of the most common reasons for specialty referrals. Despite the fact that medications have proven effective in the management of these behaviors, it is prudent to thoroughly evaluate the individual for underlying medical and non-medical causes that may be contributing to these symptoms. Some of them include conflicts with caretakers, family dysfunction, malnutrition, pain, constipation, dehydration, and urinary tract infections. It is only after this evaluation that a psychopharmacological agent should be considered to target the aggression.

Both typical and atypical antipsychotic agents have proven to be useful in managing these symptoms. Typical antipsychotic medications including haloperidol, chlorpromazine, and thioridazine are relatively safe but have immediate and long-term side effects that outweigh their benefits. In the short term, these medications are more prone to cause sedation, while long-term side effects include tremors, dystonia, and other movement disorders.

Atypical antipsychotic medications are usually preferred at the initiation of treatment. Risperidone and aripiprazole are the only two antipsychotic medications that have been approved by the US Food and Drug Administration (FDA) for the treatment of "irritability" in autistic children. "Irritability" is a broader label under which FDA has also included aggression and temper tantrums. Others medications in this category that are commonly used in clinical practice for this indication include ziprasidone, olanzapine, quetiapine, and clozapine. As a category, these medications can cause metabolic syndromes, so it is recommended to obtain baseline and follow-up height, weight, body mass index (BMI), waist circumference, fasting lipid, and glucose level along with an EKG.

Mood disorders: Mood disorders usually present as increasing irritability, withdrawal, deterioration in functioning, increase in rituals, and regression in different areas. Bipolar disorder has traditionally been difficult to diagnose in autistic children and sometimes their aggression is misleadingly labeled as bipolar disorder. Chronological history of the development of symptoms and a family history of bipolar disorder usually help clarify the diagnosis.

Depressive symptoms usually respond well to selective serotonin reuptake inhibitors (SSRIs) [19]. For varied reasons, these patients are more prone to the side effects including worsening irritability and aggression. Special focus should also be placed on the emergence of hypomanic symptoms that warrant discontinuation of the trial and re-challenge with other SSRI or non-SSRI medications. Treatment of bipolar disorders is usually focused on maintaining the safety of the patient while assessing the severity of manic or hypomanic symptoms. Atypical antipsychotics, lithium carbonate, and sodium valproate are usually the first choices.

Anxiety disorders: These disorders usually present with sudden deterioration in functioning, compulsions, rituals, phobias, and repetitive behaviors. Because of the ego-dystonic nature of these disorders, they are easier to diagnose in autistic individuals with preserved language abilities. SSRI and cognitive behavioral therapy are usually the mainstay of the treatment.

Psychotic disorders (hallucinations, agitation, aggression, delusions): A referral to child and adolescent psychiatry is usually necessary to effectively diagnose a psychotic disorder that is comorbid with autism. Both typical and atypical antipsychotic medications can be used to target these symptoms.

ADHD (hyperactivity, impulsivity, inattention). Hyperactivity and inattentive symptoms are commonly associated with autistic disorder. Behavioral management and stimulant medications are the mainstay of the treatment. Alpha agonists are also commonly used, as some children with autism are unusually sensitive to stimulant medications.

Conclusions

With better understanding of the diagnostic criteria and symptom checklists, diagnosing autism spectrum disorder is far less than a daunting task. Attention should be paid to the associated comorbid disorders and advocating for the child to receive appropriate educational and community services. Some symptoms can be better managed by behavioral interventions than by psychopharmacological management. A good working knowledge of the available services in the community is important to achieve this goal.

Acknowledgments Author gratefully acknowledges the editorial contributions by Dr Michael Liepman in the preparation of this manuscript.

References

1. Kanner L. Autistic disturbances of affective contact. Nerv Child. 1943;2:217–50.
2. Asperger H. Die 'Autistischen Psychopathen' im Kindesalter. Arch Psychiatr Nervenkr. 1944;117:76–136.
3. Wing L. Asperger's syndrome: a clinical account. Psychol Med. 1981;11:115–29.
4. Rutter M. Diagnosis and definition. In: Rutter M, Schopler E, editors. Autism: a reappraisal of concepts and treatment. New York, NY: Plenum Press; 1978.
5. American Psychiatric Association. Diagnostic and statistical manual (DSM-III). 3rd ed. Washington, DC: APA; 1980.
6. American Psychiatric Association. DSM-V development. Washington, DC: APA; 2010.
7. American Psychiatric Association. Diagnostic and statistical manual of mental disorders: DSM-IV-TR. 4th ed. Text revision. Washington, DC: APA; 2000.
8. Fombonne E. Epidemiology of pervasive developmental disorders. Pediatr Res. 2009;65: 591–8.
9. Autism and Developmental Disabilities Monitoring Network Surveillance Year 2006 Principal Investigators. Prevalence of autism spectrum disorders. Autism and Developmental Disabilities Monitoring Network, United States, 2006. MMWR. 2009;58:1–20.
10. Bailey A, Le Couteur A, Gottesman I, Bolton P, Simonoff E, Yuzda E, Rutter M. Autism as a strongly genetic disorder: evidence from a British twin study. Psychol Med. 1995;25:63–77.
11. Kumar RA, Christian SL. Genetics of autism spectrum disorders. Curr Neurol Neurosci Rep. 2009;9:188–97.
12. Landrigan PJ. What causes autism? Exploring the environmental contribution. Curr Opin Pediatr. 2010;22:219–25.

13. Watt N, Wetherby AM, Barber A, Morgan L. Repetitive and stereotyped behaviors in children with autism spectrum disorders in the second year of life. J Autism Dev Disord. 2008;38:1518–33.
14. Center for Disease Control and Prevention: Autism information center. 2010. http://www.cdc.gov/ncbddd/autism/facts.html. Accessed 23 Aug 2010.
15. Autism: Caring for children with Autism spectrum disorders: A resource toolkit for clinicians. Elk Grove Village, IL: Am Acad Pediatr; 2007.
16. American Medical Association. Special issue on autism. Arch Pediatr Adolesc Med. 2007;161:313–424.
17. Volkmar F, Cook EH Jr, Pomeroy J, Realmuto G, Tanguay P. Practice parameters for the assessment and treatment of children, adolescents, and adults with autism and other pervasive developmental disorders. J Am Acad Child Adolesc Psychiatry. 1999;38(12):32S–54S.
18. Ghaziuddin M, Weidmer-Mikhail E, Ghaziuddin N. Comorbidity of Asperger syndrome: A preliminary report. J Intellect Disabil Res. 1998;42:279–83.
19. Stewart ME, Barnard L, Pearson J, Hasan R, O'Brien G. Presentation of depression in autism and Asperger syndrome: a review. Autism. 2006;10:103–16.

Chapter 8
Attention Deficit Hyperactivity Disorder

Donald E. Greydanus

Abstract Attention deficit hyperactivity disorder (ADHD) is a common neurodevelopmental disorder that affects 4–8% of the population across the life span. Up to 90% of those with ADHD have at least one comorbid condition that may be more critical to the child's or adolescent's health than is the ADHD. Those with neurodevelopmental disorders are at high risk for ADHD. Management involves psychological therapy often in conjunction with pharmacologic treatment. Non-drug-related management strategies include appropriate educational placement, parent training, biofeedback, social skills training, support groups, psychotherapy, and/or cognitive–behavioral therapy. The emphasis in this chapter is on the pharmacologic approach that includes psychostimulants, antidepressants, alpha-2 agonists, and a norepinephrine reuptake inhibitor. Management of these patients should emphasize a multimodal approach with careful long-term follow-up by the clinician.

Introduction

It was in the nineteenth century that children were identified with features that are now classified as attention deficit disorder (ADD) or attention deficit hyperactivity disorder (ADHD) [1]. Heinrich Hoffman (1809–1894) was a physician, medical author, and illustrator in the 1800s who wrote about a young boy, Fidgety Phillip (Zappelphilipp), with characteristics of the modern day ADHD child. In the early twentieth century England, this condition was linked to hyperactivity and unruly behavior typically in boys and sometimes involved in the juvenile court system [2]. Between 1916 and 1927 such behavior was said to be due to encephalitis with

D.E. Greydanus (✉)
Department of Pediatrics and Human Development, Kalamazoo Center for Medical Studies, Michigan State University College of Human Medicine, Kalamazoo, MI 49008-1284, USA
e-mail: greydanus@kcms.msu.edu

D.R. Patel et al. (eds.), *Neurodevelopmental Disabilities*,
DOI 10.1007/978-94-007-0627-9_8, © Springer Science+Business Media B.V. 2011

consequent central nervous system injury and called encephalitis lethargica (von Economo's disease) [1].

Others terms for ADHD that were used in the twentieth century include minimum brain damage or dysfunction, hyperactive reaction of childhood, and hyperkinetic syndrome [1, 3, 4]. In 1980 it was called attention deficit disorder (ADD) and attention deficit hyperactivity disorder (ADHD) by the American Psychiatric Association's Diagnostic and Statistical Manual of Mental Disorders (DSM); these terms have continued into the twenty-first century and in this chapter, the term ADHD is used [5]. Management involves psychological and pharmacologic strategies and in 2006, 5 million persons in the United States were prescribed stimulant medication that included 3.5 million for those between 3 and 19 years of age as well as 1.5 million for those between 20 and 64 years of age [6]. This chapter emphasizes the pharmacologic approach to ADHD management in children and adolescents.

Definition

The American Psychiatric Association's Diagnostic and Statistical Manual of Mental Disorders (DSM-IV-TR, 4th ed., 2000) provide a series of detailed criteria for ADHD based on the presence of attention span dysfunction along with varying degrees of impulsivity and hyperactivity (i.e., Fidgety Philip) [5]. This is the criteria used in this chapter, though there are others, such as that used by the International Classification of Diseases, 10th ed. (ICD-10) World Health Organization (1993). The ICD-10 traditionally is used by insurance companies, allows diagnostic flexibility, and utilizes the nomenclature of attention deficit hyperkinetic disorder. Primary care clinicians may use diagnostic criteria based on the American Academy of Pediatrics' Classification of Child and Adolescent Mental Diagnoses in Primary Care: Diagnostic and Statistical Manual for Primary Care (DSM-PC): Child and Adolescent Version [7]. The diagnostic criteria for ADHD used with the DSM-PC are similar to the DSM-IV and are based on the three key elements – attention span dysfunction, hyperactivity, and impulsivity.

Epidemiology

Studies over the past several decades generally declare that 3–9% of children and adolescents meet the DRM-IV criteria for ADHD and as many as 5% of adults also meet these criteria [1, 6–11]. A lower incidence is found by some European authors using the ICD-10 or other criteria; however, using the DSM-IV, prevalence similar to that found in the United States is also noted around the world in all cultures and populations [12].

Diagnosis

As noted, the DSM-IV criteria are used in this chapter. Many decades of research have observed the potentially severe impairment in social skills attainment,

Table 8.1 Prognostic factors in ADHD

A. *Good prognosis*:
1. High intellectual functioning
2. Strong family supports
3. Good friends
4. Accepted by their peers
5. Nurtured by their teachers
B. *Poor prognosis*:
1. Low average to borderline intellectual functioning
2. Minimal family supports
3. Few friends
4. Not accepted by their peers
5. Not nurtured by their teachers
6. Have one or more comorbid psychiatric disorders

academic performance, and behavioral instability in patients with ADHD. Dopaminergic, noradrenergic, and serotonergic pathways are involved in ADHD that induce variable degrees of impairment in patients of all ages. It is a neurobehavioral and neurodevelopmental disorder as demonstrated by modern neuroimaging (i.e., PET scans) and genetic studies [1, 13, 14]. Neurobiologic research is identifying a complex, heterogeneous disorder that involves absence or paucity of connections as well as noradrenergic–dopaminergic dysfunction in various brain regions [15].

There is a 75% heritability that involves at least seven genes: DAT, DBH, 5-HTT, HTR1B, SNAP25, DRD4, and DRD5 [1, 16]. Research on the genetics of ADHD suggests there is broad heterogeneity with different genes having various effects in different families and individuals [17]. Table 8.1 lists favorable and unfavorable prognostic factors in ADHD while Table 8.2 lists the differential diagnosis for ADHD. Though there is no definitive test for ADHD, a comprehensive evaluation includes behavioral, psychological (psychiatric), and neurological testing. Previous evaluations and testing from other physicians, psychologists, and others may be useful. Commonly used ADHD rating scales include Conners Scales (www.mhs. com), ADHD Rating Scale-IV (www.guilford.com), Brown ADD Scales (psych-corp.pearsonassessments.com), CBCL (www.aseba.org), and SKAMP (www.adhd. net) [1].

ADHD Comorbidities

Table 8.3 lists conditions often comorbid with ADHD; approximately 75–90% of children and adolescents with ADHD have comorbid condition (s) including various neurodevelopmental disorders and neurological disorders (i.e., epilepsy, tic disorders) [16, 18–34]. A number of mechanisms may account for such comorbidity including shared noradrenergic system dysregulation and genetic factors. For example, pediatric patients with both ADHD and autism spectrum disorders have severe motor problems and significant impairment in executive control, adaptive

Table 8.2 Differential diagnoses of ADHD

Mental health disorders
Anxiety disorders (generalized anxiety disorder, separation anxiety)
Affective (mood) disorders
Conduct disorder
Impulse-control disorders
Mental retardation
Mood disorders
Oppositional defiant disorder
Pervasive developmental disorders; autism
Psychotic disorders: schizophrenia or other dissociative disorders
Adjustment disorders

Medical disorders
Hyperthyroidism
Early stages of progressive neurodegenerative disorders
Subclinical epilepsy, absence seizures
Frontal lobe tumor or abscess
Fetal alcohol syndrome
Klinefelter syndrome
Angelman syndrome
Velocardiofacial syndrome
Sotos syndrome
Neurobehavioral effects of lead toxicity
Sleep disorders
Obstructive sleep apnea syndrome
Effects of chronic diseases and their drug treatments (e.g., severe asthma, migraine, cancer)

Effects of drugs
Drugs of abuse (e.g., phencyclidine, cocaine, CNS stimulants)
Therapeutic drugs (e.g., phenobarbital, albuterol, corticosteroids, antihistamines)

Effects of environment
Child and adolescent abuse and neglect
Severely dysfunctional family dynamics
Highly gifted student in unchallenging curricular environment
Cognitively challenged student in regular classroom environment

functioning, and social skills [22]. Children with ADHD and parent-reported motor coordination deficits have increased levels of autistic symptoms [21]. The comorbidity may be more significant than the ADHD symptomatology; for example, patients with learning disorders and academic dysfunction may precipitate increased high-risk behavior in adolescents with or without ADHD [32]. The combination of conduct disorder or oppositional defiant disorder with ADHD results in increased high-risk behavior [5].

As noted, there is much overlap between the various comorbidities that include various neurodevelopmental disorders. For example, psychiatric disorders are common in patients with ADHD and also common with patients having autism

Table 8.3   ADHD comorbid disorders

Anxiety disorders
Autism spectrum disorders
Cerebral palsy
Communication disorders
Conduct disorder
Developmental coordination disorder
Epilepsy
Mental retardation
Mood disorders
Motor coordination disorders
Oppositional defiant disorder
Sleep disorders
Specific learning disabilities (including dyslexia)
Substance abuse disorders
Tourette syndrome and other tic disorders
Others

spectrum disorders [23]. Sleep disorders are common in a number of neurodevelopmental disorders. For example, sleep disordered breathing, restless legs syndrome (periodic limb movements of sleep), sleep-onset delay, and increased nocturnal motor activity are common in children with ADHD [24, 34]. Chronic lack of proper sleep that develops a major sleep debt will worsen or stimulate the development of various psychiatric disorders in these patients [24].

Psychiatric disorders may be found in up to 90% of ADHD pediatric patients having ADHD, while 32% have at least two and 11% have three or more psychiatric conditions [35–37]. Depression may arise several years after the diagnosis of ADHD and may in part develop from environmental problems arising from the ADHD that interact with a genetic predisposition for depression [38]. Pharmacologic treatment of ADHD may also reduce the incidence of psychiatric comorbidity in patients with ADHD [39]. Many pediatric patients with ADHD often have oppositional defiant disorder, conduct disorder, and aggressive symptomatology [27, 28, 40]. Academic dysfunction and learning disorders (i.e., dyslexia) are also commonly seen in ADHD patients [29–32].

As further research continues, ADHD may be separated into various types depending on which parts of the brain are primarily involved and which comorbidities are found in a specific patient. Thus, a careful assessment is necessary that includes information from the patient, parents, and the school to assess if the child or adolescent has ADHD and/or a comorbid condition [35, 36, 41]. It is the recommendation of various researchers that the DSM-V should reflect new research on potential sub-types of ADHD that acknowledge the various comorbidities of ADHD with similar neurogenetic qualities and the possible revision of ADHD to reflect a complex neuropsychological family of interrelated syndromes defined by an impressively wide variety of comorbid conditions, disorders, and phenomena [18, 20, 21].

Treatment

Pharmacotherapy

A plethora of management options are available for children and adolescents with ADHD that involve a combination of pharmacologic and non-pharmacologic methods [42]. Table 8.4 lists non-drug measures and the basic caveat here is that educational and psychological needs of the patient should be covered. As noted, ADHD patients often have comorbidities, as reflected in Table 8.3; attention to these comorbidities is an essential part of the overall approach to any patient with ADHD [42]. This child or adolescent should be in the proper school or class placement to help with any additional learning problems. Behavior therapy is important along with others as needed, such as speech therapy, occupational therapy, and/or physical therapy depending on the individual needs of the child or adolescent. Social skills training can be very helpful to many while the research-supported psychological therapy for ADHD is cognitive–behavioral therapy [1, 35–6]. Pediatric patients and their parents should be educated to the need for proper use of stimulants for ADHD and to avoid the unsupervised acquisition of these medications with prescription as available over the Internet [46].

The most respected research at this time evaluating treatment options for children with ADHD was conducted by the US National Institute of Mental Health (NIMN) in a well-known study called the NIMH Collaborative Multisite Multimodal Treatment Study of Children with Attention Deficit/Hyperactivity Disorder, Combined type (or the MTA study). This now classic study looked at 579 children aged 7–9.9 years of age and clearly documented the efficacy of methylphenidate (MPH) for these children as being superior to psychological therapy [47–50]. However, it also verified the efficacy of combining a pharmacologic approach with psychological therapies as well. It is the recommendation of the editors of this book and the author of this chapter that a combined and individualized approach be used for each child and adolescent with ADHD. This chapter now focuses on medications used to manage ADHD in children and youth.

Table 8.4 Non-pharmacologic management of ADHD in ADHD patients

Proper academic placement and nurturance
Psychotherapy
Cognitive–behavioral therapy (CBT)
Behavioral therapy (BT)
Psychosocial interventions:
• Support groups
• Social skills training
• Biofeedback training
• Peer mediation to resolve interpersonal conflicts
• Family therapy
• Self-management training

Stimulants

Evidence of the benefit of stimulants on children with attention span dysfunction dates back to classic studies by Bradley in 1937 on Benzedrine and Knobel in 1959 on methylphenidate [51, 52]. There are hundreds of studies that have followed these groundbreaking works that note stimulants are helpful for children, adolescents, and adults with ADHD [53–57]. Stimulants include methylphenidate and amphetamine products and they are approved by the US Food and Drug Administration (FDA) for ADHD treatment in children, adolescents, and adults. Principles of psychopharmacologic management are outlined in Table 8.5. Research has suggested that approximately three out of four ADHD patients will note benefit from stimulants and thus methylphenidates or amphetamines have become a cornerstone in drug management of this condition. Other drug classes are also beneficial, including antidepressants, alpha-2 agonists, and norepinephrine reuptake inhibitors.

Table 8.5 Principles of psychopharmacologic management for ADHD

1. Educate the patient and parents ("family") about the purpose of these medications; clarify the goals of medications (improving concentration, decreasing impulsivity, others). The clinician should avoid focusing only on medication in the clinical encounter, which implies to families that medication use alone should be the remedy to all problems. It further implies that when things are not going well, the problem must be with the choice or dose of medication. This shifts responsibility for problems completely to the clinician who must then urgently find the right medication
2. Be sure the patient and parents understand that medications are not curative
3. Correct any "myths" about medication the family may have. For example, medication will not correct family problems (i.e., alcoholism in a parent, contentious custody battles)
4. Wait for the patient/family to approve of a trial medication period before embarking on medication management. Do not force medication on a child or adolescent
5. Educate the patient/family about potential side effects of medications and how you will deal with them; follow these patients on a regular basis to monitor efficacy and adverse effects
6. Provide a thorough evaluation of the patient and family to determine possible comorbidities that may benefit from other medications
7. Be supportive of other management tools (i.e., psychoeducation strategies, behavioral therapy)
8. Begin with a low dose and increase slowly until identified target symptoms are sufficiently improved; stop the medication(s) if side effects are unacceptable or upper medication levels are reached without amelioration of target symptoms
9. Specific medications and doses may vary from patient to patient and are identified by careful trial and error. Medication(s) that are helpful may change as the child emerges to adolescence and adulthood
10. Adolescents may require a medication dose higher than needed for adults because of increased renal clearance of drugs, lower body fat percentage, increased liver metabolism, or idiosyncratic medication metabolism
11. Strive to achieve complete syndrome remission if feasible (rather than settling for symptom improvement)
12. Share responsibility explicitly by clearly stating what issues the family must work on, the school must work on, the child or adolescent must work on, and the physician must work on

Source: Modified with permission from Greydanus and Pratt et al. [117].

Current medical treatment of ADHD focuses on attenuation of dopamine and norepinephrine neurotransmission and the future of research in pharmacologic management includes identifying the specific actions of each of these medications to better match specific ADHD patients' genotypes with specific pharmacologic interventions [58]. Though there are no long-term studies establishing the safety profile for long-term use of anti-ADHD medications, such as psychostimulants, there is no evidence that predicts a negative safety record nor is there clear evidence of long-term efficacy [59].

Methylphenidate Products

Methylphenidate (MPH) is the most commonly prescribed stimulant used for patients of all ages with ADHD after its market introduction in 1957 in the United States. It is a non-amphetamine sympathomimetic chemical that has mild central nervous system stimulant effects because of brain stimulation and cortical arousal system activation [60, 61]. The reason it is so popular for ADHD is its ability to improve attention span dysfunction in varying degrees in different patients and this is due to selective binding of the presynaptic dopamine transporter in the CNS prefrontal and striatal regions that in turn induces an increase in extracellular dopamine. In addition, there is blockade of the norepinephrine transporter in the CNS norepinephrine system.

In those with ADHD, including patients with neurodevelopmental disorders, this pharmacologic action results in improved attention span with enhanced concentration; in addition, there may be varying degrees of less hyperarousal, less motor restlessness that includes reduced gross as well as fine motor movement and reduced impulsivity; there may even be lowered aggressive behavior and perhaps an improvement in antisocial behavior. A number of assessment instruments have been developed to assist in measurement of drug benefit and these include patient/parent interviews, ratings of parents or guardians, and reports of school teachers (including grades and written documents) [62]. Table 8.6 lists reasons for failure of stimulants to be effective in patients with ADHD. Current research is looking at the effect of comorbidities on the response of patients with ADHD to stimulants, as for example, those with ADHD and disruptive disorders (opposition defiant disorder or conduct disorder) responding well versus a poor response in those with ADHD and anxiety disorders [63]. Successful utilization of stimulants for adolescents with ADHD may reduce subsequent development of psychiatric disorders and academic failure [39].

A number of short-acting (immediate-release) MPH products are available as well as an increasing number of longer acting MPH preparations that have been developed over the past two decades (see Table 8.7). In all these products there is no correlation between the patient's weight and the optimal medication dose; in addition, MPH plasma levels are not helpful and not clinically used to monitor drug effects. There is no unbiased research that is currently available to guide clinicians in which of these products are best [64, 65]. They all contain MPH and this

Table 8.6 Reasons for failure of methylphenidate or amphetamines

- Inaccurate diagnosis
- Comorbid disorders that overshadow the ADHD
- Medication doses that are too high or not high enough
- Medication is diverted to others in or outside the family
- Intolerable medication side effects
- Medication is used as a drug of abuse for its euphoric effects
- Patient and/or family not accepting of medication
- Patient does not respond to MPH but does to other stimulants or alternative medications
- Patient does not respond to medications of any kind

Source: Modified with permission from Greydanus and Pratt et al. [118].

is the chemical that produces the potentially positive effects. Thus, a trial and error technique is used often based on personal clinician preference as well as insurance acceptability.

The MPH patch may be useful to give ADHD patients more control over the stimulant dosing by having the patient potentially choose when to remove the patch [66]. If the patient has problems swallowing pills (tablets or capsules), some of the longer acting products (Ritalin-LA, Metadate-CD, Focalin-SR, Adderall-XR) can be opened and then placed (sprinkled) on foods [66]. Some researchers conclude that there is better compliance with longer acting (extended-release) stimulants versus short-acting stimulants [67]. For example, studies note that at least half of adolescents prescribed stimulants are not compliant, though long-acting medications may improve adherence in these youth [15].

Amphetamine Products

Amphetamine is a non-catecholamine, sympathomimetic amine with CNS stimulant action resulting in dopamine and norepinephrine reuptake blockade into presynaptic neurons; there is also heightened release of these neurotransmitters into the synaptic cleft in the CNS. This chemical is classically produced as dextroamphetamine sulfate (the dextro isomer of D,L-amphetamine sulfate) or as mixed amphetamine salts. Table 8.8 lists currently available amphetamine products that can be short acting or long acting.

Vyvanse (lisdexamfetamine) is a long-acting formulation of dextroamphetamine that has been available since 2007 [66, 68–72]. Lisdexamfetamine dimesylate is an inactive, water-soluble prodrug in which D-amphetamine is bonded to L-lysine and after oral ingestion, it is metabolized into L-lysine and active D-amphetamine [70]. Lisdexamfetamine dimesylate is marketed as a product difficult to alter as a drug of abuse and it may lower the risk of ADHD patients abusing their medication [68]. However, as noted with other long-acting stimulants, its actual advantage or differentiation over other available long-acting products remains unclear [72]. Potential side effects of both stimulants (MPH or amphetamines) are noted in Table 8.9.

Table 8.7 Methylphenidate preparations

| Brand name (in United States) | Dosage form | Dosing regimen | | Maximum per day | Duration of effect in hours |
		Start	Titrate weekly		
Active ingredient: d,l-methylphenidate					
Ritalin; generic form available	Scored tablets: 5, 10, 20 mg	5 mg 2–3 times/day; 1 dose before breakfast, 1 before lunch	5–10 mg; give a third dose in the afternoon if needed	Not to exceed 20 mg/dose; 60 mg/day	3–4
Methylin	Scored tablets: 5, 10, 20 mg; chewable tablets: 2.5, 5, 10 mg; oral solution: 5 mg/ml, 10 mg/10 ml	5 mg 2–3 times/day; 1 dose before breakfast, 1 before lunch	5–10 mg; Give a third dose in the afternoon if needed	Not to exceed 20 mg/dose; 60 mg/day	4–8
Ritalin SR	Sustained release tablets: 20 mg	20 mg before breakfast	20 mg; Give a second dose in afternoon if needed; for desired dose and duration, short-acting form may be used	60 mg	6–8
Metadate ER	Extended-release tablets: 10, 20 mg	10 mg before breakfast	10 mg; give a second dose in afternoon if needed	60 mg	4–8
Methylin ER	Extended-release tablets: 10, 20 mg	10 mg before breakfast	10 mg; give a second dose in afternoon if needed	60 mg	4–8

Table 8.7 (continued)

Brand name (in United States)	Dosage form	Dosing regimen		Maximum per day	Duration of effect in hours
		Start	Titrate weekly		
Metadate-CD	Extended-release capsules: 10, 20, 30 mg. Can be sprinkled	20 mg before breakfast	20 mg; give a second dose in the afternoon if needed	60 mg	4–8
Ritalin-LA	Long-acting capsules: 10, 20, 30, 40 mg; can be sprinkled	10 mg before breakfast	5–10 mg; Use short-acting form (Ritalin) to titrate if needed	60 mg	4–8
Concerta	Capsules: 18, 27, 36, 54 mg; do not split or chew or crush	18 mg before breakfast	18 mg	72 mg	8–12
Daytrana	Transdermal patch: 10,15,20,30 mg	10 mg patch applied 2 h before desired effect; remove 9 h later	10 mg	30 mg	12
Active ingredient: d, methylphenidate					
Focalin	Scored tablets: 2.5, 5, 10 mg	2.5 mg 1–2 times a day	2.5 mg; give a third dose in afternoon if needed	30 mg	4–5
Focalin XR	Extended-release capsules: 5, 10 mg; can be sprinkled	5 mg before breakfast	5 mg; give a second dose in afternoon if needed; for desired dose and duration short-acting form (Focalin) may be used	30 mg	8–12

Table 8.8 Amphetamine preparations

Brand name (in United States)	Dosage form	Dosing regimen		Maximum per day	Duration of effect (h)
		Start	Titrate weekly		
Active ingredient: dextroamphetamine					
Dexedrine	Tablets: 5 mg	5 mg 1–2 times/day	5 mg	40 mg	4–6
Generic form available					
Dextrostat	Scored tablets: 5, 10 mg	2.5–5 mg 1–2 times/day	5 mg	40 mg	4–6
Generic form	Extended-release capsules: 5, 10, 20 mg	5 mg 1–2 times/day	5 mg	40 mg	4–6
Dexedrine Spansule	Spansules: 5,10,15 mg; can be sprinkled	5 mg before breakfast	5 mg	45 mg	6–10
Vyvanse (lisdexamfetamine)	Capsules: 20, 30 mg, 40 mg, 50 mg, 60 mg, 70 mg	30 mg once day	10–20 mg	70 mg	12 h
Active ingredient: mixed salts of amphetamine (dextroamphetamine plus levoamphetamine)					
Adderall	Tablets: 5, 7.5, 10, 12.5, 15, 20, 30 mg	5–10 mg 1–2 times per day; 1 dose before breakfast, second before lunch	5–10 mg	40 mg	4–6
Generic form available					
Adderall XR	Extended-release capsules: 5, 10, 15, 20, 25, 30 mg; can be sprinkled	5–10 mg before breakfast	5–10 mg	30 mg	8–12

Table 8.9   Potential side effects of stimulant drugs

Headache[a]
Nausea/vomiting[a]
Anorexia[a]
Insomnia (delayed onset of sleep)

Weight loss[a]
Moodiness (irritability)

Tachycardia
Palpitations
Sudden cardiac death
Increase in blood pressure
"Unmasking" of Tourette Syndrome
Rebound phenomenon

Reduced seizure threshold
Irritability/restlessness
Emotional lability
Appearance of psychosis or psychotic features

Growth retardation (at higher doses, over longer times, in those with short
    stature or slow axial growth)
Skin rash (rare)

---

[a]Commonly seen side effects.
Source: Modified with permission from Greydanus and Pratt et al. [119].

Contraindications for Stimulant Use

Contraindications for use of stimulants (i.e., methylphenidate or amphetamines) include sensitivity or allergy to either medication, glaucoma, psychosis, hyperthyroidism, drug (including alcohol) dependence, psychomotor agitation, or high levels of anxiety or inner tension. Monoamine oxidase inhibitors (MAOs) should not be used concomitantly with stimulants because this may lead to a severe hypertensive development; thus, one should allow 2 weeks to pass after stopping MAOs and starting stimulants.

There are rare reports of sudden death of pediatric and adult patients on stimulants, some of which seem to be due to underlying cardiovascular conditions; thus, stimulants are avoided in those patients with significant structural heart conditions, symptomatic heart disorders (i.e., angina or heart failure as noted mainly in adults), significant cardiac arrhythmias, and poorly controlled hypertension [73–77]. Based on rare but well-known reports of significant cardiovascular side effects in children, adolescents, and adults on stimulants, United States Food and Drug Administration has required the placement of a strong warning on stimulant labels that alert clinicians and patients to this possibility. An electrocardiogram is not necessary before placing a child or an adolescent on stimulants for ADHD [78]. However, patients should receive a careful cardiovascular screening before stimulant prescription occurs for ADHD; Table 8.10 lists important components to such screening.

Table 8.10 Cardiovascular screening for stimulant prescription

Personal history
Exertional chest pain
Shortness of breath
Presyncope
Syncope
Dizziness
Palpitations
Fatigue
Recent febrile illness
Congenital heart disease
Heart murmur
Hypertension
Lipid disorder or abnormalities

Past history
Kawasaki's disease
Rheumatic fever

Family history
Marfan syndrome
Cardiomyopathy
Long QT syndrome
Premature cardiac death (before age 50)
Hypertension
Lipid disorders

Cardiovascular exam
Heart rate; blood pressure; delayed femoral arterial pulses (coarctation of aorta)
Systolic ejection murmur that intensifies with standing or Valsalva maneuver and diminishes
    with squatting (hypertrophic cardiomyopathy)
Decrescendo diastolic murmur of aortic valve insufficiency (may be present in Marfan
    syndrome)
Holosystolic murmur of mitral valve insufficiency (may be present in Marfan syndrome)
Systolic ejection murmur or midsystolic clicks (mitral valve prolapse)

A history of Tourette syndrome, other chronic motor tic disorder, or epilepsy represents a relative contraindication to stimulant use. Children and adolescents with developmental disorders, ADHD, and well-controlled epilepsy may be carefully placed on stimulants if there are no stimulant contraindications, such as concomitant psychosis. Approximately 20% of children with epilepsy have ADHD and having ADHD increases risks for seizures; this bidirectional relationship may be due to shared underlying neurodevelopmental mechanisms, common genetic defects, effects of chronic seizures, and effects of antiepileptic medications leading to sleep problems or inattention [25, 79, 80].

Screening patients with ADHD who have no clinical evidence of epilepsy with an electroencephalogram (EEG) before starting stimulants is not recommended [79]. However, EEGs may be useful to distinguish between inattention due to epilepsy (i.e., absence or partial complex seizures) and inattention due to other factors, such as ADHD [81]. Some anti-seizure medications have ADHD-like side effects, including topiramate, phenobarbital, vigabatrin, and gabapentin [80]. Some anticonvulsants have beneficial anti-ADHD effects and these include carbamazepine and lamotrigine [81]. Methylphenidate appears safe for those with controlled epilepsy and clinicians should be aware of anecdotal reports of worsening of seizures in children with uncontrolled epilepsy placed on MPH [79, 81].

There are anecdotal reports of sudden deaths from lethal cardiac arrhythmias in patients placed on both tricyclic antidepressants (TCAs) and stimulants [82–83]. Drugs that inhibit cytochrome P450 2D6 isoenzyme (i.e., paroxetine and quinidine) may heighten MPH effects, while MPH can also interfere with the metabolism of some antiepileptic medications, including phenobarbital and phenytoin.

Stimulant Side Effects

Potential adverse effects of stimulants are listed in Table 8.9. A number of these side effects are transient and may be abetted by using a "start low and go slow" prescription pattern in which one starts with a low dose and gradually raises the dose seeking optimal efficacy with minimal adverse effects that are tolerable to the child or adolescent. Nausea and emesis associated with stimulant use may be relieved by taking the medication with meals. Dizziness is typically worse with short-acting versus long-acting stimulants; also, if dizziness occurs, correct for any associated dehydration and observe for blood pressure alterations. Stimulant-associated headaches may be noted at peak plasma levels or at times of medication withdrawal; switching to another formulation may be beneficial in such cases.

Research in general notes that use of stimulants does not increase the adolescent's risk for development of drug dependence on various illicit drugs; however, this may develop anyway in some patients and there is a high comorbidity of substance abuse disorders and ADHD [83]. Prescription of psychostimulants should be provided only with great care for youth with ADHD and comorbid substance abuse disorder; in this situation, longer acting stimulant formations seem to be less preferred by those with drug dependency than short-acting stimulants [84, 85].

Most children grow normally on stimulants though controversy in this regard has raged for many years [86]. Some growth delay may be due to reduced food intake due to the anorexia side effect noted with stimulants, though most will attain their genetically directed ultimate adult height. Thus, height should be carefully followed in growing children and one should remember that some children may have ADHD as well as a primary growth disorder. Children and adolescents who are not growing well and do not have a primary growth condition may benefit from taking them off stimulants for a period of time (i.e., during the summer or on weekends), providing extra calories (high calorie or fortified supplements) as the medication wears off (i.e., in the evening), and/or using other non-stimulant, anti-ADHD medications (vide infra).

Tolerance is a well-known phenomenon that may arise with use of stimulant and typically can be seen in those on high-stimulant doses or who chronically abuse these medications. If tolerance is noted, carefully taper off the specific stimulant and try another anti-ADHD drug. Rebound is another phenomenon in which heightened

ADHD symptoms are noted as the stimulant wears off; these symptoms include sadness, excitability, or irritability. If rebound occurs, try using a lower dose of immediate-release stimulant in the afternoon or prescribed a sustained-released formulation. Insomnia is a common feature in many with ADHD and also with some developmental disorders in which there is a reciprocal relationship between many neurodevelopmenal disorders and comorbid sleep disorders.

Thus, provide a thorough evaluation for sleep problems in these children or adolescents and treat any primary or secondary problems that may arise; see Chapter 11 on Sleep Disorders in this text [24, 34]. Sometimes the insomnia will improve over time if other insomniac causes are not present. Additional measures that can be considered including giving the last stimulant dose earlier in the day, reducing the amount of the last dose, or use a long-acting product in the morning only.

One should remember that most currently available long-acting stimulants exert effects for up to 12 h or more [71]. Depending what other conditions are found, judicial prescription of additional medication at night with sedative properties may be useful; these drugs include melatonin (3–6 mg at bedtime [HS]), clonidine (0.1–0.4 mg HS), trazodone (25–50 mg HS), and mirtazepine (7.5–15 mg HS) [87]. Resent research suggests that the combination of melatonin or extended-release guanfacine (see later in this chapter) with stimulants appears to be safe and potential effective in promoting sedation [61].

Studies note that half to three-quarters of patients with ADHD also have Tourette syndrome (TS) and sometimes the tics manifest after starting stimulant medications to manage the ADHD [88, 89]. There is no evidence that stimulants cause the TS and as noted before, the presence of tic or a tic disorder is a relative contraindication to use of stimulants for ADHD [90]. If both tics and ADHD are present, the stimulants may be continued if effective and anti-tic drugs may be added, such as risperidone, pimozide, or haloperidol (see Chapter 16 on Tic Disorders in this text). It should be noted that it is the ADHD and not tics themselves that cause the main cognitive and executive dysfunction; thus, it is important to treat the ADHD [91]. However, if it is concluded that the stimulants are significantly worsening the tics, stop the stimulant, and add other anti-ADHD medications that do not normally worsen tics, such as alpha-2 agonists (i.e., clonidine or guanfacine) or atomoxetine [92]. Avoid bupropion, since this medication may improve ADHD but worsen tics. Supratherapeutic doses of dextroamphetamine may also worsen tics and should be avoided [92].

Monitoring Patients on Stimulants

There is no research regarding long-term use of stimulants, though there is none to suggest this practice is harmful and is accepted practice if the medication continues to be helpful. Those on stimulants should have monitoring of blood pressure and pulse at each visit, since these are often mildly increased when on stimulants. Height and weight should be carefully monitored as well. Those on long-term stimulant use also should have a periodic complete blood count that includes a differential and platelet count.

Non-stimulant Medications

Atomoxetine

Atomoxetine is a selective norepinephrine reuptake inhibitor that blockades the presynpatic norepinephrine and dopamine transporter in the prefrontal cortex [93–96]. It may be selected for those not tolerating or wanting a stimulant medication for ADHD and also for those where stimulants are not effective as well as for those with prominent anxiety symptoms. Atomoxetine is a long-acting medication with anti-ADHD effects of 18–24 h and is an FDA-approved drug, non-stimulant drug for ADHD that may take 2–8 weeks for full anti-ADHD benefit [61, 97, 98]. Research suggests that atomoxetine has a less therapeutic effect on ADHD than stimulants [98]. However, it may be beneficial for pediatric patients with ADHD and comorbid depression [38]. There is no evidence it is harmful for patients with ADHD and epilepsy [81].

Atomoxetine can be prescribed for oral use in various capsule dosages: 10, 18, 25, 40, 60, 80, and 100 mg. The initial dose for a patient weighing 70 kg or less is 0.5 mg/kg/day that can be increased every 3 days as tolerated to 1.2 mg/kg/day in single or twice daily schedule. Recommended maximum dosage is 1.4 mg/kg/day or 100 mg/day. If the patient weighs over 70 kg, an initial dose of 40 mg/day is suggested that is titrated up to 80 mg/day (single to over two doses) not to exceed 100 mg/day.

There is no increase in tic, cardiovascular complications, drug diversion, or drug addiction for those taking atomoxetine [92, 99]. However, a number of potential side effects are noted, as listed in Table 8.11. Since there is a heightened risk for mydriasis, it should be not prescribed for patients with narrow-angle glaucoma. Children and adolescents who are on atomoxetine should be monitored for increased

Table 8.11 Atomoxetine side effects

Anorexia
Constipation
Dry mouth
Nausea
Emesis
Sedation
Fatigue
Headache
Dizziness
Mood swings
Suicidal ideations
Aggressive behavior
Dyspepsia
Stomach
Growth delay
Tachycardia
Hepatotoxicity

risks for suicidality since this medication has a US FDA Black Box warning that is similar to that found with antidepressants and other medications. There is also a warning regarding potential hepatotoxicity and thus baseline and periodic liver function testing are necessary for those taking atomoxetine. Drug–drug interactions can occur with inhibitors of the cytochrome P450, 2D6 isoenzyme, including selective serotonin reuptake inhibitors.

Alpha-2 Agonists

Clonidine

Clonidine is a presynaptic, central-acting non-stimulant that is popular with some clinicians for ADHD management. It is an alpha2-adrenergic agonist that stimulates alpha2-adrenoreceptors in the brainstem and induces a reduction in central nervous system outflow. It may take 4–6 weeks for full effect and its recommended use includes ADHD, Tourette's disorder, post-traumatic stress disorder, and severe aggressiveness seen with oppositional defiant disorder or conduct disorder [100]. In those with ADHD it is typically used as an alternative or adjunctive MPH medication; if used with MPH medication, it may be used to treat the insomnia often seen with stimulants. A long-acting clonidine formulation is undergoing current research trials [61].

Clonidine is made in tablet (0.1, 0.2, and 0.3 mg) and transdermal patch (same doses). Careful titration is needed for building up and stopping this medication and the dosage range is usually 0.1–0.3 mg/day with a maximum of 0.4 mg/day. It is given 2–3 times a day or if used for sedation, all at night. Avoid sudden cessation since this may lead to severe rebound hypertension, cerebrovascular accidents, and even sudden death.

Table 8.12 provides a list of possible clonidine adverse effects. Patients taking clonidine should be observed for hypotension and rebound hypertension. It should not be used in those with structural cardiac conditions and there are rare, unexplained reports of sudden death in children and adolescents on both clonidine and MPH [1]. Cardiovascular screening is recommended before staring clonidine as noted with MPH (see Table 8.10) and one should obtain an electrocardiogram prior to prescription.

The patch formulation provides clonidine effects over several days and may result in less sedation than noted with the oral form, thus potentially improving compliance with some patients. Dermatitis may occur as noted with any patch formulation; if dermatitis develops, local application of hydrocortisone and changing the patch site are usually effective. Stop the patch formulation if severe skin reactions occur; in such cases, do not then try oral clonidine since this may lead to a generalized dermatological reaction such as angioedema or acute urticaria.

Guanfacine

Guanfacine is related to clonidine and is an alpha2A-adrenergic agonist used in short- and long-acting forms to treat patients with ADHD [100]. One advantage of

Table 8.12 Side effects of clonidine

Sedation (50%)
Dry mouth
Headache
Nausea/vomiting
Constipation
Depression
Contact dermatitis (patch)
Erythema (patch)
Sexual dysfunction
Dizziness
Dysphoria
Fatigue/lethargy
Postural hypotension
Reduction in heart rate
Rebound phenomenon
Withdrawal effects (rebound tachycardia, severe hypertension, heart failure from sudden clonidine cessation)

Source: Modified with permission from Greydanus and Pratt et al. [120].

the short-acting form is that there is less blood pressure morbidity and less sedation than noted with clonidine. In general, side effects are similar to that seen with clonidine, though more agitation and headaches are noted with the short-acting formulation. Daily dosage range of the short-acting form is 0.5–4.0 mg.

An extended formulation for guanfacine (Guanfacine XR) was approved by the FDA in 2009 for management of those 6–17 years of age with ADHD. Research has noted benefit with regard to hyperactivity as well as inattention dysfunction [57, 101–104]. The addition of this medication to the pharmacopoeia allows one to choose from two FDA-approved, non-stimulant, anti-ADHD medications – guanfacine XR and atomoxetine. The potential adverse effects of guanfacine XR include sedation (most common), lowering (usually mild) of blood pressure as well as pulse, dry mouth, constipation, dizziness, and abdominal pain. It should be remembered that rebound hypertension is well known with immediate-release alpha-2 agents. It can lead to some cardiovascular changes (mild heart rate and blood pressure reduction); thus, vital signs should be monitored and it should be avoided in patients with significant cardiovascular disease [102].

Guanfacine XR is produced in 1-, 2-, 3-, and 4-mg tablets and it is started at 1 mg, with increase of 1 mg/week up to a maximum of 4 mg; it should not be substituted on a milligram per milligram basis with immediate-release guanfacine [102]. It should be swallowed whole and not crushed. Its therapeutic effects are 8–14 h and up to 24 h in some pediatric patients [61]. Common side effects are as noted with short-acting guanfacine and usually resolve with continued use [103].

Tricyclic Antidepressants

Table 8.13 lists indications for use of tricyclic antidepressants (TCAs). Decades of research have revealed the beneficial effects of tricyclic antidepressants (TCAs) in

Table 8.13 Indications for tricyclic antidepressants

ADHD
Aggression disorders
Anxiety disorders (as panic disorder or obsessive compulsive disorder)
Depression
Enuresis
Insomnia
Migraine prophylaxis
Tourette syndrome
Neuropathy

Table 8.14 Tricyclic antidepressant side effects

Blurred vision
Confusion
Constipation
Nausea/vomiting
Dizziness
Drowsiness and sedation

Dry mouth
ECG changes
Cardiac arrhythmias
Syndrome of inappropriate antidiuretic hormone secretion
Orthostatic hypotension
Decrease in seizure threshold

Skin rash
Sudden death
Tachycardia
Tremor
Restlessness
Urinary retention
Weight gain
Suicidal ideations
Sexual dysfunction

Source: Modified with permission from Greydanus and Pratt et al. [121].

some children and adolescents with ADHD and that TCAs can be considered as alternative psychopharmacotherapy in situations when stimulants are not working or are contraindicated [97]. TCAs may be best for some with ADHD who have comorbid prominent anxiety and addictive personalities.

Pharmacologically TCAs block reuptake of serotonin and norepinephrine into the presynaptic neurons; this blockage occurs to varying degrees that also results in considerable antihistaminic and anticholinergic effects. See Table 8.14 for a list of potential TCA side effects. TCAs prescribed for ADHD include imipramine (2–5 mg/kg/day or 50–200 mg/day), nortriptyline (1–3 mg/kg/day or 20–100 mg/day), and amitriptyline (1–1.5 mg/kg/day or 50–200 mg/day).

TCA Monitoring

Start the TCA at night (bedtime) with a low dose and then very slowly titrate the dosage with careful monitoring to achieve the best efficacy and minimal side effect ratio. Obtain a baseline electrocardiogram (ECG) and repeat ECG with each increase in dose to look for cardiac arrhythmias; watch for changes in the PR interval (not to exceed 0.21 ms), QRS interval (not to exceed over 30% of its base [not over 120 ms]), and QTc (QTc not to exceed over 0.460 ms).

Serum levels of TCAs are needed to keep acceptable therapeutic levels and these are reviewed in Table 8.15. These levels are general guidelines and efficacy may not occur in these ranges while toxicity may arise in a so-called safe or therapeutic range. As noted with other antidepressants, patients placed on TCAs must be screened for suicidality since they have the US FDA black box warning in this regard. If gynecomastia or menstrual abnormalities develop on TCAs, obtain a serum prolactin level. Check liver function tests if unexplained gastrointestinal symptoms are present.

Sedation can be severe with TCAs and is typically worse with imipramine than with nortriptyline or amitriptyline. Less rebound is noted with TCAs than with stimulants. Additional adverse effects of TCAs include blurred vision, dry mouth, diarrhea, constipation, urination difficulty, hyperprolactinemia, and blood sugar changes (hyper- or hypoglycemia). Tremor induced by a TCA may be improved by carefully lowering the dose and/or adding propranolol (10–40 mg/day). If agitation develops on the TCA, lower the dose or switch to an alternative drug. It the patient has latent bipolar disease, mania may develop and if latent schizophrenia is present, then psychosis may occur when adding a TCA.

If a TCA is withdrawn suddenly, a constellation of symptoms may arise leading to a discontinuation syndrome with nausea, emesis, fatigue, and worsening behavior. Use TCAs very cautiously in those with epilepsy since the seizure threshold can be lowered. Most antidepressants (except for mirtazapine and bupropion) can lead to hyponatremia and/or syndrome of inappropriate secretion of antidiuretic hormone (SIADH). TCAs should also be prescribed cautiously in those with a history of cardiovascular disease, anorexia, narrow-angle glaucoma, hyperthyroidism, or patients receiving thyroid supplementation. Metabolism of TCAs is with the cytochrome P450 system and thus one must be careful when adding additional medications. In this regard, adding MPH to a TCA may lead to increasing levels of the TCA while

Table 8.15 Tricyclic antidepressant therapeutic levels[a]

Amitriptyline (AMI)	120–150 ng/ml
Nortriptyline (NOR)	50–150 ng/ml
AMI and NOR	120–250 ng/ml
Imipramine (IMI)	150–300 ng/ml
Desipramine (DES)	150–300 ng/ml
IMI and DES	125–225 ng/ml

[a]Levels established for adults in management of depression.

adding a TCA with a selective serotonin reuptake inhibitor (SSRI) can lead to toxic TCA levels. Avoid using TCAs with monoamine oxidase inhibitors (MOAs) or with medications that prolong the QTc interval.

Dose-related cardiovascular effects of TCAs range from mild rise in heart rate and variable hypotension to cardiac arrhythmias, including heart block. Rare cases of sudden death in pediatric patients on TCAs are reported; the use of desipramine in children has lead to some cardiac deaths and it is not recommended, even though it seems to be one of the most beneficial TCAs for ADHD [36, 82–83]. Providing a TCA to an adolescent must be done with caution in light of death that may result from an overdose. Combining alcohol and TCAs can result in respiratory depression and death. The cardiovascular toxicity profile and the death from an overdose potential have resulted in TCAs now infrequently used for ADHD management.

Bupropion

Bupropion is an antidepressant that has been noted to improve attention span dysfunction by inhibition of norepinephrine and dopamine reuptake into the presynaptic neuron [105, 106]. It is often considered as a second-line agent in ADHD management and used to treat some conditions that are comorbid with ADHD [15, 38, 57, 83, 107–109]. For example, long-acting bupropion may also be useful for management of adolescents with substance abuse who have comorbid mood disorders and ADHD [110]. It is manufactured as immediate-release tablets (75 and 100 mg), sustained release tablets (100, 150, and 200 mg), and as extended-release tablets (150 and 300 mg). The daily dosage range for bupropion is 50–300 mg (3.0–6.0 mg/kg/day) of the immediate-release form; it is also used in a range of 100–150 mg twice daily as the sustained release form and 150 mg or 300 mg once daily with the extended-release form.

The noradrenergic/dopaminergic effects of bupropion can lower seizure threshold and also lead to tremors, weight loss, anxiety, agitation, and insomnia (see Table 8.16 for a list of potential bupropion side effects). The risk for seizures is 0.1% under 300 mg a day and 0.4% over 300 mg a day; the risk is dose dependent and is noted over 150 mg of the immediate-release formulation or over 6 mg/kg/day. Bupropion is avoided thus not only in those with seizures but also in patients with a history of head trauma and anorexia nervosa as well as bulimia nervosa, those withdrawing from a CNS depressant, and patients taking medication that lower the seizure threshold [81]. It carries the US FDA black box warning on suicidality and thus patients on this drug should be monitored for the development of suicidal ideations. The metabolism of bupropion is via the cytochrome P450 system and it can interact with various other drugs that affect the 2B6 isoenzyme, including sertraline, paroxetine, and desipramine. Bupropion should not be taken along with MOAIs.

Venlafaxine

Venlafaxine is classified an atypical antidepressant with has selective serotonin/norepinephrine reuptake inhibitory action; it also weakly inhibits dopamine

Table 8.16 Bupropion side effects

Anorexia
Weight loss
Agitation
Nausea
Constipation
Restlessness
Dizziness
Insomnia
Headache
Tics (exacerbation)
Seizures (0.1% under 300 mg/day and 0.4% over 300 mg/day)
Suicidality

update [110]. It is used as a second- or third-line agent for ADHD. It is available in pill form of varying strengths (25-, 50-, 75-, and 100-mg tablets) and its dosage is 1–3 mg/kg/day or 37.5–225 mg/day. Its side effect profile is similar to bupropion though there is a lower risk of subsequent seizures. Venlafaxine may increase blood pressure leading to a dose-related sustained hypertension; it also increases serum cholesterol. Thus, patients on this medication should have regular blood pressure monitoring as well as yearly serum cholesterol checks. Venlafaxine is contraindicated in those with heart disease.

As noted with other antidepressants, it has a FDA Black Box warning for suicidality. It is metabolized by many isoenzymes of the cytochrome P450 system and has the potential for many drug–drug interactions, including MAOIs and triptans. Thus, clinicians should be cautious adding other medications to venlafaxine. Mydriasis may occur and thus it should be avoided in patients with increased intraocular pressure or at risk for acute narrow-angle glaucoma.

Miscellaneous

Modafinil is a non-amphetamine stimulant that is approved by the FDA for narcolepsy and obstructive sleep apnea/hypopnea syndrome (OSAHS), but not for ADHD in children and adolescents [111]. It does not increase adrenergic activity though it acts in some ways as a sympathomimetic agent; it also does not bind to catecholamine receptors. It has been noted to improve attention span in those with ADHD, though its mechanism in this regard is not known [97, 112]. Typical dosing is 50–100 mg/day. Common side effects include nervousness, dizziness, anxiety (dose related), insomnia, headache, and gastrointestinal dysfunction. It should not be used in patients with a history of Tourette syndrome and cardiovascular disease, and should be used with caution in psychotic individuals. A number of drug interactions occur due to its metabolism via the cytochrome P450 system and it can serve as an inducer or an inhibitor of this system. Armodafinil is the R-enantiomer of modafanil now being promoted to management excessive daytime sleepiness and there is no evidence that it benefits those with ADHD [111].

Polyunsaturated fatty acids (fish oil; omega 3-polyunsaturated fatty acids), acetyl-L-carnitine, donepezil (central anticholinesterase), ropinirole (dopamine agonist), altropane (potent dopamine reuptake inhibitor), nicotinic acetylcholine receptor antagonists, GABA B receptor antagonists, AMPA (ampakines) receptor modulators, iron supplements (with adolescents have low serum ferritin levels), and various supplements have shown some efficacy in some studies for patients with ADHD [15, 97, 110, 113–116]. Further research is needed to determine if any of these agents are actually useful for children and adolescents with ADHD who have a variety of other medications that are known and approved by the US Food and Drug Administration [1].

Conclusions

Attention deficit (hyperactivity) disorder (ADD; ADHD) is a common neurodevelopmental and neuropsychiatric disorder that affects 3–9% of the population across the life span [1]. ADHD is a complex, heterogeneous disorder that involves absence or paucity of connections as well as noradrenergic–dopaminergic dysfunction in various brain regions. As many as 90% of those with ADHD also have one or more comorbid disorders that may profoundly affect their lives and also the overall efficacy of ADHD management options. These various conditions share many genetic and neurobiological traits that place them in a fascinating interactional dance throughout the lifetime of the ADHD patient and his/her family as well as peers.

A plethora of management options are available for children and adolescents with ADHD that involve a combination of pharmacologic and non-pharmacologic methods (see Table 8.4) [42]. After several decades of observation and research, psychostimulants remain the most effective drug treatment for most patients with ADHD. A variety of long-acting methylphenidate and amphetamine products are now available, though there are few studies to guide the patient, family, and clinician in which one is best for a particular patient. Additional drugs are also noted to benefit some ADHD patients and include a variety of antidepressants (such as bupropion), alpha-2-agonists (short- and long-acting formulations), and a norepinephrine reuptake inhibitor (atomoxetine). Other drugs are in the pharmaceutical pipeline and may prove beneficial as the twenty-first century matures.

A trial-and-error method is necessary throughout the life span to find the best agent(s) and formulation(s) that produces optimal efficacy and lowest adverse effect ratio at various times in the ADHD patient's life. Polypharmacy is a common approach to help ADHD patients with multiple and complex symptomatology, though more research is clearly needed to improve the benefits while lowering the side effect profiles of such a strategy [107]. Attention to the specific ADHD comorbidity pattern of each patient is always important in overall management plans [1]. The future of ADHD management looks promising thanks to the pioneering work of Bradley and Knobel in the twentieth century linked with the prowess of modern pharmacology [51, 52].

References

1. Greydanus DE, Pratt HD, Patel DR. Attention deficit hyperactivity disorder across the lifespan: the child, adolescent, and adult. Dis Mon. 2007;53(3):1–59.
2. Still G. The Coulstonian lectures on some abnormal physical conditions in children. Lecture 1. Lancet. 1902;1:1008–12.
3. Clements SD. Minimal brain dysfunction in children: terminology and identification. Washington, DC: United States Department of Health, Education, and Welfare; 1966.
4. Ounsted C. The hyperkinetic syndrome in epileptic children. Lancet. 1955;269(6885): 303–11.
5. American Psychiatric Association. Diagnostic and statistical manual of mental disorders. 4th ed, text rev. Washington, DC: American Psychiatric Association; 2000. pp. 85–93.
6. Greydanus DE, Pratt HD. Attention deficit hyperactivity disorder. In: Greydanus DE, Pratt HD, Patel DR, editors. Behavioral pediatrics. 2nd ed. Lincoln, NE: iUniverse Publishing; 2006. pp. 107–42.
7. Wolraich ML, Felice ME. The classification of child and adolescent mental diagnoses in primary care: diagnostic and statistical manual for primary care (DSM PC): child and adolescent version. Elk Grove Village, IL: American Academy of Pediatrics; 1986. pp. 93–110.
8. Faraone SV, Sergeant J, Gillberg C, Biederman J. The worldwide prevalence of ADHD: is it an American condition? World Psychiatry. 2003;2:104–13.
9. Kessler RC, Adler L, Barkley R, et al. The prevalence and correlates of adult ADHD in the United States: results from the National Comorbidity Survey Replication. Am J Psychiatry. 2006;163:716–23.
10. Katragadda S, Schubiner H. ADHD in children, adolescents, and adults. Prim Care Clin Office Pract. 2007;34(4):111.
11. Lara C, Fayyad J, de Graaf R, et al. Childhood predictors of adult attention-deficit/hyperactivity disorder: results from the World Health Organization World Mental Health Survey Initiative. Biol Psychiatry. 2009;65(1):46–54.
12. Biederman J, Farone SV. Attention-deficit/hyperactivity disorder. Lancet. 2005;366:237–48.
13. Biederman J. Attention-deficit/hyperactivity disorder: a selective overview. Biol Psychiatry. 2005;57:1215–20.
14. Bush G. Attention-deficit/hyperactivity disorder and attention networks. Neuropsychopharmacol. 2010;35:278–300.
15. Dopheide JA, Pliszka SR. Attention-deficit-hyperactivity disorder: an update. Pharmacotherapy. 2009;29(6):656–79.
16. Faraone SV, Khan SA. Candidate gene studies of attention-deficit/hyperactivity disorder. J Clin Psychiatry. 2006;67(Suppl 8):13–20.
17. Sharp SI, McQuillin A, Gurling HM. Genetics of attention-deficit hyperactivity disorder (ADHD). Neuropharmacology. 2009;57(7–8):590–600.
18. Rommelse NN, Altink ME, Fliers EA, et al. Comorbid problems in ADHD: degree of association, shared endophenotypes, and formation of distinct subtypes. Implications for a future DSM. J Abnorm Child Psychol. 2009;37(6):793–804.
19. Elia J, Ambrosini P, Berrettini W. ADHD characteristics: I. Concurrent co-morbidity patterns in children and adolescents. Child Adolesc Psychiatry Ment Health. 2008;2(1):15–20.
20. Gadow KD, DeVincent CJ, Schneider J. Comparative study of children with ADHD only, autism spectrum disorder + ADHD, and chronic multiple tic disorder + ADHD. J Atten Dis. 2009;12(5):474–85.
21. Reiersen AM, Constantino JN, Todd RD. Co-occurrence of motor problems and autistic symptoms in attention-deficit/hyperactivity disorder. J Am Acad Child Adolesc Psychiatry. 2008;47(6):662–72.
22. Murray MJ. Attention-deficit/hyperactivity disorder in the context of autism spectrum disorders. Curr Psychiatr Rep. 2010;Aug;12:33–40.

23. Simonoff E, Pickles A, Charman T, et al. Psychiatric disorders in children with autism spectrum disorders: prevalence, comorbidity, and associated factors in a population-derived sample. J Am Acad Child Adolesc Psychiatry. 2008;47(8):921–9.
24. Konofal E, Lecendreux M, Cortese S. Sleep and ADHD. Sleep Med. 2010;11(7):652–8.
25. LaJoie J, Miles DK. Treatment of attention-deficit disorder, cerebral palsy, and mental retardation in epilepsy. Epilepsy Behav. 2002;3(5S):42–48.
26. Bottcher L, Flachs EM, Uldall P. Attentional and executive impairments in children with spastic cerebral palsy. Dev Med Child Neurol. 2010;52(2):e42–e47.
27. Connor DF, Steeber J, McBurnett K. A review of attention-deficit/hyperactivity disorder complicated by symptoms of oppositional defiant disorder or conduct disorder. J Dev Behav Pediatr. 2010;31(5):427–40.
28. Hummer TA, Kronenberger WG, Wang Y, et al. Executive functioning characteristics associated with ADHD comorbidity in adolescents with disruptive behavior disorders. J Abnorm Child Psychol. 2010;Aug;6:21–26.
29. Trani MD, Casini MP, Capuzzo F, et al. Executive and intellectual functions in attention-deficit/hyperactivity disorder with and without comorbidity. Brain Dev. 2010;Aug;6:33–40.
30. Germano E, Gagliano A, Curatolo P. Comorbidity of ADHD and dyslexia. Dev Neuropsychol. 2010;35(5):475–93.
31. Barnard-Brak L, Sulak TN, Fearon DD. Coexisting disorders and academic achievement among children with ADHD. J Atten Dis. 2010;Jun;7:21–26.
32. McNamara J, Vervaeke SL, Willoughby T. Learning disabilities and risk-taking behaviors in adolescents: a comparison of those with and without comorbid attention-deficit/hyperactivity disorder. J Learn Disabil. 2008;41(6):561–74.
33. Forbes F. Improving recognition and management of ADHD. Practitioner. 2010;254(1728):34–38.
34. Goraya JS, Cruz M, Valencia I, et al. Sleep study abnormalities in children with attention deficit hyperactivity disorder. Pediatr Neurol. 2009;40(1):42–46.
35. Greydanus DE, Pratt HD. Attention deficit/hyperactivity disorder in adolescents. In: Greydanus DE, Patel DR, Pratt HD, editors. Essential adolescent medicine. New York, NY: McGraw-Hill Medical Publishing; 2006. pp. 751–68.
36. Greydanus DE, Calles JL Jr, Patel DR. Pediatric and adolescent psychopharmacology: a practical manual for pediatricians. Cambridge: Cambridge University Press; 2008.
37. Kunwar A, Dewan M, Faraone SV. Treating common psychiatric disorders associated with attention-deficit/hyperactivity disorder. Expert Opin Pharmacother. 2007;8(5):555–62.
38. Daviss WB. A review of co-morbid depression in pediatric ADHD: etiology, phenomenology, and treatment. J Child Adolesc Psychopharmacol. 2008;18(6):565–71.
39. Biederman J, Monteaux MC, Spencer T, et al. Do stimulants protect against psychiatric disorders in youth with ADHD? A 10-year follow-up study. Pediatrics. 2009;123(1):71–78.
40. Gau SS, Ni HC, Shang CY, et al. Psychiatric comorbidity among children and adolescents with and without persistent attention-deficit hyperactivity disorder. Aust NZ J Psychiatry. 2010;44(2):135–43.
41. Barkley RA, editor. Attention deficit hyperactivity disorder: a handbook for diagnosis. 3rd ed. New York, NY: Guilford; 2006.
42. Culpepper L. Primary care treatment of attention-deficit/hyperactivity disorder. J Clin Psychiatry. 2006;67(Suppl 8):51–58.
43. Greydanus DE, Sloane MA, Rappley MD. Psychopharmacology of ADHD in adolescents. Adolesc Med. 2002;13:599–624.
44. Greydanus DE, Pratt HD, Sloane MA, et al. Attention-deficit/hyperactivity disorder in children and adolescents: Interventions for a complex costly clinical conundrum. Pediatr Clin North Am. 2003;50:1049–92.
45. Greydanus DE:. Psychopharmacology of ADHD in adolescents: Quo vadis? Psychiatr Times. 2003;20:5–9.
46. Schepis TS, Marlowe DB, Forman FG. The availability and portrayal of stimulants over the internet. J Adolec Health. 2008;42:458–65.

47. Jensen PS, Hinshaw SP, Swanson JM, Greenhill LL, Conners CK, et al. Findings from the NIMH Multimodal Treatment Study of ADHD (MTA): implications and applications for primary care providers. J Dev Behav Pediatr. 2001;22:60–73.

48. National Institute of Mental Health (NIMH). Attention deficit hyperactivity disorder. NIMH, NIH Publication No. 01-4589, 2001. Available at: http://www.nimh.nih.gov/publicat/helpchild.cfm

49. National Institute of Mental Health. NIMH research on treatment for attention deficit hyperactivity disorder (ADHD): The multimodal treatment study. Questions and answers. Washington, DC: NIMH, 2000. Available at: http://www.nimh.nih.gov/events/mtaqa.cfm

50. MTA Cooperative Group. National Institute of Mental Health Multimodal Treatment Study of ADHD Follow-up: 24 month outcomes of treatment strategies for attention-deficit/hyperactivity disorder. Pediatrics. 2004;113(4):754–61.

51. Bradley C. The behavior of children receiving benzedrine. Am J Psychiatry. 1937;94: 577–85.

52. Knobel M, Wolman MB, Mason E. Hyperkinesis and organicity in children. Arch Gen Psychiatry. 1959;81:94–105.

53. Clarke SD. ADHD in adolescence. J Adolesc Health. 2000;127:77–8.

54. Schubiner H, Robin AL, Young J. Attention-deficit/hyperactivity disorder in adolescent males. Adolesc Med. 2003;14:663–76.

55. Pliszka SR, Crismon ML, Hughes CW, et al. The Texas Children's Medication Algorithm Project: revision of the algorithm for pharmacology of attention deficit/hyperactivity disorder. J Am Acad Child Adolesc Psychiatry. 2006;45(6):642–57.

56. Staufer WB, Greydanus DE. Attention-deficit/hyperactivity disorder psychopharmacology for college students. Pediatr Clin North Am. 2005;52:71–84.

57. Kaplan G, Newcorn JH, Ivanov IS. Pharmacologic management of ADHD in children and adolescents. Int J Child Adolesc Health. 2010;3(2):22–35.

58. Wilens TE. Mechanism of action of agents used in attention-deficit/hyperactivity disorder. J Clin Psychiatry. 2006;67(Suppl 8):32–38.

59. Gilchrist RH, Arnold LE. Long-term efficacy of ADHD: pharmacotherapy in children. Pediatr Ann. 2008;37(1):46–51.

60. Solanto MV, Arnsten AFT, Castellanos FX:. The neuroscience of stimulant drug action in ADHD. In: Solanto MV, Arnsten AFT, Castellanos FX, editors. Stimulant Drugs and ADHD. London: Oxford University Press; 2001. pp. 355–79.

61. Greydanus DE, Kaplan G, Antshel KM. Attention deficit hyperactivity disorder: neuropsychologic and pharmacologic considerations. In: Noggle CA, Dean RS, editors. The neuropsychology of psychopharmacology. New York, NY: Springer; 2010.

62. Reiff MI, Stein MT. ADHD evaluation and diagnosis: a practical approach to office practice. Pediatr Clin North Am. 2003;50:1019–48.

63. Ter-Stepanian M, Grizenko N, Zappitelli M, Joober R. Clinical response to methylphenidate in children diagnosed with attention-deficit hyperactivity disorder and comorbid psychiatric disorders. Can J Psychiatry. 2010;55(5):305–12.

64. Drugs for Treatment of ADHD. Treat Guidelines. Med Lett. 2006;4:77.

65. Focalin XR for ADHD. Med Lett. 2009;51:22–24.

66. Chavez B, Sopko MA Jr, Ehret MJ, et al. An update on central nervous system stimulant formulations in children and adolescents with attention-deficit/hyperactivity disorder. Ann Pharmacother. 2009;43(6):1084–95.

67. Marcus SC, Wan GJ, Kenmner JE, et al. Continuity of methylphenidate treatment for attention-deficit/hyperactivity disorder. Arch Pediatr Adolesc Med. 2005;159:572–8.

68. Faraone SV. Lisdexamfetamine dimesylate: the first long-acting prodrug stimulant treatment for attention-deficit hyperactivity disorder. Expert Opin Pharmacother. 2008;9(9):1565–74.

69. Findling RL, Ginsberg LD, Jain R, Gao J. Effectiveness, safety, and tolerability of Lisdexamfetamine dimesylate in children with attention-deficit hyperactivity disorder: an open-label, dose-optimization study. J Child Adolesc Psychopharmacol. 2009;19(6): 649–62.

70. Mattingly G. Lisdexamfetamine dimesylate: a prodrug stimulant for the treatment of ADHD in children and adults. CNS Spectr. 2010;15(5):315–25.
71. Brams M, Moon E, Pucci M, López FA. Duration of oral long-acting stimulant medications for ADHD throughout the day. Curr Med Res Opin. 2010;26(8):1809–25.
72. Cowles BJ. Lisdexamfetamine for treatment of attention-deficit/hyperactivity disorder. Ann Pharmacother. 2009;43(4):669–76.
73. Perrin JM, Friedman RA, Knilans TD. The Black Box Working Group and the Section on Cardiology and Cardiac Surgery. Pediatrics. 2008;122:451–53.
74. Vitiello B, Towbin K. Stimulant treatment of ADHD and risk of sudden death in children. Am J Psychiatr. 2009;166(9):955–7.
75. Wilens TE, Prince JB, Spencer TJ, Biderman J. Stimulants and sudden death: what is a physician to do? Pediatrics. 2006;118(3):1215–19.
76. Gould MS, Walsh BT, Munfakh JL, et al. Sudden death and use of stimulants in youths. Am J Psychiatry. 2009;166(9):992–1001.
77. McCarthy S, Cranswick N, Potts L, et al. Mortality associated with attention-deficit hyperactivity disorder (ADHD) drug treatment: a retrospective cohort study of children, adolescents, and young adults using the general practice research database. Drug Saf. 2009;32(11):1089–96.
78. Warren AE, Hamilton RM, Bélanger SA, et al. Cardiac risk assessment before the use of stimulant medications in children and youth: a joint position statement by the Canadian Paediatric Society, the Canadian Cardiovascular Society, and the Canadian Academy of Child and Adolescent Psychiatry. Can J Cardiol. 2009;25(11):625–30.
79. Kaufmann R, Goldberg-Stern H, Shuper A. Attention-deficit disorders and epilepsy: incidence, causative relations, and treatment possibilities. J Child Neurol. 2009;24(6): 727–33.
80. Hamoda HM, Guild DJ, Gumlak S, et al. Association between attention-deficit/hyperactivity disorder and epilepsy in pediatric populations. Expert Rev Neurother. 2009;9(12): 1747–54.
81. Schubert R. Attention deficit disorder and epilepsy. Pediatr Neurol. 2005;32(1):1–10.
82. Varley CK. Sudden death related to selected tricyclic antidepressants in children: epidemiology, mechanisms and clinical implications. Paediatr Drugs. 2001;3:613–27.
83. Wilens TE, Farone SV, Biederman J, et al. Does stimulant therapy of attention-deficit/hyperactivity disorder beget later substance abuse? A meta-analytic review of the literature. Pediatrics. 2003;111:179–85.
84. Ivanov I, Pearson A, Kaplan G, Newcorn J. Treatment of adolescent ADHD and comorbid substance abuse. Int J Child Adoles Health. 2010;3(2):45–60.
85. Kollins SH. A qualitative review of issues arising in the use of psycho-stimulant medications in patients with ADHD and co-morbid substance use disorders. Curr Med Res Opin. 2008;24(5):1345–57.
86. Swanson JM and the MTA Cooperative Group. National Institute of Mental Health Multimodal Treatment Study of ADHD follow-up: changes in effectiveness and growth after the end of treatment. Pediatrics. 2004;113:762–9.
87. Greydanus DE, Merrick J. Psychopharmacology in children, adolescents, and adults with attention deficit hyperactivity disorder. In: Gordon SM, Mitchell AE, editors. Attention deficit hyperactivity disorder. New York, NY: Nova Science Publishers; 2009. pp. 257–72.
88. Bloch MH, Leckman JF. Clinical course of Tourette Syndrome. J Psychosom Res. 2009;67(6):497–501.
89. Cavanna AE, Servo S, Monaco F, Robertson MM. The behavioral spectrum of Gilles de la Tourette syndrome. J Neuropsychiatry Clin Neurosci. 2009;21(1):13–23.
90. Jankovic J. Tourette's syndrome. N Engl J Med. 2001;345:1184–92.
91. Roessner V, Becker A, Banaschewski T, Rothenberger A. Executive functions in children with chronic tic disorders with/without ADHD: new insights. Eur Child Adolesc Psychiatry. 2007;16(Suppl 1):36–44.

92. Bloch MH, Panza KE, Landeros-Weisenberger A, Leckman JF. Meta-analysis: treatment of attention-deficit/hyperactivity disorder in children with comorbid tic disorders. J Am Acad Child Adolesc Psychiatry. 2009;48(9):884–93.

93. Atomoxetine (Strattera) for ADHD. Med Lett. 2003;45:11–12.

94. Atomoxetine: Strattera revisited. Med Lett. 2004;46:65.

95. Michelson D, Allen AJ, Busner J, et al. Once-daily atomoxetine treatment for children and adolescents with ADHD: a randomized, placebo-controlled study. Am J Psychiatry. 2002;159:1896–901.

96. Garnock-Jones KP, Keating GM. Atomoxetine: a review of its use in attention-deficit hyperactivity disorder in children and adolescents. Paediatr Drugs. 2009;11(3):203–26.

97. Waxmonsky JG. Nonstimulant therapies for attention-deficit hyperactivity disorder (ADHD) in children and adults. Essent Psychopharmacol. 2005;6(5):262–76.

98. May DE, Kratochvil CJ. Attention-deficit hyperactivity disorder: recent advances in paediatric pharmacotherapy. Drugs. 2010;70(1):15–40.

99. Spencer TJ, Sallee FR, Gilbert DL, et al. Atomoxetine treatment of ADHD in children with comorbid Tourette syndrome. J Atten Disord. 2008;11(4):470–81.

100. Scahill L. Alpha-2 adrenergic agonists in children with inattention, hyperactivity, and impulsiveness. CNS Drugs. 2009;23(Suppl 1):43–49.

101. Biederman J, Melmed RD, Patel A, et al. Long-term, open-label extension study of guanfacine extended release in children and adolescents with ADHD. CNS Spectr. 2008;13(12):1047–55.

102. Connor DF, Rubin J. Guanfacine extended release in the treatment of attention deficit hyperactivity disorder in children and adolescents. Drugs Today (Barc). 2010;46(5):299–314.

103. Sallee FR, McGough J, Wigal T, et al. Guanfacine extended release in children and adolescents with attention-deficit/hyperactivity disorder: a placebo-controlled trial. J Am Acad Child Adolesc Psychiatry. 2009;48(2):155–65.

104. Arnsten AF, Scahill L, Finding RL. Alpha-2 adrenergic receptor agonists for treatment of attention-deficit/hyperactivity disorder: emerging concepts from new data. J Child Adolesc Psychopharmacol. 2007;17(4):393–406.

105. Daviss WB. Bupropion for adolescents with attention-deficit/hyperactivity disorder. J Am Acad Child Adolesc Psychiatry. 2001;40:307–14.

106. Reimherr FW, Hedges DW, Strong RE, et al. Bupropion SR in adults with ADHD: a short-term, placebo-controlled trial. Neuropsychiatr Dis Treat. 2005;1(3):245–51.

107. Wigal SB. Efficacy and safety limitations of attention-deficit hyperactivity disorder pharmacotherapy in children and adults. CNS Drugs. 2009;23(Suppl 1):21–31.

108. Clayton AH. Extended-release bupropion: an antidepressant with a broad spectrum of therapeutic activity? Expert Opin Pharmacother. 2007;8(4):457–66.

109. Verbeeck W, Tuinier S, Bekkering GE. Antidepressants in the treatment of adult attention-deficit hyperactivity disorder: a systemic review. Adv Ther. 2009;26(2):170–84.

110. Pityaratstian N:. Advances in alternative pharmacotherapy of ADHD. J Med Assoc Thai. 2005;88(Suppl 4):S357–S62.

111. Armodafinil for wakefulness. Med Lett Dr Ther. 2010;52:61–2.

112. Turner DC, Clark L, Dowson J, et al. Modafinil improves cognition and response in adult attention-deficit/hyperactivity disorder. Biol Psychiatry. 2004;55:1031–40.

113. Keen D, Hadijikoumi I. ADHD in children and adolescents. Clin Evid (Online). 2008;Oct 2; PMID:19445793.

114. Richardson AJ, Montgomery P. The Oxford-Durham Study: a randomized, controlled trial of dietary supplementation with fatty acids in children with developmental coordination disorder. Pediatrics. 2005;115(5):1360–6.

115. Hamre HJ, Witt CM, Kienle GS, et al. Anthroposophic therapy for attention deficit hyperactivity: a two-year prospective study in outpatients. Int J Gen Med. 2010;3:239–53.

116. Olfson M. New options in the pharmacological management of attention-deficit/hyperactivity disorder. Am J Manag Care. 2004;10(4 Suppl):S117–S24.

117. Greydanus DE, Pratt HD et al. Attention-deficit/hyperactivity disorder in children and adolescents: interventions for a complex costly clinical conundrum. Pediatr Clin North Am. 2003;50:1061–1062.
118. Greydanus DE, Pratt HD et al. Psychopharmacology of ADHD in adolescents. Adolesc Med. 2002;13:604.
119. Greydanus DE, Pratt HD et al. Psychopharmacology of ADHD in adolescents. Adolesc Med. 2002;13:607.
120. Greydanus DE, Pratt HD et al. Psychopharmacology of ADHD in adolescents. Adolesc Med. 2002;13:615.
121. Greydanus DE, Pratt HD, et al. Attention-deficit/hyperactivity disorder in children and adolescents: interventions for a complex costly clinical conundrum. Pediatr Clin North Am. 2003;50:1079.

Chapter 9
Sleep in Children and Adolescents with Neurobehavioral Disorders

Bantu Chhangani and Donald E. Greydanus

Abstract Sleep disturbances are highly prevalent in children and adolescents who have neurobehavioral and neurodevelopmental disorders. Evidence also suggests a relationship between the quality of sleep and neurobehavioral symptoms. Timely recognitions and effective management are therefore essential to improve the quality of life of children with these disorders. Various behavioral techniques remain the cornerstone of management for sleep disorders in children and adolescents with very limited and selective use of pharmacotherapy. This chapter reviews sleep in children and adolescents who have attention-deficit hyperactivity disorder, autism spectrum disorder, bipolar disorder, and eating disorders.

Introduction

Sleep problems are highly prevalent in the pediatric population and there is a growing body of evidence suggesting a relationship between the sleep quality in children and adolescents and behavioral and emotional problems [1]. There is a significant amount of research that is needed in this field, given the current paucity of data and lack of clear understanding. This chapter discusses the commonly encountered behavioral problems in pediatrics and associated sleep disturbances.

Attention-Deficit Hyperactivity Disorder

Attention-deficit hyperactivity disorder (ADHD) is a neurocognitive and behavioral abnormality commonly seen in adolescence and childhood and estimated to affect 3–9% of school-aged children [2]. It is characterized by consistent symptoms of

D.E. Greydanus (✉)
Department of Pediatrics and Human Development, Kalamazoo Center for Medical Studies,
Michigan State University College of Human Medicine, Kalamazoo, MI 49008-1284, USA
e-mail: greydanus@kcms.msu.edu

D.R. Patel et al. (eds.), *Neurodevelopmental Disabilities*,
DOI 10.1007/978-94-007-0627-9_9, © Springer Science+Business Media B.V. 2011

inattention, impulsivity, and/or hyperactivity which occur before the age of 7 and result in impaired functioning in two or more settings [2].

ADHD and primary sleep disorders appear to have a complex and bidirectional relationship which has become increasingly evident over the past several years. The sleep problems that children and adolescents with ADHD experience may be multifactorial, e.g., the first-line Food and Drug Administration (FDA)-approved medications for the treatment of ADHD have been shown to cause sleep problems including increased latency to sleep, poor sleep efficiency, and total reduced sleep problems [3]. Common sleep complaints encountered include sleep onset difficulties, bedtime resistance, increased nocturnal disruptions, difficulty experienced with morning awakenings, and even daytime sleepiness [4, 5]. On the other hand, children with primary sleep disorders can present with inattention and hyperactivity. The most well-studied sleep disorders in patients with ADHD are sleep-disordered breathing or obstructive sleep apnea (OSA), periodic limb movements of sleep (PLMS), and restless legs syndrome (RLS).

Obstructive sleep apnea is a sleep-related disorder characterized by intermittent episodes of complete or partial upper airway obstruction, resulting in gas exchange abnormalities (hypoxia and hypercapnea) and fragmented sleep. It is a common disorder with a relatively high prevalence rate of 2–5% when compared to other childhood conditions such as sickle cell anemia and diabetes [6, 7]. Pediatric obstructive sleep apnea can occur at any age, but because most cases are due to adenotonsillar hypertrophy, the highest prevalence is observed to be between the ages of 2 and 6 years coinciding with peak adenotonsillar hypertrophy relative to upper airway size [8, 9]. Patients with habitual snoring and obstructive sleep apnea (OSA) may present with symptoms of ADHD which generally improve after the OSA has been treated, suggesting that while the presence of untreated OSA can certainly aggravate ADHD, perhaps untreated OSA may actually play a role in causing the symptoms of ADHD. This, however, remains far from proven and currently is at best an anecdotal observation [10, 11].

Several studies have also been carried out focusing on the relationship between ADHD and periodic limb movements in sleep (PLMS) and these have concluded that children with ADHD have a higher incidence of PLMS [12, 13].

Although not always co-morbid, a multitude of studies have also demonstrated that RLS is more common in patients with ADHD and vice versa. Restless legs syndrome is a neurologic sensorimotor disorder characterized by unpleasant paresthesias which occur primarily in the lower extremities and are accompanied by a strong and nearly irresistible urge to move. The paresthesias may include numbness, tingling, aching and can also be experienced, albeit less commonly in other parts of the body including the arms and the trunk. These symptoms are brought on during periods of inactivity and display a circadian pattern such that the paresthesias are worse in the evening and night in those with normal circadian rhythm activity. A complete or partial improvement is usually seen with movement for as long as the movement continues [14]. The association between RLS and ADHD can be explained by a number of hypotheses. First, sleep disruption in RLS leads to decreased quality and quantity of sleep and thus sleep deprivation and daytime fatigue. Tired children are usually hyperactive and inattentive and have paradoxical overactivity. Second, these disorders may share a common dopamine underactivity and or iron deficiency, and lastly, RLS and ADHD may share a genetic link [15, 16].

Objectively, results from polysomnography (PSG), actigraphy, and multiple sleep latency testing (MSLT) data have demonstrated increased rates of movements and sleep-disordered breathing but have been inconsistent with regard to sleep parameters such as sleep duration and latency to sleep onset [17, 18], indicating higher subjective reports of sleep complaints with relatively weak objective evidence.

Autism Spectrum Disorder

The autism spectrum disorder (ASD) is one of the most devastating neurobiologic disorders characterized by significant social deficits, impaired communication, repetitive behaviors, and a restricted range of interests [19]. Several recent studies have reported prevalence rates of sleep problems in patients with ASD as high as 40–85% when compared with 20–40% in typically developing children [20, 21]. Commonly reported sleep disturbances include prolonged sleep onset latency, restless sleep, and frequent nocturnal awakenings and reduced total sleep time.

There is also strong objective evidence of sleep disturbances measured by polysomnography and actigraphy. These include prolonged latency to sleep and poor sleep efficiency [22]. Studies have also demonstrated an increased level of anxiety, depression, and aggressive behavior in the children and adolescents with the sleep disturbances in comparison to the children with ASD who do not have sleep disturbances [22]. This may lead to increased stress and altered sleep quality for the parents of children with ASD and sleep disturbances [23].

Bipolar Disorder

Pediatric bipolar disorder (PBD) is a disorder characterized by the presence of thoughts of grandiosity, elation, decreased need for sleep, and high levels of activity [24]. It is thought to have a more severe presentation and course compared to adult bipolar disorder [25]. Sleep disturbances are the most common prodrome of mania with a prevalence rate of 35–45% and sleep loss may act as a precipitating factor in manic episodes. Conversely, advancing the sleep–wake schedule has been to show an improvement in mood. On polysomnography, common findings include interruption of sleep continuity and reduced rapid eye movement (REM) sleep.

Eating Disorders

Studies in adults suggest that sleep problems may play a role in the risk of obesity and the growing body of evidence indicates that sleep deprivation leads to certain metabolic and hormonal changes which in term may increase appetite, insulin intolerance and lead to weight gain [26]. The few studies in children thus far [27] indicate that this may also be true in children and adolescents. Hence, sleep disturbances, sleep deprivation, and erratic sleep wave schedules could contribute to growing epidemic of weight gain and obesity.

Anorexia nervosa and bulimia nervosa are on the other end of the nutritional spectrum but relatively little research has been conducted to investigate the effects of sleep disturbances on these disorders and most of the data available so far are correlational. Typically, adolescents with anorexia nervosa display poor sleep efficiency and increased nocturnal awakenings and a reduction in slow wave sleep [28], whereas adolescents with bulimia nervosa have been observed to have shorter total sleep duration due to later bedtime and earlier rise time due to the binging and purging [29].

Management

Given the high prevalence and chronicity within select populations and negative consequences of pediatric sleep disturbances, effective management of this condition is becoming increasingly necessary. Two main therapeutic approaches are generally utilized: cognitive–behavioral and pharmacologic therapy. While the efficacy of cognitive–behavioral therapy or behavioral therapy alone is relatively well established, there is a paucity of evidence-based data for use of pharmacologic therapy within the pediatric population. Commonly utilized behavioral therapy includes recommendations pertaining to good sleep hygiene, stimulus control, and the use of worry management.

Sleep hygiene recommendations include educating the affected children and their parents on eliminating behaviors which may aggravate the sleep disturbances. These generally include the avoidance of stimulating electronic devices in the bedroom a few hours prior to bedtime, maintenance of a structured sleep–wake schedule such that there are no erratic changes during weekends or holidays, and discouragement of caffeinated beverages or naps during the day. Children are also encouraged to have bright light exposure in the morning and avoid bright light exposure in the evenings.

Stimulus control is a behavioral technique utilized in order to reverse learned maladaptive behaviors which have occurred due to the sleep disturbances and are further aggravating these. Children are educated on engaging in sleep-compatible behaviors in bed and the bedroom. They are provided instructions on using the bed and bedroom only for sleeping with avoidance of any stimulating electronic device like television or phones. They are asked to step out of bed if unable to initiate sleep within 20 min of bedtime and go to another room where they can engage in nonstimulating activities such as reading or listening to relaxing music. Children should avoid sleeping in any other part of the home except their bedrooms and asked to return to bed when they become drowsy. This may need to be repeated if they experience sleep maintenance problems. Also, as part of this behavioral technique, they are asked to arise out of bed around the same time every morning. In general, children and adolescents are asked to avoid spending an excessive amount of time in bed lying awake as that can worsen the perception of sleep disturbances.

Behavioral techniques including a scheduled "worry time" can be utilized in patients who have a significant amount of anxiety, bedtime worry, and vigilance as these can all interfere with sleep onset. Children are instructed on scheduling a "worry time" usually in the middle of the day which is essentially a time period during which they are encouraged to process their worries or fears prior to bedtime so that these worries or ruminative thoughts are eliminated from the presleep period. Finally, the children and adolescents can be educated on relaxation techniques like breathing exercises and progressive muscle relaxation.

Conclusions

Emerging data suggest that sleep problems and behavioral or emotional and developmental disabilities may have a bidirectional relationship. Sleep disturbances are highly prevalent in this population of children and further clinical trials are necessary to investigate this relationship further as well as explore therapy.

References

1. Stein MA, Mendelsohn J, Obermeyer WH, Amromin J, Benca R. Sleep and behavior problems in school aged children. Pediatrics. 2001;107(4):e60.
2. American Psychiatric Association. Diagnostic and statistical manual of mental disorders. 4th ed. text rev. Washington, DC: APA; 2000.
3. Charach A, Ickowicz A, Schachar R. Stimulant treatment over five years: adherence, effectiveness, and adverse effects. J Am Acad Child Adolesc Psychiatry. 2004;3(5):559–67.
4. Cortese S, Faraone SV, Konofal E, Lecendreux M. Sleep in children with attention-deficit/hyperactivity disorder: meta-analysis of subjective and objective studies. J Am Acad Child Adolesc Psychiatry. 2009;48(9):894–908.
5. Surman CB, Adamson JJ, Petty C, Biederman J, Kenealy DC, Levine M, et al. Association between attention-deficit/hyperactivity disorder and sleep impairment in adulthood: evidence from a large controlled study. J Clin Psychiatry. 2009;70(11):1523–29.
6. Newacheck PW, Taylor WR. Childhood chronic illness: prevalence, severity and impact. Am J Public Health. 1992;82(3):364–71.
7. Gislason T, Benediktsdottir B. Snoring apneic episodes, and nocturnal hypoxemia among children 6 months to 6 years old. An epidemiologic study of lower limit of prevalence. Chest. 1995;107(4):963–66.
8. Fujioka M, Young LW, Girdany BR. Radiographic evaluation of adenoidal size in children: adenoidal naso-pharyngeal ratio. AJR Am J Roentgenol. 1979;133 (3):401–4.
9. Cl. M. Sleep-disordered breathing in children. Am J Respir Crit Care Med. 2001;164(1): 16–30.
10. O'Brien LM, Mervis CB, Holbrook CR, Brunner JL, Smith NH, McNally N, et al. Neurobehavioral correlates of sleep-disordered breathing in children. J Sleep Res. 2004;13(2):165–72.

11. Dillon JE, Blunden S, Ruzicka DL, Guire KE, Champine D, Weatherly RA, et al. DSM-IV diagnoses and obstructive sleep apnea in children before and 1 year after adenotonsillectomy. J Am Acad Child Adolesc Psychiatry. 2007;46(11):1425–36.
12. Chervin RD, Archbold KH, Dillon JE, Pituch KJ, Panahi P, Dahl RE, et al. Associations between symptoms of inattention, hyperactivity, restless legs and periodic leg movements. Sleep. 2002;25(2):213–8.
13. Picchietti DL, England SJ, Walters AS, Willis K, Verrico T. Periodic limb movement disorder and restless legs syndrome in children with attention-deficit hyperactivity disorder. J Child Neurol. 1998;13(12):588–94.
14. American Academy of Sleep Medicine. The international classification of sleep disorders: diagnostic and coding manual. 2nd ed. Westchester, IL: Am Acad Sleep Med; 2005. pp. 114–6.
15. Cortese S, Konofal E, Bernardina BD, Mouren MC, Lecendreux M. Sleep disturbances and serum ferritin levels in children with attention-deficit hyperactivity disorder. Eur Child Adolesc Psychiatry. 2009;18(7):393–9.
16. Konofal E, Lecendreux M, Deron J, Marchand M, Cortese S, Zaim M, et al. Effects of iron supplementation on attention-deficit hyperactivity disorder in children. Pediatr Neurol. 2008;38(1):20–6.
17. Gruber R. Sleep characteristics of children and adolescents with attention deficit-hyperactivity disorder. Child Adolesc Psychiatr Clin Am. 2009;18(4):863–76.
18. Konofal E, Lecendreux M, Bouvard MP, Mouren-Simeoni MC. High levels of nocturnal activity in children with attention-deficit hyperactivity disorder: a video analysis. Psychiatry Clin Neurosci. 2001;55(2):97–103.
19. Rapin I, Tuchman RF. Autism: definition, neurobiology, screening, diagnosis. Pediatr Clin North Am. 2008;55(5):1129–46.
20. Richdale AL. Sleep problems in autism: prevalence, cause and intervention. Dev Med Child Neurol. 1999;41(1):60–6.
21. Sadeh A, Gruber R, Sleep RA. neurobehavioral functioning, and behavior problems in school-age children. Child Dev. 2002;73(2):405–17.
22. Malow BA, Marzec ML, McGrew SG, Wang L, Henderson LM, Stone WL. Characterizing sleep in children with autism spectrum disorders: a multidimensional approach. Sleep. 2006;29(12):1563–71.
23. Meltzer LJ. Brief report: sleep in parents of children with autistic spectrum disorders. J Pediatr Psychol. 2008;33(4):380–6.
24. Geller B, Zimerman B, Williams M, Delbello MP, Frazier J, Beringer L. Phenomenology of prepubertal and early adolescent bipolar disorder: examples of elated mood, grandiose behaviors, decreased need for sleep, racing thoughts and hypersexuality. J Child Adolesc Psychopharmacol. 2002;12(1):3–9.
25. Birmaher B, Axelson D, Strober M, Gill MK, Valeri S, Chiappetta L, et al. Clinical course of children and adolescents with bipolar spectrum disorders. Arch Gen Psychiatry. 2006;63(2):175–83.
26. Spiegel K, Tasali E, Penev P, Van Cauter E. Brief communication: sleep curtailment in healthy young men is associated with decreased leptin levels, elevated ghrelin levels and increased hunger and appetite. Ann Intern Med. 2004;141(11):846–50.
27. Snell EK, Adam EK, Duncan GJ. Sleep and the body mass index and overweight status of children and adolescents. Child Dev. 2007;78(1):309–23.
28. Nobili L, Baglietto MG, De Carli F, Savoini M, Schiavi G, Zanotto E, et al. A quantified analysis of sleep electroencephalography in anorectic adolescents. Biol Psychiatry. 1999;45(6):771–5.
29. Latzer Y, Tzischinsky O, Epstein R, Klein E, Peretz L. Naturalistic sleep monitoring in women suffering from bulimia nervosa. Int J Eat Disord. 1999;26(3):315–21.

Chapter 10
Learning Disabilities

Helen D. Pratt and Donald E. Greydanus

Abstract Children, adolescents, and young adults diagnosed with a learning disability have a constellation of symptoms that result in significant functional impairments. Youth who experience learning disabilities may also have additional behavioral symptoms that complicate diagnosis. Early recognition and intervention may have significant impact on long-term positive outcomes. Interventions include behavioral academic, psycho-educational, as well as individual and family therapy. This chapter briefly reviews terminology, definitions, epidemiology, diagnosis, treatment, and management of symptoms of learning disabilities in children, adolescents, and young adults.

Introduction

Adolescents diagnosed with a learning disability have a constellation of symptoms that result in a discrepancy between their intellectual abilities and academic performance. Complaints of symptoms may come from teachers and parents, or from the adolescent/young adult patients themselves. Neurodevelopmental impairments can lead to youth developing learning disabilities [1]. During the growth and maturation of the nervous system and the progressive development of sensory and perceptual abilities, various deficits or impairments may develop and manifest in terms of learning disabilities [1] that become apparent in one or more developmental domains (see Table 10.1) [1, 2]. Youth who do not have the ability to exhibit age-appropriate learning skills both in relevant settings (school, home, work) and in demand situations experience learning problems (see Table 10.2) [3–13]. Learning disabilities may occur in youth with superior, average, or low intellectual functioning [3]. The intent of this chapter is to discuss learning disabilities in children and adolescents.

H.D. Pratt (✉)
Department of Pediatrics and Human Development, Kalamazoo Center for Medical Studies, Michigan State University College of Human Medicine, Kalamazoo, MI 49008-1284, USA
e-mail: pratt@kcms.msu.edu

D.R. Patel et al. (eds.), *Neurodevelopmental Disabilities,*
DOI 10.1007/978-94-007-0627-9_10, © Springer Science+Business Media B.V. 2011

Table 10.1 Domains of function development

Physical or somatic growth
Neurological
Motor (gross and fine)
Visual
Cognitive
Auditory
Language
Perceptual motor
Kinesthetic
Psychosocial
Integrative and adaptive

Table 10.2 Types of impairments by domains of function

Problems with cognitive functioning
Academic failure (overall difficulty achieving or maintaining age-appropriate skills such as reading, writing, arithmetic, spelling, task completion, compliance, instruction following)
Inability to acquire or retain new information
Inability to engage in higher order thinking skills
Inability to follow instructions or directions
Inability to execute tasks in order to complete an assigned task
Inability to organize time, tasks, or projects in a manner that allows satisfactory completion
Inability to sustain and focus attention on relevant or essential stimuli
Inability to become aroused to danger or essential stimuli (alertness)
Poor impulse control

Problems with communicating
Oral language
 Problems with oral language (production, articulation)
 Problems with written language (spelling, production/graphomotor)
Auditory language
 Inability to hear relevant stimuli
 Inability to process auditory stimuli (comprehension)
 Inability to detect and discriminate between sounds or spoken language in a manner that allows appropriate cognitive, motor, or emotional responses

Problems with motor functioning
Fine motor
 Inability to write legibly
 Inability to cut paper designs with scissors, inability to button, fasten, sew, draw, and match to sample designs
 Inability to control motor responses (tics, tremors, fidgeting, jerky motions, uncontrolled motions)
Gross motor
 Inability to hop, skip, jump, walk, run, walk a balance beam 6 in. off the ground, walk straight line toe to toe – forward and backward
 Inability to control motor responses (tics, tremors, fidgeting, jerky motions, uncontrolled motions)
 Problems with perceptual–motor functioning

Table 10.2 (continued)

Inability to coordinate neurological signals to motor, neurological, cognitive, visual, auditory domains, to plan and/or execute motor responses (such as maintaining or regaining balance, or producing motor response requiring manual dexterity to write, catch, throw, wave, walk, run)

Inability to integrate domains adequately to respond appropriately to environmental stimuli

Problems with visual–motor functioning

Inability to detect and process visual information or to copy homework from the board or from a text to a paper, reproduce object/word from visual cue (visual motor processing, eye–hand coordination)

Problems with psychosocial functioning
Inability to regulate emotions
Inability to calm down after being upset
Lack of confidence in skills or abilities
Inability to respond appropriately to affective stimuli
Inability to control or regulate behavior
Lack of motivation
Low frustration tolerance
Inability to initiate friendships
Inability to sustain positive peer relationships
Inability to sustain positive family relationships
Inability to develop and sustain interpersonal relationships
Problems with overestimating their scholastic competence, social acceptance, or behavioral conduct
Integrative and adaptive
Inability to integrate all domains so that age- and developmentally appropriate tasks can be executed, evaluated, and adjusted to meet performance and learning needs of the individual

Terminology

In the International Classification of Functioning (ICF) manual the World Health Organization (WHO) uses three major terms to describe all "disabilities," physical, mental, and functional [10]. The following terms are used in this chapter to discuss intellectual disability:

- Adaptive function is the ability to detect stimuli, recognize the function of a stimulus, process the condition in which the stimulus occurs, determine the appropriate reaction, and execute that action to minimize dangers as well as maximize rewards to experience the world in a positive manner [8].
- Disorder is associated with words like chaos, disarray, confusion, turmoil, mayhem, and syndrome. This is both a medical and a mental health term; a disorder can be diagnosed when the criteria for labeling are met.
- Disability is the functional consequence of impairment (e.g., inability, restricted capability). It is an umbrella term covering impairments, activity limitations, and participation restrictions in the general society in which a person lives [10]. According to the Americans with Disabilities Act (ADA), the term "disability" means, with respect to an individual, a physical or a mental impairment that

substantially limits one or more major life activities of such individual; a record of such an impairment; or being regarded as having such an impairment [14].

- Handicap is the social consequence of impairment (e.g., isolation, loss of job, or having to make career changes because of communication difficulties) [10, 14].
- Impairment is defined as an abnormality of a structure or a function (e.g., an abnormality of the ear or auditory system). It is important to remember that not all impairments result in disabilities and that not all individuals with disabilities are handicapped [14]. Contextual factors (i.e., interaction between features of a person's body and features of the environment) significantly influence the impact of a child's or an adolescent's impairment (environmental, social, medical, or biological) and affect the person's deficits and functioning [10].
- Neurodevelopment encompasses various domains that can be categorized as physical or somatic, neurological, sensory–perceptual, cognitive, and psychosocial or emotional [1].
- Intellectual disability refers to significant limitations in intellectual functioning, and adaptive function is not at the individual's expected level of function for his or her age or culture. Skill, performance, and adaptive mastery represent one type of intellectual function. Two additional areas of intellectual function include the ability to express conceptual thinking and the ability to employ social skills effectively [1, 9, 15].
- Intellectual functioning (intelligence) refers to general mental capacity that involves the ability to learn, reason, problem solve, manipulate information, apply that information, and use it to navigate successfully through various situations, circumstances, and life in general [12].

Definition of Learning Disabilities

Learning disabilities (LD) are described in the literature as (a) a neurological disorder, (b) representing complex groups of functional impairments, (c) a constellation of interdependent symptoms that result in functional impairments, and (d) representing a discrepancy between academic potential and achievement. Learning disabilities occur in the presence of adequate overall intelligence and may be present in youth with low or high intellectual functioning. The term "learning disability" is simply a label [3, 16]. Terminology is sometimes confusing, because the terms "learning disability" and "learning disorder" are often used interchangeably in the literature and share an acronym (LD). Learning disorder is often described in the literature as a group of "disorders," and both learning disorder and learning disability require a difference between academic ability and performance. These shared factors add to the confusion [10]. Learning disability is a medical and academic term, while learning disorder is a mental health term.

Learning disability is defined by the federal law entitled IDEA (Individuals with Disabilities Education Improvement Act of 2004) [17] as a "…. group of disorders in one or more basic psychological processes involved in understanding or in using language, spoken or written that may manifest itself in an imperfect ability to listen, think, speak, read, write, spell or to do mathematical calculations, including conditions such as perceptual disabilities, brain injury, minimal brain dysfunction, dyslexia, and developmental aphasia…" [3, 10, 16, 18, 19]. The term does not include learning problems that are primarily the result of visual, hearing, or motor disabilities, of mental retardation, of emotional disturbance, or of environmental, cultural, or economic disadvantage [14, 16]. Other definitions by organizations that work to help individuals with learning disabilities also use the word "disorder" to define and describe the term "learning disability" [10, 17, 19, 20]. Internationally it is also confusing, because in the United Kingdom, for example, learning disability is used as the term for intellectual disability.

Types of Learning Disabilities

Reading

Reading involves several components, such as the basic skills needed to read, the ability to read accurately, comprehension of the material read, and the ability to understand as well as use the information that is read [7, 11, 19]. Impaired reading ability can result in substantially lower reading performance than is expected for the individual's age, intelligence, and educational levels. Impairment that severely interferes with a person's academic achievement, resulting in performance deficits (poor phonological processing or word recognition), may be diagnosed as a reading disability (formerly called dyslexia) [11, 16, 21–23].

Language

Language (spoken or written) includes expression and comprehension skills as represented by the ability to (a) understand language or use words to decode and synthesize information, and to apply that information to learning and performance skills (receptive and expressive); (b) read or discriminate the meanings and use of words, and understand those words in sentences, apply that knowledge to paragraphs, stories, and other texts (oral or written); and (c) understand the semantic differences and syntax (word order), learn new words, and use expressive language to communicate effectively with others. Disabilities in language skills can result in frustration, stress, failed interpersonal relationships, and academic problems (i.e., reading, writing, and spelling). Impairments in oral language should be screened to detect potential learning problems [16, 21, 24].

Written Expression

Written expression is significantly affected by the individual's reading and language skills. Issues with writing ability can result in problems with spelling, understanding syntax or sequence of language, decoding language, or composing grammatically correct sentences in written documents [5, 16, 21].

Mathematics

Mathematics skills include calculation; reasoning; understanding or naming mathematical terms, operations, or concepts; decoding or recognizing mathematical symbols or signs; copying numbers or figures; following sequences of mathematical steps (counting; strategic counting or memorizing and recalling multiplication tables, comparisons); concepts such as magnitude comparisons; fluency in estimating; the ability to recognize unreasonable results; flexibility when mentally computing; and the ability to move among different number representations and use the most effective representation. Impairments in mathematical functioning are easily caused by mild to severe deficits in the other functional domains [1, 4, 9, 11, 19, 20, 25].

Etiologic Concepts

Although the specific causes of deficits in learning, cognition, and attention are not known, current research indicates that etiology is diverse as well as complex and typically directed toward the roles of genetic factors, neuroanatomy, neurotransmitters, and the association between neurological and familial–hereditary factors. Evidence suggests that most learning disabilities do not stem from a single, specific area of the brain but from difficulties in coordinating information from various brain regions and their interconnections [8]. Some scientists believe that disturbances begin before birth and include effects of the following: errors in fetal brain development; genetic factors; maternal tobacco, alcohol, and other drug use (such as cocaine); complications during pregnancy or delivery; toxins in the child's environment (such as exposure to cadmium); chemotherapy; or radiation [8]. Adolescents who have experienced normal development transition through the complex process of maturation while attaining mastery and integration of learning, cognition, and attention by late adolescence [1, 2].

Epidemiology

Research notes that two-fifths of youth in the United States have learning disabilities [2]. Five of every 100 students in the United States are diagnosed with learning disabilities and this number predominately affects males [19]. Of the children who have learning disabilities, a significant number also have reading problems, 50% have math deficits, and 75% have social skills deficits [10, 19]. Specific reading disability is common, with up to 17.5% of all children being affected [20].

Diagnosis

The mnemonic IDEA prescribes a specific evaluation procedure and criteria for diagnosing learning disabilities [10]. A child has learning disabilities if he/she has been provided with learning experiences appropriate for age and ability level, has been evaluated via observation by a qualified professional, and is found to have a severe discrepancy between achievement and intellectual ability in one or more of the following areas: oral or written expression of language, listening, comprehension, basic reading skill, reading comprehension, mathematics calculation, and/or mathematics reasoning [10, 16, 20, 26]. The impairments in learning must be significant and be the primary cause of problems in functioning, even in the presence of other disabilities (i.e., physical, mental, behavioral). Significance is defined as standard scores on achievement tests that are more than two standard deviations below scores obtained in intelligence tests. However, the concept of IDEA mandates that the scores on standardized tests and difference between those scores and performance cannot be the only factors considered by Individual Educational Planning Committees (IEPC) [11, 19, 17, 26].

Diagnosing learning disabilities is often difficult. Some impairments are subtle and not readily apparent; however, in combination with other disabilities or disorders, they have a synergistic effect on an individual's functional ability to learn at a developmentally and age-appropriate level [11, 20, 26]. Special education services in most states in the United States use IDEA rules to govern provision of early intervention, special education, and related services [16]. Public agencies must use the state criteria in determining whether a child has a specific learning disability [20]. This determination is carried out by a multidisciplinary team.

Differential Diagnosis

IDEA mandates that the term "learning disability" does not include learning problems that are primarily the result of visual, hearing, or motor disabilities, mental retardation, emotional disturbance, or of environmental, cultural, or economic disadvantage [3, 11, 26]. Some associated problems include cognitive processing deficits, co-morbid mental disorders, general medical conditions, or the individual's ethnic or cultural background. The presence of a sensory deficit does not preclude diagnosis if the learning problems are in excess of those usually associated with the deficit.

Distinction between a learning disability and attention-deficit hyperactivity disorder (ADHD) is often difficult because of overlapping features and these two disorders often co-exist because of similar neurobehavioral and genetic traits. In

Table 10.3 Differential diagnosis of learning disabilities

Attention-deficit hyperactivity disorder (ADHD)
Normal academic variation in attainment
Impairment in vision and hearing or motor skills
Mental retardation
Emotional disturbance
Cultural factors
Environmental or economic disadvantage
Limited English proficiency
Pervasive developmental disorders
Chromosomal anomalies/genetic disorders
Neurological disorders
Congenital malformations
Inborn errors in metabolism
Developmental disorders
Severe toxic exposure
Chronic mental illness
Severe infectious illness
Chronic disease
Side effects of medication used to treat other conditions
Psycho-emotional trauma
Psychological trauma

addition, children diagnosed with learning disabilities show higher rates of anxiety. Youth with learning disabilities, by contrast, characteristically demonstrate phonologic, logic, and language problems not seen in children with anxiety disorders (see Table 10.3) [10, 12, 17].

Co-morbidity

Children and adolescents with learning disabilities can manifest problems in attention, communication, language, behavior, emotions, self-confidence, adjustment, inappropriate social behavior, and poor social skills [19].

Assessment

IDEA mandates that the evaluating agency must obtain parental consent to evaluate the child to determine if the child needs special education and related services, and must adhere to prescribed timeframes (unless extended by mutual written agreement of the child's parents and a group of qualified professionals). The assessment must include a pre-referral documented observation of the child's or adolescent's academic performance and behavior (in the areas of impairment) in his or her learning environment (i.e., classroom setting or for children of preschool age in an environment appropriate for a child of that age) [10, 15, 17, 26]. The child's or adolescent's medical home professional should be included in this pre-referral data gathering and that information included in the documentation.

The physician or the medical home professional should also conduct a comprehensive assessment that begins with a physical examination (including neurological screening and mental status exams) and obtain the following histories: medical, psychosocial, family demographics, academic, substance use/abuse, violence exposure, mental health, abuse, and neglect. Data on familial history of mental illness, substance use/abuse, physical or sexual abuse, domestic violence, child abuse/neglect, and incarceration are also essential to seek in this comprehensive assessment.

Behavioral observation is an important tool as well. At the very least, the child should be observed at school in several different activities or classes and in the physician's or psychologist's office. Ideally, home observations should also be scheduled. This data gathering should include three additional types of information: (a) the onset, frequency, duration, and intensity of problem issues or behaviors; (b) anecdotal information (parental and teacher observations); and (c) school records in addition to teacher observations. Evidence of deficits in any of the functional domains that impede optimal learning warrants a referral to a "qualified professional" [19, 17, 26].

Multidisciplinary Assessment Team

IDEA mandates that a group of "qualified professionals" be convened to evaluate an individual who has met its mandates to receive a special education service evaluation. Assessment teams include the child's parents, the child or the adolescent, and a group of qualified professionals. According to the IDEA, the team of qualified professionals must include the following:

- The child's regular teacher (if there is no "regular teacher," a regular classroom teacher qualified to teach a child of his or her age; or for a child of less than school age, an individual qualified by the state educational agency (SEA) to teach a child of his or her age).
- At least one person qualified to conduct individual diagnostic examinations of children, such as a school psychologist, a speech–language pathologist, or a remedial reading teacher [11, 26].

School districts have strict guidelines for inclusion created by the federal Education for All Handicapped Children Act, or as it was renamed, the IDEA (PL 94–142) [17]. Youth who meet criteria for a learning disability are mandated to receive special accommodation services in the school. Multidisciplinary teams (comprised of educators, school psychologists and social workers, the involved parents, speech therapists, occupational therapists, and other specialists) are mandated by IDEA to evaluate eligibility for special education services or special accommodation in the school [10, 15, 19].

The multidisciplinary assessment team is charged with providing documentation to prove that the underachievement is not due to lack of appropriate instruction in reading or math. The group must consider documentation demonstrating that prior to a referral for evaluation, the child has received appropriate instruction in regular education settings delivered by qualified personnel and that repeated assessments of achievement at reasonable intervals, reflecting formal assessment of student's progress during instruction, were provided to the child's parents [11, 26]. Assessment must be based on the child's responses to standardized and alternative scientific research-based interventions.

The relevant qualified professionals may include any of the following, depending on the functional impairments of the individual patient and relevant state guidelines: teachers (classroom, reading, etc.) and psychologists (school, clinical, child, developmental, neuro-psychologist, occupational therapists, speech pathologists/audiologists, physical therapists, social worker, or other qualified persons). Psychologists can conduct assessments that are especially useful for detecting multiple deficits which cause impairments with outcomes that are specifically related to learning. Recommendations are made to the patient's school; the physician can ask that the school consider convening an Individual Educational Planning Committee.

Treatment

Treatment includes a range of adjunctive aides to facilitate the individual's ability to function successfully and master all age- and grade-appropriate skills in each domain of function (see Table 10.4) [1, 9, 11, 23, 24, 27]. Psycho-pharmacological interventions are discussed in other chapters. Interventions for strengthening abilities and minimizing disabilities for youth with learning disabilities change from early childhood (i.e., remediating deficits, minimizing or eliminating negative impact of impairments) to adolescence (i.e., accommodation designed to minimize impairments and maximize strengths) to young adulthood (i.e., accommodation to maximize performance) [10, 27].

Management

Management of learning disabilities is based on various educational interventions [11]. The educational system generally welcomes physician input and support. By providing updates on medications or medical conditions (with parental consent), physicians can better prepare educators to meet the needs of the child, the adolescent, or the young adult. IDEA describes the physician's role as a qualified professional who can diagnose and evaluate the disability [19].

Outcomes

Learning disabilities are not cured, but accommodations can be made; learning impairments can be eliminated in some cases and minimized in others. As a child matures, he or she will have the greatest chance of being successful if given early,

Table 10.4 Tools to assist youth who have learning disabilities

---

Skills enhancement
Teaching higher order thinking skills employing some of the tools listed in Table 10.3
Problem-solving skills courses
Vocabulary comprehension
Critical thinking skills
Intensive direct instructional courses
Reading classes
Tutoring

Interventions that enhance communication and performance skills
Written directions
Cue cards
Job aides (visual stepwise cues that instruct how to perform a task or job coaches who model
each step of a task to complete a job function)
Administer instructions and tests orally (audio recording and/or job coach)
Allowing alternative communication tools (use of typewriters or computers)
Placeholders for eye tracking problems
Untimed tests
Repetition of new and old materials
Breaking information into smaller chunks

Distraction techniques
Playing music
Allowing youth to move or manipulate, hold or squeeze a soft object while reading or listening
to oral information
Memory joggers

---

consistent, effective, and lifelong treatment. Children who are forced to grow up in the absence of effective continuous treatment may develop symptoms severe enough that impairments escalate into the diagnosis of specific disorders [11].

Conclusions

Children and youth who present with impairments in learning benefit from early detection, intervention, and support if they are to navigate the maturational process successfully. Early intervention improves outcomes for the majority of children with learning disabilities. Early and continuous supportive interventions can even be effective with individuals who have severe learning disabilities [28]. Delayed detection often results in greater problems in academic, social, emotional, and psychological functioning, and can even result in a child or an adolescent dropping out of school. Most researchers agree that learning disabilities are enduring. Parental attitudes and commitment, availability of resources, and the presence of associated neurological deficit or medical disorder can also significantly impact outcomes. However, with support and appropriate intervention (designed according to individual instructional requirements), affected youth can develop the ability to compensate or master appropriate coping mechanisms that allow them to function effectively in the world and greatly minimize the overall negative outcomes of learning disabilities [22].

The physician plays a critical role in the detection, identification, referral, and management of youth who present with symptoms of learning disabilities. The severity of the child's problems and the impact those impairments have on the individual's functioning at school determine if that individual is eligible for services through the school system. When youth do not qualify for special education or special accommodation services, the physician can assist the families by providing referral to community professionals who can evaluate the student's functional impairments. The type and specificity of the referral questions governs the type of assessments the community professional will conduct.

References

1. Pratt HD, Greydanus DE. Learning disabilities. In: Greydanus DE, Patel DR, Pratt HD, Calles JL, editors. Behavioral pediatrics. 3rd ed. New York, NY: Nova Science; 2009. pp. 51–60.
2. Pratt HD, Patel DR, Greydanus DE. Sports and the neurodevelopment of the child and adolescent. In: Delee JC, Drez DD, Miller MD, editors. Orthopaedic sports medicine. 2nd ed. Philadelphia, PA: WB Saunders; 2002. pp. 624–43.
3. Herr CM, Bateman BD. Learning disabilities and the law. In: Swanson HE, Harris KR, Graham W, editors. Handbook of learning disabilities. New York, NY: Guilford; 2003. pp. 57–75.
4. Butterworth B. The development of arithmetical abilities. J Child Psychol Psychiatr. 2005;46:3–18.
5. Katusic SK, Colligan RC, Weaver AL, Barbaresi WJ. The forgotten learning disability: epidemiology of written-language disorder in a population-based birth cohort (1976–1982), Rochester, Minnesota. Pediatrics. 2009;123:1306–13.
6. National Joint Committee on Learning Disabilities website. 2010. Accessed 1 Aug 2010. http://www.ncld.org/resources1/njcld-position-papers
7. Shelley-Tremblay J, O'Brien N, Langhinrichsen-Rohling J. Reading disability in adjudicated youth: prevalence rates, current models, traditional and innovative treatments. Aggress Violent Behav. 2007;12:376–92.
8. Patel DR, Greydanus DE, Calles JL Jr, Pratt HD. Developmental disabilities across the lifespan. Dis Mon. 2010;56(6):299–398.
9. Metfessel NS, Michael WB, Kirsner DA. Instrumentation of Bloom's & Krathwohl's taxonomies for writing of educational objectives. Psychol Sch. 1969;6:227–31.
10. World Health Organization. The International Classification of Functioning, Disability and Health (ICF). 2010. http://www.who.int/en/. Accessed 1 Aug 2010.
11. US Department of Education, Office of Special Education Programs' (OSEP's) website, 2010.
12. Pratt HD. Neurodevelopmental issues in the assessment and treatment of deficits in attention, cognition, and learning during adolescence. Adolesc Med State Art Rev. 2002;13(3):579–98.
13. Seidman LJ, Biederman J, Monuteaux MC, Doyle AE, Faraone SV:. Learning disabilities and executive dysfunction in boys with attention-deficit/hyperactivity disorder. Neuropsychology. 2001;15(4):544–56.
14. The American with Disabilities Act. 2010. http://www.ada.gov. Accessed 1 Aug 2010.
15. American Association of Intellectual and Developmental Disabilities (AAIDD). 2010. Definition of intellectual disability. http://www.aamr.org/content_100.cfm?navID=21. Accessed 1 Aug 2010.
16. National Joint Committee on Learning Disabilities. The NJCLD Definition of LD. 2010. http://www.ncld.org/resources1/njcld-position-papers. Accessed 1 Aug 2010.

17. The Individuals with Disabilities Education Improvement Act of 2004. 2010. 20 USC 1400 HR 1350 PL 108-446. http://idea.ed.gov. Accessed 1 Aug 2010.
18. American Psychiatric Association. Diagnostic and statistical manual of mental disorders. 4th ed. Text rev. Washington, DC: APA; 2000. pp. 39–84.
19. American Academy of Pediatrics. Council on children with disabilities. Provision of educationally related services for children and adolescents with chronic diseases and disabling conditions policy statement. Identification of specific learning disabilities. Pediatrics. 2007;119(6):1218–23.
20. Horowitz SH Identifying math learning disabilities early. National Center for Learning Disabilities (NCLD), 2007. http://www.ncld.org/ld-basics/ld-aamp-language/ld-aamp-math/identifying-math-learning-disabilities-early. Accessed 1 Aug 2010.
21. American Speech–Language–Hearing Association. Language-based learning disabilities Website. Rockville, MD. http://www.asha.org/public/speech/disorders/LBLD.htm#one. Accessed 1 Aug 2010.
22. Shaywitz SE, Shaywitz BA. Dyslexia (specific reading disability). Biol Psychiatry. 2005;57:1301–9.
23. Goldston DB, Walsh A, Arnold EM, Reboussin B, Daniel SS, Erkanli A, et al. Reading problems, psychiatric disorders, and functional impairment from mid- to late adolescence. J Am Acad Child Adolesc Psychiatry. 2007;46:25–32.
24. American Speech–Language–Hearing Association Early Identification of Speech–Language Delays and Disorders. 2010. Learning disabilities online 2000. http://www.ldonline.org/article/Early_Identification_of_Speech-Language_Delays_and_Disorders. Accessed 1 Aug 2010.
25. Shalev RS, Gross-Tsur V. Developmental dyscalculia. Pediatr Neurol. 2001;24:334–42.
26. US Department of Education Office of Special Education and Rehabilitative Services (OSERS). 2010. Identification of specific learning disabilities. Washington DC: US Department of Education, Office of Special Education Programs. http://idea.ed.gov/explore/view/p/%2Croot%2Cdynamic%2CTopicalBrief%2C23%2C. Accessed 1 Aug 2010.
27. Wilder R, Williams JP. Students with severe learning disabilities can learn higher order comprehension skills. J Educ Psychol. 2001;93(2):268–79.
28. American Association of Intellectual and Developmental Disabilities. 2010. Intellectual disability: Definition, classification, and systems of supports. Washington, DC: American Association of Intellectual and Developmental Disabilities.

Chapter 11
Intellectual Disability

Dilip R. Patel and Joav Merrick

Abstract Intellectual disability is characterized by deficits in cognitive and adaptive abilities that initially manifest before 18 years of age. In the United States, the prevalence of intellectual disability is estimated to be between 1 and 3 out of every 100 individuals in the general population. Most individuals have mild intellectual disability and the cause is generally not identified. A small percentage of individuals have severe deficits and will need lifetime supports. The diagnosis of intellectual disability requires formal psychometric testing to assess the intelligence quotient and adaptive functioning. The management of individuals who have intellectual disability is based on providing general medical care, treatment of specific behavioral symptoms, early intervention, special education, and variable degrees of community-based supports.

Introduction

Intellectual disability is now a more internationally accepted term used to describe deficits in cognitive and adaptive functioning. The term cognitive–adaptive disability is also used by some authors in this context. The evolution of the terminology from idiocy to mental retardation to intellectual disability is a reflection of a better understanding of the concept of cognition and cognitive deficits within the scientific and sociocultural contexts. Although intellectual disability is initially identified in infancy and early childhood years, it has lifelong implications for growth and development, education, ability to live independently, health care, finding employment, and need for community-based supports. In the United States, various Federal and State laws provide the framework and funding for intervention services, educational services, and other support services for individuals who have intellectual disability.

D.R. Patel (✉)
Department of Pediatrics and Human Development, Kalamazoo Center for Medical Studies, Michigan State University College of Human Medicine, Kalamazoo, MI 49008-1284, USA
e-mail: patel@kcms.msu.edu

D.R. Patel et al. (eds.), *Neurodevelopmental Disabilities*,
DOI 10.1007/978-94-007-0627-9_11, © Springer Science+Business Media B.V. 2011

In addition to medical evaluation and management, the physician plays a vital role in facilitating and coordinating the overall long-term management for individuals who have intellectual disability. This chapter reviews the definition, epidemiology, clinical features, diagnosis, and treatment of intellectual disability.

Definition

According to the American Association on Intellectual and Developmental Disabilities (AAIDD), intellectual disability "is a disability characterized by significant limitations both in intellectual functioning and in adaptive behavior as expressed in conceptual, social, and practical adaptive skills" [1]. The assessment of intellectual functioning and adaptive behavior must take into consideration the expectations based on individual's age and culture. The influence of sensory, motor, communication, or behavioral factors on cognitive assessment should also be appropriately considered in administration of assessment instruments and interpretation of their results.

In the United States, a widely used definition is the one from the Individuals with Disabilities Education Act that defines intellectual disability as "significantly sub-average general intellectual functioning, existing concurrently with deficits in adaptive behavior and manifested during the developmental period that adversely affects a child's educational performance."

According to the Diagnostic and Statistical Manual of Mental Disorders [2], intellectual disability (or mental retardation) is defined as an intelligence quotient (IQ) of approximately 70 or below on an individually administered standardized test of intelligence concurrent with deficits in adaptive functioning in two of the following areas: communication, self-care, home living, social or interpersonal skills, use of community resources, self-direction, functional academic skills, work, leisure, health, and safety. All definitions stipulate that the onset of disability must occur before the age of 18 years.

It is generally agreed that, although not perfect, appropriately measured IQ provides the best estimate of intellectual functioning. Based on the mean value for IQ of 100, the upper limit of 70 as the cutoff represents the value that is two standard deviations below the mean. Because there is a five-point standard error of measurement, it is argued that a range of 70–75 should be considered as the upper limit of IQ as the cutoff value for intellectual disability. Based on the typical bell-shaped curve of distribution of IQ scores, raising the IQ score from 70 to 75 as the upper limit of cutoff will double the number of individuals with intellectual disability from 2.27 to 4.85%. An individual with an IQ score of 75 with significant adaptive disability will be considered to have intellectual disability, whereas an individual with no adaptive disability and an IQ score of 65 may not be considered to have intellectual disability.

The severity of intellectual disability is further categorized based on intellectual functioning, adaptive functioning, and intensity of supports needed (see Table 11.1) [1]. When the severity of intellectual disability cannot be reliably assessed, but there is a high level of confidence based on clinical judgment, a diagnosis of intellectual disability is made without specifying the severity.

Table 11.1 Classification of intellectual disability severity [2]

Severity level	Percent of individuals who have intellectual disability	Intelligence quotient range	Intensity of supports needed in daily living activities such as school, work, or home
Mild	85	From 50–55 to 70	Intermittent: support on as needed basis, episodic or short term
Moderate	10	From 35–49 to 50–55	Limited: consistent over time, but time limited
Severe	4	From 20–25 to 35–40	Extensive: regular, consistent, lifetime support. Regular support in at least one aspect such as school, work, or home
Profound	1	Less than 20–25	Pervasive: high intensity, across all environments, lifetime, and potentially life sustaining

Based on American Psychiatric Association. DSM-IV-TR, 2000; American Association of Intellectual and Developmental Disabilities. Mental Retardation, 2002.

Epidemiology

The reported prevalence of intellectual disability reflects consideration of the definition used, method of ascertainment of the data, and the characteristics of the population studied. Based on the typical bell-shaped distribution of intelligence in the general population and two standard deviations below the mean as a cutoff point, approximately 2.5% of the population is expected to have intellectual disability. Most epidemiological studies consider those with an IQ score of 50 or less as having severe and those above that as having mild intellectual disability. Eighty-five percent of individuals with intellectual disability have mild intellectual disability. The prevalence of severe intellectual disability has remained the same over several decades at 0.3–0.5% of the population in the United States. Based on the United States National Center for Health Statistics 1997–2003 National Health Interview Survey, the prevalence of intellectual disability among children aged 5–17 years is estimated to be 7.5 per 1,000.

Intellectual disability is reported to be twice as common in males compared to females. The recurrence risk of intellectual disability in families with one previous child with severe intellectual disability is reported to be between 3 and 9%.

Mild intellectual disability is associated predominantly with environmental risk factors and a specific etiology can be identified in less than half of affected individuals. On the other hand, underlying biological or neurological etiology can be identified in more than two-thirds of affected individuals who have severe disability. The most common identified conditions in children with severe intellectual disability include chromosomal disorders, genetic syndromes, congenital brain malformations, neurodegenerative diseases, congenital infections, inborn errors of metabolism, and birth injury.

Clinical Features

Children who have intellectual disability can present with a wide range of initial clinical symptoms and signs depending up on the underlying cause and severity of the disability [3–8]. Children who have severe intellectual disability generally present early and with clinical features of underlying condition. Children with mild intellectual disability generally do not have underlying identifiable etiology and present with developmental delay or behavioral symptoms and are identified relatively later. Common presentations of intellectual disability by age are summarized in Table 11.2. The age at which intellectual disability can be recognized depends on its severity (see Table 11.3).

Other mental disorders (see Table 11.4) are three to four times more common in children with intellectual disability compared to those that do not have intellectual disability [9]. Children may present with behavioral symptoms of these disorders in addition to intellectual disability. In these children a dual diagnosis of intellectual disability and co-morbid mental disorder should be made if criteria for both are met.

Table 11.2 Common presentations of intellectual disability (a) by age [6]

Age	Area of concern
Newborn	Dysmorphic syndromes, microcephaly
	Major organ system dysfunction (e.g., feeding and breathing)
Early infancy (2–4 months)	Failure to interact with the environment
	Concern about vision and hearing impairments
Later infancy (6–18 months)	Gross motor delay
Toddlers (2–3 years)	Language delays or difficulties
Pre-school (3–5 years)	Language difficulties or delays
	Behavioral difficulty, including play
	Delays in fine motor skills: cutting, coloring, drawing
School age (older than 5 years)	Academic underachievement
	Behavior difficulties (attention, anxiety, mood, conduct, and so on)

Used with permission from Shapiro and Batshaw [6], table 38-4, p. 193.
[a]The word mental retardation from source is replaced with intellectual disability.

Table 11.3 Age at recognition of intellectual disability

Severity of intellectual disability	Most likely age at recognition
Mild	$\geq$5–6 years
Moderate	3–5 years
Severe	$\leq$3 years
Profound	$\leq$2 years

Table 11.4 Conditions
co-morbid with intellectual
disability

Mental disorders
- Attention-deficit/hyperactivity disorder
- Mood disorders
- Pervasive developmental disorders
- Stereotypic movement disorder
- Anxiety disorders
- Obsessive compulsive disorder

Medical conditions
- Seizure disorders
- Hearing impairments
- Vision impairments
- Motor impairments
- Obesity
- Type 2 diabetes mellitus
- Gastroesophageal reflux disease

Behavioral symptoms
- Self-injurious behaviors
- Aggression
- Self-induced vomiting
- Sleep disturbances
- Challenging behavior

Diagnosis

Diagnosis is suspected based on the presenting symptoms. Next step is to obtain additional history (see Table 11.5) followed by a complete general physical examination, dysmorphology examination, and neurological examination. By definition, a diagnosis of intellectual disability requires individualized cognitive and adaptive testing by qualified examiners using standardized instruments (see Table 11.6). Standardized testing should be age appropriate, take into account mental age of the child, and culturally sensitive. Appropriate accommodations should be made for any motor, behavioral, or language variations. A workup should include complete audiological and vision evaluation in all children [3–8].

Table 11.5 Key elements of history

Details of presenting symptoms
- Onset, duration, progression, severity of symptoms
- Current level of development and functioning as reported by parents or caregivers

Prenatal
- Mother's and father's age at birth of the child
- Nature of prenatal care
- Previous pregnancies: number, term, preterm, abortions, living
- Multiple gestations
- Maternal weight gain
- Fetal activity

Table 11.5 (continued)

- Maternal medical and obstetric complications
- Use of medications, drugs of abuse, alcohol, tobacco, radiation exposure
- Prenatal maternal infections

Perinatal
- Hospital or home delivery details
- Length of gestation
- Labor: spontaneous delivery, induced, vaginal, forceps, cesarean section
- Intrapartum monitoring, use of analgesia or anesthesia (epidural)
- Prolapse cord, breech, polyhydramnios, oligohydramnios, prolonged rupture of membranes
- Maternal fever, toxemia, abnormal bleeding, abnormalities of placenta
- Meconium or foul-smelling amniotic fluid

Neonatal
- Birth weight, height, head circumference
- Dubowitz score, small or large of gestational age
- Apgar scores, any resuscitation
- Duration of nursery stay
- Respiratory distress, assisted ventilation, apnea, seizures, sepsis, jaundice
- Blood type, Coombs
- Congenital anomalies, feeding problems
- Brain imaging, laboratory testing

Developmental
- Time and nature of initial parental concerns about development
- Any previous developmental evaluations
- Specific developmental diagnosis if any and at what age
- Early major milestone attainment

Medical/surgical
- Major illnesses or surgeries
- Injuries and hospitalizations
- Procedures or investigations

Family history
- Fetal wastage
- Unexplained infant or childhood deaths
- Parental and sibling health
- Medical conditions in family members: congenital, genetic, neurological, psychiatric, learning disorders, intellectual disability, speech and language disorders

Personal/social history
- Parent occupation, socioeconomic status, level of education
- Primary caregiver, living situation, school functioning
- Any current services or therapies, early intervention or other special health services
- Extracurricular activities, family adjustment, school adjustment
- Use of medications

Review of systems
- Guided by presenting symptoms

Table 11.6 Selected standardized instruments

Instrument	Age range
Measures of cognitive abilities	
Bayley Scales of Infant Development III	1–42 mo
Wechsler Pre-School and Primary Scale of Intelligence	2 y 6 mo–7 y 3 mo
McCarthy Scales of Children' Abilities	2 y 6 mo–8 y 6 mo
Stanford-Binet Intelligence Scale (5th edition)	2–85 y
Wechsler Intelligence Scale for Children (WISC-IV)	6–12 y
Leiter International Performance Scale-Revised (Leiter-R)	2–21 y
Measures of adaptive abilities	
Vineland Adaptive Behavior Scale II (VBAS II)	Birth to 19 y
Adaptive Behavior Scales II (ABAS II)	Birth to 89 y
Scales of Independent Behavior-Revised (SIB-R)	Birth to 80 y
AAMR Adaptive Behavior Scales (ABS)	3–21 y

There is no consensus regarding the need to establish an etiological diagnosis in all children who have intellectual disability. Parents or other caregivers are also divided in their need to know the cause of intellectual disability in their child. Factors that might guide the decision to pursue etiological diagnosis are summarized in Table 11.7 and some reasons offered by those who favor such an approach are summarized in Table 11.8.

In the absence of well-defined clinical symptoms and signs, an extensive workup that includes genetic testing, neuroimaging, and metabolic testing is needed to

Table 11.7 Factors that may guide decision to pursue etiological diagnosis

Severity of intellectual disability
- Biologic cause can be found in 75% of individuals with severe intellectual disability

Presence or absence of disease-specific symptoms and signs
- Disease-specific features may indicate which tests to order

Parental decision as to future pregnancy
- If more children are planned, a prenatal diagnosis and early appropriate intervention may be planned

Parental desire to know the cause of intellectual disability
- Varies. Some may want to know so that specific disease may be treated if treatment is available. Others may want to focus on services

Table 11.8 Reasons offered in support of pursuing an etiological diagnosis

Associated complications can be anticipated
Specific cause may be treatable
Aid in the development of prevention strategies
Research is facilitated
Intervention can be planned for anticipated behavioral symptoms
Genetic counseling can be provided
Helps in long-term life planning

Table 11.9 Differential
diagnosis

Developmental language disorders
Borderline intellectual functioning (IQ 71–84)
Pervasive developmental disorders
Hearing impairment
Visual impairment
Environmental deprivation
Dementia (rare)
Schizophrenia (rare)

search for potential cause of intellectual disability. Such an extensive workup should preferably be undertaken in consultation with specialists with expertise in this field. The yield of these tests in identifying a cause varies depending upon the presence or the absence of associated symptoms and signs. Newborn screening programs generally identify major inborn errors of metabolism and the yield of metabolic testing done later in infancy and childhood is reported to be ≤1%. The yield of neuroimaging in detecting brain abnormality ranges from 33 to 63%. Abnormal findings on neuroimaging may or may not help in establishing a cause of intellectual disability. The yield of genetic testing in identifying a specific genetic condition ranges from 2 to 7%.

In children who have intellectual disability, the predominant deficits are noted in cognitive abilities and language. Their social development is consistent with their mental age and generally there are no motor deficits. Children who have developmental language disorders or specific language impairments have predominant deficits in various aspects of language development, whereas their social, motor, and cognitive development progresses typically. Children who have pervasive developmental disorders have predominant deficits in social and language or communication domains, whereas their motor development is typical. In children who present with symptoms suggestive of intellectual disability, hearing and vision impairments should be ruled out. Conditions to be considered in the differential diagnosis of intellectual disability are listed in Table 11.9.

Treatment

Children who have intellectual disability are best managed by an interdisciplinary team approach in the setting of a medical home [10]. The physician should provide the general medical care similar to all children including preventive care according to established guidelines. Specific health maintenance guidelines are published by the American Academy of Pediatrics for several conditions (e.g., Down syndrome) associated with intellectual disability and can be accessed at www.aap.org.

The behavioral symptoms and co-morbid conditions seen in children and adolescents who have intellectual disability are managed most commonly by behavioral approaches. In select cases, psychotropic medications are used. Depending upon the personal expertise of the child's physician, this should preferably be done in consultation with a child psychiatrist. Various psychotropic medications used to manage behavioral symptoms include stimulants, antidepressants, mood stabilizers, and antipsychotics.

The physician should refer the child to community-based agencies and programs for appropriate intervention services primarily depending on the age of the child. The physician should have ongoing communication with local agencies that provide such intervention services to the child and should facilitate and coordinate needed medical evaluations and specialist consultations.

In the United States, several Federal and State laws provide the framework and funding for intervention programs and educational services for children with developmental disabilities including those who have intellectual disabilities. The mainstay of overall management of young children (younger than 3 years of age) who have intellectual disability is early intervention services provided by local community agencies through the development and implementation of the individualized family service plan. For children and adolescents between the ages 3 and 16 years, the main focus is on educational interventions, including special education, developed and implemented by the student's school district. This is called the individualized education plan or the IEP. An individualized transition plan is developed between 14 and 16 years of age that addresses the student's transition to adult services, vocational training, and independent living. After the completion of the high school, the individual is supported by the individualized habilitation (support)

Table 11.10 Severity of intellectual disability and adult age functioning [6]

Level	Mental age as adult	Adult adaptation
Mild	9–11 y	Reads at 4–5th grade level; simple multiplications/divisions; writes simple letters, lists; completes job application; basic independent job skills (arrive on time, stay at task, interact with co-workers); uses public transportation; may qualify for recipes
Moderate	6–8 y	Sight-word reading; copies information, e.g., address from card to job application; matches written number to number of items; recognizes time on clock; communicates; some independence in self-care; housekeeping with supervision or cue cards; meal preparation, can follow picture recipe cards; job skills learned with much repetition; uses public transportation with some supervision
Severe	3–5 y	Needs continuous support and supervision; may communicate wants and needs, sometimes with augmentative communication techniques
Profound	Less than 3 y	Limitations of self-care, continence, communication, and mobility; may need complete custodial or nursing care

Used with permission from Shapiro and Batshaw [6], table 38-6, p. 197.

plan that provides adult support services. The intensity of support services needed depends upon the severity of intellectual disability (see Table 11.1). The adult outcomes and functioning of individuals with intellectual disability are summarized in Table 11.10 [11].

Conclusions

Intellectual disability is defined as significant limitations in cognitive functioning characterized by an intelligence quotient of about 70 or below and concurrent deficits in adaptive functioning. The severity is classified as mild, moderate, severe, and profound, based on the IQ scores and the intensity of supports needed. Eighty-five percent of individuals who have intellectual disability have mild deficits. Environmental factors are predominant risk factors for mild intellectual disability, whereas biologic factors are predominant risk factors for severe intellectual disability. The age at initial presentation depends upon the severity of the deficits. Intellectual deficits can be identified in most children by 3–5 years of age. The diagnosis is based on clinical evaluation and psychometric testing for cognitive and adaptive functioning. The need to search for the cause of intellectual disability in all cases is debatable. The main strategies for management of individuals who have intellectual disability are general medical care, treatment of co-morbid conditions, treatment of behavioral symptoms, special education, vocational training, and community-based supports.

Acknowledgments This chapter is adapted with permission from Patel and Merrick [12].

References

1. Schalock RL, Borthwick-Duffy SA, Buntinx WHE, Coulter DL, editors. Intellectual disability: definition, classification, and systems of supports. 11th ed. Washington, DC: AAIDD; 2009.
2. American Psychiatric Association. Diagnostic and statistical manual of mental disorders. 4th ed. Text rev. Washington, DC: American Psychiatric Association; 2000. pp. 41–8.
3. Curry CJ, Stevenson RE, Anghton D, et al. Evaluation of mental retardation: recommendations of a consensus conference. American College of Medical Genetics. Am J Med Genet. 1997;72:468–77.
4. Moeschler JB, Shevell MI, and Committee on Genetics. Clinical genetic evaluation of the child with mental retardation or developmental delays. Pediatrics. 2006;117:2304–16.
5. Pratt HD, Greydanus DE. Intellectual disability (mental retardation) in children and adolescents. Prim Care. 2007;34:375–86.
6. Shapiro BK, Batshaw M. Mental retardation (intellectual disability). In: Kliegman RM, Behrman RE, Jenson HB, Stanton BF, editors. Nelson textbook of pediatrics. 18th ed. Philadelphia, PA: Saunders/Elsevier; 2008. pp. 191–7.
7. Shevell MI, Ashwal S, Donley D, et al. Practice parameter: Evaluation of the child with global developmental delay. Neurology. 2003;60:367–79.
8. VanKarnebeck CDH, Janswiejer MCE, Leenders AGE, et al. Diagnostic investigation in individuals with mental retardation: A systematic literature review of their usefulness. Eur J Human Genet. 2005;13:2–65.

9. Calles JL Jr.. Use of psychotropic medications in children and adolescents with cognitive–adaptive disabilities. Pediatrics Clin North Am. 2008;55(5):1227–40.
10. Rubin IL, Crocker AC, editors. Medical care for children and adults with developmental disabilities. Baltimore, MD: Paul H Brookes; 2006.
11. Kandel I, Schofield P, Merrick J. Aging and disability. Research and clinical perspectives. Victoria, BC: International Academic Press; 2007.
12. Patel DR, Merrick J. Intellectual disability. In: Greydanus DE, Patel DR, Pratt HD, Calles J Jr, editors. Behavioral pediatrics, 3rd ed. New York, NY: Nova Science; 2009.

Chapter 12
Developmental Language Disorders

Nickola Wolf Nelson

Abstract Developmental language disorders can present either as primary or as secondary disorders, depending on whether they occur alone or concurrent with other neurodevelopmental disorders. This chapter outlines classifications, definitions, and clinical features of primary and secondary neurodevelopmental language disorders and provides an overview of approaches to diagnosis and treatment.

Introduction

Children can experience language delays or unusual patterns of language and communication development for a variety of reasons, some associated with known risk factors such as low birth weight, hearing impairment, diagnosable genetic conditions, or chromosomal abnormalities, such as Down syndrome. In other cases, genetic influences are more subtle and not immediately detectable, or nurturing or environmental risk factors are involved, so that risks become apparent only as children fail to develop expected abilities on schedule. The processes of early identification, diagnosis, and treatment require alertness to signs that developmental milestones are not being met. Children with other neurodevelopmental disorders, such as hearing impairment or intellectual disability, often need extra support for language development by virtue of those other difficulties. Some children with comorbid disorders, including children with autism spectrum disorders, present with symptoms of communication impairment as key diagnostic features. When developmental milestones are not met on schedule, regardless of reason, they serve as red flags that specialized assessment and intervention procedures may be needed.

N.W. Nelson (✉)
Department of Speech Pathology and Audiology, PhD Program in Interdisciplinary Health Sciences, Western Michigan University, Kalamazoo, MI 49008-5355, USA
e-mail: nickola.nelson@wmich.edu

D.R. Patel et al. (eds.), *Neurodevelopmental Disabilities*,
DOI 10.1007/978-94-007-0627-9_12, © Springer Science+Business Media B.V. 2011

Some red flags can be detected in early infancy. Danger signs are noted, for example, when infants have difficulty establishing or maintaining eye contact, engaging in reciprocal turn taking, or calming when comforted even though their physical needs appear to have been met and their emotional needs are being addressed. Physicians can play an important role in supporting anxious parents who sense that something is wrong but are losing confidence in their ability to connect with an infant who does not seem to respond to their overtures. Healthy newborns recruit their parents' attention with their eyes, and infants soon learn how to use vocalizations and movements to engage with their parents in reciprocal interactions that are known as "protoconversations." Health-care professionals can refer parents to resources, such as early intervention programs that provide family-centered services for families with infants with developmental risks. Professionals also can reassure parents that, although it is not their fault the infant is struggling, there are things they can do to encourage the child to connect emotionally and communicate interpersonally, for example, by following their child's attentional lead, staying close, continuing to encourage social exchanges, and supporting the child to close communication circles [1].

Some children with risks for language disorder present no obvious risks at birth and establish early social connections with caregivers but are delayed in producing first words. When first words have not appeared by 18 months or when toddlers produce speech that is hard to understand (even by caregivers) and are not producing two-word combinations by 2 years, they should be referred for further assessment. For children developing typically, vocabulary and grammar expand at a remarkable pace during the preschool years. Most children are capable of formulating and comprehending complex sentences by the time they enter kindergarten. They can recount stories about events in their lives (with limited parental support) and maintain attention and ask appropriate questions when someone tells a story or reads a book to them. Children who cannot do these things should be assessed further and may be candidates for language intervention. During the preschool years, parents continue to play an important role in supporting their child's language and communication development and preparing their child to become literate. They can improve their skills for engaging their child in conversation by showing interest in and commenting on their child's focus of attention, modeling language that is only a bit beyond the child's current level, and helping their child construct associations between symbolic language, experiences, and concepts in play, everyday living activities, and books.

Some children appear to develop normally during the preschool years but experience exaggerated difficulty when they enter school and begin formal education in reading and writing. Such children may be showing risks for learning disabilities, which involve difficulty making automatic and easily retrievable connections between spoken and written language. For example, many children who later are identified as having specific reading impairment (also called dyslexia) have difficulty hearing individual sounds within words (called phonological awareness) and associating single sounds with letter, or syllables and morphemes with patterns of letters (called the orthographic principle). Children with dyslexia generally have adequate listening comprehension but problems with reading comprehension secondary to excessive difficulties with reading decoding. Spelling may be a problem for such students even after they develop sufficient reading skills to handle most texts, and intervention may be needed at transition points as they proceed through their education. Other children may learn quickly and without obvious instruction how to associate spoken words with print, but when their comprehension is probed it becomes clear that they understand little of what they are reading.

During the school-age years and adolescence, children face challenges on both the social and the academic front. They must learn to interact socially with peers using the latest social slang and understanding body language and tonal differences that signal sarcasm or other indirect meanings. They also must learn to navigate through the shark-infested waters of social maneuvering, status, and invitation into or rejection from different social groups. In the academic arena, they must acquire increasingly sophisticated self-regulatory and executive skills for paying attention, keeping notes, detecting their teachers' subtle cues about what is important, garnering the self-confidence to persist in the face of failure, and deciding what information is relevant (and likely to be on the test), so they can devote cognitive–linguistic effort to forming associations and putting information into long-term memory for later retrieval. Academic learning contexts also become increasingly linguistically complex, and discipline-specific discourses of science, math, and social studies place increasing and differential demands on language systems. Both reading comprehension and written expression bring new demands for executive skills and for dealing with complex and highly embedded syntactic forms. Children and adolescents whose language skills may have been adequate for earlier contextual experiences and who "sound okay when they talk" may begin to flounder. Professionals should remain alert to the need to investigate whether language weaknesses may be a factor in explaining learning and behavioral difficulties that first become evident during later childhood and adolescence.

The collaboration of interdisciplinary teams can increase the potential for successful early identification and ongoing alertness to potential language-related learning difficulties. A number of professional disciplines can serve as resources to families and physicians seeking to understand why language is slow to develop and how to encourage it when a disorder is suspected or confirmed. These include speech–language pathologists, audiologists, early childhood specialists, reading specialists, and special education teachers. Other personnel with expertise for differential diagnosis and treatment are developmental psychologists and occupational therapists.

The purpose of early identification is to help children and families gain access to appropriate services and possibly ameliorate the long-term effects of deficits. It is important to remember that "early identification" for some forms of language-learning difficulty, however, may be possible only during the school-age years. The goal is for timely diagnosis and access to appropriate treatment approaches to improve developmental outcomes and enhance the prognosis to acquire language and communication skills to support academic learning, social participation, and healthy transitions into adulthood.

This chapter outlines current classifications and clinical features of primary and secondary neurodevelopmental language disorders, with support from epidemiological research. It also provides a brief overview of principles guiding diagnosis and treatment of developmental language disorders. The focus is on practical considerations for medical clinicians and allied health professionals who share responsibility for identifying children at risk and for providing appropriate assessment and intervention services.

Definitions and Classification

Developmental language disorders can be specific to spoken and written language systems, in which case they are considered primary impairments, or they may be secondary to other neurodevelopmental disorders, in which case they vary with characteristics of those disorders. During toddlerhood, late language emergence may be identified as a developmental risk rather than a disorder.

Late Language Emergence

Children who exhibit delays in language acquisition as toddlers may be termed "late talkers" or classified as demonstrating late language emergence. Such classifications are not equivalent to a diagnosis of language impairment or disorder but suggest heightened risk for continuing difficulty. The term "late talker" fits cases in which children are slow to talk, yet achieve other developmental milestones on time, show no symptoms of other developmental disorders, use gestures and other nonverbal means to communicate with their family, have normal hearing, and can understand many words and sentences. Research has shown that the majority of late-talking children (up to 80%) catch up with their peers by the time they reach school age [2–5]. Some children, however, do not catch up. The problem is in predicting which late-talking children will develop into typical language/literacy learners and which will show persistent problems that might be ameliorated through early intervention services.

Language Impairment

A primary neurodevelopmental disorder of language may be classified as developmental language disorder [6] or language impairment [7]. The American Speech–Language–Hearing Association [8] defined language disorder as follows:

> impaired comprehension and/or use of spoken, written and/or other symbol systems. The disorder may involve [1] the form of language (phonology, morphology, syntax) [2], the content of language (semantics), and/or [3] the function of language in communication (pragmatics) in any combination. (p. 40)

Language disorder may be classified further as specific language impairment (SLI), if a child's nonverbal cognitive abilities are significantly higher than his/her language abilities, or as nonspecific language impairment (NLI), if both verbal and nonverbal abilities are below normal limits but nonverbal cognitive abilities are not low enough to reach criteria for diagnosing intellectual disability (i.e., nonverbal IQ above 70) [9]. Research now shows that children with NLI function much the same as children with SLI, with differences more dimensional than categorical [10].

Based on large-scale epidemiological study, in which 1,929 kindergarten children were tested (known as the "Epi-SLI study"), Tomblin and Zhang [1999] found evidence that children with articulation-only impairment (i.e., specific speech sound disorders) differed from the larger group of children with language impairment. After testing the same cohort at second, fourth, and eighth grades, Tomblin and Zhang [11] concluded that the children's difficulties were explained best by a model with two dimensions – vocabulary abilities and sentence abilities. These two dimensions explained variation better than traditional categories of reception and expression. In fact, little evidence was found for separate factors for language expression and reception, as classification in the DSM-IV [12] implied.

The DSM-IV classification actually included five categories of speech–language impairment: expressive language disorder (315.31), mixed receptive–expressive language disorder (315.32), phonological disorder (315.39; formerly "developmental articulation disorder"), stuttering (307.0), and communication disorder not otherwise specified (307.9). The "NOS" category included conditions such as voice disorder that did not fit in any of the other classifications. At the time of this writing, a work group on language disorder (of which the author was a member) was proposing a modified classification system more consistent with the research reported in this chapter. Readers may consult the web site for updates on changes (http://www.dsm5.org/ProposedRevisions).

Evidence-based systems for classifying subgroups of language impairment are currently emerging. Conti-Ramsden, Crutchly, and Botting [13], working in the UK, found evidence for a five-category system: (a) phonological alone; (b) phonological–syntactic; (c) lexical–syntactic; (d) semantic–pragmatic; and (e) verbal auditory agnosia. Bishop [14] identified a group of children, also in the UK, who did not meet the definition of classical autism but who had a profile characterized by semantic–pragmatic problems that led to socially inappropriate conversational interactions [15]. Such children might produce excessive speech but have difficulty understanding and formulating coherent connected discourse [16]. Bishop [14] suggested the term "pragmatic language impairment" to apply to this profile. Support for a fundamentally different classification called pragmatic language impairment also came from a study of 604 children in the United States who were identified in kindergarten and followed into second grade as showing pragmatic difficulties dissociated from other phonological and semantic/syntactic language skills [17].

At this point, it is premature to support any one system of subclassification for primary spoken language impairment. As boundaries between SLI and NLI begin to blur, the most defensible system may be one that acknowledges distinctions between primary and secondary language impairments and between profiles that differentially involve sound/word and sentence/discourse levels of spoken and written language. Such a system might also allow for a category of pragmatic language impairment.

Learning Disability

The term learning disability encompasses a heterogeneous group of disorders. Approximately 80% of children who are identified with learning disability have a disability in reading [18]. When diagnosed in the school-age years by interdisciplinary teams in school settings, the term used for language-based academic learning difficulties is specific learning disability. The term language-learning disability also may be used to emphasize the role of underlying language knowledge and awareness deficits in explaining children's academic learning problems that cannot be explained in other ways.

The DSM-IV did not use the term learning disability, but included a diagnostic group of "learning disorders" (formerly known as "academic skills disorders"), which included reading disorder (315.00) and disorder of written expression (315.2). The workgroup on learning disability for the DSM-5 posted on the web site (accessed October 20, 2010) a definition that described learning disability as "A group of disorders characterized by difficulties in learning basic academic skills (currently or by history), that are not consistent with the person's chronological age, educational opportunities, or intellectual abilities. Basic academic skills refer to accurate and fluent reading, writing, and arithmetic."

The use of the term learning disability was suggested by Kirk [18] to replace prior labels, such as minimal brain damage or minimal brain dysfunction (MBD). This set the stage for viewing learning disability as a problem in acquiring basic academic skills, including speech, language, reading, and writing in the absence of more general cognitive or neurodevelopmental deficits. The first definition of learning disability in the federal law in the United States now known as the Individuals with Disabilities Education Improvement Act [19] included the "need for a severe discrepancy between achievement and intellectual ability for identification as learning disabled" [20]. Numerous modified definitions of learning disability have been proposed since then. In the 2004 reauthorization of IDEA, the requirement for cognitive referencing to identify a "severe discrepancy" was specifically removed from federal policy, and the following wording was used to define the condition and specify the process.

In general, the term "specific learning disability" means a disorder in one or more of the basic psychological processes involved in understanding or in using language, spoken or written, which disorder may manifest itself in the imperfect ability to listen, think, speak, read, write, spell, or do mathematical calculations (Part A, Section 602, Definitions, Paragraph [21]).

> ... a local educational agency shall not be required to take into consideration whether a child has a severe discrepancy between achievement and intellectual ability in oral expression, listening comprehension, written expression, basic reading skill, reading comprehension, mathematical calculation, or mathematical reasoning (Section 614 (b) (6) (A)).

In determining whether a child has a specific learning disability, a local educational agency may use a process that determines if the child responds to scientific, research-based intervention as a part of the evaluation procedures... (Section 614, b, 2 & 3).

Similar to SLI, definitions of specific learning disability are based on the premise that difficulty achieving academic success in the area of spoken and written language and mathematics is "unexpected" compared to an essentially normal development in other domains. Efforts to identify subtypes or phenotypes of learning disability based on differential processing abilities (e.g., visual versus auditory learners or left-brain versus right-brain learners) have not been successful. The lack of supportive research data for subtypes has led many to abandon processing and profile models of disability "because the research could not identify interactions between interventions and information-processing modality, neuropsychological profiles, or learning styles and orientations" [22].

Dyslexia is a classification of learning disability that can be differentially diagnosed, even though boundaries are not always clear. The diagnosis of dyslexia applies when children have impaired skills for analyzing words into their phonological, syllabic, and morphemic components and for learning to read and spell, with secondary effects on reading comprehension, but whose listening comprehension skills are basically intact [23, 24]. Due to historical and sociocultural factors, the term dyslexia is more likely to be used by medically trained personnel and those in private schools than by professionals in public schools, who use the term, learning disability [23, 25]. The term specific reading impairment also applies to this constellation of features. Research points to deficits in the phonological aspects of language as a root cause of reading difficulty in dyslexia [26, 27].

In contrast to dyslexia, some children demonstrate a condition known increasingly as specific comprehension deficit [23], but which also may be termed hyperlexia. This condition involves a pattern of precocious surface level reading accompanied by problems with abstract language comprehension and pragmatic/social communication [28]. Hyperlexia may be more a symptom than a syndrome. It can co-occur with a number of diagnoses, including autism spectrum disorder, mental retardation, or schizophrenia [28], but precocious surface reading with limited comprehension is not, by itself, diagnostic of any one syndrome. Catts et al. [29], therefore, recommended the term specific comprehension deficit to avoid "the association with autism or the narrow connotation that hyperlexia sometimes denotes" (p. 27).

Rourke [21] proposed the term nonverbal learning disability to describe a phenotype that may be associated with certain genetic syndromes (e.g., Fragile X and Williams syndromes) and conditions (e.g., fetal alcohol spectrum disorder or agenesis of the corpus callosum) or occur in isolation of them. The primary symptoms of nonverbal learning disability are relative deficits in areas involving social pragmatics, tactile, and visual–spatial skills, accompanied by relative strengths in rote verbal memory, single-word reading decoding, and high volume of speech output (but with unusual prosody). Rourke hypothesized that the common set of assets and difficulties observed in this phenotype might be traced to underdeveloped, damaged, or dysfunctional white matter pathways, the largest of which, the corpus callosum, connects the two cerebral hemispheres (http://www.nlearningdisability-bprourke.ca, accessed March 24, 2007). Neither the term hyperlexia nor the term specific comprehension deficit is considered synonymous with the label nonverbal learning disability; yet, similarities can be noted among the three classifications and with the syndrome Bishop [14] termed pragmatic language impairment.

Language Impairment Secondary to Other Conditions

Complex systems support language and communication development, so any impairment that affects a critical developmental system can affect the development of speech, language, and communication as well. Consider how each of the following systems may be involved:

- Healthy neurosensory systems, particularly hearing, but also vision, are critical to reception of spoken and written language input and for supporting verbal and nonverbal communication;
- Healthy neuromotor systems are critical for speech production and for fine motor control of writing and keyboarding;
- Healthy cognitive systems are critical for language comprehension, concept development, and sensitivity to communicative context;
- Healthy social–emotional systems are critical for intra- and interpersonal sensitivity and the development of social competence; and
- Healthy family and community systems are critical for providing safe and supportive environments in which developing abilities can be nurtured.

Heightened risks for disorders of language and communication can be associated with barriers to development in any of these internal or external systems. When other neurodevelopmental disorders can be diagnosed, such as intellectual disability, hearing impairment, traumatic brain impairment, or autism spectrum disorder, co-occurring language impairment is considered "secondary." Regardless of whether language disorders are primary or secondary, however, language and communication skills should constitute priority targets for assessment and intervention.

Epidemiology

Epidemiological evidence about the prevalence and nature of neurodevelopmental language disorder is increasing. One epidemiological study [30] showed a prevalence of 13–19% of children showing symptoms of late language emergence at 24 months, with male children showing almost three times the risk of female children. A family history of late talking was a risk indicator, as was low birth weight, with children born at less than 85% of optimum birth weight showing almost twice the risk for late language emergence. Greater risk was not, however, associated with parental education level or socioeconomic status, or with parental mental health, family functioning, or parenting practices. A subsequent study [31] followed 128 of the original children who were late talkers at 24 months and compared them to 109 control children (who were epidemiologically equivalent) at age 7 years. This study showed that children with early delays were almost twice as likely as children in the control group (20% versus 11%) to be identified as below normative levels on general language ability in the early years of school.

The comprehensive prospective "Epi-SLI study" [32] involved testing of 1,929 kindergarten children in Iowa and Illinois. That study showed a prevalence rate of 7.4% (8% for boys and 6% for girls). It also showed that language impairment was likely to be underdiagnosed because 71% of kindergarten children who met criteria for a diagnosis of SLI had not been previously identified. Some language delays or disorders seem to resolve at one point only to reappear later on [33, 34]. Many children with early language delay do not progress to within normal limits for their age and can be expected to change to another diagnostic classification, such as learning disability, during their school-age years [35]. Table 12.1 shows the prevalence figures for children served in 2008 under different categories of IDEA. Whereas the highest percentage in the preschool years is speech–language impairment, the highest percentage in the later school-age years clearly shifts to the category of learning disability.

Kavale and Forness [36] expressed concern that "in place of epidemiological studies, learning disability prevalence is often established through policy statements issued by national organizations" (p. 83) [as in Table 12.1]. Kavale and Forness noted further that such processes are inherently political and may reflect advocacy to serve more students under the learning disability rubric. This may account for the fact that 52% of all children with disabilities in the United States (more than 2.5–2.8 million children) with special education needs are served under the classification of learning disability.

Clinical Features

When developmental milestones are not met on schedule, regardless of reason, they signal a need for further exploration and individualized assessment – formal and

Table 12.1 Numbers (and percentages) of children served in 2008 in the United States and territories in each disability category under Part B of the individuals with disabilities education

Disability category	Age category (years)			
	3:0–5:11	6:0–11:11	12:0–17:11	18:0–21:11
Specific learning disability	14,050 (2.0%)	819,369 (30.5%)	1,552,328 (54.3%)	154,201 (44.5%)
Speech or language impairment	330,223 (46.6%)	959,015 (35.7%)	156,628 (5.5%)	6,318 (1.8%)
Mental retardation	12,403 (1.7%)	151,594 (5.6%)	251,111 (8.8%)	73,426 (21.2%)
Emotional impairment	3,488 (0.5%)	117,968 (4.4%)	269,723 (9.4%)	30,377 (8.8%)
Multiple disabilities	7,876 (1.1%)	46,154 (1.7%)	58,938 (2.1%)	18,981 (5.5%)
Hearing impairment	8,427 (1.2%)	31,588 (1.2%)	34,335 (1.2%)	4,858 (1.4%)
Orthopedic impairment	7,695 (1.1%)	28,212 (1.1%)	28,842 (1.0%)	5,317 (1.5%)
Other health impairment	18,091 (2.6%)	252,587 (9.4%)	366,315 (12.8%)	29,496 (8.5%)
Visual impairment	3,425 (0.5%)	11,799 (0.4%)	12,131 (0.4%)	1,886 (0.5%)
Autism	44,977 (6.3%)	161,236 (6.0%)	112,972 (4.0%)	18,610 (5.4%)
Deaf–blindness	207 (0.03%)	673 (0.03%)	848 (0.03%)	224 (0.06%)
Traumatic brain injury	967 (0.1%)	8,310 (0.3%)	13,992 (0.5%)	2,564 (0.7%)
Developmental delay[a]	257,175 (36.3%)	96,923 (3.6%)		

Source: U.S. Department of Education Improvement Act (IDEA) [42].
[a]Developmental delay is applicable only to children aged 3–9 years.

informal. Milestones for typical language development and red flags signaling cause for concern are summarized in Table 12.2.

As noted previously, late language emergence, also called "late talking," resolves for approximately 80% of children who are behind initially but meet developmental milestones by school age. Clinical features that should be considered in deciding whether to provide intervention for such children include the presence of multiple risk factors, such as a family history of language problems, chronic otitis media, cognitive delay, social communication difficulties, or environmental risks. As shown in Table 12.2, other clinical features specific to language development that should be viewed as red flags include difficulty following verbal instructions, limited use of gestures and sounds to communicate, limited symbolic play, and few word combinations at 30 months and beyond [37, 38].

Table 12.2 Developmental milestones and red flags signaling cause for concern

Age	Developmental milestones	Red flags
Infants/toddlers (birth to 2:11 years)	• Responds to cuddling and quiets to comforting • Engages in mutual eye gaze and synchronous interactions • Responds to verbal and nonverbal signals, smiles reaches • Babbles canonically (bababa, mamama) by 6–8 months • Enjoys baby games (e.g., peekaboo, pattycake) • Finger point emerges around 10 months • First words around 12 months • Vocabulary spurt around 18 months • Combines two words by 24 months • Combines three words by 36 months • Begins to inflect words with -ing, plural, and possessive morphemes, uses some irregular past tense by 36 months • Shows interest in books, pointing, and trying to turn the pages	• Stiffens when held; cries when touched; feeding difficulties • Fails to meet parental eye gaze or engage in synchronous movement in first 3 months • Few early sounds or reduction of babbling at around 8 months may signal hearing problems • Limited response to "baby talk" by 4 months • Limited response to baby games at 10 months • No finger point by 15 months • Does not share focus on an object with adult when attention called • Does not recruit adult's shared attention on an object • No words by 18 months • Fewer than 50 words by 24 months • Few or no two-word combinations by 24 months • Few or no three-word combinations by 36 months • Will not stay in lap and look at age-appropriate books for more than one to two pages

Table 12.2 (continued)

Age	Developmental milestones	Red flags
Preschoolers (3:0–5:11 years)	• Produces intelligible words with consonant–vowel patterns: CV, CVC, CVCV, CVCVC • Vocabulary develops rapidly; can use abstract words for emotions by end of period • Awareness of phonological structure of words apparent in word play, rhymes, etc. • Uses past tense -ed, forms of *be*, articles *a, the* (although errors are still expected) • Sentence structure expands with more words and morphemes (-ed, -s, etc.) per utterance (called mean length of utterance or MLU) • Syntax is used to combine several ideas into one sentence by using connectors like *and, but, because, when, after* • Play shows increasing ability to represent ideas and things symbolically and to imitate adult communication scripts (talking on the phone, fast food orders, doctor's office) • Shows ability to cooperate socially with peers in pretend play and other activities • Emergent literacy for looking at books; retelling stories	• Phoneme/articulation repertoire is so limited that even caregivers cannot understand speech; produces mostly CV combinations (does not "close" syllables) • Vocabulary limited; difficulty responding to contextually supported wh-questions (*what, whose, where*) at age 4–5 years • Cannot play with rhymes by age 4–5 years • MLU less than 3.5 words by 4 years • MLU less than 4.5 words by 5 years • Unresponsive to requests for information or action • Limited expression of comments or questions • Limited symbolic use of toys to create scenes; few coordinated actions or repetitive, nonsymbolic use of toys (e.g., spinning wheels, lining up cars without turning it into a meaningful game) • Limited interest in books; difficulty listening to or telling stories or anecdotes

Table 12.2 (continued)

Age	Developmental milestones	Red flags
Middle childhood (6:0–10:11 years)	• Develops phonemic awareness for identifying initial and final sounds and the alphabetic principle for relating print symbols to speech sounds (by late grade 1) • Develops orthographic awareness for relating syllable patterns to morphemes (e.g., silent -e rule; -ough, -ight, -ing) (by grade 3) • Understands and formulates sentences with embedded and subordinated clauses representing complex temporal (*while, during*), causal (*because*), conditional (*if … then*), and logical (*whereas, however*) relationships (skills increase across grades) • Comprehends complex spoken and written texts (narrative and expository); retells, summarizes, and answers questions about them; produces stories and reports with mature organizational structures (skills increase across grades)	• Cannot identify initial and ending sounds of words; has difficulty relating letters to speech sounds; cannot generate intelligible spellings of CVC words by late grade 1 • Restricted sentence length (average of less than five words); difficulty ordering words, showing noun–verb agreement, awkward phrasing (any age) • Inadequate vocabulary for listening, speaking, reading, writing; inappropriate word choices; reliance on all-purpose words (*stuff, thing*); misunderstanding of academic relational words (*center, near, below, after*) (at grade level and lower) • Pragmatically inappropriate interactions with adults or peers; difficulty grasping subtle or indirect meanings; not accepted by peers • Difficulty with self-talk and self-regulation of attention and executive functions
Adolescence (11:0–20:11 years)	• Spells most words correctly; can read novel texts and figure out words and meanings from context, using word roots and morphological variation • Understands and produces complex sentences in spoken and written language • Develops skill for public presentation of formal oral and written discourse; revises and edits when writing; reads critically • Socially adept at forming new relationships, including with the opposite sex; varies communication style for academic, social, and vocational activities	• Ongoing difficulty with reading decoding, spelling, word analysis skills • Difficulty comprehending and producing complex sentences in spoken and written modalities • Pragmatically inappropriate interactions with adults or peers; difficulty grasping subtle or indirect meanings and reading body language and tone • Difficulty with self-talk and self-regulation of attention and executive functions

© Nelson [44], shared with permission from author.

Clinical features of specific language impairment during the preschool years include delay in meeting developmental age norms for vocabulary and syntax development. Clinical features of learning disability during the school-age years include difficulty learning to read and write. This includes difficulty with the sound/word skills needed for reading decoding and spelling, alternately or in addition to difficulty with the sentence/discourse skills needed for listening and reading comprehension and for oral and written expression. Clinical features of dyslexia may include difficulty showing awareness of the phonological structure of words, even though the child's vocabulary is basically intact and the child's auditory comprehension is strong. Because spoken and written language learning and disorders are intertwined at multiple levels and different profiles may be associated with different intervention needs, it is important for assessment activities to focus across language levels and modalities and to include social communication as well as basic language skills.

Diagnosis

Even though infants and toddlers are not expected to be competent language users, it is important to be alert to early signs of developmental difficulty and divergence from expected communicative behaviors. Observational tools that are appropriate for infants and toddlers include the MacArthur-Bates Communicative Developmental Inventories (CDIs), second edition [39]; the Ages and Stages Questionnaire (ASQ): A Parent-Completed, Child-Monitoring System, second edition [40]; and the Rossetti Infant–Toddler Language Scale [41].

Informal observations also contribute to diagnosis of early language-learning risks. This includes observing abilities such as eye gaze and gesturing to confirm that the child can engage in interpersonal attention with a caregiver (i.e., looking at each other), as well as shared attention to objects. This involves following the caregiver's gaze and gestures to look at objects or using gestures and vocalizing to gain the caregiver's attention and shared focus on objects. Developmental milestones are for first words to appear by approximately 1 year of age (at least by 18 months), two-word combinations by 2 years, and three-word combinations by 3 years – making these milestones relatively easy to remember. Delays in reaching language and communication milestones constitute some of the earliest symptoms of developmental difficulty in multiple developmental domains, not just language. They may be readily recognized by parents and other health-care providers.

Diagnosis of language impairment or learning disability during the preschool or school-age years primary language impairment also requires multiple forms of evidence, including parental report, scores from a standardized, individually administered test showing a child to be delayed significantly compared to a sample of developmentally normal children, and evidence from a communication sample gathered in a relatively naturalistic context. Assessment teams should consider whether a child's prior cultural–linguistic experiences make it appropriate to use diagnostic tests that have been standardized on a mainstream population and use alternative procedures if not. Diagnosis should never be based on a single source of input, measure, or procedure, no matter how well designed and researched the tool, but should be supported by evidence from more than one type of measure, including input from parents and teachers.

Many schools now use screening assessments to evaluate acquisition of key academic language skills at regular intervals, which may lead to a diagnosis of learning disability. The goal of such programs, called response-to-intervention (RtI) programs, is to identify children who are not achieving adequately despite receiving high-quality general education instruction [43], and, therefore, appear to need additional assistance. To further differentiate children's needs for specialized intervention, they may move systematically (guided by the decisions of a school-based child study team) through three tiers of instructional activities, conceptualized as a pyramid, with the majority of children at the bottom and only a few moving toward the top. When children have difficulty despite having received increasingly individualized intervention at each of the three tiers and when individualized assessments confirm the presence of deficits compared to typically developing peers, a special education diagnosis of learning disability may be made.

Treatment

Treatment decisions are complex. They may be influenced by theoretical points of view about language development. Some clinicians prefer approaches that are based on behaviorist principles, and others prefer approaches based on social interactionist principles [44]. Increasingly, speech–language pathologists and special educators are adopting the principles and procedures of evidence-based practice that are used in the medical field, including literature searches and appraisal of evidence both in the literature and in working with a particular child and family.

Three general principles that should guide treatment decisions and procedures are to (1) establish treatment goals that are individualized for the child and relevant to the important contexts of the child's life and age; (2) engage broader systems of families, peers, and teachers in supporting the child's language development; and (3) intensify language-learning experiences that are known to support language development when it proceeds without disorder. The first principle involves mutual goal setting and assessment that seeks to identify gaps between how the child currently functions in key communicative contexts and how the child might function differently. This allows clinicians to apply the third principle, which is to provide experiences that heighten cues in the environment the child needs to process in order to expand his/her language abilities. The second principle emphasizes that improving a child's language abilities involves more than a clinician can do in a therapeutic session.

Increasingly, research groups have been developing materials that can be used by families and teachers to support children's language and literacy development. One group at the University of Washington developed a set of videos called "Language is the Key." They include the following:

- Talking & Books: (20 min DVD or VHS), which shows parents how to use picture books to promote language development and early literacy and teaches dialogic reading strategies;
- Talking & Play: (20 min DVD or VHS), which shows parents how to promote language and literacy when children are engaged in play or everyday activities;
- Web site: http://www.walearning.com/products/language-is-the-key/.

Another group at the Hanen Centre in Toronto, Canada, has developed a series of resources and offers training workshops. Their materials include the following:

- It Takes Two to Talk®, which is a model of family-focused early language intervention for young children with expressive and/or receptive language delays;
- Learning Language and Loving It™, which is designed for teaching early childhood educators and preschool teachers to promote children's social, language, and literacy development within everyday activities and conversations;
- More Than Words, which is a family-focused program designed to provide tools for parents of children with autism spectrum disorder (ASD) to help their children communicate socially;
- TalkAbility™, which is a family-focused program designed for parents of verbal children (aged 3–7 years) on the autism spectrum that offers practical tools parents can use to help their children communicate; and
- You Make the Difference, which is designed to support parents of typically developing children (birth to 5 years), to learn how to foster their children's early language, social, and literacy development using positive everyday interactions.
- Web site: http://www.hanen.org/web/Home/tabid/36/Default.aspx.

Treatment planning also involves deciding whether children with language disorders secondary to sensory, motor, and cognitive deficits might benefit from assistive technology designed to compensate for other comorbid areas of impairment. For example, cochlear implants or traditional hearing aids can make it possible for children with profound hearing impairment to learn spoken language auditorially; children with severe neuromotor impairments may be able to communicate with support from augmentative and alternative communication devices and techniques; and children with cognitive impairments may benefit from computerized supports as they learn to read and write.

Conclusions

Children with neurodevelopmental language disorders come with a variety of labels, characteristics, and needs. This chapter has described primary language disorders, including spoken language impairment and language-based learning disabilities, as well as secondary disorders that co-occur with other neurodevelopmental conditions, discussed throughout this text. Developmental milestones and red flags for concern were outlined. Although a comprehensive overview of diagnosis and treatment methods was beyond the scope of this chapter, basic considerations were described. The need for interdisciplinary collaboration and communication was emphasized. The goal is for members of the team, including parents, as well as children and adolescents where appropriate, to apply their diverse expertise to prioritize goals and plan relevant interventions to support participation in the social and learning contexts of infancy through adolescence.

References

1. Greenspan SI, Wieder S. Infant and early childhood mental health: a comprehensive developmental approach to assessment and intervention. Washington, DC: American Psychiatric Publishing; 2006.
2. Girolametto L, Wiigs M, Smyth R, Weitzman E, Pearce P. Children with a history of expressive vocabulary delay: Outcomes at 5 years of age. Am J Speech Lang Pathol. 2001;10:358–69.
3. Paul PV. First- and second-language English literacy. Volta Rev. 1996;98(2):5–16.
4. Rescorla L. Language and reading outcomes at age 9 in late-talking toddlers. J Speech Lang Hear Res. 2002;45:360–71.
5. Rice ML, Taylor CL, Zubrick SR. Language outcomes of 7-year-old children with or without a history of late language emergence at 24-months. J Speech Lang Hear Res. 2008;51: 394–407.
6. Rice ML, Warren SF. Introduction. In: Rice ML, Warren SF, editors. Developmental language disorders: From phenotypes to etiologies. Mahwah, NJ: Lawrence Erlbaum; 2004. pp. 1–3.
7. Law J, Garrett Z, Nye C. The efficacy of treatment for children with developmental speech and language delay/disorder: A meta-analysis. J Speech Lang Hear Res. 2004;47:924–43.
8. American Speech-Language-Hearing Association. Definitions of Communication Disorders and Variations [Relevant Paper]. Available from www.asha.org/policy. 1993.
9. Catts HW, Fey ME, Zhang X, Tomblin JB. Estimating the risk of future reading difficulties in kindergarten children: A research-based model and its clinical implementation. Lang Speech Hear Serv Sch. 2001;32:38–50.
10. Tomblin JB, Zhang X, Weiss A, Catts H, Ellis WS. Dimensions of individual differences in communication skills among primary grade children. In: Rice ML, Warren SF, editors. Developmental language disorders: from phenotypes to etiologies. Mahwah, NJ: Lawrence Erlbaum; 2004. pp. 53–76.
11. Tomblin JB, Zhang X. Are children with SLI a unique group of language learners? In: Tager-Flusberg H, editor. Neurodevelopmental disorders: contributions to a new framework from the cognitive neurosciences. Cambridge, MA: MIT Press; 1999. pp. 361–82.
12. American Psychiatric Association. Diagnostic and statistical manual of mental disorders. 4th ed. Text Revision (DSM-IV-TR). Washington, DC: American Psychiatric Association; 2000.
13. Conti-Ramsden G, Crutchly A, Botting N. The extent to which psychometric tests differentiate subgroups of children with SLI. J Speech Lang Hear Res. 2003;40:765–77.
14. Bishop DVM. Pragmatic language impairment: A correlate of SLI, a distinct subgroup, or part of the autistic continuum? In: Bishop DVM, Leonard LB, editors. Speech and language impairments in children: Causes, characteristics, intervention, and outcome. Hove: Psychology Press; 2000. pp. 99–113.
15. Bishop DVM, Norbury CF. Exploring the borderlands of autistic disorder and specific language impairment: A study using standardized diagnostic instruments. J Child Psychol Psychiatr. Allied Disciplines. 2002;43:917–29.

16. Bishop DVM, Adams C. Conversational characteristics of children with semantic-pragmatic disorder. 2. What features lead to a judgment of inappropriacy? Br J Disord Commun. 1989;24:241–63.
17. Tomblin JB, Zhang X, Weiss A, Catts H, Ellis WS. Dimensions of individual differences in communication skills among primary grade children. In: Rice ML, Warren SF, editors. Developmental language disorders: from phenotypes to etiologies. Mahwah, NJ: Lawrence Erlbaum; 2004. pp. 53–76.
18. Kirk SA. Educating exceptional children. Boston, MA: Houghton Mifflin; 1962.
19. Individuals with Disabilities Education Improvement Act of 2004. Pub. L. No. 108–446, 118 Stat. 2647. 2004.
20. Hallahan DP, Mock DR. A brief history of the field of learning disabilities. In: Swanson HL, Harris KR, Graham S, editors. Handbook of learning disabilities. New York, NY: Guilford; 2003. pp. 16–29.
21. Rourke BP. Syndrome of nonverbal learning disabilities. New York, NY: Guilford; 1995.
22. Fletcher H, Buckley S. Phonological awareness in children with Down syndrome. Down Syndr Res Pract. 2002;8(1):11–18.
23. Catts HW, Kamhi AG. Classification of reading disabilities. In: Catts HW, Kamhi AG, editors. Language and reading disabilities. 2nd ed. Boston, MA: Allyn Bacon; 2005. pp. 72–93.
24. Snowling MJ. Dyslexia. Oxford: Blackwell; 2000.
25. Kamhi AG. A meme's eye view of speech-language pathology. Lang Speech Hear Serv Sch. 2004;35:105–11.
26. Snowling MJ. Phonological processing and developmental dyslexia. J Res Read. 1995;18(2):132–8.
27. Stanovich KE, Siegel LS. Phenotypic performance profile of children with reading disabilities: A regression-based test of the phonological-core variable-difference model. J Educ Psychol. 1994;86:24–53.
28. Aram D, Healy JM. Hyperlexia: A review of extraordinary word recognition. In: Obler LK, Fein D, editors. The exceptional brain: Neuropsychology of talent and special abilities. New York, NY: Guilford; 1988. pp. 70–102.
29. Catts HW, Hogan TP, Adlof SM. Developmental changes in reading and reading disabilities. In: Catts HW, Kamhi AG, editors. The connections between language and reading disabilities. Mahwah, NJ: Lawrence Erlbaum; 2005. pp. 25–40.
30. Zubrick SR, Taylor CL, Rice ML, Slegers D. Late language emergence at 24 months: An epidemiological study of prevalence and covariates. J Speech Lang Hear Res. 2007;50: 1562–92.
31. Rice ML, Taylor CL, Zubrick SR. Language outcomes of 7-year-old children with or without a history of late language emergence at 24-months. J Speech Lang Hear Res. 2008;51:394–407.
32. Tomblin JB, Records NL, Buckwalter P, Zhang X, Smith E, O'Brien M. Prevalence of specific language impairment in kindergarten children. J Speech Lang Hear Res. 1997;40:1245–60.
33. Rescorla L. Language and reading outcomes at age 9 in late-talking toddlers. J Speech Lang Hear Res. 2002;45:360–71.
34. Scarborough HS, Dobrich W. Development of children with early language delays. J Speech Hear Res. 1990;33:70–83.
35. Mashburn AJ, Myers SS. Advancing research on children with speech-language impairment: An introduction to the early childhood longitudinal study – longitudinal cohort. Lang Speech Hear Serv Sch. 2010;41:61–9.
36. Kavale KA, Forness SR. Learning disability as a discipline. In: Swanson HL, Harris KR, Graham S, editors. Handbook of learning disabilities. New York, NY: Guilford; 2003. pp. 76–93.
37. Watt N, Wetherby A, Shumway S. Prelinguistic predictors of language outcome at three years of age. J Speech Lang Hear Res. 2006;49:1224–37.
38. Wetherby A, Goldstein H, Cleary J, Allen L, Kublin K. Early identification of children with communication delays: Concurrent and Predictive Validity of the CSBS Developmental Profile. Inf Young Child. 2003;16:161–74.

39. Fenson L, Marchman V, Thal D, Dale P, Reznick J, Bates E. MacArthur-Bates Communicative Developmental Inventories-second edition (CDIs). Baltimore, MD: Paul H Brookes; 2007.
40. Bricker D, Squires J. Ages and Stages Questionnaire: a parent-completed, child-monitoring system – second edition (ASQ). Baltimore, MD: Paul H Brookes; 1999.
41. Rossetti L. Rossetti Infant-Toddler Language Scale. East Moline, IL: LinguiSystems; 2005.
42. U.S. Department of Education, Office of Special Education Programs, Data Analysis System (DANS), OMB #1820–0043: "Children with Disabilities Receiving Special Education Under Part B of the Individuals with Disabilities Education Act," 2008. Data updated as of August 3, 2009. Data downloaded and summarized October 19, 2010 from https://www.ideadata.org/arc_toc10.asp#partbCC
43. Snow CE, Burns MS, Griffin P, editors. Preventing reading difficulties in young children. national research council, committee on the prevention of reading difficulties of young children. Washington, DC: Natl Acad Press; 1998.
44. Nelson NW. Language and literacy disorders: Infancy through adolescence. Boston, MA: Allyn Bacon/Pearson Education; 2010.

Chapter 13
Disorders of Speech and Voice

Helen M. Sharp and Stephen M. Tasko

Abstract Speech is a learned behavior that requires rapid coordination of respiratory, phonatory, and articulatory systems coupled with intact language, cognition, and hearing functions. Speech is often divided into sub-domains that include speech sound production (articulation), fluency, resonance, and voice quality. Children develop control of each of these sub-domains over a period of years, often raising questions for parents and pediatricians about whether a child's speech is typical or of concern. Speech disorders can be caused by structural anomalies, neuromotor problems, developmental mislearnings, or a combination of these etiologies. Assessment by a speech–language pathologist often provides insight into the etiology and allows an appropriate plan of care. Speech services are often coordinated with other medical, dental, or allied health professional services to provide comprehensive care.

Introduction

Speech is a learned neuromotor behavior that requires voluntary, rapid, and fine coordination of the respiratory, phonatory, resonance, and articulatory systems. Speech requires adequate breath support with rapid inhalation followed by sustained, controlled exhalation. The muscles of the larynx bring the vocal folds together and the flow of air from the lungs creates a vibration in the vocal folds that the listener hears as voice. The sound produced by the vocal folds is shaped through movements of the articulators to yield the variety of consonants and vowels that comprise any spoken language. The articulators include the tongue, mandible, lips, and soft palate as well as immobile structures of the oral and pharyngeal cavities including the palatal vault, the tonsils, adenoids, and teeth. Thus, in order to say "mama" the speaker must generate a positive expiratory lung pressure, approximate

H.M. Sharp (✉)
Department of Speech Pathology and Audiology, Western Michigan University, Kalamazoo, MI 49008, USA
e-mail: helen.sharp@wmich.edu

D.R. Patel et al. (eds.), *Neurodevelopmental Disabilities*,
DOI 10.1007/978-94-007-0627-9_13, © Springer Science+Business Media B.V. 2011

the vocal folds to initiate and sustain vibration, vary the position of the soft palate to allow some of the audible speech signals to escape through the nose, approximate and release lip closure, and maintain the appropriate tongue posture for the vowel "a." Individual speech sounds are produced through the coordinated movements of these systems that alter the shape of the oral–pharyngeal spaces. Figure 13.1 shows the relationships of anatomic structures and spaces that are involved in speech production.

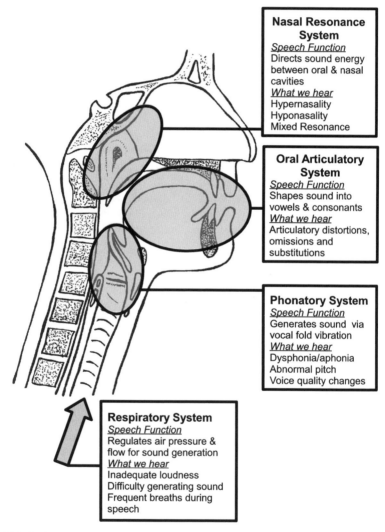

Nasal Resonance System
Speech Function
Directs sound energy between oral & nasal cavities
What we hear
Hypernasality
Hyponasality
Mixed Resonance

Oral Articulatory System
Speech Function
Shapes sound into vowels & consonants
What we hear
Articulatory distortions, omissions and substitutions

Phonatory System
Speech Function
Generates sound via vocal fold vibration
What we hear
Dysphonia/aphonia
Abnormal pitch
Voice quality changes

Respiratory System
Speech Function
Regulates air pressure & flow for sound generation
What we hear
Inadequate loudness
Difficulty generating sound
Frequent breaths during speech

Fig. 13.1 Mid-sagittal view of the head and neck highlighting regions important for speech and voice production. Perceptual characteristics of disordered speech associated with each region of the vocal tract are described

Definitions

Speech is the term often used to describe the entire process of coordinated function of the respiratory, phonatory, resonance, and articulatory systems to produce sounds that when sequenced together fluently represent the words of a language. Speech is one means of expressing language and should be differentiated from language itself. Chapter 12 addresses language development and disorders. Speech sounds in a language are typically categorized as vowel sounds, in which the vocal tract is relatively open or has limited constriction, and consonant sounds that are produced by narrowing the vocal tract through movement of the articulators. This process of shaping the airflow and vocal sound is called articulation. The system of linguistic rules that govern the way in which sounds in a language can be combined is called phonology.

Speakers combine individual speech sounds to form words and then combine words into sentences. Therefore, in addition to how specific speech sounds are articulated, speech production is also described according to the qualities of fluency, prosody, resonance, voice, and overall speech intelligibility. Fluency is used to describe the smoothness or fluidity of speech. Significant repetitions or hesitations of sounds and words can reduce speech intelligibility, decrease efficiency of information transfer, or distract the listener from the message, thus impairing communication. Prosody refers to the typical intonation patterns of a language or regional dialect that includes the stresses on syllables or words or the "melody" of speech. Resonance is used to describe a quality of nasality within the speech signal that is most often perceived as normal, excessively nasal (hypernasal), or insufficiently nasal (hyponasal). Resonance is largely controlled through the timing and function of the velopharynx which acts as a valve and closes to direct sounds through the oral cavity for most speech sounds (e.g., "sh") or opens to allow for nasal speech sound production in which the sound escapes through the nose (e.g., "m"). Voice or phonation is the tone that is the produced from periodic vibration of the vocal folds. Establishing vocal fold vibration requires coordination of the respiratory system, to provide the necessary positive airway pressure, and laryngeal muscle activity, to tense and approximate the vocal folds so they vibrate as air flows past them. Voice is the prominent sound energy source used when articulating vowels and many consonants. The listener's ability to understand the speaker, or speech intelligibility, is influenced by the combination of articulatory precision, prosody, fluency, resonance, and vocal quality.

The Development of Speech

For most children, intelligible speech is acquired over the first 3 years of life with continued development of articulatory precision through the early school-aged years [1]. Speech development requires that the infant is exposed to adult speakers, has intact cognition for language representation, and has intact hearing together with the motor capability to control and coordinate the respiratory, laryngeal, and articulatory systems. Speech production is a function that is overlaid on a number of structures that, from an evolutionary perspective, originally served other roles. However, control of these structures appears to be task specific. Therefore, the capacity to use articulatory, laryngeal, or respiratory structures for other functions such as vegetative breathing, gagging, coughing, chewing, or swallowing does not mean that the child also has the capacity for normal speech and voice [2].

Development of Speech Sounds

Infants begin to vocalize with cries, then as they gain more control they start to produce vowel-like cooing sounds at about age 2–4 months. Babbling is defined as strings of repeated consonants and vowels ("babababababa") and typically emerges in the 3–6 month age range [3]. Babbling requires coordination of respiratory pressure, vocal fold movement, lip, tongue, soft palate (velum), and jaw movements for sequencing two speech sounds. Infants hear their own babbling sounds and are reinforced by hearing themselves as well as by the reactions of others. Infants with significant hearing loss are more likely to exhibit significant delays in the onset of babbling often beyond 11 months of age [4]. By 8 or 9 months infants should imitate babbled sequences and begin to produce strings of speech-like sounds with intonation that mimics adult forms of speech called jargon [3–5].

A child's first true word is usually produced between 10 and 13 months of age. A true word is considered any consistent production of a sound sequence that carries a consistent meaning. An infant may, for example, reliably use the highly simplified sound sequence "gam" when referring to her grandmother, although at this stage of development the infant does not have adequate neuromotor control to produce a word like "grandma" in full.

The infant typically produces the sounds of a language in a somewhat predictable sequence that varies according to the child's primary language exposure. In English, for example, vowels emerge early, followed by bilabial consonant sounds such as "m, b, and w" [5]. Nasals are often produced early, while sounds that require the child to hold an articulatory posture with continuous air pressure tend to appear later in the acquisition sequence. In English, "l" and "r" and the voiced and voiceless fricative sounds "th, s, z, sh, and zh" emerge relatively late and remain inconsistent for months or even years. These sounds are often referred to as "the late 8" because they are often absent, substituted, or distorted through 5 or 6 years of age [3]. Similarly, among Spanish speakers the trilled "r" remains inconsistent beyond 5 years of age [1].

There is considerable variation in the timing of development for specific consonant sounds in children's speech, but typically developing children who are acquiring English or Spanish produce a representation of most speech sounds in the language by 4 years of age. However, children will continue to perfect speech sound productions well beyond this age [1–5]. It is typical for young children to produce later developing speech sounds in some word positions or contexts, but be unable to produce those same sounds in other words.

Children often simplify adult word productions, particularly multisyllabic words or words containing late developing speech sounds. These simplifications most often follow systematic rules called phonological processes. Examples of typical phonological processes include dropping the final consonant of a word (e.g., "bath" becomes "ba"), reduction of consonant clusters to one consonant (e.g., "skate" becomes "kate"), or eliminating a syllable from a multisyllabic word (e.g., "elephant" becomes "efunt"). These simplifications are normal for very young children, but should gradually disappear over time. Most simplification patterns diminish by age 3, allowing the child to be understood by others. However, some simplification patterns persist through age 4 or 5 and a few, most notably "r" and "l" distortions may linger until about age 7 years of age [6].

Development of Fluency

Children and adults exhibit typical disfluencies in connected speech such as short pauses or hesitations; interjections (e.g., "um"); abandoning an utterance; and revising words, phrases, or sentences. Occasional repetitions of longer words, phrases, or sentences also occur in normal communication. Young children who are grappling with the challenges of speech and language learning will often exhibit these disfluent patterns with greater frequency than older children or adults.

Development of Resonance

Resonance quality is heard mainly in the vowel sounds of speech because the vowels take on the characteristics of nearby consonants. Early infant vowel productions have a nasal quality because the velopharynx is not closed. Nasal speech sounds "m" and "n" are among the first consonant sounds infants learn as they are produced anteriorly in the mouth and do not require velopharyngeal closure. Over time the infant begins to achieve the velopharyngeal closure required to produce oral consonants such as "b."

Most people lack adequate nasal resonance, or are hyponasal, when the nasal airway is obstructed due to upper respiratory infection or allergies. Many very young children use velum-to-adenoid closure, rather than velum-to-pharyngeal wall closure because adenoid tissue occupies much of the nasopharyngeal space [7], thus it is common for very young children to have slightly hyponasal speech.

Development of Voice

The infant's first vocal function is often a cry and gradually the infant gains control of her voice exhibited through cooing and then babbling. Infants gain control of vocal loudness and pitch variations through squealing and other vocal play. The vibratory frequency of the vocal folds largely dictates what we hear as the pitch of the voice. People speak at a characteristic or habitual pitch which varies with factors such as age and gender. Additionally, speakers vary pitch to produce a variety of intonation patterns (prosody) to enhance meaning and interest to speech. Vocal pitch is higher in pre-pubescent children than in adults. Typically boys and girls do not speak at markedly different pitches until puberty. During puberty the larynx expands in size, resulting in a lowering of habitual pitch for both genders, but this is most pronounced in boys due to a disproportionately large growth of the larynx.

Disorders of Speech and Voice

A speech disorder is defined by the American Speech–Language Hearing Association (ASHA) as "an impairment of the articulation of speech sounds, fluency and/or voice" [8]. The etiologies of communication disorders are often categorized as organic disorders that negatively affect the structures needed for speech (e.g., cleft palate) or voice production (e.g., laryngeal web); neuromotor disorders that reduce strength, movement, or coordination of one or more of the systems or structures involved in speech production (e.g., cerebral palsy); or idiopathic or functional disorders that occur in the absence of either organic or neurologic conditions sufficient to explain the observed speech or voice production deficits. These classifications can be helpful in diagnosis and treatment planning. For example, two children with repaired cleft palate may both present with hypernasal speech, but one due to a residual tissue deficit (organic) and the other related to mislearning of the distinction between nasal and non-nasal/oral speech sounds (functional). Although each of these children may have similar medical histories and similar sounding speech, one child will require physical management combined with speech therapy while the other will likely benefit from speech therapy alone.

Many children who exhibit speech and voice disorders have co-occurring organic, neuromotor, and functional causes. For example, Annie, a child with cerebral palsy secondary to significant prematurity, may exhibit reduced speech intelligibility which could be related to dental malocclusion, mild neuromotor discoordination, persistent speech sound simplification patterns, high-frequency hearing loss, or a combination of these. Although there may be uncertainty about the etiology of Annie's speech disorder, it is clear that her speech production is not within the expected range. Therefore, it is likely that Annie and her family could benefit from a speech–language assessment and possible intervention. The speech–language pathologist must address each possible etiology as a contributing factor in making a diagnosis, constructing an appropriate plan for intervention, and recognizing structural and neurologic limitations to speech production that may require coordinated treatment with other medical or dental specialists.

Clinical Assessment of Speech and Voice

Developmental checklists should include milestones for speech and language acquisition so that speech, voice, and language disorders are not overlooked. However, there are no "gold standards" for screening children for speech and language development in the pediatric office [9]. Evaluation of speech, voice, and language skills in young children may be particularly difficult in the pediatrician's office given that other developmental assessments and routine medical care such as vaccinations need to be completed. Also, very young or shy children may not speak during a well-child or other medical office visit so pediatricians need to may rely on parental report. Fortunately, parents are often excellent reporters of early speech and language acquisition including number and variety of words [10], fluency [11, 12], and delayed language development [13]. Many parents have recorded their child's speech on mobile phones which can also serve as a useful tool.

When children have a known diagnosis, for example, cerebral palsy, hearing loss, or cleft palate, there is some expectation that speech and language skill development may be affected so parents and pediatricians may detect concerns early. However, speech and voice disorders often occur in the absence of a known diagnosis. In order to assist the pediatrician in describing and understanding cases in which the articulation, fluency, resonance, or voice concern is the presenting symptom we describe the general problem that parents or other caregivers are likely to notice, possible causes to consider, and specific characteristics to look or listen for in the child's speech. The organizational structure follows the typical clinical decision-making approach, first to rule out organic or neurologic causes and then to consider developmental, functional, or combined etiologies. A summary of general causes and example characteristics is presented in Table 13.1.

Table 13.1 Summary of observed speech, fluency, resonance, and voice characteristics, the common causes associated with the clinically observed behavior, and specific examples of what to look for or listen for in the child's speech

Observation	Possible causes	Look or listen for
Speech is difficult to understand	Malocclusion or other oral structural anomaly	Jaw or dental misalignments Distortions of specific speech sounds
	Neuromotor disorders Dysarthria	Reduced precision with vowel or consonant production, increases as length of utterance increases Short utterances with frequent or irregular pauses for breathing Abnormally slow speech rate Unusual prosody
	Apraxia	Groping oral movements during speech Difficulty repeating multisyllabic words Inconsistent ability to say certain sounds or words

Table 13.1 (continued)

Observation	Possible causes	Look or listen for
	Phonological disorders	Simplification patterns persist longer than expected
		Simplification patterns are unusual
		Specific sounds, groups of sounds, or sounds in specific positions of words are absent
Disfluent speech	Developmental stuttering	Repeats speech sounds, words, or phrases
		Prolongs speech sounds
		Blocking or "freezing" on speech sounds
		Extraneous movements of the head, neck, or limbs
		Avoids words and speaking situations
	Cluttering	Rapid or irregular speaking rate
		Articulatory imprecision
		Difficult for the listener to follow the narrative
		Lack of awareness of the listener's ability to understand the message
Hypernasality	Submucous cleft palate	Bifid uvula
		Blue-appearing midline raphe
		V-shaped notch at border of hard and soft palates
		May have excessively nasal speech
	Velopharyngeal dysfunction (structural)	Hypernasality
		Nasal air emission
	Velopharyngeal dysfunction (neuromotor)	Intermittent hypernasality, hyponasality, or mixed resonance
Hyponasality	Adenoid enlargement	Mouth breathing, difficulty with nasal airflow
	Sinus or nasal obstruction	Reduced nasality, sounds "stuffy"
Vocal quality is abnormal	Vocal fold pathology	Persistent hoarseness
		Complaint of vocal fatigue
		Visible lesions on the vocal folds
	Vocal fold paralysis	Persistent breathy voice or aphonia
		Respiratory stridor
		Short utterances or frequent pauses for breathing
		Difficulty projecting voice
		Complaint of vocal fatigue
		Swallowing difficulties including aspiration
	Functional voice disorders	Persistent hoarseness, breathiness, or aphonia
		Strained or tight voice
		Neck or jaw tension
		Complaint of vocal fatigue
		Excessive or inappropriate voice use patterns

Disorders of Speech Sound Production

Perceptual Characteristics of Speech Sound Disorders

Speech sounds disorders are a large class of conditions that include problems with articulation or learning the phonological rules that guide word assembly in a language. These may have structural, neurologic, or language-based etiologies. As a class of disorders, speech sound disorders reduce accuracy in production of speech sounds that negatively impacts the child's speech intelligibility. The child's speech may include omissions, substitutions that follow predictable patterns, "slurred," or "slushy" speech sound production, and each characteristic has implications related to underlying cause. Differentiating among these disorders becomes important for treatment planning. When grouped together it is estimated that speech sound disorders occur among 15% of preschool-aged children [3].

Organic Causes of Speech Sound Disorders

Intelligible speech production requires accurate placement of the articulators and there are a variety of congenital conditions that may interfere with the structural integrity of these articulators including cleft palate, micro- or macro-glossia, and maxillary or mandibular hypoplasia. Normal dental and jaw relationships are critical to typical articulation patterns. For example, a child with a significant open bite may have difficulty achieving an adequate lip seal for "m, b, and p" production. Dental malocclusion may cause distortions of speech sounds, particularly consonant sounds that use the teeth, for example, "th, f, and v."

Ankyloglossia (also known as tongue tie) occurs in approximately 5% of newborns [14]. While often implicated in feeding and speech difficulties, ankyloglossia has negative effects for a relatively small proportion of infants and children with this condition. Messner and colleagues [14] report that 83% of infants with ankyloglossia were breastfed successfully, while 25% of mothers reported difficulties. If feeding is not affected, ankyloglossia can be left untreated until speech develops. Like feeding, speech is negatively affected for only a small portion of individuals with ankyloglossia. When speech is affected, tongue tip sounds such as "l, n, t, d, and th" may be "slushy" or "slurred."

On oral examination, a child with significant ankyloglossia will most often demonstrate limited range of motion for the tongue tip together with a heart-shaped appearance of the tongue tip on protrusion [15]. However, there is no clear relationship between oral appearance and functional outcome [15], thus treatment decisions should most often incorporate an assessment of speech sound production to determine whether speech (or feeding) is affected.

Neurologic Causes of Speech Sound Disorders

A child who has sustained any insult to the central or peripheral nervous system is at risk for diminished strength, movement precision, or coordination among the respiratory, phonatory, resonance, and articulatory systems. A disorder of speech

motor movement is called dysarthria. Like cerebral palsy, dysarthria can be classified as flaccid, spastic, ataxic, hypokinetic, hyperkinetic, or mixed [16]. Neurologic
signs of motor impairment such as weakness, slowness, inaccuracy, altered muscle
tone, tremor, and discoordination can help define the specific clinical features of a
dysarthria. Children with dysarthria may experience control abnormalities in any
or all of the respiratory, phonatory, articulatory, resonance, or prosodic elements of
speech production, often significantly diminishing speech intelligibility.

Childhood apraxia of speech (CAS; also called developmental apraxia of speech
or dyspraxia) is a poorly understood condition that remains somewhat controversial with respect to clear diagnostic criteria, cause, and approaches to intervention
[17, 18]. CAS is typically categorized as a neuromotor disorder, primarily related to
its similarity to adult forms of apraxia which are most often associated with lesions
in the frontal and parietal lobes of the dominant hemisphere [19]. While some children with CAS exhibit neural lesions, in the majority of cases the etiology is not
well understood.

The speech of children with CAS is characterized by "groping" oral movements
and inconsistency in speech sound production [18–20]. For example, the child
may say a speech sound in a word, but is then unable to repeat just the sound in
isolation when asked. Unusual prosody, poor intelligibility, increased errors with
longer utterances, and unusual developmental trajectory for speech are also often
associated, but not required to make the diagnosis of CAS [18–20]. CAS occurs
most often "in the absence of identified neuromotor deficits," with no clear evidence
of weakness, paralysis, absent, or abnormal reflexes [20, pp. 3–4]. While CAS is
considered idiopathic for many children associated social, behavioral, cognitive,
and learning anomalies may co-occur which suggests the need for interdisciplinary
assessment [21].

Developmental, Functional, Idiopathic, or Behavioral Causes of Speech Sound Disorders

If phonological simplifications persist past age expectation or are atypical, the child
may be identified as having a speech sound disorder referred to as a phonological
disorder. Phonological disorders are characterized by patterns of error that follow
the simplification rules used by younger children or by unusual patterns of error
that are not typical of younger children [6]. Some children mislearn certain speech
sounds or whole classes of speech sounds. For example, the child may produce all
fricative (continuous) sounds ("f, s") as stop consonants ("p" and "t") and then persist in this pattern. It may not be possible to discern whether the child's speech sound
errors follow a predictable pattern without collecting a comprehensive inventory of
speech sounds the child produces in various speaking contexts.

Disorders of Speech Fluency

Perceptual Characteristics of Fluency Disorders

Stuttering is a relatively common fluency disorder in children. Like normally developing children, children who stutter also exhibit a range of typical disfluencies,

such as hesitations and interjections. However, children who stutter also exhibit disfluencies and other behaviors atypical of normal development. Primary stuttering behaviors consist of frequent repetitions of speech sounds, syllables, words and phrases (e.g., "t-t-t-top"), prolongation of speech sounds (e.g., "mmmmany"), and a sudden blocking or freezing of the articulatory or vocal mechanism resulting in tension and silence. The frequent use of interjections such as "um" or "ah" or word revisions is also common. Stuttering episodes are intermittent but typically occur near the beginning of utterances and words. Additionally, children who stutter often exhibit a range of extraneous head, neck, and body movements that co-occur with speaking. Common behaviors are eye blinking, aversion of eye gaze, facial grimaces, jaw and face tremor, head jerking, and foot tapping. As the child becomes more aware of her speech difficulties, she may begin avoiding difficult sounds, words, and speaking situations and develop fear, embarrassment, and other negative emotions associated with talking. The full constellation of stuttering features can be highly variable from individual to individual making it challenging for the clinician to identify and manage.

Cluttering is a developmental fluency disorder that is distinct from, but often co-occurs with stuttering. The speech of children who clutter can be quite difficult to understand due to a combination of rapid and irregular speech rate, a general lack of articulatory precision, poor thought and language formulation, diminished conversational skills, and an apparent lack of awareness of communication problems [22].

Neurologic Causes of Fluency Disorders

Although rare, cases of stuttering resulting from brain injury do occur. The basal ganglia is the most common site of lesion associated with neurologic stuttering [23]. Other neurologic and/or developmental language disorders can mimic fluency disorders. For example, if a child has difficulty with word retrieval, this can appear as hesitations, revisions, or interjections in his speech. Therefore, children who have sustained central nervous system injuries or who exhibit developmental delays may appear to stutter, but careful diagnostics may reveal an underlying language disruption or disorder.

Developmental, Functional, Idiopathic, or Behavioral Causes of Fluency Disorders

For the vast majority of cases, stuttering is considered a developmental speech disorder with no clear organic or neurologic cause. The onset of symptoms tends to first appear around the time of rapid expansion of speech and language skills, between 2 and 3.5 years of age with an average age of onset of around 2.5 years [11]. Although recovery from stuttering can occur, approximately 1% of the general population experiences chronic, lifelong stuttering [24], making it a relatively common communication disorder. Stuttering is much more common in boys. It also tends to occur in families suggesting a genetic factor for at least some individuals. Recent studies have begun to identify specific genetic anomalies associated with familial stuttering [25]. Current theories of developmental stuttering generally consider it to be a complex, multi-factorial disorder with genetics, behavior, and environment serving as contributing factors [11].

Resonance Disorders

Perceptual Characteristics of Resonance Disorders

Resonance disturbances alter the quality of speech often in a way that is described as "nasal." However, this term is often applied to two conditions with quite different implications. Reduced nasal energy in speech (hyponasality) is heard during an acute upper respiratory infection, with allergies, or with enlarged adenoids that block speech energy from escaping through the nasal cavity. Excessive nasal energy in speech, or hypernasality, is heard on non-nasal speech sounds and associated vowels [7]. Hypernasal speech may be accompanied by audible nasal air emission, heard most often on high pressure oral speech sounds such as "s or sh." Nasal air emission can also be seen on a laryngeal mirror held under the nose on repetition of syllables such as "papapa" or "sasasasa." Chronic velopharyngeal dysfunction may be accompanied by secondary behaviors, such as facial grimace, or by compensatory articulation patterns. For example, the child may use the vocal folds to produce "k" instead of using his tongue against the soft palate. Compensatory articulation patterns significantly reduce intelligibility. Some children present with both hypo- and hypernasal speech. Perceptual discrimination of hypo-, hyper-, and mixed resonance can be very difficult, particularly in connected speech. Hypernasal speech is never normal and this should trigger further investigation and assessment.

Organic Causes of Resonance Disorders

Cleft palate is the most common cause of structural disruption to the velopharyngeal complex. Oral clefts occur in 1 in 600 live births in the United States [26] with similar rates worldwide. Ideally, cleft palate should be repaired by 12 months of age [7] in order to allow the child to acquire speech sounds with an intact palate and functioning velopharyngeal mechanism. Of children with repaired cleft palate, approximately 25% will require some additional physical management [7].

Submucous cleft palate is a form of cleft palate that is often undetected at birth. The cardinal signs of submucous cleft palate are a bifid uvula, blue-appearing midline of the velum, and visible or palpable V-shaped notch at the border of the hard and soft palates [7]. Submucous clefts are often detected in association with a complaint about hypernasal speech, although many individuals with submucous cleft palate have asymptomatic speech. Submucous cleft palate is a contraindication for full adenoidectomy and may be associated with an underlying syndrome in a child with other observable developmental or congenital anomalies [7].

Neurologic Causes of Resonance Disorders

Any condition that involves diminished motor coordination for speech, such as dysarthria, can cause difficulties that affect velopharyngeal timing and yield a perception of hypernasality or mixed resonance. Sensorineural hearing loss can also yield resonance disturbances.

Functional Causes of Resonance Disorders

Occasionally a child mislearns a speech sound or family of speech sounds and persists in producing the sound with nasal air emission. This is called phoneme-specific nasal air emission and is most often observed in fricative sounds ("s and z") and is very amenable to treatment through speech therapy [7].

Voice Disorders

Perceptual Characteristics of Voice Disorders

As noted earlier, pitch is a prominent perceptual attribute of the voice. Abnormally high or low pitch or abnormal pitch variation can be indicative of a voice disorder. The respiratory–phonatory system is also largely responsible for controlling vocal intensity. It is not uncommon for young children to speak at greater loudness levels when compared to adults. Persistently loud voice can be an indication for preventive intervention because louder voice requires greater collision forces of the vocal folds and is associated with the development with benign lesions of the vocal folds, including vocal nodules and polyps [27]. Inadequate habitual loudness or a reduced ability to voluntarily vary loudness to meet communication demands can also be indicators for abnormality.

Pitch and loudness often fail to adequately capture the essence of a vocal disturbance. Often there is a deviation in the quality of voice production. A voice quality abnormality is termed dysphonia. Aphonia is a lack of any vocal tone and is perceptually equivalent to a whisper. While voice quality is a somewhat difficult to define, standard terminology has been adopted to help specify changes in voice quality including breathiness, strain, and roughness. In some cases, these perceptual features help determine etiology.

It is also common for a child with a voice disorder to report other symptoms associated with the voice disturbance. Depending on the underlying etiology, these symptoms can include vocal fatigue or change in vocal function through the day, limited vocal range, frequent coughing and throat clearing, excess mucus production, respiratory stridor, swallowing difficulties, and soreness and other sensations in and around the larynx.

Temporary voice problems are commonly associated with upper respiratory infections. However, approximately 4% of preschoolers and between 6 and 9% of primary school children experience chronic voice problems [27–29]. Longitudinal studies suggest that most school age children with voice problems do not experience symptom resolution simply with maturation and therefore require some professional management [30].

Organic Causes of Voice Disorders

Children can exhibit a range of congenital and acquired organic conditions that result in voice and laryngeal disturbances. Congenital laryngeal abnormalities include subglottic stenosis, laryngocele, laryngomalacia, laryngeal webbing, and, less frequently, laryngeal clefts [31]. Acquired conditions include laryngeal papillomatosis, intubation-related laryngeal trauma, and lesion formation secondary to uncontrolled gastroesophageal reflux [31]. In addition to causing vocal disturbances, many of these conditions are often associated with respiratory and swallowing problems.

Neurologic Causes of Voice Disorders

The most common neurologically based voice disorder observed in children is paresis or paralysis of a vocal fold. Vocal fold paralysis can be a congenital or acquired during surgical injury, neck trauma, vascular lesions, tumors, or inflammatory illness [32]. Unilateral vocal fold paralysis can result in weak, breathy voice production, problems with aspiration during drinking, and respiratory stridor. Bilateral vocal fold paralysis can cause aphonia, breathiness, and significant difficulties with airway protection during swallowing. Bilateral paralyzed vocal folds can also obstruct the airway, requiring surgical management. Finally, dysphonia can be an important perceptual feature of dysarthria that arises from neurological trauma or disease.

Developmental, Functional, Idiopathic, or Behavioral Causes

Children can also present with range of functional voice disorders that occur in the absence of any laryngeal abnormality. One example of this type of voice disturbance is muscle tension dysphonia, which is thought to result from speaking with inappropriately high levels of laryngeal muscle tension. Another example of a purely functional voice disorder is puberphonia, a relatively rare condition where, in spite of normal anatomical change, an adolescent boy maintains a pre-pubescent high-pitched speaking voice. More commonly, inappropriate vocal use patterns such as excessive talking, shouting, growling can contribute toward the development of benign vocal fold lesions such as vocal fold nodules, polyps, and contact ulcers. Finally, in an attempt to compensate for the presence of an organic or neuromotor disturbance, the child may develop maladaptive behaviors that serve to worsen the voice disturbance.

When to Refer

A speech–language evaluation is typically a non-invasive, relatively inexpensive mechanism through which to provide assurance that the child is developing as expected or to identify areas of concern related to speech production. If one or more of the features of speech, fluency, resonance, or voice presented in Table 13.1 are present, the child should be referred for assessment.

Suspected Speech Sound Disorders

It is typical for parents to be able to understand the speech of very young children more easily than others. The child should be able to convey in-context messages by age 3 and be understood by an unfamiliar adult by age 4 years. If parents or others express concern that the child's speech cannot be understood, even at younger ages, the child may benefit from referral.

Suspected Fluency Disorders

If a child is demonstrating features of stuttering (and/or cluttering), a referral to a speech–language pathologist for a formal speech evaluation is recommended. While recovery from stuttering is not uncommon, the speech–language pathologist is in the best position to diagnose a fluency disorder, determine the risk for persistence [11], and develop the most effective management plan for the child. Although there is no known cure for stuttering, effective treatment approaches are available, even for very young children [33].

Suspected Resonance Disorders

Abnormal quality of speech resonance is never expected, although transient periods of hyponasality occur in association with upper respiratory infections and allergies. Although seemingly disparate, it can be quite difficult to differentiate hypo- from hypernasality in connected speech. Thus, careful assessment of oral versus nasal speech sounds is critical together with ruling out other distortions and voice disturbances that can mimic resonance disorders. Most often, children with suspected resonance disturbances should be seen by otolaryngology and/or speech–language pathology. When a submucous cleft palate is suspected or when a child with a known repaired cleft exhibits speech, hearing, or dental occlusion concerns, the family should be encouraged to pursue assessment and treatment through a coordinated interdisciplinary cleft palate team.

Suspected Voice Disorders

Persistent voice abnormalities are not expected during typical speech and language development. However, short-lived changes in voice quality are not an unusual event for young children. Upper respiratory infections of viral or bacterial origin are relatively common and frequently result in transient hoarseness and other vocal symptoms. A vocal abnormality that lasts longer than typically expected from upper respiratory infection warrants a referral for an otolaryngology and speech–language pathology evaluation. Many large medical centers have dedicated multi-disciplinary teams devoted to assessment and management of voice disorders.

Evaluation of Speech and Voice Disorders

When a child is referred for assessment of vocal or speech function, the speech–language pathologist will first establish the nature of the concern. Across conditions, the speech–language pathologist will benefit from understanding the child's medical history, known medical diagnoses, and be provided with other developmental concerns or assessments that have been conducted. It is typical to talk with a parent or guardian before the assessment to establish the nature of the concern and the caregivers' primary concerns and goals.

A typical speech or voice assessment requires about a 1 h evaluation and includes eliciting a conversational sample of spoken language through play as well as through standardized test procedures. Often these techniques are combined in order to observe how the child uses voice and speech as a social communication tool and to narrow the observation of specific speech sounds, voice, resonance characteristics, or fluency.

Evaluation of Speech Production

Although the primary reason for concern may be the child's speech intelligibility or capacity for production, it is often important to establish the child's language comprehension and expression skills, because delays and disorders of language can yield concomitant delays and disorders of speech intelligibility.

Articulation is assessed using standardized measures that allow the child to produce every consonant sound in every word position across 30–50 words. This approach allows the speech–language pathologist to determine which sounds or classes of sounds are absent or distorted in single word productions. This is often extended to short sentences through story repetition tasks. Additionally, the speech–language pathologist will provide some trial instruction or demonstration to assess how easy or difficult it is for the child to modify his or her speech production. This assessment of stimulability assists with determining appropriate goals for therapy.

Evaluation of Speech Fluency

Speech fluency is assessed by evaluating the frequency, type and severity of disfluent events across a variety of speech tasks including conversation, reading (if child is literate), and during situations known to cause difficulties (such as the telephone). Extraneous movements of the head and body are also noted. A frank discussion with the child's parents as well as self-report questionnaires help provide information about the child's reactions and attitudes about stuttering specifically and communication in general. Typically, screening of speech and language skills are performed to rule out any co-existing speech sound, voice, or language-based communication disorder.

Evaluation of Speech Resonance

Resonance is assessed perceptually in conversation as well as across specific oral and nasal speech sounds, noting sound substitutions or patterns of compensatory articulation, observing for behavioral signs, such as facial grimace (wrinkling the nose or face during production of specific speech sounds). An oral examination is conducted to rule out patent oral–nasal fistulae, submucous cleft palate, asymmetries or deviations in palatal movements, or other neurologic or structural changes in the oral cavity. It should be noted that visual inspection of palate length is not related to velopharyngeal function. Perceptual and oral examination data are then used to determine whether an instrumental assessment of velopharyngeal function is appropriate. Several instrumental methods are available and allow measurements of oral–nasal balance in speech relative to norms, pressure flow or nasometry, or direct visualization of the velopharyngeal structures during speech production, nasoendoscopy, and videofluoroscopy [7].

Evaluation of Vocal Function

Given the wide range of etiologies of voice disorders, a comprehensive evaluation is required prior to developing an appropriate management plan. At a minimum, management of voice disorders in children will involve an otolaryngologist and a speech–language pathologist. As with any clinical evaluation, the assessment typically begins with a careful symptom, health, and social history. In addition, the clinician will also carefully scrutinize the vocal use patterns to determine if the child engages in excessive and/or inappropriate vocal behaviors. During clinical evaluation phase of the assessment, it is critical to obtain a laryngoscopic examination to determine the structure and basic function of the larynx. A formal evaluation of vocal function will include a perceptual analysis of voice for a variety of speaking tasks. In some instances, additional instrumental analysis of the voice using acoustic and aerodynamic analyses may be indicated.

Management

If speech or voice therapy is indicated through evaluation, a variety of models for delivery of service may be used. Traditionally, speech and voice therapy is conducted in outpatient clinical settings with one-on-one direct service. Very young children often qualify for home-based early intervention that incorporates a great deal of parent and family education and intervention in a familiar setting for the child. For children with speech sound disorders, small group sessions are often available and allow children to use speech in a naturalistic setting with their peers. Services are offered through early infant, toddler, and preschool programs, the public schools, as well as hospital-based outpatient clinics, private practices, and university teaching clinics.

Intervention for speech and voice disorders is designed to accommodate the child's age and interests. Most children perceive speech therapy as fun because it is centered around the child and is often structured using play-based approaches with behavioral reinforcement for accurate production of the target goals.

Assessments may yield uncertainty about whether the child is a candidate for speech therapy. For example, a trial of therapy may be proposed for a child with a fluency, resonance, or voice disorder. In some cases, the child may exhibit "borderline" function that is not suggestive of an immediate need for intervention, but may yield some concern. In such cases, parent education about expectations for continued development is critical. Parents are provided with suggestions to implement at home together with a planned re-evaluation to monitor the child's development of speech, voice, fluency, and language skills.

Structural disorders such as malocclusion, significant ankyloglossia, or visible lesions on the vocal folds may require coordinated medical, dental, and speech services. Children with significant neurological impairments often require coordination of services with physical and occupational therapy for wheelchair positioning or limb control for access to communication devices.

Conclusions

Speech is an efficient mechanism for communication and requires cognitive representation of language together with finely controlled coordination of respiration, vocal, and articulatory movements. Children develop the fundamental control for speech beginning in infancy and continue to fine tune articulation through about age 7 years. During this period of development children may exhibit speech disorders related to hearing, anatomic, neurologic, linguistic, or idiopathic problems. Underlying causes of speech disorders often co-occur.

The speech–language pathologist evaluates the child's voice, speech production mechanism, coordination, fluency, and intelligibility relative to chronological age and language comprehension and production skills. Thus, the speech–language pathologist's role is to ascertain primary disorders and develop an appropriate plan of treatment based on an understanding of the likely causes of the concerns.

Parents may be the first to identify a concern about their child's speech intelligibility, voice quality, or fluency, although they may not differentiate among these terms. Consultation with a speech–language pathologist may provide assurances to parents and pediatricians regarding expected disruptions in speech production or help to identify a child who could benefit from early intervention. Early intervention appears to reduce later complications associated with social communication barriers for children with unintelligible speech. Evidence suggests that children with speech sound disorders, particularly with associated language impairments, are at risk for difficulties with acquisition of reading [34, 35], thus early identification and intervention can assist in prevention and appropriate education planning.

References

1. Fabiano-Smith L, Goldstein BA. Early, middle, and late-developing sounds in monolingual and bilingual children: an exploratory investigation. Am J Speech Lang Pathol. 2010;19: 66–77.
2. Weismer G. Philosophy of research in motor speech disorders. Clin Linguist Phon. 2006;20(5):315–49.
3. Robb MP. Intro: a guide to communication sciences and disorders. San Diego, CA: Plural; 2010.
4. Eilers RE, Oller DK. Infant vocalizations and the early diagnosis of severe hearing impairment. J Pediatrics. 1994;125(5 Pt 1):844.
5. Owens RE. Development of communication, language, and speech. In: Anderson N, Shames G, editors, Human communication disorders: an introduction. 8th ed. Upper Saddle River, NJ: Pearson; 2011. pp. 16–53.
6. Bernthal JE, Bankson NW. Articulation and phonological disorders. 5th ed. Boston, MA: Pearson Allyn Bacon; 2004.
7. Peterson-Falzone SJ, Hardin-Jones MA, Karnell MP. Cleft palate speech. 4th ed. St. Louis, MO: Mosby-Elsevier; 2010.
8. American Speech Language Hearing Association. Definitions of communication disorders and variations, 1993. www.asha.org/policy. Accessed 09Aug 2010.
9. Nelson HD, Nygren P, Walker M, Panoscha R. Screening for speech and language delay in preschool children: systematic evidence review for the US preventive services task force. Pediatrics. 2006;117(2):e298–e319.
10. Marchman VA, Martine-Sussman C. Concurrent validity of caregiver/parent report measures of language for children who are learning both English and Spanish. J Speech Lang Hear Res. 2002;45(5):983–97.
11. Yairi E, Ambrose NG. Early childhood stuttering: for clinicians by clinicians. Austin, TX: Pro-Ed; 2005.
12. Einarsdottir J, Ingham R. Accuracy of parent identification of stuttering occurrence. Int J Lang Commun Disord. 2009;44(6):847–63.
13. Sachse S, Von Suchodoletz W. Early identification of language delay by direct language assessment or parent report? J Dev Behav Pediatr. 2008;29(1):34–41.
14. Messner AH, Lalakea K, Aby J, Macmahon J, E B. Ankyloglossia: incidence and associated feeding difficulties. Arch Otolaryngol Head Neck Surg. 2000;126:36–39.
15. Lalakea ML, Messner AH. Ankyloglossia: does it matter? Pediatr Clin North Am. 2003;50:381–97.
16. Murdoch BE. Neurogenic disorders of speech in children and adults. In: Anderson N, Shames G, editors, Human communication disorders: an introduction. 8th ed. Upper Saddle River, NJ: Pearson; 2011. pp. 272–304.
17. Morgan AT, Vogel AP. Intervention for childhood apraxia of speech. Cochrane Database Syst Rev. 2008;16(3):CD006278.
18. Shriberg LD, Aram DM, Kwiatkowski J. Developmental apraxia of speech: i. descriptive and theoretical perspectives. J Speech Lang Hear Res. 1997;40(2):273–85.

19. Duffy JR. Motor speech disorders: substrates, differential diagnosis, and management. St. Louis, MO: Elsevier Mosby; 2005.
20. American Speech-Language-Hearing Association. Childhood apraxia of speech [Technical Report], 2007. www.asha.org/policy. Accessed 09 Aug 2010.
21. Teverovsky EG, Bickel KO, Feldman HM. Functional characteristics of children diagnosed with childhood apraxia of speech. Disabil Rehabil. 2009;31(2):94–102.
22. Ward D. Stuttering and cluttering: frameworks for understanding and treatment. New York, NY: Psychol Press; 2006.
23. Ludlow CL, Stuttering: LT. a dynamic motor control disorder. J Fluency Disord. 2003;28: 273–95.
24. Bloodstein O, Ratner NB. A handbook on stuttering. 6th ed. Clifton Park, NY: Thomson/Delmar; 2008.
25. Kang C, Riazuddin S, Mundorff J, Krasnewich D, Friedman P, Mullikin JC, Drayna D. Mutations in the lysosomal enzyme-targeting pathway and persistent stuttering. N Engl J Med. 2010;362(8):677–85.
26. National Institutes of Dental and Craniofacial Disorders: prevalence (number of cases) of cleft lip and cleft palate. Author, 2010. http://www.nidcr.nih.gov/DataStatistics/FindDataByTopic/ CraniofacialBirthDefects/PrevalenceCleft+LipCleftPalate.htm. Accessed 18 Aug 2010.
27. Andrews ML, Summers AC. Voice treatment for children and adolescents. San Diego, CA: Singular; 2002.
28. Carding PN, Roulstone S, Northstone K. ALSPAC Study Team. The prevalence of childhood dysphonia: a cross-sectional study. J Voice. 2006;20(4):623–30.
29. Duff MC, Proctor A, Yairi E. Prevalence of voice disorders in African American and European American preschoolers. J Voice. 2004;18(3):348–53.
30. Powell M, Filter MD, Williams B. A longitudinal study of the prevalence of voice disorders in children from a rural school division. J Commun Disord. 1989;22(5):375–82.
31. Sapienza CM, Ruddy BH, Baker S. Laryngeal structure and function in the pediatric larynx: clinical applications. Lang Speech Hear Serv Sch. 2004;35:299–307.
32. Wilson DK. Voice problems in children. 3rd ed. Baltimore, MD: Williams Wilkins; 1987.
33. Jones M, Onslow M, Packman A, Williams S, Ormond T, Schwarz I, Gebski V. Randomised controlled trial of the Lidcombe programme of early stuttering intervention. BMJ. 2005;331:659–66.
34. Peterson RL, Pennington BF, Shriberg LD, Boada R. What influences literacy outcome in children with speech sound disorder? J Speech Lang Hear Res. 2009;52(2):1175–88.
35. Schuele CM. The impact of developmental speech and language impairments on the acquisition of literacy skills. Ment Retard Dev Disabil Res Rev. 2004;10(3):176–83.

Chapter 14
Tic Disorders

Donald E. Greydanus

Abstract Tics are movements that are sudden, brief, stereotyped, purposeless, and involuntary. They are often identified as motor tics, vocal tics, and sensory tics. Tic disorders are one of the most common neuropsychiatric and neurodevelopmental abnormalities in children and adolescents that are mostly genetic or idiopathic in origin. Tic disorders are classified as transient tic disorder, chronic motor or vocal tic disorder, Tourette's disorder, and tic disorder not otherwise specified. They are diagnosed with classic features that begin before 18 years of age and are not the result of stimulants or disorders such as Huntington's disease or post-viral encephalitis. Treatment involves psychopharmacology as reviewed in this chapter. Cognitive and behavior therapies are also beneficial for these patients. Therapy should seek to improve the quality of life for children, adolescents, and adults with tic disorders.

Introduction

Tic disorders are among the most common neuropsychiatric and neurodevelopmental abnormalities in children and adolescents that may also extent into the adult population. Current classification usually is based on the terms as defined by the American Psychiatric Association's Diagnostic and Statistical Manual of Mental Disorders, 4th edition, Text Revision [DSM-IV-TR], published in 2000 [1]. This chapter reviews the definition, clinical features, epidemiology, and pharmacologic treatment of tic disorders. Cognitive and behavior therapies are also important with attention to improvement of the quality of life for these children and adolescents. Treatment of comorbidities is also a critical part of the overall management plan.

D.E. Greydanus (✉)
Department of Pediatrics and Human Development, Kalamazoo Center for Medical Studies,
Michigan State University College of Human Medicine, Kalamazoo, MI 49008-1284, USA
e-mail: greydanus@kcms.msu.edu

D.R. Patel et al. (eds.), *Neurodevelopmental Disabilities,*
DOI 10.1007/978-94-007-0627-9_14, © Springer Science+Business Media B.V. 2011

Definition

Tic or habit spasms are movements that are sudden, brief, highly stereotyped, involuntary, and purposeless. Tics are usually identified as motor tics, vocal tics, and a rare-type sensory tics. The traditional manner of tic disorder classification is based on that of the DSM-IV-TR by the American Psychiatric Association: transient tic disorder, chronic motor/vocal tic disorder, Tourette's syndrome (disorder), and tic disorder not otherwise specified [1].

In order to meet the definition of a tic disorder in this system, the onset is before age 18 years and the underlying etiology is not based on such conditions as substance abuse disorder, Huntington's disease, or post-viral encephalitis. It is anticipated that the publication of DSM-V in 2012 or 2013 will result in further changes to the specific nosology of tic disorders [2]. The etiology of tic disorders remains unclear at present, and Table 14.1 lists current theories [3–5]. Tic disorders are essentially genetic or idiopathic in nature. Clearly further research is needed to establish underlying etiologic mechanisms in various tic disorders.

Clinical Features

Clinical features are based on the type of tic disorder that is present, and classification includes transient tic disorder, chronic motor or vocal tic disorder, Tourette's disorder (syndrome), and tic disorder not otherwise specified.

Transient Tic Disorder

Those with transient tic disorder develop one or multiple tics (motor or vocal) that are present for at lease 4 weeks but not longer than 12 consecutive months [6]. Typically there is a positive family history for tics. Tics may include shrugging of shoulders, blinking of eyes, facial grimaces, and other types of tics; however, vocal tics are not found. The child or youth may voluntarily suppress their tics for minutes to hours until the tic reoccurs. The tics may worsen with stress and multiple motor

Table 14.1 Etiologic theories of tic disorders [3–5]

1. Circuitry abnormalities (inhibitory dysfunction) in such areas of the central nervous system as the globus pallidus, thalamus, striatum, and frontal lobe (frontal–subcortical circuits)
2. Effects of PANDAS (pediatric autoimmune neuropsychiatric disorders associated with streptococci) due to infection with group A beta-hemolytic streptococcus
3. Prefrontal-dopaminergic dysfunction
4. Dopaminergic abnormality (noted by improvement in tics often seen with use of neuroleptic medications)
5. Increase in numbers of dopamine receptors and increased levels of dopamine transporters
6. Basal ganglia dysfunction

tics may sometimes be seen as well. Fortunately, transient tic disorder lives up to its name, and the condition usually spontaneously resolves, typically within weeks of its onset, though some may last up to 12 months.

Chronic Motor or Vocal Tic Disorder

Those with this diagnosis develop one or multiple tics (motor or vocal), and these tics last longer than 1 year and there is no period absent of tics for more than 3 months [6]. Motor and vocal tics are not found at the same time.

Tourette's Disorder (Syndrome)

There is a 3–4:1 male to female ratio in Tourette's syndrome (disorder), and its onset is usually between 2 and 15 years of age; the average age of onset is 7 years, and, by established definition, the end age of onset is 21 years of age. A positive family history is usually found for tic disorders (transient or chronic) and/or Tourette's disorder.

Symptomatology in Tourette's disorder includes the development of multiple motor tics and one (or more) vocal tic lasting longer than 1 year but with no tic-free period of more than 3 months [6–10]. Table 14.2 lists the many types of tics that may occur in children and adolescents with Tourette's disorder. A tic builds up an unpleasant sensation that must eventually be relieved and then leads to more tics

Table 14.2 Tics noted in Tourette's syndrome

Simple or complex tics involving	Head
	Neck
	Trunk
	Extremities (upper or lower)
Motor tics	Eye blinking
	Lip smacking
	Shoulder shrugging
	Head tossing
	Grimacing
	Others
Simple vocal tics	Coughing
	Grunting
	Shouting
	Crying
	Barking
	Throat clearing
	Sniffing
Complex vocal tics	Echolalia (repeating words)
	Palilalia (repeating the last sound)
	Coprolalia (swearing)

Modified with permission from Greydanus and Tsitsika [6, ch. 12, p. 226]

Table 14.3 Conditions associated with Tourette's syndrome

Condition	Frequency (estimated %)
Attention-deficit hyperactivity disorder	50–60
Obsessive–compulsive disorder	25–50
Other anxiety disorders	30–40
Mood disorders	30–40
Learning disorders (±ADHD)	20–30
Disruptive behavior disorders	Common, but more related to ADHD
Explosive anger ("rage"), including intermittent explosive disorder	Common, related to ADHD and mood disorders
Substance use disorders	Unknown, but increases with age
Pervasive developmental disorders	Unknown, but likely low

Modified with permission from Greydanus and Tsitsika [6, p. 227]

via a complex restimulation mechanism [11]. Various conditions associated with Tourette's syndrome are noted in Table 14.3. Attention-deficit hyperactivity disorder (ADHD) is noted in 30–50% of pediatric patients while 30–60% also have obsessive–compulsive disorder.

In the usual presentation motor tics begin before vocal tics and one tic is the presenting scenario in about half of patients while many tics may initially occur in the other half. The first tic is an eye tic in 37% of cases versus a head tic in 16% and a vocal tic in 18% [6–10]. A sensory tic is found in 3% and is characterized by an unpleasant feeling or sensation developing around a muscle group or joint that is relieved by a tic. Coprolalia is the initial feature in 0.1% of those with Tourette's disorder; however, it may eventually be seen in about one-third of these patients. It is characteristic that voluntary tic suppression for a brief amount of time can occur that eventually leads to a tic because of the buildup of a feeling of unpleasantness. Some children with Tourette's disorder note improvement during adolescence while some continue as adults with potential major disability due to the tic disorder.

Tic Disorder Not Otherwise Specified

Situations that do not meet criteria for Tourette's syndrome, transient tic disorder, or chronic motor or vocal tic disorder are classified in the American Association of Psychiatry system as Tic Disorder Not Otherwise Specified [1].

Epidemiology

Transient tic disorder is found in 4–20% of children and young teenagers with a 2–3:1 male to female ratio. Chronic motor tic disorder (chronic tic disorder) is found in 1–2% of the general population, and experts typically relate it to Tourette's syndrome, and a positive family history for Tourette's disorder is often present;

its etiology is typically linked to dysfunction of CNS dopamine metabolism (see Table 14.1). Gilles de la Tourette's syndrome (Tourette's syndrome or disorder) is found in 5 per 10,000, and it is 10 times more common in children versus adults [12]. A recent report based on data from the 2007 National Survey of Children's Health of US children and adolescents aged 6–17 years of age concludes that the estimated prevalence of Tourette's syndrome by parent report is 3.0 per 1,000; 79% had at least one comorbid condition (see Table 14.3) [13].

Diagnosis

The diagnosis is made in the individual who presents with classic features, and Table 14.4 presents a differential diagnostic system for involuntary muscle movements [14–16]. As noted, tics are not due to medications (as stimulants) or to such illnesses as post-viral encephalitis or Huntington's disease [15].

Treatment

Management of tics and tic disorders involves a variety of strategies ranging from education of the patient (family) about the specific condition that is present to behavioral–cognitive therapy that can be intensive and also various pharmacologic therapies [15, 17–19]. The web site of the Tourette Syndrome Association from the United States (http://www.tsa-usa.org) contains useful information for patient and parent education.

Table 14.4 Involuntary muscle movements

Athetosis	Slow, sinuous, writhing, involuntary movement that most frequently involves distal extremities; frequently increased by voluntary movements
Ballismus	Wild, flinging, coarse, irregular, involuntary movements beginning in proximal limb muscles
Chorea	Rapid, irregular, non-repetitive, sudden movement that may involve any muscle or muscle group; these movements generally interfere with voluntary movements
Dystonia	Slow, twisting, involuntary movements associated with changes in muscle tone; movements generally involve trunk and proximal extremity muscles
Myoclonus	Involuntary rapid, shock-like muscular contractions that are generally non-repetitive; can be increased by voluntary actions
Spasm	Slow and prolonged involuntary contraction of a muscle or group of muscles
Tic	Involuntary, repetitive movement of related groups of muscles; movements do not interfere with voluntary muscle movements
Tremor	Involuntary movement that may be a slow or rapid vibration of the involved body art; tremors may get worse with movement (intentional tremor) or may occur only at rest

Used with permission from Kuperman [53]

Transient tic disorder typically resolves spontaneously within 12 months, often within a number of weeks. Thus, specific medical management of transient tic disorder is not necessary unless unusual or comorbid conditions arise. Management of tic disorders should also include attention to the quality of life of these patients including how well they are doing with respect to their families, schools, and peers. Clinicians should note that complete tic suppression with pharmacology is usually not possible. Attention should also be carefully paid to comorbid conditions found with Tourette's syndrome such as attention-deficit hyperactivity disorder and obsessive–compulsive disorder (see Table 14.3).

Pharmacotherapy

A wide variety of pharmacologic agents have been used to manage the tics of Tourette's syndrome or chronic motor tic disorder, as noted in Table 14.5 [3, 4, 6, 10, 20–24]. Traditional medications have included pimozide, clonidine, and haloperidol while many other drugs have been used to reduce tics but with less research and anecdotal support behind them.

The majority of the drugs noted in Table 14.5 are linked to letters A, B, or C categories designed to provide information about empirical research support [6]. Category A signifies that the medication has good supportive evidence for safety and efficacy based on two randomized, placebo-controlled studies while Category B signifies fair supportive evidence based on at least one placebo-controlled study supporting it. Finally, Category C drugs have minimal supportive evidence based on less rigorous support such as case reports or open-label studies indicating some efficacy in tic amelioration. This table and these categories will provide helpful information in drug selection for tic control. Figure 14.1 provides a suggested algorithm for management of Tourette's syndrome. Further discussion is now provided regarding alpha-agonists, antipsychotics, and miscellaneous drugs.

Alpha-Agonists

Alpha-agonists include clonidine and guanfacine, and though they lessen CNS adrenergic outflow, their mechanism in reducing tic frequency is not clear at present. Table 14.6 lists indications for use of these drugs. Clonidine is a central-acting, presynaptic, alpha2-adrenergic agonist prescribed two to four times a day with a daily dose range of 0.05–0.3 mg; sometimes it is given only at bedtime [3, 4, 10, 25]. Clonidine is available in a pill or patch formulation; the patch which enhances compliance in some is changed every 7 days.

Guanfacine is an alpha2A-adrenergic agonist that is related to clonidine and used by some clinicians for tic amelioration in patients with Tourette's disorder or chronic motor tic disorder. Guanfacine is prescribed three times a day, and its daily dose ranges from 0.5 to 1 mg. There are no known specific contraindications (i.e., severe drug interactions) linked with these medications.

Table 14.5 Medications used in persons with Tourette's syndrome and comorbid disorders and ages at which use may be appropriate[a]

Class	Agent (A–C)[b]	Doses[a]	Ages[c]
Antipsychotics			
First generation			
Phenothiazines	Fluphenazine (B)	1.5–10 mg/d	≥18
Butyrophenones	Haloperidol (A)	1–4 mg/d	≥18; ≥3[d]
Other	Pimozide (A)	0.05–0.2 mg/kg/d	≥12
Second generation	Risperidone (A)	0.25–2 mg, 1–2×/d	≥18
	Ziprasidone (B)	5–40 mg/d	≥18
	Olanzapine (C)	2.5–12.5 mg/d	≥18
	Quetiapine (C)	25–150 mg/d	≥18
Partial DA agonist	Aripiprazole (C)	10–20 mg/d	≥18
Alpha-agonists	Clonidine (B)	0.05–0.3 mg/d	≥12
	Guanfacine (B)	0.5–1 mg, 3×/d	≥12
Anticonvulsants	Topiramate	50–200 mg/d	≥2
	Levetiracetam	1–2 g/d	≥16
Antidepressants	Fluoxetine (A)	10–60 mg/d	≥7
SSRIs (for OCD)	Sertraline (A)	50–250 mg/d	≥6
	Fluvoxamine (A)	50–350 mg/d	≥6
	Paroxetine (B)	10–60 mg/d	≥18
	Citalopram (B)	20–60 mg/d	N/A
	Escitalopram (B)	10–20 mg/d	N/A
Other (for ADHD)	Atomoxetine	0.5–1.2 mg/kg/d	≥6
DA receptor agonists	Pergolide (B)	0.1–0.4 mg/d	≥18
Muscle relaxants	Baclofen (C)	5–20 mg, 3×/d	≥12
Miscellaneous	Nicotine patch (C)	7–21 mg/d	≥18
	Mecamylamine (C)	2.5–7.5 mg/d	≥18
	Tetrabenazine (C)	12.5–25 mg, 1–3×/d	≥18
Psychostimulants: see Chapter 5 for details			

Modified with permission from Greydanus and Tsitsika [6, ch. 12, p. 228]

DA, dopamine

[a]Dosing is clinically based, unless stated otherwise

[b]Empirical support categories

[c]Ages (years) are for FDA-approved indications; use for other indications and/or at other ages is based on clinical judgment

[d]For "severe behavioral problems"

Table 14.7 lists potential side effects of alpha-agonists, the most common of which are drowsiness, sedation, dizziness, dry mouth, and constipation. Sedation is a major problem for many pediatric patients with these medications, especially clonidine. Less sedation is noted by some with the patch form of clonidine. Orthostatic hypotension is noted but fortunately is not a common adverse effect. Some experts note that rebound hypertension seen with sudden withdrawal of an alpha-agonist is more common in children versus adults [6]. Gradual buildup and withdrawal when using clonidine are recommended to avoid rebound hypertension. Less sedation and

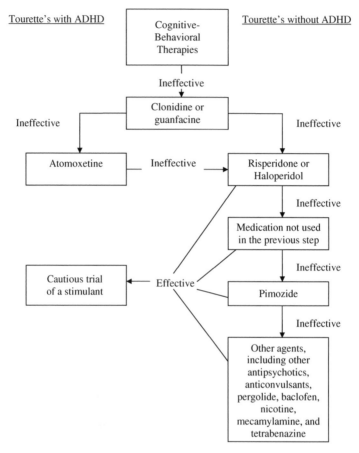

Fig. 14.1 Treatment algorithm for Tourette's syndrome, with/without ADHD. Modified with permission from Greydanus and Tsitsika [6, p. 239]

Table 14.6 Suggested indications for use of clonidine [6]

1. First-line drug for management of tics in Tourette's disorder
2. Alternative or adjunctive drug to stimulants for ADHD (sedative effects may offset insomniac effects of stimulants)
3. Post-traumatic stress disorder
4. Severe aggressiveness seen with conduct disorder or oppositional defiant disorder

blood pressure issues but more headaches and agitation are reported with guanfacine versus clonidine. Gradual titration or buildup is suggested when using clonidine, and abrupt stopping can induce rebound hypertension.

Baseline data are suggested when using clonidine, such as blood pressure, pulse, blood sugar, and electrocardiogram (ECG). These studies can be repeated periodically including an ECG every 6 months. There have been reports of very rare

Table 14.7 Potential side effects of clonidine [6]

1. Sedation (50%) and drowsiness
2. Dizziness
3. Dry mouth
4. Constipation
5. Headache
6. Postural hypotension
7. Withdrawal effects: rebound tachycardia, severe hypertension, and even heart failure from sudden clonidine withdrawal
8. Nausea/emesis
9. Fatigue/lethargy
10. Depression
11. Dysphoria
12. Rebound phenomena
13. Sexual dysfunction
14. Erythema (with the patch)
15. Contact dermatitis (with the patch)

cardiac-related deaths in children and adolescents who were taking both clonidine and methylphenidate (see Chapter 8 on ADHD medications). The mechanism of these rare sudden deaths is not clear, but alpha-agonists should be avoided in those with known structural heart disease.

Antipsychotics

If the tic disorder becomes severe, troubling to the patient, and has not improved with use of intensive behavioral therapy and use of the alpha-agonists, then experts suggest a trial of an antipsychotic medication [3, 4, 6–10, 15, 20, 22, 24–29]. Though the exact method of tic amelioration is not clear, it is presumed to involve dopamine blockade of post-synaptic receptors or dopamine receptor blockade in the CNS cortico-striato-thalamic-cortical circuitry [6]. Full tic suppression may not occur even with high-dose or intensive antipsychotic coverage, and thus, tic frequency reduction along with intensive behavioral management and patient/family education about tic disorders may be the best plan in such refractory cases.

Haloperidol and pimozide are first-generation antipsychotics that have been popular antipsychotics in the past while risperidone (second-generation antipsychotic) is more popular with many clinicians more recently [6, 15, 26, 29, 30] (see Table 14.5). Haloperidol is a butyrophenone and research has noted a 70% reduction in tic frequency in 25% of patients with haloperidol at a dose that avoids major side effects [6]. Approximately half of the patients with tic disorders note tic reduction with haloperidol only if a high enough dose is used that leads to major adverse effects while 25% do not improve with haloperidol [6].

Pimozide leads to tic reduction in 70–80% of children and adolescents at a dose that avoids severe side effects. Pimozide is recommended for Tourette's syndrome and not for chronic motor tic disorder. Experience with risperidone is being accumulated in regard to the amount of tic frequency reduction at a dose that avoids severe adverse effects. Thus, a low dose for any of these agents should be the starting dose with slow and careful titration to a high dose as needed to find the best balance between amelioration of the tics with minimal side effects. Use a "start low and go slow" rule in such prescriptions and monitoring [6].

If haloperidol is chosen by the clinician, begin at an oral dose of 0.25 mg/day and increase to 2 mg/day (divided into a twice a day dosing scheme) as tolerated by the patient. Tic reduction usually occurs at doses lower than that needed to treat psychosis; however, some may need these higher doses as 4–5 mg daily (see Table 14.5). If using pimozide, begin with a 1 mg daily dose and increase up to 4 mg given two times per day. In children start with 0.05–0.2 mg/kg/day and do not exceed a 10 mg daily dose. If risperidone is used for tic suppression, dosing is similar to that noted for haloperidol – start with 0.25 mg a day and slowly increase if needed up to 2 mg twice a day (see Table 14.5).

Though antipsychotics may be effective (partial or full) when used for tic disorders, the concern is the potential for severe side effects that are well known with these medications, such as extrapyramidal symptoms (EPS), neuroleptic malignant syndrome (NMS), cognitive impairment, and lethargy [31, 32] (see Chapter 8 by Greydanus and Chapter 10 by Pratt and Greydanus, this book). The atypical antipsychotics (also called second-generation antipsychotics) cause increase in blood sugar to varying amounts. Also, some atypical antipsychotics (AAs) tend to induce weight gain, and these, in increasing order, include risperidone, quetiapine, and olanzapine (see Table 14.5). The AAs also can cause increase in serum prolactin, except for aripiprazole and quetiapine.

Fluphenazine and haloperidol are contraindicated in those with liver disease, subcortical brain damage, mental obtundation, and blood dyscrasias. If one concludes that use of stimulants and not Tourette's disorder is the cause of the patient's tics, do not combine antipsychotics with stimulants. Pimozide may cause QTc interval prolongation, and it should not be combined with other medications that prolong the QTc interval, including chlorpromazine, thioridazine, nefazodone, sertraline, fluoxetine, fluvoxamine, citalopram, and ziprasidone.

Measure height, weight, and body mass index (BMI) when starting antipsychotics and measure these parameters at each follow-up visit. Check the blood pressure and pulse at the initial visit and then every 3 months at a minimum. Check fasting serum glucose and lipids when starting AAs and then repeat at 3 months and then every 6 months thereafter while on this medication. The clinician should always be observant for the development of extrapyramidal signs (such as dystonic reactions, see Table 14.4) and check for as well record such observations at dose initiation, once every 3 months, and at any increase in the dose [33]. Tardive dyskinesia often starts with abnormal buccal–lingual movements which may also include chorea [33]. If pimozide or ziprasidone is used for tic suppression, obtain a baseline and follow-up ECGs, especially when increasing the dosage. Be aware of the potential rise in serum prolactin and check if clinically warranted, such as when symptoms of menstrual disorders arise in adolescent females.

Miscellaneous Drugs

A variety of other drugs are used in attempts to suppress tic, including muscle relaxants, anticonvulsants, dopamine receptor agonists, and others (see Table 14.5) [34, 35]. Unlike alpha-agonists and antipsychotics that have been considered, these other medications are not the first ones used in pharmacologic management of tic disorders and are best used in consultation with experts in pediatric tic disorders – as pediatric neurologists or child psychiatrists. Treatment of comorbid conditions is important. For example, approximately half of the pediatric patients with Tourette's syndrome also have obsessive–compulsive symptomatology that may improve with such drugs as the tricyclic antidepressant clomipramine or various selective serotonin reuptake inhibitors (SSRIs): fluoxetine, fluvoxamine, sertraline, and citalopram [6, 36] (see Chapter 10).

Stimulants

As noted, it is important to treat conditions found along with tic disorders, such as obsessive–compulsive symptomatology. Another example is that of ADHD (attention-deficit hyperactivity disorder) that is found in 50% or more of those with Tourette's disorder. A child or adolescent with Tourette's disorder and ADHD can be prescribed both anti-tic drugs (such as haloperidol or pimozide) and anti-ADHD drugs (as methylphenidate or amphetamine preparations) if these medications are effective for the pediatric patient [37–41] (see Chapter 8). There is no clear evidence that stimulants cause Tourette's disorder and a patient with ADHD on stimulants that are helpful for the ADHD who then develops tics can be placed on anti-tic medications as noted.

Continuous and careful monitoring by the clinician is important in this "start low and go slow" approach. If the tics seem to be worsened by stimulant medication, other anti-ADHD medications (see Chapter 8) can be used instead of the stimulants – such as alpha2-agonists (clonidine or guanfacine) or atomoxetine (selective norepinephrine reuptake inhibitor) [42, 43]. A dose range of 0.5–1.2 mg/kg/day for atomoxetine may be used; see Chapter 8 for a discussion of potential adverse effects with this medication. Research suggests that methylphenidate and alpha2-agonists are an effective combination of medications for children with both ADHD and tic disorders; in such cases, avoid high ("supratherapeutic") doses of dextroamphetamine which may worsen the tics [43]. Bupropion is an antidepressant that may improve ADHD symptomatology but may also worsen tic frequency.

Other Treatments

Research is also focusing on a variety of other drugs including glutamate modulators, nicotinic agents, antiandrogens, and if a few, very dysfunctional tics are present – botulinum injection [44, 45]. Additional measures under research include habit reversal therapy, electroconvulsive therapy (ECT), deep brain simulation, and repetitive transcranial magnetic stimulation [44–46].

Conclusions

Tics are movements that are sudden, stereotyped, purposeless, and involuntary; they include motor tics, vocal tics, and sensory tics. Tic disorders are one of the most common neuropsychiatric and neurodevelopmental abnormalities noted in children and adolescents that may continue on to adulthood. Current classification of tic disorders includes transient tic disorder, chronic motor or vocal tic disorder, Tourette's syndrome, and tic disorder not otherwise specified. By definition tic disorders are diagnosed before age 18 years and not due to such medications (as stimulants) or conditions such as Huntington's disease or post-viral encephalitis. Tic disorders can result in considerable behavioral stress and sequelae to the patient, and these issues should be carefully evaluated as well as managed. A variety of comorbid conditions may also be found including obsessive–compulsive disorder, ADHD, other anxiety disorders, mood disorders, and others (see Table 14.3).

Management of tic disorders includes patient/family education about these conditions, cognitive and behavioral management, treatment of comorbid conditions, and judicious use of psychopharmacology [47–52]. Management seeks to reduce or remove the tics to improve the patient's quality of life and psychosocial functioning [47–50]. Figure 14.1 provides a suggested algorithm for Tourette's syndrome management. The first line of medication management usually includes alpha2-agonists (clonidine and guanfacine) and antipsychotics (haloperidol, pimozide, and risperidone); a variety of other medications are also used in selective situations (see Table 14.5). Consultation with experts in pediatric tic disorders, such as pediatric neurologists and child psychiatrists, is recommended for patients with difficult-to-control tic disorders.

References

1. American Psychiatric Association. Diagnostic and statistical manual of mental disorders. 4th ed. text rev. Washington, DC: American Psychiatric Association; 2000. pp. 100–5.
2. Walkup JT, Ferrao Y, Leckman JF, et al. Tic disorders: some key issues for DSM-V. Depress Anxiety. 2010;27(6):600–10.
3. Greydanus DE, Patel DR, Olipra D. Tic disorders in children and adolescents: principles of psychopharmacologic management. Int J Child Adolesc health. 2010;3:271–80.
4. Greydanus DE, Van Dyke DH. Neurologic disorders. In: Greydanus DE, Patel DR, Pratt HD, editors. Essential adolescent medicine. New York, NY: McGraw-Hill Medical Publications; 2006. pp. 235–79.
5. Swedo SE, Leonard HL, Rapport JL. The pediatric autoimmune neuropsychiatric disorders associated with streptococcal infections (PANDAS) Subgroup. Pediatrics. 2004;113:907–11.
6. Greydanus DE, Tsitsika AK. Tic disorders in children and adolescents. In: Greydanus DE, Calles JL Jr, Patel DR, editors. Pediatric and adolescent psychopharmacology. Cambridge: Cambridge University Press; 2008. pp. 223–40.

7. Pina-Garza JE. Tic disorders in children and adolescents. In: Greydanus DE, Patel DR, Pratt HD, editors. Behavioral pediatrics. 2nd ed. New York, NY: iUniverse; 2006. pp. 497–507.
8. Leckman JF. Tourette's syndrome. Lancet. 2002;360:1577–86.
9. Jankovic J. Tourette's syndrome. N Engl J Med. 2001;345:1184–92.
10. Kuperman S. Tic disorders in the adolescent. Adolesc Med. 2002;13:537–51.
11. Turtle L, Robertson MM:. Tics, twitches, tales: the experiences of Gilles de la Tourette's syndrome. Am J Orthopsychiatry. 2008;78(4):449–55.
12. Bloch MH, Peterson BS, Scahill L, et al. Adulthood outcomes of tic and obsessive-compulsive symptom severity in children with Tourette syndrome. Arch Pediatr Adolesc Med. 2006;160:65–69.
13. Centers for Disease Control and Prevalence (CDC). Prevalence of diagnosed Tourette syndrome in persons aged 6–17 years-United States, 2007. MMWR. 2009;58(21):581–5.
14. Delgado MR, Albright AL. Movement disorders in children: definitions, classifications and grading systems. J Child Neurol. 2003;18(Suppl 1):S.
15. Greydanus DE, Tsitsika AK, Disorders. T. In: Greydanus DE, Patel DR, Pratt HD, Calles JL Jr, editors. Behavioral pediatrics. 3rd ed. New York, NY: Nova Science; 2009. pp. 121–30.
16. Sanger TD. Pathophysiology of pediatric movement disorders. J Child Neurol. 2003;18 (Suppl 1):S9–S24.
17. Pratt HD. Principles of psychological management. In: Greydanus DE, Calles JL Jr, Patel DR, editors. Pediatric and adolescent psychopharmacology. Cambridge: Cambridge Univ Press; 2008. pp. 1–24.
18. Weisz JR, Jensen-Doss A, Hawley KM. Evidence-based youth psychotherapies versus usual clinical care: a meta-analysis of direct comparisons. Am Psychologist. 2006;61(7):671–89.
19. Piacentini J, Woods DW, Scahill L, et al. Behavior therapy for children with Tourette disorder: a randomized controlled trial. JAMA. 2010;303(19):1929–37.
20. Edgar TS. Oral pharmacotherapy of childhood movement disorders. J Child Neurol. 2003;18(Suppl 1):S40–S49.
21. Gilbert D. Treatment of children and adolescents with tics and Tourette syndrome. J Child Neurol. 2006;21:690–700.
22. Rampello L, Alvano A, Battaglia G, Bruno V, Raffaele R, Nicoletti F. Tic disorders: from pathophysiology to treatment. J Neurol. 2006;253:1–15.
23. Tourette Syndrome Study Group. Treatment of ADHD children with tics: a randomized controlled trial. Neurology 2004;58:527–36.
24. Scahill L, Erenberg G, Berlin CM Jr, Budman C, Coffey BJ, Jankovic J, et al. Contemporary assessment and pharmacotherapy of Tourette syndrome. NeuroRx. 2006;3:192–206.
25. Cohen DJ, Young JG, Nathanson JA, Shaywitz BA. Clonidine in Tourette's syndrome. Lancet. 1979;2:551–3.
26. Gaffney GR, Perry PJ, Lund BC, Bever-Stiller KA, Arndt S, Kuperman S. Risperidone versus clonidine in the treatment of children and adolescents with Tourette's syndrome. J Am Acad Child Adolesc Psychiatry. 2002;41:330–6.
27. Budman C, Coffey BJ, Shecter R, et al. Aripiprazole in children and adolescents with Tourette disorder with and without explosive outbursts. J Child Adolesc Psychopharmacol. 2008;18(5):509–15.
28. McCracken JT, Suddath R, Chang S, et al. Effectiveness and tolerability of open label olanza-pine in children and adolescents with Tourette syndrome. J Child Adolesc Psychopharmacol. 2008;18(5):501–8.
29. Pringsheim T, Marras C. Pimozide for tics in Tourette's syndrome. Cochrane Database Sys Rev. 2009;15(2):CD006996.
30. Chevreuil C, Reymann JM, Frémaux T, et al. Risperidone use in child and adolescent psychiatric patients (French). Therapie. 2008;63(5):359–75.
31. Gudmundsen GR, McClellan JM. Schizophrenia in childhood and adolescence. In: Greydanus DE, Patel DR, Pratt HD, Calles JL Jr, editors. Behavioral pediatrics. 3rd ed. New York, NY: Nova Science; 2009. pp. 349–68.

32. Calles JL Jr. Schizophrenia in childhood and adolescence. In: Greydanus DE, Calles JL Jr, Patel DR, editors. Pediatric and adolescent psychopharmacology. Cambridge: Cambridge Univ Press; 2008. pp. 133–54.

33. Greydanus DE, Feinberg AN, Patel DR, Homnick DN, editors. The pediatric diagnostic examination. New York, NY: McGraw-Hill Medical Publications; 2008. p. 371, 616.

34. Kuo SH, Jimenez-Shahed J. Topiramate in treatment of Tourette syndrome. Clin Neuropharmacol. 2010;33(1):32–4.

35. Fernández-Jaén A, Fernández-Mayoralas DM, Munoz-Janeno N, et al. An open-label, prospective study of levetiracetam in children and adolescents with Tourette syndrome. Eur J Paediatr Neurol. 2009;13(6):541–5.

36. Wehr AM, Namerow LB. Citalopram for OCD and Tourette's syndrome. J Am Acad Child Adolesc Psychiatry. 2001;40:740–1.

37. Greydanus DE, Pratt HD. Attention-deficit/hyperactivity disorder in children and adolescents: interventions for a complex costly clinical conundrum. Pediatr Clin North Am. 2003;50: 1049–92.

38. Greydanus DE, Nazeer A, Patel DR. Psychopharmacology of ADHD in pediatrics: current advances and issues. Neuropsychiatr Dis Treat. 2009;5:171–81.

39. Greydanus DE, Pratt HD, Patel DR. Attention deficit hyperactivity disorder across the lifespan. Dis Mon. 2007;53(2):65–132.

40. Greydanus DE, Pratt HD. Attention deficit hyperactivity disorder. In: Greydanus DE, Patel DR, Pratt HD, editors. Behavioral pediatrics. 2nd ed. New York, NY: iUniverse Publishers; 2007. pp. 107–42.

41. Greydanus DE, Merrick J. Psychopharmacology in children, adolescents, and adults with attention deficit hyperactivity disorder (ADHD). In: Gordon SM, Mitchell AE, editors. Attention deficit hyperactivity disorder (ADHD). New York, NY: Nova Science; 2009. pp. 257–72.

42. Spencer TJ, Sallee FR, Gilbert DL, et al. Atomoxetine treatment of ADHD in children with comorbid Tourette syndrome. J Atten Dis. 2008;11(4):470–81.

43. Bloch MH, Panza KE, Landeros-Weisenberger A, Leckman JF. Meta-analysis: treatment of attention-deficit/hyperactivity disorder in children with comorbid tic disorders. J Am Acad Child Adolesc Psychiatry. 2009;48(9):884–93.

44. Bestha DP, Jeevarakshagan S, Madaan V. Management of tics and Tourette's disorder: an update. Expert Opin Pharmacother. 2010; 12 May.

45. Shprecher D, Kurlan R. The management of tics. Mov Disord. 2009;24(1):15–24.

46. Bloch MH. Emerging treatments for Tourette's disorder. Curr Psychiatry Rep. 2008;10(4):323–30.

47. Kenney C, Kuo SH, Jimenez-Shahed J. Tourette's syndrome. Am Fam Phys. 2008;77(1): 651–8.

48. Eapen V, Crncec R. Tourette syndrome in children and adolescents: special considerations. J Psychosom Res. 2009;67(6):525–32.

49. Cutler D, Murphy T, Gilmour J, Heyman I. The quality of life of young people with Tourette syndrome. Child Care Health Dev. 2009;35(4):496–504.

50. Pringsheim T, Lang A, Kurlan R, et al. Understanding disability in Tourette syndrome. Dev Med Child Neurol. 2009;51(6):468–72.

51. Burd L, Li Q, Kerbeshian J, et al. Tourette syndrome and comorbid pervasive developmental disorders. J Child Neurol. 2009;24(2):170–5.

52. Debes NM, Hjalgrim H, Skov L. The presence of comorbidity in Tourette syndrome increases the need for pharmacological treatment. J Child Neurol. 2009;24(12):1504–12.

53. Kuperman S. Tic disorders in children and adolescents. In: Greydanus DE, Wolraich ML, editors. Behavioral Pediatrics. New York, NY: Springer; 1992. Chap. 33. p. 452.

Chapter 15
Medical Management of Cerebral Palsy

Nancy N. Dodge

Abstract Cerebral palsy is a disorder of motor control due to a static lesion of the developing brain. It was described almost 150 years ago and is quite familiar to both the lay and the medical communities. Continuing advances in our understanding of the causes and treatment of this heterogeneous disorder, when broadly understood and applied, will allow more children and adults with cerebral palsy to reach their full potential. This chapter reviews the definition, clinical presentation, and medical management of cerebral palsy.

Introduction

Cerebral palsy is a common neuromotor disorder affecting infants and children worldwide. In addition to primary motor deficits, children with cerebral palsy have many other associated and secondary conditions that need a multidisciplinary approach to diagnosis and medical management. Most children who have cerebral palsy now survive into adulthood and require long-term care planning. This chapter reviews the definition, epidemiology, clinical features, diagnosis, and management of cerebral palsy. The emphasis is on medical management in the primary care setting.

Definition

The definition of cerebral palsy has evolved over the years, reflecting changing understanding of the causes and consequences of this disorder. A recent definition, put forward by the American Academy for Cerebral Palsy and Developmental Medicine, is

N.N. Dodge (✉)
Michigan State University, Lansing, MI, USA; Neurodevelopmental Pediatrics, Helen DeVos Children's Hospital, Grand Rapids, MI 49503, USA
email: nancy.dodge@devoschildrens.org

D.R. Patel et al. (eds.), *Neurodevelopmental Disabilities*,
DOI 10.1007/978-94-007-0627-9_15, © Springer Science+Business Media B.V. 2011

Cerebral palsy describes a group of disorders of the development of movement and posture, causing activity limitations that are attributed to non-progressive disturbances that occurred in the developing fetal or infant brain. The motor disorders of cerebral palsy are often accompanied by disturbances of sensation, cognition, communication perception and/or by a seizure disorder [1].

This definition emphasizes the associated conditions, but retains key elements of previous definitions:

- Cerebral palsy is a disorder of motor function.
- Although the manifestations may change over time, the causative lesion is static.
- The cause originates from the brain sometime during its developmental period.

Explaining the definition of cerebral palsy to families can prevent unnecessary grief, as it is not unusual for families to confuse the condition with muscular dystrophy or to presume cognitive impairment.

Epidemiology

The incidence of cerebral palsy has remained virtually unchanged over the past 40 years at approximately 2.5 per 1,000 live births [2]. This represents a great disappointment to those who anticipated that advances in perinatal care would eliminate many cases of cerebral palsy, but a relief to those that feared a drastic increase in numbers due to improved survival of critically ill newborns. This is best understood in the context of our current understanding that the etiology of most cases of cerebral palsy is prenatal in origin. The etiology of cerebral palsy can be thought of using the four P's: prenatal, perinatal, postnatal, and prematurity (see Table 15.1).

Although physicians and parents have traditionally thought of hypoxic or ischemic white matter damage as "causing" cerebral palsy, that view does not take into account the contribution of prenatal risk factors, such as maternal illness, or late risk factors, such as chronic lung disease [3]. These instead point to a role for inflammatory mediators either causing damage or affecting brain development at critical periods [4]. Although perinatal causes received the most attention in the

Table 15.1 Common prenatal, perinatal, and postnatal causes of cerebral palsy

Prenatal	Brain malformations
	In utero stroke
	Congenital cytomegalovirus infection
Perinatal	Hypoxic ischemic encephalopathy
	Viral encephalitis
	Meningitis
Postnatal	Accidental and inflicted head trauma
	Anoxic insult
	Child abuse

past, they actually represent a small minority of cases. In most preterm infants, no single "cause" of their cerebral palsy can be identified, and we focus instead on risk factors. If we are someday going to be able to reduce the incidence of cerebral palsy, the areas most amenable to intervention are those related to preventing postnatal brain injury to infants and those for reducing preterm births [5]. Both will require societal change.

Clinical Features

The essential clinical findings of cerebral palsy include delayed motor milestones, abnormal muscle tone, hyperreflexia, and absence of regression or evidence of a more specific diagnosis. These clinical findings should be present to the degree that the child appears unlikely to "outgrow" these findings. The potential to "outgrow" the manifestations of cerebral palsy is best recognized in the preterm population, who may have transient abnormalities in tone and reflexes that may seem to interfere with motor progress, but these clinical findings resolve by 1–2 years of age [6]. Term infants as well sometimes "outgrow" the manifestations of cerebral palsy [7, 8], so clinical judgment is needed for determining how long to "watch" before labeling. Community factors, such as pressure to label so services can be obtained, may also arise. However, two principles should be kept in mind [9]: Intervention should never be delayed awaiting diagnosis or etiologic assessment and [1] families do best when informed up front that cerebral palsy is a possibility.

The etiologic evaluation plays several roles, including identification of the cause of the child's disability and exclusion of alternative diagnoses. Of particular importance is exclusion of disorders that might be treated differently if a specific diagnosis is known, such as dopa-responsive dystonia [10] which responds dramatically to dopamine supplementation. Inborn errors of metabolism may present with motor impairment and abnormal tone and should be suspected if there is a suggestion of loss of skills (motor regression) or if the motor impairment and abnormal tone have unusual accompanying symptoms, such as unexplained hypoglycemia, recurrent emesis, or progressively worsening seizures [11]. A family history of unexplained neurologic symptoms or infant deaths would also raise the possibility of an underlying metabolic disorder. There is no consensus that metabolic screening of children with suspected cerebral palsy is indicated in the absence of other suggestive signs of symptoms [12]. Those following children with cerebral palsy "of unknown etiology" should, however, be vigilant for the appearance of a late symptom that might suggest a more specific diagnosis (see Table 15.2).

Diagnosis

Despite advances in technology, cerebral palsy remains a clinical diagnosis and represents a continuing role for the "art" of medicine. MRI of the brain is currently the

Table 15.2 Mimics of cerebral palsy

Disorder	Clue
Familial spastic paraplegia	Family history
Transient toe walking	Normal deep tendon reflexes
Muscular dystrophy	Calf hypertrophy, positive Gower's sign
Metabolic disorders	Regression, lethargy, unusual vomiting
Sjogren–Larrson	Ichthyosis
Lesch–Nyhan	Severe self-mutilation
Mitochondrial disorders	Recurrent stroke, cardiomyopathy, hypoglycemia
Genetic disorders	Multiple anomalies
Miller–Dieker	Lissencephaly
Rett syndrome	Acquired microcephaly, hand wringing

evaluation of choice for the vast majority of children with suspected cerebral palsy and will show an abnormality in about 90% of cases [13, 14]. These may include major and minor brain malformations, in utero strokes, and white matter loss. White matter abnormalities, including periventricular leukomalacia, are strongly associated with cerebral palsy in very low birth weight infants, but can be seen in full-term infants as well [15, 16]. As the resolution of MRI scanning improves, we also see more nonspecific white matter abnormalities, the meaning of which, it is hoped, will be clarified in the coming few years.

Classification

The broad and inclusive nature of the term cerebral palsy limits it usefulness in both clinical and research settings: How much does a child with a localized motor deficit due to a small prenatal stroke have in common with a child who had a global brain insult due to herpes encephalitis? This has been traditionally addressed using a classification system combining the predominant type of motor abnormality with the distribution of this abnormality (see Table15.3). This classification system has recently been complemented by a functionally based classification system, the Gross Motor Functional Classification System [17], detailed in Table 15.4. Each system continues to have its own role. Clear characterization of the type of motor involvement guides certain aspects of treatment. For example, certain medications that reduce spasticity are of no help with dystonia and may make athetosis worse. The Gross Motor Functional Classification System has shown particular utility in clarifying prognosis, as functional levels have been shown to be fairly stable over time [18, 19] and are very helpful in research.

Prognosis

Most parents ask, "Will my child walk?" An often unspoken question is, "Will my child be able to have a long life?" The majority of children with cerebral palsy do

Table 15.3 Types of cerebral palsy

Spastic
Hemiplegia (unilateral involvement)
Diplegia (disproportionate lower extremity involvement)
Quadriplegia (total body involvement)
Dyskinetic
Choreoathetoid
Dystonic
Hypotonic
Mixed

Table 15.4 Gross motor functional classification system

Level	Function
I	Ambulatory in all settings
II	Walks without aides but has limitations in community settings
III	Walks with aides
IV	Mobility requires wheelchair or adult assist
V	Dependent for mobility

walk. Historically, the outlook for walking in a particular child was based on either their subtype of cerebral palsy or their age of sitting. Children with hemiplegic and diplegic cerebral palsy usually walk, while those with quadriplegia rarely do, and those with dyskinetic cerebral palsy have an intermediate chance of ambulation. Looking at the age of sitting, most children who sit independently by age 2 years will walk, while only rarely will those who are unable to sit by 4 years of age eventually walk. Given the documented stability of Gross Motor Functional Classification System over time [7], Gross Motor Functional Classification System level is increasingly being used to help answer questions about walking. In regard to survival, only the most severe degrees of cerebral palsy are associated with shortened survival. For the group defined by the need for tube feedings and the inability to lift the head in prone, they have a median survival of 17 years [20]. Death due to respiratory problems is much more common than it is in the general population. However, death due to accident or injury is less likely to occur than would be expected in the general population [21].

Management

For optimal care, the child with cerebral palsy must not be viewed in isolation, but rather considered in the context of his or her family and community. Family-centered care is considered the optimal model of care for all children, but is especially important for children with special needs [22]. The essence of family-centered care is the recognition that, while we as medical professionals bring knowledge, training, and experience to the team, parents bring specific knowledge about their child and past care received, as well as a perspective of their child in the settings of school, home, and community in which the child actually lives out his or her life. Parents can help us see how medical recommendations we might make would impact the child's participation at school and might foresee barriers to a treatment plan that we might not anticipate. Establishing open communication and a collaborative approach maximizes adherence and sets the stage for optimal care.

A major component of community participation for most children is school. Optimally, children are referred for early intervention services when developmental concerns are first recognized, without waiting for specialty assessment or diagnosis. Children with cerebral palsy or another qualifying educational diagnosis are then transitioned from early intervention to the school system at 3 years of age. Parents often have questions about school services and procedures. To be of assistance, medical professionals need a basic working knowledge of relevant legislation, such as the Individuals with Disabilities Education Act, the US federal legislation that governs special education, or similar legislation in other countries. Schools may also need our input as to how various aspects of the child's medical condition and its treatment have an impact on the child's ability to function at school.

Therapies, which may be applied both inside and outside the school setting, are considered a cornerstone of treatment for children with cerebral palsy. Many studies compare different types of therapies or document progress with a certain therapy [23], but few studies have included a control group or longitudinal follow-up that allows clear demonstration that therapy changes the natural history of the disorder [24]. Different therapy disciplines address different aspects of cerebral palsy. The physical therapist focuses on posture and mobility, the occupational therapist on hand skills and adaptive equipment, and speech and language therapists on communication, whether verbal or nonverbal. Oromotor or feeding therapy is an area of overlap between occupational and speech therapy. Adjunctive therapies, such as hippotherapy (therapeutic horseback riding) [25] and aquatic exercise [26], have been supported by small, uncontrolled studies and are appealing to many in the field because they involve activities that children without disabilities enjoy as well. Strengthening activities, whether in the context of therapy or physical activity, have been shown to improve function in controlled trials [27] and can, as in any other child, improve cardiovascular fitness and mood. [28].

Orthotics may be used for multiple purposes in the child with the foot in a more functional position for gait or be used to slow the development of contractures at the ankles. The most common, the ankle-foot orthosis, can provide stability at the ankle. Spinal orthoses can be used in an attempt to slow progression of scoliosis [29]. Optimal orthotic management requires collaboration among the patient's physical therapist, orthotist, and, if involved, orthopedic surgeon or physiatrist.

Schools and other community agencies can be valuable sources of information about many topics pertinent to certain individuals with cerebral palsy, such as social security income, respite care, and, for young people with cognitive impairment, guardianship. In the USA, United Cerebral Palsy and its local affiliates can be a valuable source of information and support, and comparable organizations exist in other countries. A significant number of individuals with cerebral palsy enjoy good general health and experience challenges limited to motor functions. Others have some or many of the associated problems discussed by body systems in the following sections.

Seizures

Approximately 30% of persons with cerebral palsy have a seizure disorder [30]. Just like seizures in the general population, seizures in persons with cerebral palsy may come on at any age and be of any type. In other words, there is nothing "unique" about seizures in children with cerebral palsy. Choice of anticonvulsants, when required, is guided as usual by seizure type and side effect profile. Also like other children, a child with cerebral palsy may be able to be tried off such medicines once the child has been seizure-free for at least 2 years [31]. What warrants special consideration in this population, however, is monitoring for anticonvulsant side effects, as these children may have other medical issues that could be exacerbated by side effects of anticonvulsant medications. For example, a child with feeding problems and gastroesophageal reflux may suffer further nutritional compromise if she develops anorexia as a side effect of an anticonvulsant, such as topiramate [32]. Likewise, children with associated learning problems may do better with some of the newer generation anticonvulsants, which appear to have less impact on cognition, although complete data are lacking [33].

Cognition and Learning

Roughly half of individuals with cerebral palsy have associated cognitive impairment, with others having overall cognitive skills in the normal range but with specific deficits in learning or attention that could be classified as learning disabilities or attention deficit/hyperactivity disorder [30]. The risk of associated cognitive or learning difficulties varies somewhat with the type of cerebral palsy, with those with quadriplegic cerebral palsy having the highest risk of cognitive impairment and those with hemiplegic cerebral palsy the lowest. This makes sense given that children with spastic quadriplegia have had a more global brain insult, while those with hemiplegia have had a quite localized one. Those with other cerebral palsy subtypes have an intermediate risk of impaired cognition. What is perhaps more important for the clinician to remember is that there are clearly exceptions, and that it is crucial that persons with extensive physical involvement be given the opportunity to demonstrate their mental abilities. This may require the intervention of a skilled speech and language pathologist to appreciate nonverbal communication potential and a willingness to listen to families who feel that their child understands more than he or she can demonstrate.

For individuals whose motor impairment hinders verbal communication, augmentative communication and other rehabilitation technologies can allow them to communicate and learn at their cognitive level. The clinician may need to advocate for patients with cerebral palsy to receive such technology, especially to have access to it in all settings – at home, in school, and within the community.

Nutrition and Growth

Children with cerebral palsy face multiple challenges to normal growth and are more likely to be underweight and short compared with peers [34]. Most evidence in regard to stature [35], however, points to the short stature as a consequence of being chronically underweight. Even adequate assessment of growth status can be a challenge in this population. Medical offices may lack scales for older children who cannot stand, and length measures may be difficult to reliably obtain in a child with joint contractures or a child who is in constant motion due to choreoathetosis. The latter can be addressed by using segmental measures, such as upper arm or tibial length, for which standards are available [36]. Use of such measures requires staff training, as even small errors in these measurements can result in misclassification of the child's growth status.

In the past, these children's poor nutritional status was accepted as part of the condition, but it has been shown that these children can grow normally [37] and benefit from being adequately nourished [34]. Although being underweight is the most common nutritional problem among those with cerebral palsy, some with cerebral palsy are overweight. Excess weight in a person with cerebral palsy should be reduced to prevent respiratory compromise [38] and to facilitate maximal mobility and ease of care [39].

The evaluation of the underweight child with cerebral palsy begins with the diet history, which means looking at what foods and drinks are offered, how long meals take, and how the child eats. Children with cerebral palsy may have impaired control of oromotor musculature, impairing their ability to handle food and drink, resulting in prolonged mealtimes, increased spillage, or delayed transition to more calorically dense table foods [40]. Some families restrict dairy products because of concerns about constipation or about the development of excessive mucous with milk. An occupational therapist may be able to offer suggestions and adaptations, such as improved seating and adaptive cups, to make eating and drinking more efficient. Interventions to increase the caloric density of the diet can help the child consume more calories and other nutrients. A registered dietitian can be very helpful in this regard, but, if this resource is not available, clinicians can recommend such strategies as adding extra butter or sauces to foods, incorporating high-calorie beverages in the diet, such as milkshakes, drinkable yogurts, and commercially available complete nutrition drinks.

The accompanying step is a careful history and physical examination looking for medical factors that might interfere with intake. The possibilities are numerous and include sources of discomfort, such as constipation or hip pain, and abnormal losses, such as emesis due to gastroesophageal reflux or as a medication side effect. Medication side effects are common contributors to nutritional problems in this group of patients and should always be considered. It is also helpful to keep in mind uncommon presentations of common problems. For instance, practitioners may only consider the possibility of clinically significant gastroesophageal reflux when parents report chronic vomiting, but discomfort after meals, early satiety, or unexplained respiratory problems [41] may also be presenting signs.

Swallowing

Persons with cerebral palsy are at increased risk for dysphagia, which can affect their health in several ways. Dysphagia with aspiration may result in or contribute to recurrent pulmonary infections or reactive airway disease. It can limit food choices and compromise the efficiency of intake, contributing to impaired nutrition. However, just as in the discussion of gastroesophageal reflux earlier, dysphagia may not always present as clinicians might expect. When documented to aspirate, most individuals with cerebral palsy do so silently, meaning they do not cough at the time of aspiration [42]. Thus, practitioners must have a high index of suspicion for dysphagia and seek indirect signs and symptoms of aspiration, such as congestion or wet vocal quality with meals. Prolonged feeding times are also associated with dysphagia [43]. Dysphagia should also be sought in persons with recurrent pneumonia or reactive airway disease of unexplained cause or severity.

Reliable assessment of swallowing coordination requires fluoroscopic visualization of swallow during intake of barium-containing foods and beverages. These studies are performed with the individual seated in a neutral position and are done in conjunction with a speech pathologist or occupational therapist with feeding experience. The therapist reviews a videotape of the study before interpretation, as aspiration can be missed at the time in a busy fluoroscopic suite. Bedside assessments and upper gastrointestinal series studies cannot substitute for a formal videofluoroscopic study, and ultrasound assessment remains investigational [44]. A thorough report will comment on risk factors for aspiration, such as residue in the valleculae and pyriform sinuses and laryngeal penetration, as well as the presence and frequency of aspiration. It should also discuss what compensations, if any, were seen to be effective, such as thickness and rate of flow of liquids given. If no liquid consistency can be found to be safe, alternative modes of nutrition and hydration need to be considered.

Gastrointestinal

Just as control of the muscles of the limbs and trunk is affected in cerebral palsy, so is the smooth muscle of the gastrointestinal tract. Persons with cerebral palsy have a high incidence of gastroesophageal reflux and constipation and may have altered gut motility as well, resulting in delayed gastric emptying and intestinal dysmotility [45]. Disorders here may have an impact on many aspects of a child's life. Both gastroesophageal reflux and constipation can impair nutritional intake and be sources of pain. Reflux can contribute to acute and chronic pulmonary problems [46] and can be a source of blood loss leading to chronic anemia and to dental erosions [47].

Gastroesophageal reflux in persons with cerebral palsy differs from those in the general population in incidence more than treatment. Medications to decrease gastric acid production are the first-line therapies. Those that directly effect motility may also be helpful, but their use is limited by their side effect profiles. Other interventions that can be considered include upright (but not slumped) position after meals, avoidance of reported dietary triggers and high osmolarity medications and supplements, and relief of any constipation. Surgical treatment of gastroesophageal reflux with fundoplication is considered in cases of clinically significant but medically refractory gastroesophageal reflux or in conjunction with gastrostomy placement when gastroesophageal reflux is present or suspected (to be discussed further below).

Gastrostomy placement is contemplated in the setting of insufficient intake or excessive feeding times despite intervention or in persons who, due to risk of aspiration, pose a danger to themselves if they eat and drink orally. This is an emotionally laden step for most families, as feeding one's child is intimately connected with the parental role, and the inability to meet this most basic need of the child can be seen as a failure. The gastrostomy is also a marker of how "different" the child is and that the child's differences are not going to go away. Families may need some time to make this decision and may benefit greatly from talking with another parent who has faced a similar choice. The ability of gastrostomy to facilitate more normal growth and to improve the child's quality of life is well documented, although its impact on family quality of life and the child's longevity is less clear [48]. Finally, the circumstances under which the gastrostomy should be accompanied by a fundoplication to prevent reflux remain a matter of experience and opinion, with no controlled studies to provide guidance [49]. Children should be followed closely after gastrostomy placement to address issues of feeding intolerance promptly when they arise and to prevent excessive weight gain.

Constipation is estimated to occur in 80% of individuals with cerebral palsy. The cause is multifactorial and for any given child may include low fluid or fiber intake, decreased activity, and difficulty sitting comfortably on the toilet. There are likely skeletal muscle contributors as well, such as difficulty relaxing the pelvic floor musculature and with pushing. For many, intestinal motility is also abnormal [50]. Constipation for these individuals is more than a nuisance. It can adversely affect appetite, continence, and comfort. Just as in typically developing individuals, it can predispose to urinary tract infections [51].

There are many potential interventions for constipation in this population as well. For some, the first step is getting them sitting on the toilet. For those already using the commode, better positioning on the toilet, including foot support, can help assessment and intervention in fluid and fiber intake may provide some avenues for improvement, keeping in mind that increased fiber in the face of low fluid intake is likely to make matters worse. For many, medications are needed. These include osmotic agents, such as polyethylene glycol, and laxatives, such as senna. Mineral oil should be used with caution, if at all, in this population because of the risk of lipoid pneumonia if aspirated [52].

Respiratory

Respiratory compromise in children with cerebral palsy is a major source of morbidity and mortality, especially among those with severe motor involvement. Cerebral palsy is associated with an increased risk of upper airway obstruction, which can cause chronic obstructive sleep apnea, as well as acute airway obstruction, especially when illness or sedation compound underlying airway issues [53]. Snoring in association with apneic pauses or gasping respirations is a clear indication for polysomnography, as is unexplained daytime somnolence [54]. Parenchymal lung disease may be caused by chronic aspiration of food, secretions, or refluxed gastric contents. Severe scoliosis [55] and obesity [39] can both cause restrictive lung disease.

Orthopedic

Orthopedic surgeons experienced in the care of children with cerebral palsy are integral members of the treatment team for all but those most mildly affected. They can monitor for the secondary musculoskeletal complications of cerebral palsy, which include contractures, joint dislocations (especially at the hips), and bony deformities, such as scoliosis. Orthopedic surgeons can also suggest interventions to prevent such complications. Through prescription of therapy and bracing, they can direct interventions to help an ambulatory child walk more efficiently. Thus, their role goes beyond that of surgery, although they also have much to contribute through surgery as well. Unfortunately, the research base supporting the role of orthopedic surgery in care of these children is limited, although a recent evidence-based review of the role of surgical adductor releases for hip subluxation in cerebral palsy found guarded support for the procedure [56]. Tools at the disposal of the orthopedist include gait analysis, which can guide clinical decision making by breaking down the gait into its components, indicating the muscle activity pattern and the alignment of the body in each phase of gait.

Areas of particular concern in the child with cerebral palsy include the hips [57] and spine [58]. A consensus statement published in *Developmental Medicine and Child Neurology* in 2006 [59] recommended baseline hip films at 30 months of age in all children who can walk fewer than 10 steps and that these films should be repeated every 6–12 months until age 7 years. The statement also recommends spinal radiographs at ages 5 and 10 years in nonambulatory children with cerebral palsy and otherwise as clinically indicated.

Goals of orthopedic treatment include prevention of deformity, as well as treatment of deformity when such treatment will improve comfort and quality of life. Decisions about surgical interventions must take into account the natural history of the disorder, about which we still know little. Children with dislocated hips may develop pain later, but which ones? The decision to surgically treat scoliosis in the most severely involved persons with cerebral palsy is a particularly complex one. Will the benefits for preventing progressive pulmonary compromise and loss of sitting outweigh the risks of a major surgery? This decision is best made by an experienced team with input from family and those who know the patient well.

Thorough preoperative preparation can significantly decrease the risk of postoperative morbidity and mortality. This assessment should include a careful evaluation that looks for all the associated problems discussed in this issue. Particular emphasis should be placed on nutritional status and proactive management of gastroesophageal reflux and dysphagia, as poor nutrition, reflux, and aspiration are clearly shown [60, 61] to correlate with postoperative morbidity and mortality. Other pertinent areas to consider are the child's airway and pulmonary status, the child's risk for bleeding problems, and the child's dental health. Assessment of bone density should be considered in those who have had significant nutritional problems, have had recurrent or pathologic fractures, or who take medications that could interfere with bone health [62]. Preliminary steps to improve bone density include ensuring optimal intake of calcium, phosphorus, and vitamin D. Use of such medications as the bisphosphonates has received preliminary study [63].

Abnormal Tone

Spasticity affects most people with cerebral palsy, and a significant minority have dystonia, either in addition to or instead of the spasticity. Despite the clear difference in definitions, dystonia and spasticity are commonly confused in practice. Developing the skills to differentiate the two is important for patient care, as different treatment approaches are often needed. Spasticity is defined as a velocity-dependent increase in tone. Dystonia involves involuntary muscle contractions that cause twisting, repetitive movement, and abnormal postures [64]. The second major challenge to the clinician is determining where the abnormal tone fits in with the child's "big picture," as we do not want to treat the tone abnormalities for their own sake, but to improve the child's function, comfort, or ease of care. Therapists working with the child have helpful input in this regard.

Interventions for spasticity usually start with passive stretching and other physical therapy interventions [65]. The choice of which steps to take next depends on whether the spasticity is generalized or localized. Localized spasticity, such as in the heel cords or hamstrings, can respond well to injections of botulinum toxin [66] or phenol [67]. In more generalized spasticity, considerations include oral medications, such as baclofen [68], dorsal rhizotomy [69], and intrathecal baclofen by implanted pump [70]. These options are best explored by an experienced interdisciplinary team. For the generalist, what is most important is to realize that treatment options do exist and to help families find them when appropriate. Also important for those who care for children with intrathecal baclofen pumps is awareness of the signs and symptoms of both baclofen withdrawal and overdose, as both situations can be life threatening. Symptoms of baclofen withdrawal include fever, itching, and increased stiffness, while lethargy, seizures, and respiratory suppression can be seen with excessive doses. All patients with baclofen pumps are instructed to carry emergency procedure information with them at all times.

Dystonia is even more of a challenge to treat. In general, it responds less robustly and predictably to a narrower spectrum of medications, such as trihexyphenidyl [71]. Dystonia may also respond to intrathecal baclofen [72], but usually requires higher doses [73].

Vision

Individuals with cerebral palsy have a high incidence of eye disorders, which range from refractive errors and strabismus to visual impairment [74]. There is some relationship to the etiology of the child's cerebral palsy, as prematurity is associated with retinal abnormalities that may affect vision [75] and also cause a high incidence of severe myopia [76]. Those with a severe global central nervous system insult or disproportionate occipital involvement are at more risk of cortical visual impairment, and the severity of visual deficits increases with increasing severity of motor impairment. Other lesions may be associated with optic nerve hypoplasia [77]. Regardless of cause, ophthalmologic problems are important to identify, as they are often treatable. In situations where no direct treatment exists, such as optic nerve hypoplasia, a better understanding of the child's visual status will affect educational and therapy interventions. All children with cerebral palsy should be evaluated by a pediatric ophthalmologist as soon as vision concerns are suspected. Many recommend such evaluation even if the child is asymptomatic [78]. Children with confirmed visual impairment qualify for and should receive specialized vision services through the schools [79].

Hearing

The incidence of hearing impairment in persons with cerebral palsy is estimated to be 10–15% [80]. Just as in the case of vision, preterm infants are at increased risk, as are those who suffered a hypoxic or infectious insult. Former premature infants, as well as infants treated with extracorporeal membrane oxygenations [81] and those with intrauterine cytomegalovirus infections [82], may experience late-onset or progressive hearing loss and thus require periodic hearing assessment over the first several years of life.

Urologic

A poorly defined subset of individuals with cerebral palsy may experience voiding dysfunction [83]. This possibility should be considered in those with recurrent urinary tract infections, unexplained irritability, or failure to achieve continence when otherwise expected based on the child's level of cognitive and motor functions. Studies have indicated that, on average, children with cerebral palsy achieve continence later than their peers [84], but the data were not controlled for cognitive level.

Dental

Persons with cerebral palsy are at high risk for dental issues [85]. These include malocclusion due to the abnormal forces in the oromotor musculature [86]. Some children with cerebral palsy have a hyperactive gag reflex or oral aversion, which makes dental hygiene difficult. The child's positioning needs may be difficult to accommodate in the usual dental office, and the individual may have difficulty cooperating with dental procedures because of motor or cognitive issues [87]. Finally, dental care sometimes seems to "get lost" among the child's many other care needs. There is also the mistaken assumption that persons who receive all their nutrition by gastrostomy, because they are not eating, do not need regular dental cleaning. The converse is actually true: Persons who are exclusively fed via gastrostomy have a high risk for calculus deposition and gingivitis [88].

Sialorrhea

Individuals with oromotor impairment may experience drooling past the age considered socially acceptable or many do so to a degree that interferes with activities. Complications of chronic drooling may include odor, chapping, and, rarely, pulmonary compromise. Like many other issues, a spectrum of interventions exists from least to most invasive, with treatment decisions guided more by the degree to which sialorrhea is interfering with the individual's life than by the amount or frequency of drooling. Options include oromotor therapy [89], intraoral appliances [90], and such medications as glycopyrrolate [91], botulinum injections [92], and surgery [93]. The first two address deficits in mouth closure and swallowing frequency, while the latter interventions help indirectly by decreasing saliva production. Those who undergo surgery for drooling need careful dental follow-up, as the incidence of caries appears to increase following surgery [94].

Pain

Pain is a common problem for individuals with cerebral palsy, with more than half of adults [95] and children [96] with cerebral palsy reporting pain as an ongoing health concern. Common sources are musculoskeletal and gastrointestinal. Particularly challenging is the nonverbal child with severe cerebral palsy who is excessively irritable or who cries with discomfort. Parents are sometimes desperate to find someone who will take responsibility for working through the problem as opposed to

Table 15.5 Possible sources of pain

Systems	Source
Cranial	Increased intracranial pressure
	Migraines and other headaches
Ophthalmologic	Corneal abrasions
	Glaucoma
Dental	Abscesses
	Temporomandibular joint pain
Gastrointestinal	Gastroesophageal reflux
	Constipation
Musculoskeletal	Patella alta
	Hip dislocation
	Scoliosis
Neuromuscular	Muscle spasms
Urologic	Urolithiasis
	Bladder spasms
Other	Decubitus ulcers

ruling out the causes in their area of specialization. Often a thorough history and physical examination, with attention to the time course and temporal association (worse after meals or diaper changes, for example), can suggest a potential cause and intervention. Several possibilities may have to be explored and empiric interventions tried before the child finally becomes more comfortable. Parents are usually remarkably patient with this "trial and error" process as long as it moves in a timely manner and they are kept involved and informed. Table 15.5 lists some potential sources of pain to which this population is predisposed.

Sleep

Children with cerebral palsy are prone to sleep problems, with an incidence recently reported to be 23% [97]. These difficulties may include difficulty falling asleep, frequent night awakening, and a sleep schedule that does not fit the needs of school or family. For any given child, there are potential behavioral, neurologic, and physical causes. Some parents of children with special needs may have difficulty with the limit setting that is necessary for children to develop good sleep habits, such as falling asleep in their own bed and putting themselves back to sleep after a normal night awakening. In some children, the "biologic clock" or other neural mechanisms involved with sleep initiation and maintenance may be abnormal. Physical causes may include difficulty with position changes during the night as well as the myriad potential sources of discomfort mentioned in the previous section. When behavioral concerns and sources of discomfort have been addressed but sleep problems persist, medication may be considered. Studies with grade B evidence support the use of melatonin [98], particularly to help the child fall asleep, with some studies showing the additional benefit of fewer night awakenings and longer duration of sleep. Antihistamines, the melatonin receptor agonist ramelteon, and a variety of other medications are used, though they lack supportive research, and no medications approved by the Food and Drug Administration for insomnia in adults have been studied adequately in children.

Transition

The vast majority of individuals with cerebral palsy live into adulthood and thus need to make the transition to adult medical care. Numerous barriers to this transition have been identified [99], including insufficient knowledge and training in childhood-onset disabilities among adult health-care providers, as well as funding issues. The American Academy of Family Medicine, the American College of Physicians, and the American Academy of Pediatrics [100] have agreed on steps to ease the transition of persons with special needs from pediatric to adult health care. One of these steps addresses the training issue. They also recommended three concrete steps that pediatric practitioners can take now to improve transition: Identify a health-care provider who will take responsibility for working with the patient and family on transition; work with the individual and family to develop a written transition plan; and facilitate development of a portable health-care summary. Fortunately, many transition checklists and medical summary templates are available to facilitate these tasks. Many are available through the National Center of Medical Home (www.medicalhomeinfo.org).

Conclusions

Making the diagnosis of cerebral palsy is only the beginning. The role of the pediatric health-care provider is also to help families manage the ongoing health issues that may arise and to give the families the confidence they are doing all that they can and should do to help their child reach his or her potential.

Acknowledgments The author wishes to thank her colleagues for their constructive comments and Terri Shoemaker for assistance with the references. This chapter is adapted with permission from author's previous work, Dodge [101].

References

1. Bax M, Goldstein M, Rosenbaum P, Leviton A, Paneth N, Dan B, et al. Proposed definition and classification of cerebral palsy. Dev Med Child Neurol. 2005;47:571–6.
2. Paneth N, Hong T, Korzeniewski S. The descriptive epidemiology of cerebral palsy. Clin Perinatol. 2006;33(2):251–67.
3. Paneth N. Cerebral palsy in term infants – birth or before birth? J Pediatr. 2001;138:791–2.

4. Back S. Perinatal white matter injury: the changing spectrum of pathology and emerging insights into pathogenic mechanisms. Ment Retard Dev Disabil Res Rev. 2006;12(2): 129–40.
5. Nelson K. Can we prevent cerebral palsy? N Engl J Med. 2003;349(18):1765–9.
6. D'Eugenio D, Slagle T, Mettelman B, Gross SJ. Developmental outcome of preterm infants with transient neuromotor abnormalities. Am J Dis Child. 1993;147:570–4.
7. Nelson KB, Ellenberg JH. Children who "outgrew" cerebral palsy. Pediatrics. 1982;69(5):529–36.
8. Wu YW, Lindan CE, Henning LH, Yoshida CK, Fullerton HJ, Ferriero DM, et al. Neuroimaging abnormalities in infants with congenital hemiparesis. Pediatr Neurol. 2006;35(3):191–6.
9. Little WJ. On the influence of abnormal parturition, difficult labour, premature birth, and asphyxia neonatorum on the mental and physical conditions of the child, especially in relation to deformities. Trans Obstet Soc Long. 1862;3:293–344.
10. Jan M. Misdiagnoses in children with dopa-responsive dystonia. Pediatr Neurol. 2004;31:298–303.
11. Bass N. Cerebral palsy and neurodegenerative disease. Curr Opin Pediatr. 1999;11:504–7.
12. Ashwal S. Practice parameter: diagnostic assessment of the child with cerebral palsy: report of the quality standards subcommittee of the American academy of neurology and the practice committee of the child neurology society. Neurology. 2004;62(6): 851–63.
13. Yin R. Magnetic resonance imaging findings in cerebral palsy. J Paediatr Child Health. 2000;36(2):139–44.
14. Krägeloh-Mann I, Petersen D, Hagberg G, Vollmer B, Hagberg B, Michaelis R. Bilateral spastic cerebral palsy – MRI pathology and origin. Analysis from a representative series of 56 cases. Dev Med Child Neurol. 1995;37(5):379–97.
15. Woodward LJ, Anderson PJ, Austin NC, Howard K, Inder TE. Neonatal MRI to predict neurodevelopmental outcomes in preterm infants. N Engl J Med. 2006;355:685–94.
16. Miller SP, Shevell MI, Patenaude Y, O'Gorman AM. Neuromotor spectrum of periventricular leukomalacia in children born at term. Pediatr Neurol. 2000;23(2):155–9.
17. Palisano R, Rosenbaum P, Walter S, Russell D, Wood E, Galuppi B. Development and reliability of a system to classify gross motor function in children with cerebral palsy. Dev Med Child Neurol. 1997;39:214–23.
18. Palisano RJ, Cameron D, Rosenbaum PL, Walter SD, Russell D. Stability of the gross motor function classification system. Dev Med Child Neurol. 2006;48:424–8.
19. McCormick A, Brien M, Plourde J, Wood E, Rosenbaum P, McLean J. Stability of the gross motor function classification system in adults with cerebral palsy. Dev Med Child Neurol. 2007;49:265–9.
20. Strauss D, Shavelle R, Reynolds R, Rosenbloom L, Day S. Survival in cerebral palsy in the last 20 years: signs of improvement? Dev Med Child Neurol. 2007;49:86–92.
21. Hemming K, Hutton J, Pharoah P. Long-term survival for a cohort of adults with cerebral palsy. Dev Med Child Neurol. 2006;48:90–5.
22. Arango P. Families, clinicians, and children and youth with special healthcare needs: a bright future. Pediatr Ann. 2008;37(4):212–22.
23. Stanger M, Oresic S. Rehabilitation approaches for children with cerebral: overview. J Child Neurol. 2003;18:S79–88.
24. Charles JR, Wolf SL, Schneider JA, Gordon AM. Efficacy of a child-friendly form of constraint-induced movement therapy in hemiplegic cerebral palsy: a randomized control trial. Dev Med Child Neurol. 2006;48:635–42.
25. Sterba J. Does horseback riding therapy or therapist-directed hippotherapy rehabilitate children with cerebral palsy? Dev Med Child Neurol. 2007;49:68–73.
26. Kelly M, Darrah J. Aquatic exercise for children with cerebral palsy. Dev Med Child Neurol. 2005;47:838–42.

27. Dodd K, Taylor N, Graham H. A randomized clinical trial of strength training in young people with cerebral palsy. Dev Med Child Neurol. 2003;45:652–7.

28. Morris C. Orthotic management of cerebral palsy. Dev Med Child Neurol. 2007;49:791–6.

29. Terjesen T, Lange J, Steen H. Treatment of scoliosis with spinal bracing in quadriplegic cerebral palsy. Dev Med Child Neurol. 2000;42:448–54.

30. Odding E, Roebroeck M, Stam H. The epidemiology of cerebral palsy: incidence, impairments and risk factors. Disabil Rehabil. 2006;28(4):183–91.

31. Delgado MR, Riela AR, Mills J, Pitt A, Browne R. Discontinuation of antiepileptic drug treatment after two seizure-free years in children with cerebral palsy. Pediatrics. 1996;97(2):192–7.

32. Ajlouni A, Shorman A, Daoud AS. The efficacy and side effects of topiramate on refractory epilepsy in infants and young children: a multi-center clinical trial. Seizure. 2005;14(7): 459–63.

33. Loring DW, Measor KJ. Cognitive side effects of antiepileptic drugs in children. Neurology. 2004;62(6):872–7.

34. Stevenson R, Conaway M, Chumlea W. Growth and health in children with moderate-to-severe cerebral palsy. Pediatrics. 2006;118(3):1010–8.

35. Cronk C, Stallings V. Growth in children with cerebral palsy. Ment Retard Dev Disabil Res Rev. 1997;3:129–37.

36. Spender QW, Cronk CE, Charney EB, Stallings VA. Assessment of linear growth of children with cerebral palsy: use of alternative measures to height of length. Dev Med Child Neurol. 1989;31:206–14.

37. Sanders K, Cox K, Cannon R. Growth response to enteral feeding by children with cerebral palsy. JPEN J Parenter Enteral Nutr. 1990;14(1):23–6.

38. Bar-Or O. Pathophysiological factors which limit the exercise capacity of the sick child. Med Sci Sports Exerc. 1986;18(3):276–82.

39. Lazarus R, Colditz G, Berkey CS, Speizer FE. Effects of body fat on ventilatory function in children and adolescents: cross-sectional findings from a random population sample of school children. Pediatr Pulmonol. 1997;24(3):187–94.

40. Reilly S, Skuse D, Poblete X. Prevalence of feeding problems and oral motor dysfunction in children with cerebral palsy: a community survey. J Pediatr. 1996;129:877–82.

41. Spiroglou K, Xinias I, Karatzas N. Gastric emptying in children with cerebral palsy and gastroesophageal reflux. Pediatr Neurol. 2004;31(3):177–82.

42. Rogers B, Arvedson J, Buck G, Smart P, Msall M. Characteristics of dysphagia in children with cerebral palsy. Dysphagia. 1994;9(1):69–73.

43. Wright RE, Wright FR, Carson CA. Videofluoroscopic assessment in children with severe cerebral palsy presenting with dysphagia. Pediatr Radiol. 1996;26(10):720–2.

44. Yang WT, Loveday EJ, Metreweli C. Ultrasound assessment of swallowing in malnourished disabled children. Br J Radiol. 1997;70(838):992–4.

45. Del Giudice E, Staiano A, Capano G. Gastrointestinal manifestations in children with cerebral palsy. Brain Dev. 1999;21(5):307–11.

46. El-Serag HB, Gilger M. Extraesophageal associations of gastroesophageal reflux disease in children without neurological defects. Gastroenterology. 2001;121(6):1294–9.

47. Su JM, Tsamtsouris A, Laskou M. Gastroesophageal reflux in children with cerebral palsy and its relationship to erosion of primary and permanent teeth. J Mass Dent Soc. 2003;52(2):20–4.

48. Samdon-Fang L, Buter C, O'Donnell M. Gastrostomy for CP 20. Dev Med Child Neurol. 2003;45(6):415–26.

49. Vernon-Roberts A, Sullivan PB. Fundoplication versus post-operative medication for gastroesophageal reflux in children with neurological impairment undergoing gastrostomy. Cochrane Database Syst Rev. 2007;(1):CD006151.

50. Park ES, Park CI, Cho SR, Na SI, Cho YS. Colonic transit time and constipation in children with spastic cerebral palsy. Arch Phys Med Rehabil. 2004;85(3):453–6.

51. Loening-Baucke V. Urinary incontinence and urinary tract infection and their resolution with treatment of chronic constipation of childhood. Pediatrics. 1997;100:228–32.
52. Bandla HP, Davis SH, Hopkins NE. Lipoid pneumonia: a silent complication of mineral oil aspiration. Pediatrics. 1999;103(2):E19.
53. Wilkinson DJ, Baikie G, Berkowitz RG, Reddihough DS. Awake upper airway obstruction in children with spastic quadriplegic cerebral palsy. J Paediatr Child Health. 2006;42:44–8.
54. Kushida CA, Littner MR, Morgenthaler T, Alessi CA, Bailey D, Coleman J Jr, et al. Practice parameters for the indications for polysomnography and related procedures: an update for 2005. Sleep. 2005;28(4):499–521.
55. Banjar HH. Pediatric scoliosis and the lung. Saudi Med J. 2003;24(9):957–63.
56. Stott NS, Piedrahita L. Effects of surgical adductor releases for hip subluxation in cerebral palsy: an AACPDM evidence report. Dev Med Child Neurol. 2004;46:628–45.
57. Morton RE, Scott B, McClelland V. Dislocation of the hips in children with bilateral spastic cerebral palsy, 1985–2000. Dev Med Child Neurol. 2006;48:555–8.
58. McCarthy JJ, D'Andrea LP, Betz RR, Clements DH. Scoliosis in the child with cerebral palsy. J Am Acad Orthop Surg. 2006;14(6):367–75.
59. Gericke T. Postural management for children with cerebral palsy: consensus statement. Dev Med Child Neurol. 2006;48:24–4.
60. Drvaric DM, Roberts JM, Burke SW, King AG, Flaterman K. Gastroesophageal evaluation in totally involved cerebral palsy patients. J Pediatr Orthop. 1987;7(2):187–90.
61. Jevsevar DS, Karlin LI. The relationship between preoperative nutritional status and complications after an operation for scoliosis in patients who have cerebral palsy. J Bone Joint Surg Am. 1993;75(6):880–4.
62. Henderson R, Kairall J, Abbas A. Predicting low bone density in children and young adults with quadriplegic cerebral palsy. Dev Med Child Neurol. 2004;46:416–9.
63. Plotkin H, Coughlin S, Kreikemeier R. Low doses of pamidronate to treat osteopenia in children with severe cerebral palsy: a pilot study. Dev Med Child Neurol. 2006;48:709–12.
64. Sanger T, Delgado M, Gaebler-Spira D. Classification and definition of disorders causing hypertonia in childhood. Pediatrics. 2003;11:e89–97.
65. Pin T, Dyke P, Chan M. The effectiveness of passive stretching in children with cerebral palsy. Dev Med Child Neurol. 2006;48:855–62.
66. Jefferson R. Botulinum toxin in the management of cerebral palsy. Dev Med Child Neurol. 2004;46:491–9.
67. Gooch JL, Patton CP. Combining botulinum toxin and phenol to manage spasticity in children. Arch Phys Med Rehabil. 2004;85(7):1121–4.
68. O'Donnell M, Armstrong R. Pharmacologic interventions for management of spasticity in cerebral palsy. Ment Retard Dev Disabil Res Rev. 1997;3:204–11.
69. McLaughlin J, Bjornson K, Temkin N, Steinbok P, Wright V, Reiner A, et al. Selective dorsal rhizotomy: metaanalysis of three randomized controlled trials. Dev Med Child Neurol. 2002;44:17–25.
70. Hoving M, van Raak E, Palmans LJ, Sleypen FA, Fles JS, et al. Intrathecal baclofen in children with spastic cerebral palsy: a double-blind, randomized, placebo-controlled, dose-finding study. Dev Med Child Neurol. 2007;49:654–9.
71. Sanger TD, Bastian A, Brunstrom J. Prospective open-label clinical trial of trihexyphenidyl in children with secondary dystonia due to cerebral palsy. J Child Neurol. 2007;22(5):530–7.
72. Motta F, Stignani C, Antonello CE. Effect of intrathecal baclofen on dystonia in children with cerebral palsy and the use of functional scales. J Pediatr Orthop. 2008;28(2):213–7.
73. Albright AL. Intrathecal baclofen in cerebral palsy movement disorders. J Child Neurol. 1996;11(Suppl 1):S29–35.
74. Kozeis N, Anogeianaki A, Mitova DT, Anogianakis G, Mitov T, Klisarova A. Visual function and visual perception in cerebral palsied children. Ophthalmic Physiol Opt. 2007;27(1):44–53.

75. O'Connor AR, Fielder AR. Visual outcomes and perinatal adversity. Semin Fetal Neonatal Med. 2007;12(5):408–14. [Epub 2007 Aug 20]
76. Ghasia F, Brunstrom J, Gordon M, Tychsen L. Frequency and severity of visual sensory and motor deficits in children with cerebral palsy; gross motor function classification scale. Invest Ophthalmol Vis Sci. 2008;49(2):572–80.
77. Garcia ML, Ty EB, Taban M, David Rothner A, Rogers D, Traboulsi EI. Systemic and ocular findings in 100 patients with optic nerve hypoplasia. J Child Neurol. 2006;21(11):949–56.
78. Lawrence L, Trower J, Ward S. Ophthalmic evaluation and intervention for young children with cerebral palsy. Dev Med Child Neurol. 2000;83(42):13.
79. Sonksen PM, Petrie A, Drew KJ. Promotion of visual development of severely visually impaired babies: evaluation of a developmentally based program. Dev Med Child Neurol. 1991;33:320–35.
80. Murphy C, Yeargin-Allsopp M, Decouflé, Drews CD. Prevalence of cerebral palsy among ten-year-old children in metropolitan Atlanta, 1985 through 1987. J Pediatr. 1993;123: S13–9.
81. Fligor B, Neault M, Mullen C, Feldman HA, Jones DT. Factors associated with sensorineural hearing loss among survivors of extracorporeal membrane oxygenation therapy. Pediatrics. 2005;115:1519–28.
82. Williamson WD, Demmler G, Percy AK, Catlin FI. Progressive hearing loss in infants with asymptomatic congenital cytomegalovirus infection. Pediatrics. 1992;90:862–6.
83. Edby K, Mårild S. Urinary tract dysfunction in children with cerebral palsy. Acta Paediatr. 2000;89:1505–6.
84. Roijen LE, Postema K, Limbeek VJ, Kuppevelt VH. Development of bladder control in children and adolescents with cerebral palsy. Dev Med Child Neurol. 2001;43(2):103–7.
85. Rodrigues dos Santos MT, Masiero D, Novo NF, Simionato MR. Oral conditions in children with cerebral palsy. J Dent Child (Chic). 2003;70(1):40–6.
86. Winter K, Baccaglini L, Tomar S. A review of malocclusion among individuals with mental and physical disabilities. Spec Care Dentist. 2008;28(1):19–26.
87. Russell GM, Kinirons MJ. A study of the barriers to dental care in a sample of patients with cerebral palsy. Community Dent Health. 1993;10(1):57–64.
88. Jawadi AH, Casamassimo PS, Griffen A, Enrile B, Marcone M. Comparison of oral findings in special needs children with and without gastrostomy. Pediatr Dent. 2004;26(3):283–8.
89. Domaracki L, Sisson L. Decreasing drooling with oral motor stimulation in children with multiple disabilities. Am J Occup Ther. 1990;44(8):680–4.
90. Johnson HM, Reid SM, Hazard CJ, Lucas JO, Desai M, Reddihough DS. Effectiveness of the Innsbruck sensorimotor activator and regulator in improving saliva control in children with cerebral palsy. Dev Med Child Neurol. 2004;46(1):39–45.
91. Bachrach S, Walter R, Trzcinski K. Use of glycopyrrolate and other anticholinergic medications for sialorrhea in children with cerebral palsy. Clin Pediatr. 1998;37:485–90.
92. Banerjee KJ, Glasson C, O'Flaherty SJ. Parotid and submandibular botulinum toxin A injections for sialorrhoea in children with cerebral palsy. Dev Med Child Neurol. 2006;48: 883–7.
93. Burton M. The surgical management of drooling. Dev Med Child Neurol. 1991;33:1110–6.
94. Arnrup K, Crossner C. Caries prevalence after submandibular duct retroposition in drooling children with neurological disorders. Pediatr Dent. 1990;12(2):98–101.
95. Hilberink SR, Roebroeck MD, Nieuwstraten W. Health issues in young adults with cerebral palsy: towards a life-span perspective. J Rehabil Med. 2007;39(8):605–11.
96. Russo RN, Miller MD, Haan E, Cameron ID, Crotty M. Pain characteristics and their association with quality of life and self-concept in children with hemiplegic cerebral palsy identified from a population register. Clin J Pain. 2008;24(4):335–42.
97. Newman C, O'Regan M, Hensey O. Sleep disorders in children with cerebral palsy. Dev Med Child Neurol. 2006;48:564–8.
98. Stores G. Medication for sleep-wake disorders. Arch Dis Child. 2003;88:899–903.

99. Scal P. Transition for youth with chronic conditions: primary care physicians' approaches. Pediatrics. 2002;110(6):1315–21.
100. American Academy of Pediatrics, American Academy of Family Physicians, American College of Physicians–American Society of Internal Medicine. A consensus statement on health care transitions for young adults with special health care needs. Pediatrics. 2002;110(6):1304–6.
101. Dodge N. Cerebral palsy: medical aspects. Pediatr Clin North Am. 2008;55(50):1189–208.

Chapter 16
Myelomeningocele

Dilip R. Patel

Abstract Neural tube defects result from failure of neurulation during the early development of the central nervous system. Although any segment of the developing CNS can be involved, most cases affect the lumbosacral level. Multiple factors have been identified that increase the risk for neural tube defects. Dietary supplementation with folic acid has been shown to reduce the incidence of neural tube defects in many parts of the world. Most individuals, who have myelomeningocele, survive into adulthood and live a very functional life. Medical care of individuals with myelomeningocele is lifelong and requires neurological, orthopedic, urological, and other disciplines to work together to manage not only primary conditions but also many secondary and associated conditions. This chapter provides a brief review of epidemiology, clinical features, diagnosis, and treatment principles for myelomeningocele.

Introduction

Neural tube defects (NTDs) result from failure of the neurulation, that is failure of the closure of the neural tube during development of central nervous system as expected between the third and fourth week of in utero development [1, 2]. Although any segment of spinal level can be affected, 75% of cases involve the lumbosacral level [3]. Myelomeningocele is the most severe type of NTD in which there is a defect in the vertebral column through which the meninges and the spinal cord protrude at the level of the defect [2].

D.R. Patel (✉)
Department of Pediatrics and Human Development, Kalamazoo Center for Medical Studies, Michigan State University College of Human Medicine, Kalamazoo, MI 49008-1284, USA
e-mail: patel@kcms.msu.edu

D.R. Patel et al. (eds.), *Neurodevelopmental Disabilities*,
DOI 10.1007/978-94-007-0627-9_16, © Springer Science+Business Media B.V. 2011

Epidemiology

The prevalence of NTDs varies in different regions of the world [3]. In the United States, the incidence of NTDs is 1 in 4,000 live births [1, 3]. In Wales and Ireland, the prevalence is 3–4 times higher, whereas in Africa it is much lower [3]. The variability in prevalence rates of NTDs in different regions of the world is believed to be due to a combination of genetic and environmental factors. Lumbar myelomeningocele, which is 3–7 times more common in females than in males, accounts for most cases of myelomeningocele [1]. Risk factors for NTDs are listed in Table 16.1 [1–4]. A significant decrease (50%) in the prevalence of NTDs has been reported over the past four decades [3]. Some of the reasons believed to have contributed to the decrease in prevalence of NTDs include routine and widespread supplementation with folic acid, prenatal diagnosis and subsequent decision to terminate pregnancy by some couples, and improved nutrition as well as general health of women [1, 3].

Clinical Features

The primary neurological manifestations in infants and children who have myelomeningocele are owing to the motor and sensory loss, Chiari type 2

Table 16.1 Risk factors for neural tube defects

Risk factor	Evidence of risk
Nutritional	Incidence of neural tube defects peaks after famine
	Seasonal variations
	Preventive effect of acid in case-controlled and randomized studies
Environmental	East-to-west trend in the United States
	Decreased risk among Irish who migrate to the United States
	Seasonal variations
Genetic	Familial risk
	2–4% recurrence after one affected child
	11–15% recurrence after two affected children
	Ethnic differences
	Prevalence in US populations: Hispanic > white > African American
	Great Britain: highest risk in Celtic population
	India: highest risk in Sikh population
	Chromosomal abnormalities
	Genetic disorders (Waardenburg syndrome; 22p11 microdeletion)
	Variant form of methylenetetrahydrofolate dehydrogenase (677C-T)
Physical	Association with maternal fever during pregnancy
	Association with maternal use of hot tubs or sauna during pregnancy
Maternal	Obesity
	Diabetes mellitus
Teratogenic	High vitamin A intake
	Valproic acid
	Alcohol

Used with permission from Wolraich [13, table 14-10].

malformation, and hydrocephalus [3–6]. Generally, the motor and sensory function is lost below the level of the lesion in the spinal cord. However, such a loss is neither uniform nor complete in all cases. Therefore, predicting the patient's functional abilities, such as walking, based primarily on the anatomic level of lesion is often unreliable [3, 7]. Functional abilities are often affected by associated and secondary conditions. Sensory loss involving external genitalia and anus is found in most persons who have myelomeningocele. Chiari type 2 malformation is present in almost all cases of myelomeningocele. Downward displacement of the brainstem and portion of the cerebellum through the foramen magnum can result in spinal cord compression in Chiari type 2 malformation [5].

The symptoms and signs of spinal cord compression include dysphagia, choking, hoarseness, weak cry, breath-holding spells, apnea, bradycardia, disordered breathing during sleep, stiffness in the arms, and opisthotonos [1–6]. Older children may also have unsteady gait with frequent falls. Rarely sudden deaths from cardiorespiratory arrest owing to progressive cord compression in Chiari type 2 malformation have been reported [3]. Chiari type 2 malformation is associated with hydrocephalus in most cases of thoracolumbar myelomeningocele. Signs and symptoms of increased intracranial pressure (ICF) due to progressive hydrocephalus should be recognized and monitored. Hydrocephalus is treated with surgical implantation of a ventriculoperitoneal shunt [5].

In infants, signs of a blocked shunt include an increase in head circumference and a tense anterior fontanel [3]. In children older than 2 years, because the skull bones are fused, shunt obstruction or malfunction presents with signs and symptoms of increased ICP [3]. In addition to signs and symptoms of increased ICP, a child with an infected shunt will also have a fever. Signs and symptoms of a blocked shunt are often difficult to distinguish from those of tethered cord syndrome or cord compression related to Chiari type 2 malformation. A blocked or infected shunt should be suspected in a patient who develops a change in baseline functions or new neurological signs and symptoms. Change in behavior, deterioration in academic function, or weakness in extremities can be signs of shunt malfunction. The clinical features in older children, adolescents, and adults also include signs and symptoms of complications and associated and secondary conditions (see Table 16.2) [1–4]. The extent of motor and sensory deficits and stability of shunted hydrocephalus are primary factors that influence adult functioning and health.

Diagnosis

NTDs can be diagnosed prenatally. Maternal serum alpha-fetoprotein (MSAFP) is measured during the 16th–18th week of pregnancy [1, 3]. AFP is normally present in fetal cerebrospinal spinal fluid (CSF). In the presence of an open NTD, the CSF AFP leaks into the amniotic fluid and enters the maternal circulation. Measurement of MSAFP is used as a screening test to detect the presence of open NTDs. A positive MSAFP screen is followed by a high-resolution ultrasonography to detect fetal anatomic anomalies suggestive of NTDs [1–3]. If fetal anomalies are detected, an

Table 16.2 Associated and secondary conditions in myelomeningocele

Neurological	Arnold–Chiari malformation
	Hydrocephalus
	Tethered cord
	Syringomyelia
	Seizures
	Autonomic dysreflexia
Cognitive/behavioral	Intellectual disability
	Learning disability
	Nonverbal learning disability
	Attention-deficit hyperactivity disorder
Urological/renal	Neurogenic bladder
	Vesicoureteral reflux
	Hydronephrosis
	Frequent urinary tract infections
	Urinary incontinence
	Urinary retention
	Secondary chronic kidney disease and failure
	Nephrolithiasis
Gastrointestinal/nutritional	Neurogenic bowel
	Bowel incontinence, rectal prolapse
	Constipation
	Obesity
Skin	Pressure sores
	Ulcers
Endocrine	Growth hormone deficiency
	Precocious puberty
	Metabolic syndrome
Cardiovascular	Congenital heart disease
	Secondary hypertension
	Reduced aerobic capacity
	Deep venous thrombosis
	Lymphedema
Ophthalmological	Strabismus
	Esotropia
	Papilledema
	Nystagmus
Allergic	Latex
	Sensitivities to certain foods such as bananas, water chestnuts, avocados, and kiwi fruit
Sexual	Sexual dysfunction in some males

Patel et al. [11].

amniocentesis is performed. A diagnosis of NTD is made on the basis of the presence of acetylcholinesterase (AChE) and AFP in the amniotic fluid in combination with anomalies detected on ultrasonography [1–3].

Chromosomal analysis of the amniotic fluid is performed to exclude any chromosomal syndromes associated with NTDs. Prenatal diagnosis is helpful to guide parental decision to carry on with the pregnancy and for the team of physicians to anticipate and plan for medical complications associated with delivery and neonatal care of the infant with NTD [1–3].

Treatment

Folic acid (4 mg/day) supplementation starting before conception and continued through for the first 3 months of the pregnancy reduces the risk for recurrence of NTD by 70% [1]. Women who have an NTD or have a first-degree relative with an NTD also should take 4 mg/day around the time of conception. Ongoing management of associated and secondary conditions (see Table 16.2) needs primary care physician working with appropriate subspecialists; management requires neurosurgical, urological, and orthopedic interventions [1, 3, 4, 8–10, 12].

Conclusions

Most children who have thoracolumbosacral myelomeningocele survive into adulthood [1, 9]. This trend requires planning transition of medical care from pediatrics to adult health-care systems. Adults need ongoing surveillance for secondary conditions and their management. Overall mortality for a child born with myelomeningocele and who is aggressively treated is approximately 10–15% with most deaths occurring before 4 years of age [1, 3]. Approximately 70% of children who survive have normal intelligence; however, subtle neurocognitive deficits are common. Progressive deterioration in renal function is the most significant determinant of mortality in patients who have myelomeningocele [3, 9].

Acknowledgments This chapter is adapted with permission from author's previous work: Patel et al. [11].

References

1. Mitchell LE, Adzick NS, Melchionne J, Pasquariello PA, Sutton LN, Whitehead AS. Spina bifida. Lancet. 2004;364:1885.
2. Dias MS, Partington M. Embryology of myelomeningocele and enencephaly. Neurosurg Focus. 2004;16(2):1–16.
3. Liptak GS. Neural tube defects. In: Batshaw ML, Pellegrino L, Roizen NJ, editors. Children with developmental disabilities. 6th ed. Baltimore, MD: Paul H Brookes; 2007. pp. 419–38.
4. Herring JA. Disorders of the spinal cord. In: Herring JA, editor. Tachdjian's pediatric orthopaedics. 3rd ed. Philadelphia, PA: Saunders; 2002. pp. 1249–98.
5. Tubbs RS, Oakes WJ. Treatment and management of the Chiari II malformation: an evidence-based review of literature. Child Nerv Syst. 2004;20:375–81.
6. Lew SM, Kothbauer KF. Tethered cord syndrome: an updated review. Pediatr Neurosurg. 2007;43:236–48.
7. Beeker TW, Scheers MM, Faber JAJ, Tulleken CAF. Prediction of independence and intelligence at birth in meningomyelocele. Child Nerv Syst. 2006;22:33–7.

8. Simeonsson RJ, McMillen JS, Huntington GS. Secondary conditions in children with disabilities: spina bifida as a case example. Ment Retard Dev Disabil Res Rev. 2002;8(1):198–205.
9. Dicianno BE, Kurowski BG, Yang JMJ, Chancellor MB, Bejjani GK, Fairman AD, et al. Rehabilitation and medical management of the adult with spina bifida. Am J Phys Med Rehabil. 2008;87:1026–50.
10. Joyner BD, McLorie GA, Khoury AE. Sexuality and reproductive issues in children with myelomeningocele. Eur J Pediatr Surg. 1998;8(1):29–34.
11. Patel DR, Greydanus DE, Calles J Jr, Pratt HD. Developmental disabilities across the life span. Dis Mon. 2010;56(6):299–398.
12. Posner JC, Cronan K, Badaki O, Fein JA. Emergency care of the technology –assisted child. Clin Ped Emerg Med. 2006;7:38–51.
13. Wolraich M, editor. Developmental and behavioral pediatrics: evidence and practice. Philadelphia, PA: Elsevier Saunders; 2008. p. 496.

Chapter 17
Pain in Individuals with Intellectual and Developmental Disabilities

Lynn M. Breau, Meir Lotan, and Jeffrey L. Koh

Abstract Pain assessment and management is a challenging task in most populations, but individuals with intellectual and developmental disabilities (IDD) display specific barriers to adequate pain management, mostly due to the fact that they may not be able to give valid self-reports. Despite enhanced interest in the pain of children and adults with IDD in recent years, the characteristics of pain behavior and pain management in this group have scarcely been examined. This chapter will provide an overview of the current status of pain assessment for individuals with IDD and suggest psychological and pharmacological approaches to pain management for this population.

Introduction

Pain is referred to by the International Association for the Study of Pain as "an unpleasant sensory or emotional experience associated with actual or potential tissue damage or described in terms of such damage" [1]. Pain can have a negative effect on the individual's functional ability, mobility, emotional status, ability to work, interpersonal relationships, and social activities, leading to increased use of health-care services and an accompanying increase in health-care costs [2]. In addition, in the definition for pain the IASP also notes, "The inability to communicate verbally does not negate the possibility that an individual is experiencing pain and is in need of appropriate pain-relieving treatment." Adopting such a concept becomes imperative when the individual suffering from pain cannot voice discomfort, as in the very young, the very old, and persons with intellectual and developmental disabilities (IDD). Unequal access to pain relief and failure to treat pain are viewed

L.M. Breau (✉)
School of Nursing and Departments of Psychology and Pediatrics, Dalhousie University, 5869, University Avenue, Halifax, Nova Scotia, Canada B3H 3J5; Pediatric Complex Pain Team, IWK Health Centre, Halifax, Nova Scotia, Canada
e-mail: lbreau@dal.ca

D.R. Patel et al. (eds.), *Neurodevelopmental Disabilities*,
DOI 10.1007/978-94-007-0627-9_17, © Springer Science+Business Media B.V. 2011

as poor medicine, unethical practice, and an abrogation of fundamental human rights [3].

Available findings suggest that pain in people with severe intellectual disability is common, yet rarely actively treated [4]. Studies in this field also indicate that people with IDD have 2.5 times more health problems compared to people without IDD [5]. Individuals with severe or profound levels of IDD are more likely to have additional disabling conditions or multiple complex medical problems coupled with communication difficulties. Such medical problems, whether directly or indirectly linked to the disability, often necessitate painful procedures, including physical therapy treatments and various medical interventions. Recent data reveal that "sick days" in this population were associated with higher levels of pain and discomfort than were "well days" [6] and that people with severe IDD and low communication abilities are likely to experience the most pain over time [7].

The prevalence of pain in the IDD population is unclear, mainly due to communication problems that make the recognition of pain difficult [8]. People with IDD are vulnerable to the same range of pain-inflicting procedures as the non-IDD population, but in addition they are also vulnerable to experiencing pain from falls, leg braces, and ill-fitting wheelchairs [9]. A study investigating the frequency, duration, intensity, and location of pain, as well as the interference of pain with activities, in adults with cerebral palsy (CP) and IDD, found that pain was a significant problem for the majority of participants [10]. Of the 93 participants (with an average age of 38), the majority had quadriplegia (84%) and were non-ambulatory (94%). One or more areas of chronic pain (minimum of 3 months duration) was reported by 67% of the participants, and moderate to severe pain on an almost daily basis was experienced by 53%. Lower extremity pain (66%) and back pain (63%) were the most common complaints. The duration of pain ranged from a mean of 7.5 years for upper extremity pain to a mean of 20 years for hip or buttock pain. Likewise, Breau et al. [7] studied pain in 94 children aged 3–18 years with moderate to profound IDD, 44 (47%) with CP. Over four 1-week periods, 73 (78%) had pain at least once and 35–52% had pain each week. Children spent an average of 9 h per week in pain and most pain was related to musculoskeletal or gastrointestinal problems [7].

Thus, accumulating evidence suggests that individuals with IDD at all ages suffer from more pain than the general population and can be considered as a population at risk in regard to pain. Most researchers recommend that additional research is needed to carefully examine how pain can be better managed in people with IDD and multiple disabilities [10]. However, it is clear that better pain management should start with proper pain assessment and that it is essential for the clinician to use reliable evaluation tools to initiate the pain assessment and intervention processes.

Assessing Pain in Individuals with IDD

Assessing pain in individuals with IDD is a challenging task and can become extremely difficult at the levels of severe and profound IDD, the ability to verbally communicate pain experience being severely compromised [11]. Without objective assessment, pain can be misinterpreted or underestimated, which might lead to inadequate management and undermine quality of life [12].

The Complexity of Assessing Pain in Individuals with IDD

Given the constant hindrance of pain to quality of life among individuals with IDD, there is an urgent need to develop sound pain assessment tools for this population. However, the scientific world has lagged behind when it comes to pain assessment in individuals with IDD, and there are several reasons for this situation. First, many individuals with IDD have neurological problems that may affect their ability to comprehend and effectively communicate pain, thus complicating evaluation of the qualitative and quantitative aspects of their pain experience [13]. Typical cognitive difficulties among this population involve abstract thinking and spatial orientation. Therefore, individuals with IDD may be unable to give valid reports of the features of their pain sensation, such as location, intensity, or quality. They also may not be able to respond to questions about their pain or they may respond in a way that is not meaningful to caregivers [14]. These circumstances make pain measurement in these patients highly difficult or in some cases impossible [15]. Thus, due to this reduced ability to verbally communicate pain, the gold standard of pain assessment, namely self-report, cannot be used with this population.

Second, individuals with IDD often have multiple handicaps and form an extremely heterogeneous group in terms of functional and behavioral repertoires. Functional limitations, such as paralysis and inability to move, may mask expressions of pain [16]. To further complicate the issue of unclear communicative signals, challenging behaviors such as aggression, self-injury, and tantrums can be observed in this population [6]. Such behaviors not only have been connected with painful medical problems [17, 18] but can also mask pain in individuals with IDD [19, 20]. This makes it difficult to ascertain whether the behavior is attributable to pain or another source of distress or whether it is simply part of the individual's regular aberrant behavior.

Third, behavioral indicators of pain in the general population, such as facial grimaces, groaning, or altered sleep patterns [21], may well appear in individuals with IDD at times when they are not in pain [16]. It is therefore not surprising that such behaviors are attributed to the intellectual level of the individual rather than to pain [22], potentially resulting in underdiagnosis of pain.

Finally, assessing and managing pain in people with IDD can be clouded by the effects of the amount of medication consumed by this population [23], as well as the lack of appropriate pain assessment tools. Despite the increased research attention focused on expressive behavior related to pain in individuals with IDD [4, 24–27], research on this topic is still scarce and there are but a few pain assessment scales available for use in this specific population.

Existing Pain Scales

Several scales for pain assessment in individuals with IDD have been developed, the majority over recent years, and mostly for the pediatric population. One scale was developed for the general population, but has been used for individuals with IDD in the past. The following scales are ordered chronologically and their main features are summarized in Table 17.1.

The Facial Action Coding System (FACS)

The FACS is a list of facial actions (action units – AUs) based on movements of specific muscles or groups of muscles in the face [28]. FACS was repeatedly found to be highly reliable for adults without IDD by Craig and associates [29–32], as well as by other researchers [33, 34]. This scale has been used with adults with cognitive impairment (IDD) due to dementia [35, 36] and with a group with mild to moderate IDD undergoing influenza injection [11]. An adaptation, the Child Facial Coding System (CFCS; [37]), has also been used for postoperative pain in children with IDD [38]. Unfortunately, the FACS and CFCS are cumbersome to use and, although suitable for research, not yet feasible in a clinical setting.

The Evaluation Scale for Pain in Cerebral Palsy (ESPCP)

The ESPCP consists of 22 items derived from physicians' reports of cues considered to be indicative of pain during a medical examination [39]. The items include various facial expressions: crying, movements, and posture (increase in muscular tone and/or involuntary movements, analgesic postures); protective reactions (movement toward painful areas); and social behaviors (e.g., reduced interest in surroundings). Although a set of behaviors was found to reflect pain in people with cerebral palsy and severe IDD, the importance of the different items in determining pain appeared dependent on the individual's level of development.

Using the ESPCP, Collignon et al. [40] developed a 10-item observational pain scale for children with severe handicaps and adults with cerebral palsy. They then further developed the tool to better fit an adolescent population with IDD [41]. They studied 100 individuals, aged from 2 to 33 years (mean 16 years) who had multiple physical disabilities and profound IDD and lacked speech and symbolic communication. The authors report that pain could only be detected by observing global behavioral changes, rather than by the presence of a single sign. In addition, each combination of disabilities within their sample appeared to evoke a specific set of behaviors. For instance, voluntary protection of painful areas was more likely to be seen in individuals with a lesser degree of motor impairment. This tool has not been further investigated for psychometric properties. Thus, further research is needed before it can be established as a psychometrically sound tool for clinical use.

Table 17.1 A comparative summary of existing pain scales for individuals with IDD

Name	FACS	ESPCP	NCCPC	PICIC	PPP	PADS	NCAPC
No. of items	8	10,22	42	6	20	18	18
Source	Lachapelle, et al. [11]	Giusiano et al. [39]; Collignon, et al. [40]	McGrath, et al. [16]; Breau, et al. [42]; Breau, et al., 2002	Stallard, et al. [4]; Stallard, et al. [47]	Hunt, et al. [48]	Bodfish et al. [21] Phan et al. [49]	Lotan et al., 2009; Lotan, et al. [53].
Population	Adults with mild–moderate IDD	Adolescents with CP and IDD	Children with cognitive impairment	Non-communicating children	Children with severe neurological and cognitive disability	Adults with severe and profound MR	Adults at all levels of IDD
Age range (mean)	(49.6)	2–33 (16)	6–29 (14.5); 3–9; 3–18	2+ (9,4); 2–21 (7.8)	1–18 (9.9)	–	
N	40	100	20; 24; 71	49; 34	140	22; 8	228
Type of pain	Procedural	Not specified	Needle pain; long-lasting pain	Nonspecific – severe pain	Not specified	Procedural; chronic	Procedural; chronic
Psycho-metric properties — Reliability			0.78–0.82		0.74–0.89	0.86	0.94–091
Internal consistency			0.91–0.93		0.75–0.89	–	0.77
Validity	Have not been tested	Have not been tested	–	Have not been tested	Construct validity	Content validity	Content validity Construct validity
Specificity			0.81–0.74		1.00	–	–
Sensitivity			0.88–0.84		0.91	–	–

The Non-communicating Children's Pain Checklist (NCCPC)

The collection of pain items for this scale was generated by McGrath and associates [16]. They interviewed 20 parents or caregivers of children with severe IDD, aged 6–29 years, regarding cues they considered to be indicative of pain in their children. The interviews included instances of short, sharp pain, such as needle pain, as well as longer-lasting pain, such as headache or injury. A list of 31 cues was elicited. While specific behaviors often differed from one child to another, classes of behaviors (vocal, eating/sleeping, social/personality, facial expressions, body and limbs activity, and physiological reactions) were common to almost all children.

The NCCPC was developed from this initial study [42]. It was comprised of 30 items and was tested in a home setting. Parents and caregivers assessed whether the pain cues were "present" or "absent" in four situations: acute pain, long-term pain, a non-painful but distressing situation, and a non-painful, calm situation. On average, more than four times as many pain cues were present in painful situations than in calm (no-pain) situations. The total number of present cues did not differ between painful and distressed states, but scores for the "eating/sleeping" and "body/limb" subscales were higher during acute pain than during distress.

A second version, the NCCPC-PV (PV = postoperative version), was evaluated in a postoperative setting [43]. In this study, items related to eating and sleeping were omitted and each of the remaining items was scored on a four-point ordinal scale according to frequency of occurrence. Twenty-four children, aged 3–19 years, were observed by a caregiver and a researcher for durations of 10 min both before and after surgery. When available, nurses also provided their assessments. Each observer completed the NCCPC-PV independently in addition to giving a global rating of the intensity of the child's pain using a Visual Analogue Scale (VAS). The NCCPC-PV was found to show very high internal consistency (Cronbach's $\alpha = 0.91$) and good inter-rater reliability (ICC 0.78–0.82). A score of 11 on the NCCPC-PV provided 0.88% sensitivity and 0.81% specificity for classifying children who were rated at a moderate-severe level of pain postoperatively, equivalent to a rating of 3 or greater on the VAS of pain intensity.

A third version of this scale, the NCCPC-R (R = revised), used ordinal ratings according to frequency of occurrence as above, but this time included the items related to eating and sleeping. This version was evaluated in home settings [44]. Caregivers of 71 children with severe IDD, aged 3–18 years, conducted observations of their child during pain and pain-free periods. The NCCPC-R was found to have high internal consistency (Cronbach's $\alpha = 0.93$), as well as a moderate correlation with the pain intensity ratings provided by caregivers (Pearson's $r = 0.46$). Sensitivity (0.84) and specificity (0.77) for pain were optimized at a cutoff point of 7 out of a possible total score of 90. A recent adaptation of this scale, the Batten's Observational Pain Scale (BOPS), has been developed for those with IDD due to neuronal ceroid lipofuscinosis [45] and the Chronic Pain Scale for Nonverbal Adults with Intellectual Disabilities (CPS-NAID) was recently generated from the NCCPC-R for chronic/recurrent pain in adults with IDD [46].

The Pain Indicator for Communicatively Impaired Children (PICIC)

The PICIC uses six items to assess the expression of chronic pain in non-communicative children with significant IDD. A significant relationship was demonstrated between five of the six items and the presence and severity of pain [47]. However, further research is needed before the PICIC can be established as a psychometrically sound tool.

The Pediatric Pain Profile (PPP)

The PPP is a 20-item behavior rating scale designed to assess pain in children with severe neurological and cognitive disability [48]. The validity and reliability of the scale were assessed in 140 children, aged 1–18 years, who were unable to communicate through speech or augmentative communication. Parents used the PPP to retrospectively rate their child's behavior when "at their best" and when in pain. Children displayed significantly higher scores when in pain and scores were related to global evaluations of pain. Inter-rater reliability, using an intraclass correlation coefficient, ranged from 0.74 to 0.89. In order to assess the construct validity and responsiveness of the scale, the behavior of 41 children was rated before and 4 h after the administration of an analgesic. PPP scores were significantly higher before than after analgesic administration. Internal consistency ranged from 0.75 to 0.89 (Cronbach's α), and sensitivity (1.00) and specificity (0.91) were optimized at a cutoff point of 14 on a 60-point scale. Although there was no significant difference between the mean preoperative and postoperative scores, the highest PPP score occurred in the first 24 h after surgery in 14 (47%) of 30 children for whom scores were collected before surgery and up to 5 days after surgery. The authors claim that the PPP should be considered as reliable and valid and suggest that it has potential for both clinical and research purposes.

Despite such claims, it seems that more rigorous psychometric properties need to be established for the PPP and that further research is required in order to evaluate the acceptability, feasibility, and usefulness of the PPP as a tool in clinical settings for children with severe to profound neurological and cognitive disabilities. It has also yet to be determined whether the PPP is also useful for pain assessment in adults with similar degrees of disability [48].

The Pain and Discomfort Scale (PADS)

This scale was derived from the NCCPC-R [44]. It was developed to be used during a physical examination and training is required for its use. Bodfish et al. [21] conducted a set of three studies on PADS. In the first, 22 adults with severe and profound IDD were assessed before and during acute medical procedures known to produce pain and discomfort (i.e., a gastrostomy tube insertion or a toenail removal). In the second study, scores for a group with painful chronic medical conditions and physical disabilities were compared to those of a group with IDD alone and were significantly higher. In the last study, eight adults with profound IDD and medical conditions were assessed before and after pain treatment. In all cases, there was a significant reduction in PADS score from baseline to treatment, which the authors interpreted as indicative of treatment effects and reduced pain [21].

The PADS [21] was later used to detect pain and discomfort during a dental scaling procedure [49]. Twenty-eight subjects with cognitive and communication deficits were assessed at multiple baselines as well as during and after the procedure. The scores on the PADS were significantly higher during the procedure. An optimal cutoff point for sensitivity and specificity has not yet been demonstrated for the PADS [49] and the three studies conducted by Bodfish have not been published. However, the evidence suggests that the PADS has potential as a measure of pain in adults with IDD (21;49).

The Non-communicating Adult's Pain Checklist (NCAPC)

The NCAPC is a recently developed scale, based on previous research on facial expressions and body movements as indicators of acute pain and discomfort in children [44]. In the initial stage of the project [50], behaviors of 121 individuals with IDD and 38 with normal cognition (comparison group) were rated by two raters, using the FACS [28] and the NCCPC-R [44], before and during an influenza vaccination. The findings suggested that level of cognition affected baseline behavior as well as pain behavior and that the FACS might provide a false impression, suggesting that individuals with severe or profound IDD are less reactive to pain. The NCCPC-R was a more sensitive measure of pain behavior in this sample. In a subsequent study [51], videotape of 228 adults with varied levels of IDD before and during an influenza vaccination was scored using the NCCPC-R. Each of the 30 items was examined for sensitivity to change for internal consistency and to sensitivity to change of the total scale. As a result a new scale was constructed, the Non-communicating Adults Pain Checklist (NCAPC). When the new scale was re-scored and in a random subsample of 89 participants, all remaining items were sensitive to pain, internal consistency ($\alpha = 0.77$) was satisfactory, and high sensitivity to pain was found at all levels of IDD (SRM ranging between 1.20 and 2.07). Thus, the NCAPC provided better psychometrics for acute pain in this adult sample than did the NCCPC-R. In a further study, inter-rater reliability (ICC 1/1) of the NCAPC ICC (1, 1) for caregivers and physical and occupational therapists was 0.92 and 0.91, respectively [52].

In the most recent study, 58 adults at all levels of IDD were observed before and during a dental hygiene treatment and an influenza vaccination. The results suggest the NCAPC was able to significantly differentiate between pain and non-pain situations, as well as between different pain incidents. It was also sensitive to pain at all levels of IDD. Evidence for the clinical utility of the NCAPC was also generated because the data were collected in a clinical setting [53]. Scores collected with the NCAPC recently enabled the construction of a model for pain of individuals with IDD [54], further attesting to the construct validity of this set of pain cues.

To date, no articles could be found presenting the ongoing use of the above-listed scales in clinical settings, although data for several studies were collected in clinical settings. Despite early evidence of psychometrics for the scales, and for the NCCPCs and NCAPC in particular, for which multiple studies have been published, clinical feasibility and utility studies would be of benefit. There is also no data to date indicating how common use of these scales is in clinical settings worldwide to provide a sense of whether their use is aiding professionals in providing more knowledgeable management in this population.

Pain Management for Individuals with IDD

Research into pain assessment for persons with IDD has grown slowly since the 1990s. In contrast, almost no studies exist regarding pain management in this population. This does not mean that pain care cannot be delivered to this group. The consensus of most authors in this field is that most strategies developed for those without IDD can be used for those with IDD, albeit modifications may be needed in some cases. Most treatments for pain can be grouped as physical, pharmacological, or psychological. It should be noted that the International Association for the Study of Pain Core Curriculum for Professional Education in Pain (3rd ed.) indicates multidisciplinary treatment is important for those with IDD [55]. Thus, failure of any single approach or technique to fully relieve pain should not be taken as a sign that pain is untreatable. Rather, it should be taken as an indication that a multi-pronged strategy may be required in that case. They also recommend that treatment take into account that mental age may not match chronological age in this group of clients.

Physical Therapies

Physical therapy interventions for pain relief encompass a large group of treatments including exercise, acupuncture, massage, and transcutaneous electric nerve stimulation (TENS). One of the first studies to document the pain behavior of children with IDD focused on physical therapy after surgery [56], and physical therapies are a common activity in the life of many with IDD, especially those with concomitant physical disabilities such as cerebral palsy. Physical therapies not only appear to offer some pain relief for those with cerebral palsy [57] but can also be a source of pain [58, 59]. This chapter will not elaborate on physical therapy as means to reduce pain in this population. However, physical therapies are recommended in the set of treatments provided for many chronic pain conditions [60, 61], and the reader is encouraged to seek further information regarding the many physical therapies available and their effectiveness for specific pain problems. The Snoezelen environment has been found efficient in reducing pain in NIDD individuals [62, 63] and is present in many facilities for individuals with IDD, therefore it might be found useful within the IDD population as well.

Pharmacological Treatments

Acute/postoperative pain management: Individuals with IDD often have underlying musculoskeletal or neurologic abnormalities that may require more frequent surgical interventions than their non-impaired counterparts. Common operations performed in patients with IDD include tendon release, osteotomy, posterior spinal fusion, vagal nerve stimulator placement, and baclofen pump placement. As a result, these patients can have a more frequent need for pharmacological treatment of acute postoperative pain.

Although there is limited research in this area, evidence does suggest that patients with IDD are, and should be, treated similarly to those without IDD undergoing similar procedures. Koh et al. [64] showed that patients with IDD had very similar opioid requirements to a matched non-impaired group undergoing surgery of similar severity [64]. Of interest, this group also showed that IDD patients received somewhat less opioid intraoperatively as compared to their non-IDD counterparts. This finding was also shown in a study by Long et al. [65]. It is possible that anesthesiologists are somewhat conservative intraoperatively since the clinical experience of many suggests variability in response to opioids for patients with IDD. This has not been supported in the literature as of yet.

Methods of treatment of postoperative pain include intravenous (IV) opioids, patient controlled analgesia (PCA) with IV opioids, and regional anesthesia [66, 67]. All of these modalities have been used safely in patients with IDD with no evidence that these patients are at higher risk of complications as compared to their counterparts without IDD. Licht et al. showed that adult patients with IDD do well with PCA [68]. This study suggests that a subpopulation of patients with IDD do have the cognitive ability to effectively use a PCA. As with all patients, an evaluation preoperatively of the ability to understand the concept of PCA will be helpful in determining if a patient is a good candidate for this treatment modality. For those not able to safely use a PCA, PCA by proxy (a nurse or parent activates the PCA bolus when needed) is an alternative. Voepel-Lewis et al. [69] showed that PCA by proxy has a similar side effect profile as PCA and similar analgesia as measured by pain scores. In addition, Brenn showed that epidural anesthesia with a continuous infusion of bupivacaine and fentanyl provided safe and effective analgesia in patients with CP undergoing either lower extremity orthopedic procedures or Nissen fundoplications [70].

In summary, the treatment of acute postoperative pain in IDD patients can and should be managed similarly to patients without IDD. Although originally developed by the World Health Organization (WHO) for the management of cancer pain [71], the analgesic ladder approach to pain management is equally effective for acute pain management. For mild to moderate pain, oral acetaminophen and non-steroidal anti-inflammatory drugs (NSAIDs) ± an oral opioid will usually be sufficient. For more severe pain, IV opioid will be needed and can be safely used. Acetaminophen or NSAIDs may be useful supplements to IV opioids, and just as with non-IDD patients, medication should be titrated to analgesic effect while watching for side effects. Regional anesthesia, including epidural blocks and peripheral nerve blocks, can be especially useful in this population when there is a concern about the sedation effect of opioids. Anatomic abnormalities, such as severe scoliosis, may make placement of these blocks more challenging or even impossible. Nonetheless, they should be considered when medically indicated (coinciding with close respiratory follow-up). It is important to note that there is absolutely no evidence that IDD patients have any different pain perception than NIDD patients and therefore should be treated with a similar approach.

Chronic pain: Patients with IDD are at higher risk for a variety of chronic pain complaints, especially as they get older. Most commonly, patients with CP will develop musculoskeletal pain, such as hip and back pain, severe enough to require treatment. Senaran et al. [72] have also reported anterior knee pain as a common pain complaint in patients with CP. As noted above, these problems may require surgical intervention and thus overlay acute pain on top of chronic pain. However, many patients will not be good candidates for surgery and will benefit from a more comprehensive approach to their pain management.

Spasticity is seen in many patients with IDD, especially those with CP, and can contribute to chronic pain. Even everyday positioning in this group of clients might be difficult and potentially painful. Targeted treatment for spasticity, and related pain, if present, has focused on either systemic muscle relaxants or intrathecal administration of baclofen via implanted pump. An alternative approach may be the use of botox injections, despite its short-term effect (about 3 months). In a study of 34 patients with CP who had spasticity-related pain, Symons et al. [73] showed that botox injections resulted in a significant reduction in parent report of pain compared to pre-injection levels. Similarly, Lundy [74] performed botox injections in 26 patients with CP and significant hip pain.

Summary: There is still very little research examining the pharmacological treatment of pain in individuals with IDD. In the absence of research-based recommendations specific to this population, medication choices should be dictated by the patient's symptoms based on the same principles applied to those without IDD, while taking into account their previous medication consumption, which in some cases might be high and varied. There may be a role for medications commonly used for neuropathic pain, such as gabapentin and tricyclic antidepressants [75]. Gabapentin, an antiepileptic medication, has been found to be useful in a wide variety of chronic pain syndromes that are not typically neuropathic in origin. We have found it especially useful for chronic hip pain in this population. Chronic oral opioid use may be useful for some patients with diffuse pain and can be helpful in facilitating physical therapy. Extended release medications such as single-ingredient oxycodone or methadone are preferred for chronic pain and have proven effective in clinical use. The goal of medical interventions is not only to decrease pain but also more importantly to improve function and tolerance of interventions, such as physical and psychological therapies, which are critical to long-term improvements in quality of life.

Psychological Techniques

Psychological pain management techniques fall within two broad categories, behavioral and cognitive approaches. However, the terms are frequently used interchangeably and the term "cognitive behavioral" is often used to describe many of these techniques. Generally speaking, behavioral methods are simpler to perform, involving changes in behavior to reduce pain, while cognitive techniques require changing thought patterns which are expected to then result in changed behavior. Both are considered within the broad grouping of complementary and alternative medicine (CAM) treatments, which are a common part of multidisciplinary pain management and emerging as the most effective pain management approach [76].

Because behavioral techniques do not require the same level of cognitive ability, they are more often used with young children and may be more appropriate for individuals with IDD. Some forms of relaxation fall within this group, such as progressive muscle relaxation, breathing exercises, and behavioral relaxation training [77]. Operant conditioning, modeling, and some forms of distraction also fit in this category. Although there is some evidence that cognitive treatments can be effective for pain [78], Sturmey [79, 80] suggests there is little evidence for the effectiveness of this approach with individuals with IDD. He posits that those studies indicating effectiveness have generally incorporated behavioral techniques and primarily relaxation strategies that may have confounded the effects of purely cognitive aspects of the treatments. Nonetheless, some relaxation strategies, such as guided imagery and hypnoanalgesia, do incorporate simple cognitive exercises that can be effective when learned through instruction and modeling. Some of these may be possible with those with IDD, as they have been used with typically developing children, with some evidence that those under age 12 are most susceptible to the effects of hypnosis and that hypnosis is possible with children as young as 5–6 years [81]. This suggests that there is a possibility that those with IDD who have similar mental age equivalents might be capable of performing some of these techniques with appropriate instruction and guidance, yet this assumption awaits future testing.

The sections below describe the psychological treatment options that may be effective for some with IDD. Similar to pharmacological approaches, these should be personalized to the client. Individuals may have disparate skills that make one specific approach more enjoyable and/or effective than another. It is highly recommended that more than one approach be attempted and that effectiveness be assessed prior to treatment and once proficiency is reached using an appropriate validated pain tool. These techniques may also be used in combination with or as an addition to pharmacological or physical treatments.

Operant Techniques

Operant techniques involve using reinforcement from the environment to change behavior. They are most often used to change overt behaviors and may focus on reducing maladaptive behaviors that increase pain or increasing positive behaviors that reduce pain. For example, a client may complain when required to perform physical exercises, which results in caregivers reducing demands or abbreviating sessions. This could lead to slower recovery or de-conditioning, which can increase pain. In this case, reinforcement of complaining (reduced demands) may need to be removed and reinforcement for performing the desired behavior (exercises) may need to be put in place. Care must be taken when initiating operant techniques that an attempt is not being made to reduce complaints that do reflect underlying pain that has not been detected. Some research suggests that observers may feel those with IDD display exaggerated pain behavior [82]. Although some with IDD may exhibit more intense reactions than expected to pain, this may reflect reduced social inhibition, commonly seen in younger children, or these with poorer coping abilities [83], or appropriate attempts to seek help in coping with pain when they do not have the resources to manage pain independently [84]. Positive reinforcement may also be used to encourage behaviors that may reduce pain such as adherence to medical regimes and physical therapies. As with any behavior modification plan for those with IDD, care must be taken to develop reinforcements and demands that are suited to the individual's capabilities and interests.

Modeling

Those with IDD may need more guidance than NIDD individuals in performing adaptive reactions and responses to pain and in performing activities to reduce pain. Involvement of a parent or a caregiver in activities such as physical therapy, distraction, or relaxation techniques may be necessary to ensure that learning occurs. Modeling should also be used in teaching distraction or relaxation techniques to ensure the client has visual and auditory stimuli to emulate. In some cases, active positioning of the individual into relaxed postures or manual guidance of movements may also be helpful in addition to modeling and successive approximations may be needed to achieve the desired action.

Distraction

Distraction refers to activities aimed at moving an individual's attention away from pain through presentation of other stimuli. It is commonly used during procedural pain with children [85], with some evidence it may be more effective for those who are younger [86], which suggests it may be particularly useful for those with IDD. Distraction is most effective when it actively engages the person with pain. Studies indicate merely watching television or a cartoon do not reduce pain during procedures [87, 88]. Thus, activities such as playing with a toy or a videogame may be more effective than simply listening to a story. Activities can be personalized to the interests of the individual. In the case of chronic or longer lasting pain, several activities may be used interchangeably to avoid boredom and loss of attention to the task. Activities should not include movement that may exacerbate pain. However, distraction with young children frequently combines deep breathing, which can induce relaxation, via activities such as blowing bubbles or toy whirligigs.

Relaxation Techniques

Behavioral relaxation training (BRT): The only report we could locate of relaxation techniques being used for pain in an individual with IDD [89] utilized BRT. An adult with severe IDD, who was experiencing headaches, had a 48% reduction in headache complaints and a 51% reduction in analgesic use at 2 months post-training.

BRT was developed by Poppen [77, 90]. This highly structured training is suitable for individuals with IDD because it incorporates modeling of 10 relaxed postures and requires little verbal control. The success of this technique appears to be due, in part, to that fact that the training provided for individuals with IDD is geared to their level of intellectual functioning. BRT may be appropriate for individuals with some physical limitations. However, some adaptations may be needed if the individual cannot achieve some positions or experiences spasticity. BRT requires that the individual follow very specific instructions. Thus, it may be difficult to use with those who are noncompliant. Because it requires the individual to stay still for periods, it is less suited to those with symptoms of hyperactivity.

Breathing exercises: Breathing exercises, and abdominal or deep breathing in particular, have a long history of use for procedural pain relief for children [91], but are most often combined with other techniques. Only one study has studied breathing exercises in isolation from other relaxation techniques for chronic pain in children [92]. It was less effective than a combination of guided imagery and progressive muscle relaxation for recurrent abdominal pain. Nonetheless, 21% of children had fewer days with pain at 1-month follow-up and 45% by the end of 2 months. Thus, this technique may be an option for people with IDD who are not capable of other techniques. Breathing may be possible even for those with severe physical limitations, but contraindicated if respiratory conditions are present.

Guided imagery/self-hypnosis: The terms "guided imagery" and "self-hypnosis" are often used interchangeably. Guided imagery requires an individual to imagine a safe comfortable place. Hypnoanalgesia is very similar to guided imagery, but differs in that it typically includes suggestion that pain is reduced or removed from the person. Common scripts involve imagining that pain is leaving the body, that the person controls a switch to turn down the pain, or that the pain is replaced by numbness. Self-hypnosis has been shown to reduce abdominal pain [93, 94] and headache [95, 96] in children. Guided imagery has been used for functional abdominal pain in children [97], for postoperative pain in children as young as age 7 years [98], and for recurrent abdominal pain as young as 5 years [99]. These techniques have a natural appeal to those who enjoy "daydreaming" or story-telling. For those with IDD, a coach would be needed to talk the individual through the scenes or changes in pain in most cases, although those functioning at higher levels may be able to learn scripts that they can later use independently after repeated practice with coaching.

Guided imagery and self-hypnosis are suitable even for individuals who have severe physical limitations or who lack voluntary muscle control.

Progressive muscle relaxation: Progressive muscle relaxation (PMR) involves systematically relaxing body parts, sometimes after a brief period of tensing the part. It has been used for pediatric migraine [100], juvenile primary fibromyalgia [102], juvenile rheumatoid arthritis [103], and functional abdominal pain [97]. Cautela and Groden [101] have published the only manual for PMR that addresses use with children with disabilities. PMR has been taught by parents or professionals without extensive formal education in psychology, such as school nurses. PMR is not appropriate for those with severe physical limitations, who have little voluntary control over movement, or for whom movement exacerbates pain. However, it may be more appealing to those with hyperactive tendencies than other relaxation techniques because it involves active movement rather than stillness.

Biofeedback: Biofeedback refers to the use of one of the above techniques or to autogenic training (deliberate reversal of physiological arousal through self-suggestion and awareness of the body) to induce relaxation, combined with physiological feedback to assist in reaching and maintaining a relaxed state [104]. Modern software has led to development of a number of programs that are appealing to children for biofeedback training [105]. Biofeedback has shown efficacy for pediatric headache in many studies on its own or in combination with other psychological techniques [106], as well as for juvenile rheumatoid arthritis [107]. In one study, a reduction in headache pain in children was seen after only one training session [108]. Engel et al. [109] conducted a study of biofeedback with three adults with cerebral palsy who had only mild intellectual impairments and reported mixed results. Although the participants reported some decrease in pain, physiological measures did not correspond. The authors suggest that spasticity during biofeedback lead to disruptive feedback from the equipment and complicated evaluation of the physiological changes. Thus, although biofeedback may be possible for those with IDD, use with individuals with cerebral palsy may be complex. This approach may be effective for clients with IDD who enjoy computers and are able to focus on visual stimuli. In the case of those with IDD, training in simpler methods of relaxation first may be helpful, with the biofeedback component being added as a positive reinforcement. One drawback of this technique is the expense of computer equipment and software.

Use of Psychological Treatments During Acute Versus Chronic/Recurrent Pain

Most psychological techniques can be applied to acute or chronic/recurrent pain, although more evidence is available for acute situations, in part due to the easier logistics in studying pain during these short, scheduled pain events. For procedural pain, difficulties can include the fact that less in vivo practice may be possible if procedures are infrequent. Use of doll play and practice, including modeling, may be necessary to prepare individuals for procedures and repeating practice when procedures are infrequent, such as for yearly immunizations, may improve performance. In chronic/recurrent pain situations, the difficulty may lie in learning the skill in the face of pain if it is ongoing. Pain reduces our ability to learn, so practice during pain-free periods will improve an individual's skill set to be used when pain does occur. Further, many techniques have some immediate pain-reducing effects, especially distraction and relaxation techniques. However, it also appears that regular use of these approaches can lead to reduced chronic/recurrent pain through reducing baseline stress and sympathetic arousal. Thus, regular daily practice is recommended when an individual has ongoing pain. This may require use of positive reinforcement to motivate clients to practice. Scheduling practice at regular times, such as just prior to meals, can also help to maintain adherence. This may also have benefits as relaxation sessions conducted throughout the day may reduce the increase in pain most chronic pain sufferers experience over the day.

A note about psycho-education: A common component of psychological management for pain in NIDD individuals is education about their pain and the treatments that can help it, including procedures that may themselves induce pain. To date, no research has examined the effects of psycho-education regarding pain for individuals with IDD, although many individuals with IDD who have cancer feel they are not provided with information about their disease [110] and those with mild to moderate IDD appear capable of understanding information about their cancer [111]. Drahota and Malcarne [112] compared the illness concepts of 11 children with mild to moderate IDD with two control groups, one matched for chronological age and one matched for developmental level. They found that the children with IDD did not differ from the developmentally matched control group on measures of illness causation, symptom recognition, treatment, or prevention. This suggests that if information is provided at a level appropriate for an individual's developmental level [113], it should be understood. Research indicates that anxiety and fear increase the physical sensation of pain in those with IDD [114], which suggests education and preparation may help reduce pain levels. Research also indicates that having a sense of control reduces pain [115]. Thus, providing education and offering individuals choices may also help during pain. This may be as simple as a choice as to which arm a needle is inserted or which pill is taken first. Unfortunately those with IDD are often not informed about their pain, their treatments, or how to reduce their pain, meaning that they often have more fear and anxiety and may feel helpless in the face of pain.

Implementing Pain Assessment and Management in Clinical Practice

Our knowledge about pain in individuals with IDD has grown over the past 20 years, but remains incomplete. Nonetheless, all indications are that this population suffers more pain than those without IDD and that their pain is undermanaged. This has the potential to affect the individual, causing not only suffering but also reduced function [116] and maladaptive behavior [6, 20, 117]. Pain is also a major cause of concern for parents and caregivers [24], a source of frustration for health-care professionals [27], and medical problems that cause pain are a common reason for admission to hospital [118], resulting in an increased burden on those close to the person with IDD and society as a whole.

Although the literature regarding this topic is scarce, there is information to guide clinical practice. Appropriate assessment tools should be used and pain should be monitored regularly. This may require assistance from caregivers in collecting pain ratings at home because those with IDD may be inhibited during medical visits and not show obvious signs of pain. Pain assessment tools should be used in conjunction with clinical observation and proxy reports regarding function and maladaptive behavior such as self-injury or aggression. Because those with IDD may have multiple sources of pain, detailed records of pain ratings in relation to possible pain triggers may be necessary to distinguish the previous pain causality from the current source of pain in question. Because some of these clients may not be independent, pain should be assessed within a broad context, taking into account the individual, the environment, and ongoing development and experience which can alter pain perception and behavior [119]. Frameworks such as the International Classification of Functioning, Disability and Health may be helpful in doing this [120].

Conclusions

Pain is a subjective and a complex phenomenon which is hard to evaluate especially in populations with limited communication abilities such as individuals with IDD. Research suggests that even when pain is assessed in those with IDD, it may be undertreated relative to those without IDD. This suggests that professional's biases, concerns over the appropriateness of treatments, and lack of self-efficacy regarding implementation may be at play. To date, most experts in this area suggest that almost all treatments offered for pain to those without IDD can be used for the individual with IDD if delivered in a developmentally appropriate manner or adapted for their physical limitations, health status, current medication consumption, and concurrent health conditions. The complexity and issues in delivering pain care do not differ substantially from those regarding other vulnerable populations such as infants and the elderly. Multidisciplinary care is highly recommended for this group, both to increase the likelihood of synergistic effects of multiple therapies and to provide support for professionals. Pain relief for this group should be a priority and must be attempted as part of a full health management program. Individuals with IDD suffer the burden of intellectual and, frequently, physical limitations. Pain should not be an additional burden in their efforts to reach their full potential.

References

1. International Association for the Study of Pain – IASP. IASP pain terminology. Accessed 2010 Aug 14. URL: http://www.iasp-pain.org/AM/Template.cfm?Section=Pain_Defi... isplay.cfm&ContentID=1728

2. Latham J, Davis BD. The socioeconomic impact of chronic pain. Disabil Rehabil. 1994;16 (1):39–44.
3. Cousins MJ, Brennan F, Carr DB. Pain relief: a universal human right. Pain. 2004;112 (1–2):1–4.
4. Stallard P, Williams L, Lenton S, Velleman R. Pain in cognitively impaired, non-communicating children. Arch Dis Child. 2001;85 (6):460–62.
5. van Schrojenstein Lantman-De Valk HM, Metsemakers JF, Haveman MJ, Crebolder HF. Health problems in people with intellectual disability in general practice: a comparative study. Fam Pract. 2000;17 (5):405–07.
6. Carr EG, Owen-Deschryver JS. Physical illness, pain, and problem behavior in minimally verbal people with developmental disabilities. J Autism Dev Disord. 2007;37 (3):413–24.
7. Breau LM, Camfield CS, McGrath PJ, Finley GA. The incidence of pain in children with severe cognitive impairments. Arch Pediatr Adolesc Med. 2003;157 (12):1219–26.
8. Reid BC, Chenette R, Macek MD. Prevalence and predictors of untreated caries and oral pain among Special Olympic athletes. Spec Care Dentist. 2003;23 (4):139–42.
9. Regnard C, Mathews D, Gibson L, Clarke C. Difficulties in identifying distress and its causes in people with severe communication problems. Int J Palliat Nurs. 2003;9 (4):173–76.
10. Schwartz L, Engel JM, Jensen MP. Pain in persons with cerebral palsy. Arch Phys Med Rehabil. 1999;80 (10):1243–46.
11. LaChapelle DL, Hadjistavropoulos T, Craig KD. Pain measurement in persons with intellectual disabilities. Clin J Pain. 1999;15:13–23.
12. Malviya S, Voepel-Lewis T, Tait AR, et al. Pain management in children with and without cognitive impairment following spine fusion surgery. Paediatr Anaesth. 2001;11:453–58.
13. Oberlander TF, O'Donnell ME, Montgomery CJ. Pain in children with significant neurological impairment. J Dev Behav Pediatr. 1999;20:235–43.
14. Breau LM, Camfield CS, McGrath PJ, Finley GA. Risk factors for pain in children with severe cognitive impairments. Dev Med Child Neurol. 2004;46:364–71.
15. Mafrica F, Schifilliti D, Fodale V. Pain in Down's syndrome. ScientificWorldJournal. 2006;6:140–47.
16. McGrath PJ, Rosmus C, Camfield C, et al. Behaviours caregivers use to determine pain in non-verbal, cognitively impaired individuals. Dev Med Child Neurol. 1998;40:340–43.
17. De Lissovoy V. Head banging in early childhood. Child Dev. 1962;33:43–56.
18. Hart H, Bax M, Jenkins S. Health and behaviour in preschool children. Child Care Health Dev. 1984;10:1–16.
19. Clements J. I can't explain…"Challenging behaviour." Towards a shared conceptual framework. Clin Psychol Forum. 1992;39:29–37.
20. Bosch J, Van Dyke DC, Smith SM, Poulton S. Role of medical conditions in the exacerbation of self-injurious behavior: an exploratory study. Ment Retard. 1997;35:124–30.
21. Bodfish JW, Harper VN, Deacon JR, Symons FJ. Identifying and measuring pain in persons with developmental disabilities: a manual for the pain and discomfort scale. Morganton, NC: Western Carolina Center; 2001.
22. Mason J, Scior K. Diagnostic overshadowing amongst clinicians working with people with intellectual disabilities in the UK. J Appl Res Intellect Disabil. 2004;17:75–90.
23. Turk DC, Melzack R, editors. Handbook of pain assessment. 2nd ed. New York, NY: Guilford; 2001.
24. Carter B, McArthur E, Cunliffe M. Dealing with uncertainty: parental assessment of pain in their children with profound special needs. J Adv Nurs. 2002;38:449–57.
25. Donovan J. Learning disability nurses' experiences of being with clients who may be in pain. J Adv Nurs. 2002;38:458–66.
26. Fanurik D, Koh JL, Schmitz ML, et al. Pain assessment and treatment in children with cognitive impairment: a survey of nurses' and physicians' beliefs. Clin J Pain. 1999;15:304–12.
27. Oberlander TF, O'Donnell ME. Beliefs about pain among professionals working with children with significant neurologic impairment. Dev Med Child Neurol. 2001;43:138–40.

28. Ekman P, Friesen WV. Investigator's guide to the facial action coding system. Palo Alto, CA: Consult Psychol Press; 1978.

29. Craig KD, Grunau RVE. Judgement of pain in newborns: facial activity and cry as determinants. Can J Behav Sci. 1988;20:442–51.

30. Craig KD, Hyde SA, Patrick CJ. Genuine, suppressed and faked facial behavior during exacerbation of chronic low back pain. Pain. 1991;46:161–71.

31. Craig KD. The facial expression of pain. In: Turk DC, Melzack R, editors. Handbook of pain assessment. New York, NY: Guilford; 1992. pp. 257–76.

32. Craig KD, Korol CT, Pillai RR. Challenges of judging pain in vulnerable infants. Clin Perinatol. 2002;29:445–57.

33. LeResche L, Dworkin SF. Facial expression accompanying pain. Soc Sci Med. 1984;19:1325–30.

34. Prkachin KM, Berzins S, Mercer SR. Encoding and decoding of pain expressions: a judgement study. Pain. 1994;58:253–59.

35. Hadjistavropoulos T, Craig KD, Martin N. Towards a research outcome measure of pain in frail elderly in chronic care. Pain Clinician. 1997;10:71–90.

36. Hurley BAC, Volier BJ, Harnahan PA. Assessment of discomfort in advanced Alzheimer patients. Res Nurs Health. 1992;15:369–77.

37. Chambers CT, Cassidy KL, McGrath PJ, et al. Child facial coding system: a manual. Halifax: Dalhousie University, University British Columbia; 1996.

38. Breau LM, Finley GA, Camfield CS, McGrath PJ. Facial expression of pain in children with intellectual disabilities following surgery. J Pain Manage. 2009;2:51–62.

39. Giusiano B, Jimeno MT, Collignon P, Chau Y. Utilization of a neural network in the elaboration of an evaluation scale for pain in cerebral palsy. Methods Inf Med. 1995;34: 498–502.

40. Collignon P, Giusiano B, Boutin AM, Combes JC. Utilisation d'une echelle d'heteroevaluation de la douleur chez le sujet severement polyhandicape. Doul et Analg. 1997;10:27–32 [French].

41. Collignon P, Giusiano B. Validation of a pain evaluation scale for patients with severe cerebral palsy. Eur J Pain. 2001;5:433–42.

42. Breau LM, McGrath PJ, Camfield C, et al. Preliminary validation of an observational pain checklist for persons with cognitive impairments and inability to communicate verbally. Dev Med Child Neurol. 2000;42:609–16.

43. Breau LM, Finley GA, McGrath PJ, Camfield CS. Validation of the Non-communicating Children's Pain Checklist-Postoperative Version. Anesthesiology. 2002a;96:528–35.

44. Breau LM, McGrath PJ, Camfield CS, Finley GA. Psychometric properties of the non-communicating children's pain checklist-revised. Pain. 2002b;99:349–57.

45. Breau LM, Camfield C, Camfield P. Development and initial validation of the Batten's Observational Pain Scale. J Pain Manage, in press.

46. Burkitt C, Breau LM, Salsman S, et al. Pilot Study of the Feasibility of the Non-Communicating Children's Pain Checklist Revised for Pain Assessment for Adults with Intellectual Disabilities. J Pain Manage. 2009;2:37–49.

47. Stallard P, Williams L, Velleman R, et al. The development and evaluation of the pain indicator for communicately impaired children (PICIC). Pain. 2002;1–2:149.

48. Hunt A, Goldman A, Seers K, et al. Clinical validation of the paediatric pain profile. Dev Med Child Neurol. 2004;46:9–18.

49. Phan A, Edwards CL, Robinson EL. The assessment of pain and discomfort in individuals with mental retardation. Res Dev Disabil. 2005;26 5:433–39.

50. Defrin R, Lotan M, Pick CG. The evaluation of acute pain in individuals with cognitive impairment: a differential effect of the level of impairment. Pain. 2006;124:312–20.

51. Lotan M, Ljunggren EA, Johnsen TB, et al. A modified version of the non-communicating children pain checklist-revised, adapted to adults with intellectual and developmental disabilities: sensitivity to pain and internal consistency. J Pain. 2009;10:398–407.

52. Lotan M, Moe-Nilssen R, Ljunggren AE, Strand LI. Reliability of the Non-communicating Adult Pain Checklist (NCAPC) assessed by different groups of healthworkers. Res Dev Disabil, 2009;30:735–45.
53. Lotan M, Moe-Nilssen R, Ljunggren AE, Strand LI. Measurement properties of the Non-communicating Adult Pain Checklist (NCAPC): a pain scale for adults with Intellectual and Developmental Disabilities, scored in a clinical setting. Res Dev Disabil. 2010;31:367–75.
54. Lotan M, Ljunggren AE, Strand LI, Kvale A. Understanding pain behavior in individuals with intellectual and developmental disabilities, through construction of a model. Pain, in press.
55. Seers K, Breau LM, Closs J, et al. Core Curriculum for Professional Education in Pain. 3rd ed. Seattle, WA: Int Assoc Stud Pain; 2005.
56. Reynell JK. Post-operative disturbances observed in children with cerebral palsy. Dev Med Child Neurol. 1965;7:360–76.
57. Engel JM, Kartin D, Jensen MP. Pain treatment in persons with cerebral palsy: frequency and helpfulness. Am J Phys Med Rehabil. 2002;81:291–96.
58. Hadden KL, von Baeyer CL. Global and Specific Behavioral Measures of Pain in Children with Cerebral Palsy. Clin J Pain. 2005;21:140–46.
59. Miller AC, Johann-Murphy M, Pit-ten Cate IM. Pain, anxiety, and cooperativeness in children with cerebral palsy after rhizotomy: changes throughout rehabilitation. J Pediatr Psychol. 1997;22:689–705.
60. Rakel B, Barr JO. Physical modalities in chronic pain management. Nurs Clin North Am. 2003;38:477–94.
61. American Society of Anesthesiologists Task Force on Chronic Pain Management and the American Society of Regional Anesthesia and Pain Medicine. Practice guidelines for chronic pain management: an updated report by the American Society of Anesthesiologists Task Force on Chronic Pain Management and the American Society of Regional Anesthesia and Pain Medicine. Anesthesiology. 2010;112:810–33.
62. Schofield P. The effects of Snoezelen on chronic pain. Nurs Stand. 2000;15:33–4.
63. Schofield P. Evaluating snoezelen for relaxation within chronic pain management. Br J Nurs. 2002;11:812–21.
64. Koh JL, Fanurik D, Harrison RD, et al. Analgesia following surgery in children with and without cognitive impairment. Pain. 2004;111:239–44.
65. Long LS, Ved S, Koh JL. Intraoperative opioid dosing in children with and without cerebral palsy. Paediatr Anaesth. 2009;19:513–20.
66. Yaster M, Kost-Byerly S, Maxwell LG. Opioid agonists and antagonists. In: Schechter NL, Berde CB, Yaster M, editors. Pain in infants, children, and adolescents. 2nd ed. Philadelphia, PA: Lippincott Williams Wilkins; 2003. pp. 181–224.
67. Desparmet JP, Hardart RA, Yaster M. Central blocks in children and adolescents. In: Schechter NL, Berde CB, Yaster M, editors. Pain in infants, children, and adolescents. 2nd ed. Philadelphia, PA: Lippincott Williams Wilkins; 2003. pp. 339–62.
68. Licht E, Siegler EL, Reid MC. Can the cognitively impaired safely use patient-controlled analgesia? J Opioid Manag. 2009;5:307–12.
69. Voepel-Lewis T, Marinkovic A, Kostrzewa A, et al. The prevalence of and risk factors for adverse events in children receiving patient-controlled analgesia by proxy or patient-controlled analgesia after surgery. Anesth Analg. 2008;107:70–75.
70. Brenn BR, Brislin RP, Rose JB. Epidural analgesia in children with cerebral palsy. Can J Anaesth. 1998;45:1156–61.
71. Goldman A, Frager G, Pomietto M. Pain and palliative care. In: Schechter NL, Berde CB, Yaster M, editors. Pain in infants, children, and adolescents, second ed. Philadelphia, PA: Lippincott Williams Wilkins; 2003. pp. 539–62.
72. Senaran H, Holden C, Dabney KW, Miller F. Anterior knee pain in children with cerebral palsy. J Pediatr Orthop. 2007;27:12–16.
73. Symons FJ, Rivard PF, Nugent AC, Tervo RC. Parent evaluation of spasticity treatment in cerebral palsy using botulinum toxin type A. Arch Phys Med Rehabil. 2006;87:1658–60.

74. Lundy CT, Doherty GM, Fairhurst CB. Botulinum toxin type A injections can be an effective treatment for pain in children with hip spasms and cerebral palsy. Dev Med Child Neurol. 2009;51:705–10.
75. Krane EJ, Leong MS, Golianu B, Leong YY. Treatment of pain with nonconventional analgesics. In: Schechter NL, Berde CB, Yaster M, editors. Pain in infants, children, and adolescents. 2nd ed. Philadelphia, PA: Lippincott Williams Wilkins; 2003. pp. 225–40.
76. Becker N, Sjogren P, Bech P, et al. Treatment outcome of chronic non-malignant pain patients managed in a Danish multidisciplinary pain centre compared to general practice: a randomised controlled trial. Pain. 2000;84:203–11.
77. Poppen R. Behavioral relaxation training and assessment. 2nd ed. Thousand Oaks, CA: Sage; 1998.
78. Vlaeyen JW, Morley S. Cognitive-behavioral treatments for chronic pain: what works for whom? Clin J Pain. 2005;21:1–8.
79. Sturmey P. Cognitive therapy with people with intellectual disabilities: a selective review and critique. Clin Psychol Psychother. 2004;11:222–32.
80. Sturmey P. Against psychotherapy with people who have mental retardation. Ment Retard. 2005;43:55–57.
81. Olness KN, Kohen DP. Hypnosis and hypnotherapy with children. 3rd ed. New York, NY: Guilford; 1996.
82. Breau LM, MacLaren J, McGrath PJ, et al. Caregivers' beliefs regarding pain in children with cognitive impairment: relation between pain sensation and reaction increases with severity of impairment. Clin J Pain. 2003;19:335–44.
83. Burkitt C, Breau LM, Zabalia M Stratégies de faire face à la douleur chez des enfants atteints de déficience intellectuelle: une approche qualitative par l'entretien. Douleurs: Évaluation, Diagnostic, Traitement 9[S4], 50. 2008 [French].
84. Burkitt C, Breau LM, Zabalia M Evaluation parentale des stratégies de faire-face à la douleur des enfants et adolescents atteints de déficience intellectuelle. Douleurs: Évaluation, Diagnostic, Traitement 9[S4], 50. 2008 [French].
85. Cohen LL. Behavioral approaches to anxiety and pain management for pediatric venous access. Pediatrics. 2008;122 Suppl 3:S134–S39.
86. Piira T, Hayes B, Goodenough B, von Baeyer CL. Effects of attentional direction, age, and coping style on cold-pressor pain in children. Behav Res Ther. 2006;44:835–48.
87. Cassidy KL, Reid GJ, McGrath PJ, et al. Watch needle, watch TV: audiovisual distraction in preschool immunization. Pain Med. 2002;3:108–18.
88. Landolt MA, Marti D, Widmer J, Meuli M. Does cartoon movie distraction decrease burned children's pain behavior? J Burn Care Rehabil. 2002;23:61–65.
89. Michultka DM, Poppen RL, Blanchard EB. Relaxation training as a treatment for chronic headaches in an individual having severe developmental disabilities. Biofeedback Self Regul. 1988;13:257–66.
90. Schilling DJ, Poppen R. Behavioral relaxation training and assessment. J Behav Ther Exp Psychiatry. 1983;14:99–107.
91. Powers SW. Empirically supported treatments in pediatric psychology: procedure-related pain. J Pediatr Psychol. 1999;24:131–45.
92. Weydert JA, Shapiro DE, Acra SA, et al. Evaluation of guided imagery as treatment for recurrent abdominal pain in children: a randomized controlled trial. BMC Pediatr. 2006;6:29.
93. Anbar RD. Self-hypnosis for the treatment of functional abdominal pain in childhood. Clin Pediatr (Phila). 2001;40:447–51.
94. Sokel B, Devane S, Bentovim A. Getting better with honor: individualized relaxation/self-hypnosis techniques for control of recalcitrant abdominal pain in children. Fam Systems Med. 1991;9:83–91.
95. Engel JM. Relaxation training in treating recurrent non-malignant pediatric headaches. Phys Occup Ther Pediatr. 1990;10:47–71.
96. McGrath PJ, Humphreys P, Goodman JT, et al. Relaxation prophylaxis for childhood migraine: a randomized placebo-controlled trial. Dev Med Child Neurol. 1988;30:626–31.

97. Youssef NN, Rosh JR, Loughran M, et al. Treatment of functional abdominal pain in childhood with cognitive behavioral strategies. J Pediatr Gastroenterol Nutr. 2004;39:192–96.
98. Huth MM, Broome ME, Good M. Imagery reduces children's post-operative pain. Pain. 2004;110:439–48.
99. Ball TM, Shapiro DE, Monheim CJ, Weydert JA. A pilot study of the use of guided imagery for the treatment of recurrent abdominal pain in children. Clin Pediatr (Phila). 2003;42:527–32.
100. Fichtel A, Larsson B. Relaxation treatment administered by school nurses to adolescents with recurrent headaches. Headache. 2004;44:545–54.
101. Cautela JR, Groden J. Relaxation: a comprehensive manual for adults, children, and children with special needs. Champaign, IL: Research Press Company; 1978.
102. Walco GA, Ilowite NT. Cognitive-behavioral intervention for juvenile primary fibromyalgia syndrome. J Rheumatol. 1992;19:1617–19.
103. Walco GA, Varni JW, Ilowite NT. Cognitive-behavioral pain management in children with juvenile rheumatoid arthritis. Pediatrics. 1992;89:1075–79.
104. Critchley HD, Melmed RN, Featherstone E, et al. Volitional control of autonomic arousal: a functional magnetic resonance study. Neuroimage. 2002;16:909–19.
105. Schwarz MS, Andrasik F. Biofeedback: a practitioner's guide. 3rd ed. New York: Guilford; 2003.
106. Holden EW, Deichmann MM, Levy JD. Empirically supported treatments in pediatric psychology: recurrent pediatric headache. J Pediatr Psychol. 1999;24:91–109.
107. Lavigne JV, Ross CK, Berry SL, et al. Evaluation of a psychological treatment package for treating pain in juvenile rheumatoid arthritis. Arthritis Care Res. 1992;5:101–10.
108. Powers SW, Mitchell MJ, Byars KC, et al. A pilot study of one-session biofeedback training in pediatric headache. Neurology. 2001;56:133.
109. Engel JM, Jensen MP, Schwartz L. Outcome of biofeedback-assisted relaxation for pain in adults with cerebral palsy: preliminary findings. Appl Psychophysiol Biofeedback. 2004;29:135–40.
110. Tuffrey-Wijne I, Bernal J, Jones A, et al. People with intellectual disabilities and their need for cancer information. Eur J Oncol Nurs. 2006;10:106–16.
111. Tuffrey-Wijne I, Bernal J, Hollins S. Disclosure and understanding of cancer diagnosis and prognosis for people with intellectual disabilities: findings from an ethnographic study. Eur J Oncol Nurs. 2010;14:224–30.
112. Drahota A, Malcarne VL. Concepts of illness in children: a comparison between children with and without intellectual disability. Intellect Dev Disabil. 2008;46:44–53.
113. Iacono T, Johnson H. Patients with disabilities and complex communication needs. The GP consultation. Aust Fam Physician. 2004;33:585–89.
114. Benini F, Trapanotto M, Gobber D, et al. Evaluating pain induced by venipuncture in pediatric patients with developmental delay. Clin J Pain. 2004;20:156–63.
115. Turk DC, Okifuji A. Psychological factors in chronic pain: evolution and revolution. J Consult Clin Psychol. 2002;70:678–90.
116. Breau LM, Camfield CS, McGrath PJ, Finley GA. Pain's impact on adaptive functioning. J Intellect Disabil Res. 2007;51:125–34.
117. Breau LM, Camfield CS, Symons FJ, et al. Relation between pain and self-injurious behavior in nonverbal children with severe cognitive impairments. J Pediatr. 2003;142:498–503.
118. Mahon M, Kibirige MS. Patterns of admissions for children with special needs to the paediatric assessment unit. Arch Dis Child. 2004;89:165–69.
119. Breau LM. A bio-ecological approach to pediatric pain assessment. J Pain Manage. 2008;1:247–55.
120. O'Donnell ME. Using the WHO's International Classification of Functioning, Disability and Health: a framework in the management of chronic pain in children and youth with developmental disabilities. In: Oberlander TF, Symons FJ, editors. Pain in children and adults with developmental disabilities. Baltimore, MD: Paul H Brooks; 2006. pp. 139–48.

Chapter 18
Vision Impairment

Katherine Bergwerk

Abstract Neurodevelopmental disorders may occur in association with alterations in all aspects of the visual system. These vision issues can then have severe detrimental effects on the overall development of the child with decreased social emotional and communication skills in addition to the educational impact. While an all encompassing review of vision impairment in children with neurodevelopmental disabilities is daunting in scope, the varied causes of decreased vision in children with neurodevelopmental disabilities are presented. Although the difficulties in screening and evaluating these patients are obvious, nevertheless the need to do so is crucial to their well-being. New tools for assessment of vision which are easy and effective need to be developed for use in this population.

Introduction

Vision impairment of some type is common in the general pediatric population and is one of the more prominent reasons for referral to a health clinic. More specifically, refractive errors may be noted in up to 20% of the pediatric population, and strabismus [1] and amblyopia occur in approximately 2–5% in US children or have a prevalence of 10 million children [2]. These issues can result in social, behavioral, and educational difficulties, all of which can affect development. These problems tend to be more prevalent in the intellectually impaired population, both in adults [3] and in children, although exact statistics depends on the population studied. A recent study comparing children with intellectual disability to controls demonstrated that 77% of children with ID (intellectual disability) had ocular findings as compared to 42.4% of the age-matched control group. These anomalies consisted primarily of refractive errors such as hyperopia and astigmatism, as well as

K. Bergwerk (✉)
Private Prictice, Nof Ayalon, IL-99785 Israel
e-mail: bergwerk@bezeqint.net

strabismus and nystagmus. These findings were increased in accordance with the level of ID [4]. Severe visual impairment or blindness occurs at an incidence of approximately 2.5/100,000 children, with increased incidence in the first year of life and in premature infants or infants with medical comorbidities [5].

Children in general, and children with intellectual disabilities (ID) or developmental issues may not realize that their vision is abnormal, and very few children verbalize these concerns. Therefore the responsibility for the identification of patients with vision issues falls on the shoulders of the parents, caregivers, and health professionals. To this end, screening programs for school-age children to elucidate and eliminate causes of vision loss, such as amblyopia, have existed for many years [6].

In the last few years, the National Institutes of Health and other vision care organizations have tried to encourage pediatricians and primary care providers to screen children at earlier intervals for treatable causes of vision impairment, as previous studies have shown that pediatricians may not routinely test children prior to their starting school at age 5–6 years [7].

While it is more difficult to examine younger children, the benefits of early identification of vision abnormalities and their treatment are clear. These issues are more pressing in children with special needs, who may have multiple medical and educational issues. Even intellectually disabled adults who have a high incidence of visual problems are frequently unable to communicate their visual difficulties. In a study of adults with moderate to profound ID evaluated for vision impairment, 71% could perform an assessment of visual acuity using a picture chart, while methods of preferential looking were used for those unable to participate with the charts. This study found that moderate vision impairment was encountered in 10.8% of patients, severe low vision in 1.2%, and blindness in 3.8%. Over 50% had uncorrected refractive states. This demonstrated that patients with ID can generally complete some aspect of vision assessment and have a high prevalence of treatable visual impairment. Structured guidelines for screening and follow-up with optometric and ophthalmic professionals are essential to provide needed care to this community [8].

There are further impediments in the evaluation of patients with ID and in their treatment as well, due to issues such as accessibility or physical limitations, which cause difficulty in performing an evaluation.

Furthermore, the need definitely exists for improved screening tools for testing and therapy in this special needs population. This is of greater importance now, as lifespan is increasing in general and for persons with ID as well, such as Down syndrome. Down syndrome is one of the more common causes of neurodevelopmental disabilities and will be covered in greater depth later in this chapter. Furthermore, advances in techniques of in vitro fertilization and neonatology have led to the survival of younger, smaller babies who may be born in or prior to the seventh month of gestation. These babies also tend to have a significantly higher incidence of neurologic, vision, and other sensory issues which require identification and treatment. Issues such as cortical visual impairment are prominent in this population, as will be described later in the chapter.

Moreover as persons with ID are increasingly integrated into schools and workplaces and medical advances have enabled them to live longer and with greater quality of life, assisting them to maximize their potential is of the greatest importance, despite the challenges.

Categorization of Visual Impairment

There are varying definitions of the term blind and low vision. The World Health Organization (WHO) criteria for blindness and low vision are generally accepted parameters. Occasionally different local definitions are used, such as the North American definitions. According to the WHO, blindness is characterized by best corrected vision worse than 20/400 (3/60) in the better eye, or of a field of vision less than 10° [9]. These correspond to the ICD-10 classification. The North American system classifies legal blindness as best corrected vision in the better eye worse than 20/400 (6/60) or a visual field of less than 20°. The normal visual field is approximately 180°.

Low vision can be classified into severe and moderate vision impairment. Severe vision impairment is defined as best corrected vision worse than 6/60 or 20/200 feet, but better than 20/400. The definition of moderate visual impairment is best corrected vision better than 6/60 or 20/200, but less than 6/18 or 20/60.

There are numerous etiologies for impaired vision in patients with neurodevelopmental disorders and multiple methods of classification of visual impairment.

Anatomic or Descriptive Classification

Overall, uncorrected refractive errors are the most common cause of vision impairment worldwide. Approximately 12 million children aged 5–15 years worldwide have impaired vision due to refractive disorders, which are correctable with spectacles [10]. In addition to refractive errors, which are generally correctable with spectacles or vision aids, there are numerous causes of vision impairment depending on which aspect of the eye is affected [5].

The first ocular structure to encounter an image or light is the cornea. Abnormalities of the cornea, such as keratoconus found in people with Down syndrome, can cause distortion of vision. However, anomalies of the lens, such as congenital cataracts or age-related cataracts, are the most common cause of decreased vision worldwide. Glaucoma in which increased intraocular pressure causes changes in the optic nerve and thereby affects the visual field used to be a very common cause of vision loss in the middle aged and elderly populations. Now with increased screening and earlier treatment with more successful regimens, glaucoma is no longer a primary cause of vision loss in the developed world. This demonstrates the efficacy of screening programs in early detection and treatment, in the general adult population. Abnormalities of the cornea, lens, and glaucoma are areas where treatment is generally efficacious.

Retinal abnormalities such as macular degeneration account for a significant amount of vision loss worldwide especially in the elderly, while infections or dystrophies affecting the retina are a cause of vision loss in children. Children with extreme prematurity suffer from retinopathy of prematurity (ROP) in which changes in oxygen and vascular supply compromise the development of the retinal blood vessels. This can lead to distortion and even detachment of the retina. While advances have been made in the treatment of the "wet" type of macular degeneration, there is no current medical treatment available for dry macular degeneration. Retinopathy of prematurity is treated with laser therapy or surgically if there is evidence of detachments. These complicated procedures still have not been perfected and patients who have these levels of alterations to the retina often do not tend to recover full vision. Therefore stringent screening protocols exist in the neonatal setting to screen for ROP and to treat at the earliest signs of onset so that deterioration to the level of retinal detachment does not occur.

Although effective treatments for reduction of scarring or severe detachment of the retina do not yet prevail and are a source of frustration for both physicians and patients alike, nevertheless early detection of retinal abnormalities is still advised. This enables more effective counseling and allows patients to maintain more independence and a better quality of life.

Intracranial, neurologic, or higher visual pathway disorders are a complex entity. Any severe insult along the visual pathway, such as tumors or cortical visual impairment due to hypoxia, can cause impairment of vision.

An example of a descriptive classification summarizing some of the causes of decreased vision in children is presented in Table 18.1. The causes of decreased vision in children access the world vary according to region and socioeconomic status which determines availability of medical care. Hereditary retinal diseases are found throughout the world, whereas retinopathy of prematurity is only found in developed countries who have high levels of neonatal care. In contrast, vision loss due to corneal scarring is more prominent in less developed countries [11]. Simulations of the effects of myopia, cataract, glaucoma, and retinitis pigmentosa on the vision of child are presented in Fig. 18.1.

Classification According to Severity

Vision impairment can be defined according to severity as described above. Refractive errors if treated early and adequately generally result in good vision. Alternatively high myopia, hyperopia, or astigmatism which is left uncorrected can also be a cause of visual impairment.

Structural lesions in any part of the visual system described above (cornea, lens, vitreous, retina, or optic nerve) can result in low vision or blindness. Partial vision defects such as a visual field defect due to glaucoma, a lack of central vision due to macular degeneration or tunnel vision due to retinitis pigmentosa can constrict

Table 18.1 Common causes of visual impairment or blindness in children

Congenital
- Ocular
  - Optic nerve: hypoplasia/aplasia, morning glory disc, coloboma of the optic nerve
  - Lens: cataract, persistent primary vitreous
  - Congenital glaucoma
  - Anterior segment anomalies
  - Microphthalmia/anophthalmia

Complications of retinopathy of prematurity, including retinal detachment
Neurologic/neurodegenerative disease
- Cortical visual impairment
- Systemic: storage diseases, hydrocephalus or microcephaly, demyelinating diseases, phakomatoses
- Ocular
  - Retinal degenerative diseases, e.g., retinitis pigmentosa and Leber's congenital amaurosis
  - Optic atrophy

Tumors: ocular, neurologic, metastatic
Infectious/inflammatory disorders
- Systemic: encephalitis due to prenatal infection, meningitis
- Ocular: keratitis, trachoma, chorioretinitis, endophthalmitis, optic neuritis

Vascular disorders: retinal artery occlusions, arteriovenous malformations, collagen vascular diseases
Shaken baby syndrome, contusion of optic nerves or avulsion, retinal detachment, cerebral hemorrhage

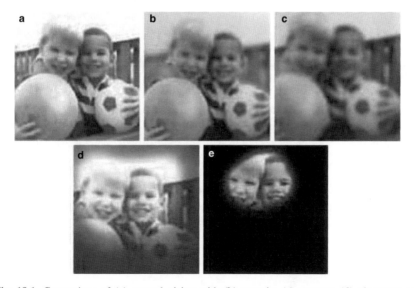

Fig. 18.1 Comparison of (**a**) normal vision with (**b**) myopia, (**c**) cataract, (**d**) glaucoma, and (**e**) retinitis pigmentosa. Photographs courtesy of National Eye Institute, National Institutes of Health

a patient's visual field and cause impairment. Vision can also be affected in different situations, such as syndromes which include impaired night vision, where the patient can have adequate function in normal daytime lighting but cannot navigate without assistance in low lighting or at night. Some patients are impaired by very poor contrast or by severe light sensitivity or deficient color vision. In children with severe visual impairment, approximately 70% have additional handicaps including 10% with dual sensory issues of hearing and vision impairment [12].

Classification According to Etiology

Vision impairment may be classified by etiology as well, such as infectious, developmental, and metabolic, or by location: intraocular, periocular, orbital, or intracranial neurologic. Causes of vision can be either static or progressive degenerative, which has impact on prognosis.

Causes of Vision Impairment Can Be Classified as to Onset

Prenatal causes of vision impairment include genetic disorders, with autosomal recessive being the most common type. Perinatal causes include complications of prematurity, infectious etiologies, and hypoxia or ischemia. Postnatal causes of vision impairment in children are frequently due to trauma but may include disorders of the central nervous system, infections, tumors, or neurodegenerative disease, or complications of medical treatment for systemic diseases. Again, these problems all occur in the general population but occur in greater frequency in persons with other anomalies including ID.

Causes of visual impairment in adults differ significantly from the causes of visual impairment in children, with cataract being the most prominent cause worldwide. Age-related macular degeneration is a most significant cause in the elderly, while diabetic retinopathy, trauma, and glaucoma tend to be found in younger adults. Vision loss due to ocular trauma is more common in young males than in young female adults. Vision loss may be due to complications of systemic diseases, most notably diabetic retinopathy. In addition, tumors are known to metastasize to the eye and its adnexa.

In summary, there are myriad causes of vision loss which differ in accordance with the age of the patient. Therefore the age and underlying systemic medical status of the patient with intellectual disability must be considered.

Examination

There are many aspects of the ocular examination and the assessment of vision (see Table 18.2). Examination techniques must be tailored to the age and level of ability of a person with ID. In addition, developmental milestones dictate segments

Table 18.2   Clinical Examination Techniques

1. History
2. Observation

Strabismus evaluation
1. Bruckner reflex: gross evaluation of red reflex, allows comparison of media opacities, strabismus, and significant refractive errors
2. Hirschberg reflex: tests ocular alignment for strabismus
3. Motility evaluation: evaluates integrity or symmetry of extra-ocular movements
4. Cover tests: for ocular alignment and ocular preference
5. Stereopsis test (Titmus or Randot types) of depth perception to evaluate degree of strabismus

Visual acuity
1. Reaction to light
2. Fix/follow toys, objects, or faces
3. Preferential looking using Teller Acuity Cards with contrasting black and white stripes of varying gradation
4. Picture/preliterate charts: Tumbling E, Allen Kindergarten chart
5. Matching tests: HOTV or Lea symbols; do not require verbal responses
6. Letter charts: Snellen letters or numbers, ETDRS

Ophthalmoscopy
1. Direct ophthalmoscope
2. Slit lamp examination
3. Dilated fundus examination

Other
Photoscreening methods

of the examination, as described in Table 18.3. In standard examination settings, a pediatric examination differs significantly from an adult examination, and this again is true in persons with ID. Particularly in the examination of this subgroup of patients, the examiner must be flexible and attentive to the special needs of the

Table 18.3   Milestones in development of vision

Age	Behavior	Approximate vision
Preterm (32 weeks)	Reacts to bright light	
	Pupils react	
Birth	Occasional fixation but poor following	20/400
	May have intermittent strabismus	
6 weeks	Can fixate on face; social smile	20/100–200
3–4 months	Follows objects well, eyes should be generally aligned	
6 months	Normal ocular alignment	20/40–20/150
1 year	Normal visual fields	
	Congenital strabismus best treated by this time	20/20–20/60
1–6 years	Hyperopic refraction most common	
6–12 years	Myopic refractive status ensues	20/20
Age 10–12	End of risk period for amblyopia	
	due to end of neuronal plasticity	

child. It is almost always possible to complete most aspects of an examination, but occasionally, due to patient cooperation, or other issues such as intermittent findings in strabismus, more than one visit may be necessary to gain a total understanding of the patient's issues. Rarely but especially in some patients with severe behavioral issues which limit cooperation, examinations of the ocular structures and refraction may have to be performed under sedation. When possible it is best to coordinate this with the patient's other care providers to limit the amount of anesthesia and hospitalizations required.

History taking is an important part of the ophthalmic examination, as in any field. Family history of ocular abnormalities must be reviewed as many conditions are familial. Medical history is important in elucidating issues of dual sensory impairment and has an impact on the examination. A child told to match pictures or follow an object may not comply with the request if they cannot adequately hear or interpret the request. This could mistakenly be construed as an abnormality of the visual system, but in fact the lack of cooperation may be due to the hearing impairment.

Manifestations of decreased vision vary with age. Children generally cope well with decreases in vision and therefore visual defects may go undetected for significant amounts of time, especially in unilateral cases. In an infant, new onset strabismus or nystagmus requires urgent evaluation. In the toddler age range, increase in falling, increased timidity, or apprehension, especially in new surroundings, may be encountered. Behavioral changes can occur as well, such as a child who is misdiagnosed as being hyperactive for leaving a seat in a classroom where in fact he is severely myopic and cannot see the board from beyond the first row of seats.

Deterioration in classroom work or inattention may also be due to decrease in vision. Some children are not even aware that their vision is not normal and therefore do not express a change in vision to their family or teachers. In cases of night blindness, children may have fear of the dark or other behavioral problems which occur only at night due to their fear of being unable to navigate independently at night.

Therefore a discussion of the child's habits with the parents or caretaker is essential to note how the child's behavior or development is progressing or decreasing in their home setting. A parent may be unable to articulate what a child's vision is but maybe able to give examples, such as child can see his mobile but has no interest in small items such as cheerios on a high chair. Parents will frequently report if a child has started to recently get closer to a television or computer screen or has no interest in such items. Eye contact is also a useful marker. Even very young infants like to watch the face of their parent or family member. Some parents will report that a child makes less eye contact or does not seem to smile as well as their previous children. A parent may also note that the child responds to him up close but does not tend to smile until he gets within a few feet of his crib or play area.

In addition it is useful to see how a child navigates into the examination room or even to watch them in the waiting room, while they are more comfortable. For example, while they are watching television in a waiting area, one can see how close the child tends to come to the screen and whether they have a head turn or head tilt which would be indicative of strabismus or ocular preference. If a child has interest in the books in the waiting area or how they play with toys such as Lego or blocks also gives some useful information especially in the preverbal ages. Once in the examination area, it is useful to have a variety of toys of different sizes and degrees of color contrast to see how a child relates to different stimuli. As children tend to lose interest quickly, it is a gain of benefit to have a variety of toys to regain their attention with a new object. Penlights should be avoided as the stimulus lacks spatial orientation. Very young babies prior to 3 months of age will preferentially follow a human face. Rattles, musical toys, or other noisemakers should not be used as testing objects as it is then unclear if the child is tracking using the visual clues or auditory input.

Prior to age 3 years, visual behavior is more subjective and can be assessed by confrontation with small toys while occluding the contralateral eye. In visual acuity testing, vision can be tested by an eye chart from age 3 years approximately and up. The opposite eye is occluded and the child is asked to identify numbers or pictures on a chart or to perform matching for the nonverbal child.

Occasionally only binocular vision is able to be assessed. Near vision should also be examined at a distance of 40 cm. Children's visual acuity can be measured using matching techniques at a slightly closer distance. Persons with severe ID may tend to be more dependent on their near vision than distance vision.

Children who are unable to perform standard visual acuity testing may be tested using the preferential looking method. In this method, the child is shown cards with gradations of white and black stripes compared with a homogenous gray background. An examiner sitting behind the cards notes when the patient is attentive to the side of the card with the gradations. The vision is determined by the last card that draws the child's attention, until the child has no visual preference. Due to the complexity of testing in this method and the lack of availability, this test is used in specialized centers only.

Screening can be done using an ophthalmoscope to test the "red reflex." This should be performed both individually and binocularly. When performed binocularly (known as the Bruckner reflex), comparison of the red reflex enables detection of items causing decreased red reflex. These include primarily cataracts, colobomas, tumors, or retinal detachments, but may rarely include clouding of the cornea as well as refractive errors and ocular misalignment. The intensity of the red reflex may depend not only on opacities, or refractive status, but there may be significant differences in the red reflex due to the varying levels of retinal pigmentation in different ethnic groups. Examination of the red reflex is a crucial part of the medical care of infants and children, recommended during all routine health visits at the pediatrician by the American Academy of Pediatrics [13]. Corneal red reflex using a penlight is directed at the patient, while maintaining his fixation in primary gaze. Location of the corneal light reflex centrally in both pupils demonstrates that the patient is orthophoric, i.e., has no ocular deviation.

If the light is displaced nasally, the eye demonstrates exotropia. Conversely, if the reflex is found laterally on the iris, the eye demonstrates esotropia. Strabismus can be elucidated by using a small toy or an object and having the patient follow the object. If there is a limitation in one field of gaze or another, then the asymmetry of the function of the extraocular muscles causes strabismus, which decreases the binocular function of the child.

Children who have decreased vision on screening examinations or any findings of strabismus or reduction in the quality of the red reflex should be referred for complete examinations by an ophthalmologist. This examination will then include examination of the anterior segment and dilated fundus examination for a more detailed examination of the intraocular structures.

In the last decade there has been increased use of vision screening devices. These devices make use of the red reflex and are able to evaluate a child from a distance. This tends to eliminate the child's fear of examination. The other advantage is the speed of the measurement which only requires a few seconds. Finally these devices as a screening tool do not necessitate the instillation of dilating drops, thereby making the exam faster for the patient and less discomfort is encountered since the patient does not have residual dilation of the pupils for the ensuing few hours. Generally one can get even a child with developmental delay to fixate or cooperate for the few seconds that photoscreening devices require. These machines are useful then in screening for strabismus and significant opacities in the visual system as well as significant refractive errors.

Occasionally subjective measurements of vision are impossible and the examination must rely primarily on objective measurements such as the physical examination of the ocular structures with particular attention to the cornea, lens, refractive status, motility status, the optic nerve, and retina.

When the ophthalmic examination alone does not provide adequate explanation for a degree of visual impairment, further testing must be done. These additional testing modalities can include imaging such as ultrasound of the eyes or more commonly, CT or MRI of the eyes, orbits, and head. Finally especially in the young infant with decreased vision without obvious intraocular abnormality evident on clinical examination, electrophysiologic testing such as the electroretinogram (ERG) or electrooculogram (EOG) or visual evoked potentials (VEP) is helpful. Visual evoked potentials can provide quantitative information useful in predicting visual acuity.

Examinations must be performed at birth or at the time of initial diagnosis, and repeated periodically to review findings (see Table 18.4). This must be done frequently especially during the amblyopic age range. Recommendations for screening schedules and content vary in the general population and are still less defined in the population of patients with ID. However, consistent follow-up is of utmost importance, and guidelines are being developed [14].

Common Causes of Vision Impairment

Refractive errors include hyperopia, myopic, and astigmatic errors. Ametropia or uncorrected refractive errors are common in the general population and in children with neurodevelopmental disorders even more so. Guidelines exist as to when spectacle correction is indicated. While mild hyperopia is the normal refractive state

Table 18.4 Vision screening schedule

Age	Examination technique
Birth	Penlight examination of pupils and external ocular anatomy
	Ocular alignment using corneal reflexes
	Red reflex using ophthalmoscope
Neonate/Toddler	Ability to follow objects light or faces
	Penlight examination of pupils and external ocular anatomy
	Ocular alignment using corneal reflexes or cover testing
	Red reflex using ophthalmoscope
Preschool years	Visual acuity by methods as above, performed monocularly
	External ocular examination using penlight or slit lamp
	Ocular alignment and motility using corneal reflexes or cover test
	Stereopsis
	Ophthalmoscopy for red reflexes and examination of the ocular fundus
School-age children	Visual acuity, Snellen method, performed monocularly
	External ocular examination using penlight or slit lamp
	Ocular alignment and motility using corneal reflexes or cover test
	Stereopsis
	Ophthalmoscopy for red reflexes and examination of the ocular fundus

for a young child, hyperopia of more than +1.5 diopters is generally treated to prevent ocular fatigue, reading difficulties, and headaches. More than three diopters of hyperopia may lead to esotropia and amblyopia. Eyes with extreme hyperopia may tend to have shallow anterior chambers and crowded optic nerves, which is occasionally mistaken for papilledema.

Myopia is less frequently encountered in preschool children, but tends to increase in school-age children, as the eye enlarges. Children with myopia have less amblyopia than hyperopic children. Myopia of greater than 2–3 diopters requires treatment even at a young age. Children with exotropia or convergence issues tend to benefit even from mild myopic prescriptions. High myopia can be found in patients who had retinopathy of prematurity. High myopia is also associated with retinal detachments and can be associated with certain syndromes.

Astigmatism may be due to irregularity in the cornea or lens. Severe astigmatism is not a common finding in early childhood, but irregularities of the cornea due to birth trauma or congenital malformations of the cornea can cause astigmatism. Mild ptosis and mild cataracts may cause astigmatism as well. Toddlers who have more than two diopters of astigmatism should have glasses, even in the early nonverbal period, in order to prevent amblyopia. Older children who are symptomatic or have more than 1.5 diopters of astigmatism should have full correction.

Finally the situation in which there are significant differences in the refraction of the two eyes is known as anisometropia. This is generally caused by a difference of more than 1.5 diopters between the two eyes, and it must be corrected in order to minimize the chances of amblyopia.

Amblyopia

Amblyopia is caused by the lack of a clear image falling on the retina of a young child. This can be either unilateral or bilateral. Amblyopia may be due to a few factors. Strabismic amblyopia occurs where an eye is deviated and therefore the image does not fall on the fovea. Deprivation amblyopia is due to a blockage of the transmission of light to the retina. This can be due to an opacity in the visual axis, such as congenital clouding of the cornea, or a congenital cataract. Refractive amblyopia can be divided into anisometropic amblyopia or ametropic amblyopia. Anisometropic amblyopia is unilateral in which there is a significant difference in the refraction of the eyes, and ametropic amblyopia is due to a high refractive error in both eyes. As visual acuity develops rapidly in the first few years of life, anything that interferes with the development of a clear retinal image can cause amblyopia. After the first decade of life, a child is no longer at risk for amblyopia as cortical plasticity is generally over by that age. The younger a child is, the more he is at risk for amblyopia. Conversely, the younger amblyopia is discovered and treated, the better the result.

Strabismus

Strabismus is a common ocular problem in children and should be addressed as early as possible. In the general population esotropia is much more common than exotropia and vertical types of strabismus are much rarer. Over half of the children who have strabismus will develop amblyopia. Strabismus may occur sporadically or there may be a familial tendency. Children with hypotonia, cerebral palsy, or other neurodevelopmental issues have a higher incidence of strabismus. Premature children even without retinopathy of prematurity have a higher incidence of strabismus as well. Prior to age 6 months intermittent or mild deviations of the ocular alignment may be within the range of normal, but by age 6 months any misalignment requires evaluation and treatment. Parents tend to notice significant strabismus and bring it to the attention of their primary care provider. Occasionally children with very wide epicanthal folds have pseudostrabismus or pseudoesotropia, where they appear esotropic, but as the nose develops, the patient will appear normal. This does not require intervention. These children still require close follow-up to rule out the development of true strabismus.

Children with congenital esotropia present early due to the generally large angle of their strabismus. The treatment for congenital esotropia is surgical with follow-up afterward, as frequently glasses are needed to maintain the surgical alignment results.

Strabismus may also result from deprivation, e.g., from presence of a tumor or cataract on one eye or both. Addressing the cause of the deprivation is vital, prior to repair of the strabismus. Accommodative esotropia is due to the presence of high hyperopic refraction and this may be ameliorated by the use of hyperopic glasses.

If this alone is not sufficient, surgery may again be indicated. Amblyopia must be corrected prior to surgical intervention. Neurologic conditions such as cranial nerve VI palsy of any etiology, such as infectious, idiopathic, or due to raised intracranial pressure, cause esotropic deviations as well.

Exotropia is rare in childhood but may present congenitally as well. Children with developmental delays or neurologic impairment tend to have more frequent exotropia. Large angle exotropia is generally treated surgically to prevent amblyopia. Untreated strabismus not only affects visual function but also is a cosmetic issue which may affect a child's social interactions.

Cataract

Cataracts can be congenital, syndromic, age related, traumatic or occur with medical conditions such as diabetes or medications, and treatment such as steroids or radiation. The treatment for cataracts is surgery in which the cloudy lens which is obstructing the visual axis is replaced with a synthetic lens. In very young ages even minor cataracts can sometimes lead to amblyopia. While extraction of the cataract and implantation of an intraocular lens is the standard treatment in older children and adults, an intraocular lens may not be implanted in very small children. This is due to the small size of the eye and the rapid growth that ensues in the toddler years, making not only the surgery but also the refractive needs challenging. In these cases an aphakic contact lens or aphakic spectacles are used. From approximately age 5 years and upward, there is no controversy and a lens is implanted. Occasionally spectacles are still needed to correct residual refractive needs including presbyopia. Cataract is the leading cause of blindness worldwide, therefore screening for cataracts and making surgery available is a high priority.

Examples of Specific Clinical Entities

Down Syndrome

Down syndrome is the most common chromosomal anomaly accounting for intellectual disability occurring at a prevalence rate of 9.2 per 10,000 live-born infants according to the Center for Disease Control [15]. The prevalence of Down syndrome is increasing, especially in children born to mothers over age 35 [16].

Down syndrome children have a variety of systemic and neurologic issues. Recent studies have shown that even in university hospital setting with specific DS clinics, patients tend to have inadequate medical surveillance which can affect their vision needs as well as their overall medical health.

Down syndrome children have myriad of eye problems (see Table 18.5), similar to those found in the general population but with greater prevalence and increased severity with earlier age of onset. Variations in the exact prevalence of findings occur depending on the study population involved; however, all studies demonstrate

Table 18.5 Common ocular manifestations in Down syndrome

Significant refractive errors, primarily astigmatism
Epicanthal folds
Blepharitis
Strabismus, primarily esotropia
Keratoconus
Nasolacrimal duct obstruction
Cataract
Retinal abnormalities
Nystagmus

increase in ocular abnormalities. Ocular findings were found in 97.4% of children with Down syndrome vs. 42.4% of control subjects [17]. Although exact statistics vary according to the population studied, Down syndrome children of school age have a high percentage (43%) of significant refractive errors [18]. These include astigmatism (60%), hyperopia (26%), and myopia (13%). Strabismus was found in 23–47% and amblyopia in 10–26% [19, 20]. Significant levels of refractive errors tend to increase with increasing age and doubled in school-age children [21]. Screening for this and providing spectacle correction can assist in maintaining a child's interest in reading and school. As stated previously, these issues can all be potentially treated to provide increased visual performance.

Children with Down syndrome were found to tolerate their spectacle correction well including bifocals as needed for issues of accommodation. In addition conditions such as nasolacrimal duct obstruction or blepharitis which both occur in approximately 30% can be treated as well. Cataracts occurred in 13–86 % and surgery should be made available to these patients when the need presents. The presence of cataract and strabismus increased with age, and therefore screening methods and examination must include regular assessment of vision, motility disturbances, and examination of the red reflex or fundus.

Finally retinal abnormalities, which occurred in up to 38% and nystagmus in 5–30%, are conditions that cannot be ameliorated either by spectacles or by surgery. However, their presence affects the child's vision and ability to perform, and the knowledge of the presence of these issues and their ensuing limitations is of importance to the patients, their parents, and educators.

In England, The United Kingdom Down Syndrome Medical Interest Group saw that with increased stringency of screening according to published guidelines, screening efficacy improved from 66 to 100%, with the advantages of earlier correction of refractive errors found. By enforcing screening at age 3 years, Down syndrome had refractive correction at age 3.5 rather than 5.5 years of age [18]. In a US study at a teaching facility, 61% of DS children had disorders which required treatment or monitoring. The percentage of children with abnormalities increased from 38% in the first year of life to 80% in school-aged children. They recommend examination at birth or at earliest diagnosis in the first 6 months of life followed by annual examination by a pediatric ophthalmologist [22]. These results demonstrate that clear guidelines to the medical community result in improved care which can definitely assist in the child's development. Finally adults with Down syndrome are at increased risk of premature age-related changes from issues such as cataract and keratoconus. Therefore screening should continue actively even in the adults years.

Cortical Visual Impairment

Cortical visual impairment (CVI) is a leading cause of visual loss in the developed world. This is primarily due to increased survival rates of preterm infants. There are multiple causes for cortical visual impairment. The damage depends on at what age the insult occurred, as different areas of the brain are affected at these time intervals (i.e., whether there was preterm or term insult). As well the degree of hypoxic/ischemic injury is also crucial in determining the extent of damage. These causes can occur singly or there may be multiple etiologies (69%) as seen in a study of children with CVI at a tertiary care referral center. Perinatal hypoxia is the most common cause in 35%, while prematurity (29%), hydrocephalus (19%), anatomic abnormalities of the central nervous system (11%), and seizures (10%) are other primary causes, with encephalitis, meningitis, and trauma being other causes [23].

Children with cortical visual impairment have a wide range of visual disability ranging from mild vision loss with cognitive visual dysfunction due to damage to the prestriate cortex, to the severe extent which may have total blindness or no light perception vision [24].

Many patients with cortical visual impairment have difficulty performing classic Snellen visual acuity due to associated neurologic impairment. Therefore vision may be assessed using alternate methods such as preferential looking (Teller type) cards or visual-evoked potentials (VEP) testing. Recent studies have shown that VEP vernier acuity type testing gave the best approximation of visual behavior [25].

Multiple ocular anomalies may be found in this patient group (see Table 18.6). Vision impairment due to cortical visual impairment is bilateral. Strabismus was found in the majority of patients, with exotropia (40%) being more common than esotropia (19%). Optic atrophy was present in almost half of the patients (42%). In addition nystagmus and high refractive errors were found in approximately 20% each. A recent study performed in 98 children with CVI followed for up to 10 years demonstrated that while the vast majority of these patients never see well, 34% did demonstrate some improvement with 17% showing mild improvement and 6% demonstrating significant improvement. The patients who had better prognosis were those who had initial better visual function.

Table 18.6 Common ocular manifestations in cortical visual impairment

Significant refractive errors
Strabismus, primarily exotropia
Nystagmus
Optic atrophy

In a contrasting study performed in 39 children with CVI followed from 0.6 to 13.7 years with a mean of 6.5 years, 49% did show significant improvement of vision with average improvement from 20/205 to 20/76 (0.43 log units). A significant percentage (47%) demonstrated improvement in contrast sensitivity. No association was found between etiology of CVI and improvement, so further studies require elucidation [26].

A significant portion of patients in both studies did demonstrate some improvement in vision. While many patients with CVI do not have ocular conditions which can be treated, it is still relevant to elucidate their degree of function and to attempt whatever rehabilitation is possible, especially in light of the multiple attendant medical conditions such as cerebral palsy, seizures, and hearing loss.

Additional Aspects of Treatment

Identification of visual impairment is a crucial to ensure optimal development and functioning. Once patients have been identified as having a diagnosis, treatment should be instituted immediately. Congenital lesions such as congenital cataracts or congenital glaucoma must be addressed as early as possible, even in the first few weeks of life as soon as anesthesia is medically appropriate. However, even with successful surgical outcomes, the development of adequate vision will not develop unless there is consistent follow-up and treatment in a team-oriented manner. The "team" approach includes not only adequate follow-up with the ophthalmologist but also significant parental involvement, understanding, and cooperation.

In addition the primary physician must be involved for issues such as antibiotic regimen consultation or for follow-up if medications such as steroids are indicated after surgery. An optometrist and optician trained specifically in pediatric issues are crucial as well to deal with issues of spectacles and patching. As an example, a child who had congenital cataract surgery and requires glasses which should sit properly. If the glasses are uncomfortable or improperly fit, i.e., too tight on a wide face or not sitting properly on a child with a flat nasal bridge, the glasses will be a source of discomfort or distraction, and the child may develop apprehension or animosity toward the glasses. Appropriate fit for spectacles is crucial as well in children who in addition to ocular issues have hearing aids or abnormalities of the ears, or facial asymmetry, which may be of consideration in syndromic children or adults.

Amblyopia therapy requires again a team approach with the ophthalmologist/optometrist/orthoptist team as well as with the family members or caretakers and the educational institution in which the child is schooled. First, opacities in the visual system must be addressed. Then appropriate glasses must be fit so that a well-focused image falls on the retina. Finally, once a child has adjusted to wearing spectacles, occlusion of the intact eye must be performed to encourage use of the amblyopic eye. This is generally done by patching the better eye on a schedule set by the ophthalmologist. Some children do not tolerate patching and then penalization with blurred glasses or atropine drops is instituted. Patching used to be prescribed on a full-time basis, but recent evidence by the Amblyopia Treatment

Studies demonstrates that adequate results may be obtained with part-time patching such as 6 h daily for severe amblyopia [27] and that 2 h daily may be sufficient in mild to moderate amblyopia [28]. These studies also discussed that recurrence is common and it is better to taper patching than to stop abruptly. Treatment success is inversely related to age, therefore early detection and initiation of treatment is vital to developing normal vision [29].

Lack of compliance is a very common issue even in children without intellectual disability or other medical issues and is more of an issue for a child with multiple sensory issues such as hearing loss or intellectual disability. Families need encouragement as frequently children are initially very resistant to patching therapy.

Ideally strabismus and amblyopia in children are best addressed as soon as identified, due to the plasticity of the neurologic system. For example, unilateral amblyopia in a 1-year old can be corrected in early infancy in 1 week of consistent patching, whereas a 7-year old who refuses to wear a patch during school and is only patched for an hour or so after school at home may require extended months of treatment to reach the endpoint of equal visual acuity or free alternation of fixation. Classically refractive amblyopia is best treated prior to 8–10 years of age, unless precluded by more pressing medical needs.

Occasionally patching treatment fails due to poor cooperation on the part of the child. This can occur in children who remove the patch in the "terrible twos " toddler period or even in later years such as 5–8 years, if the child is sensitive to the social issues of patching and therefore may refuse to wear the patch at school or in public. Generally these obstacles are surmountable. Occasionally in the early 1–3-year-old age range, it may require a period of waiting, following which treatment should be reinitiated once this especially challenging age is passed. In children with developmental delays or intellectual disability this period may last longer. Young children in the 3–6-year-old range generally respond well to initiatives such as sticker charts, prizes, or decorative patches which are now widely available. Part-time patching or optical degradation such as putting tape over the glasses in front of the stronger eye are less effective but sometimes may allow better cooperation. Maintenance therapy has been showed to be of high value according to recent results of the Amblyopia Therapy Study. Finally in extremely difficult childhood cases, results may occasionally still be achieved in the adolescent years albeit with prolonged efforts.

In all cases, close follow-up is necessary and the parents and teachers must know to watch for recurrence of strabismic deviations or change in fixation preference of the eyes. Maintenance therapy sometimes can continue for long periods of time. Recurrence or backsliding occurs not infrequently and then resumption of therapy is indicated. This can usually be reversed with resumption of therapy.

In older children and adults, cataracts should be addressed when found to be visually significant. Occasionally it is difficult to assess the degree of cataract related impairment and tools as a questionnaire of the impact on the activities of daily living are useful. Occasionally caretaker's or family members' subjective assessments make an impact on when to approach surgery, such as noting that the patient is less attentive than previously, seems to have less interest in television or food, or has more glare and tends to avoid sunlight, or is falling more than usual and having difficulty navigating stairs.

Surgery can be very successful even in patients with significant degrees of ID. Close coordination needs to occur between the surgeon, the primary medical physician, and the care givers or family member to insure the success of the surgery. It is not infrequent to find that a patient had successful surgery but then adequate results were not achieved or complications ensued due to difficulties with instilling medications, maintaining patching, preventing a patient from itching, head banging, or difficulty in follow-up.

Conclusions

Neurodevelopmental disorders may occur in association with alterations in all aspects of the visual system. These vision issues can then have severe detrimental effects on the overall development of the child with decreased social, emotional, and communication skills in addition to the educational impact. While an all encompassing review of vision impairment in children with neurodevelopmental disabilities is daunting in scope, the varied causes of decreased vision in children with neurodevelopmental disabilities have been discussed. As well the difficulties in screening and evaluating these patients are obvious; nevertheless the need to do so is crucial to their well-being. New tools for assessment of vision which are easy and effective need to be developed for use in this population.

Screening programs in clinics or residential settings have been shown to be effective. These are crucial for monitoring vision as most patients with ID do not report their change in vision. A study among residents at a facility in Scotland demonstrated that prior to initiation of a comprehensive screening, only 11% of patients had been offered vision assessment in the previous 5 years. Other than profoundly impaired patients, an assessment of vision using the variety of methods discussed earlier was achieved. In this screening, 23/63 patients required new refractive correction. Nine of the 73 (14%) had cataracts and were referred for surgical consultation. In another study of 710 adult patients with ID ranging from moderate to profound, significant refractive errors were found in 51%. These studies are examples of how screening programs can identify issues and provide appropriate treatment to enhance the vision of patients with ID. These issues are even more crucial in children with ID in which there is still potential for correction of issues of amblyopia, which are not readily amenable to treatment in the adult population.

It is important to recall that even low vision is useful vision. Resources now are becoming more available in the developed world for persons with decreased vision. Vision rehabilitation serves are best provided by a multidisciplinary team which may include the primary care physician, ophthalmologist, optometrist, orthoptist, social worker, nurses, rehabilitation therapists or counselors, and orientation and mobility specialists. Resources such as Lighthouse International, Prevent Blindness America, or the Helen Keller Foundation can provide resources such as online materials or support groups of national or local nature. There are at least 1,400 such groups in the United States alone. There are also online catalogues as well with numerous products such as closed circuit television (CCTV), large print libraries, talking books, and devices which enable patients to maintain their levels of independence at home, including talking watches, medication reminders, or glucose monitors for diabetics with low vision.

Research must continue to provide further detailed information on epidemiologic data in the population with intellectual disability. Checklists for caretakers to assess vision or questionnaires to assist in assessing vision need to be developed for this population and schedules for effective and screening need to be implemented. The goal is to help all children with or without developmental disabilities to maximize their potential and enjoy a fully active life.

References

1. Granet DB Vision development, testing, and visual screening. In: Hertle RW, Schaffer DB, Foster JA, editors. Pediatric eye disease: color atlas and synopsis. New York, NY: McGraw Hill; 2002. pp. 197–204.
2. American Academy of Ophthalmology. Amblyopia. San Francisco: Am Acad Ophthalmology, 2002.
3. McCulloch DL, Sludden PA, McKeown K, Kerr A. Vision care requirements among intellectually disabled adults: a residence-based pilot study. J Intellect Disabil Res. 1996;40: 140–50.
4. Akinci A, Oner O, Bozkurt OH, Guven A, Degerliyurt A, Munir K. Refractive errors and ocular findings in children with intellectual disability. JAAPOS. 2008;12:477–81.
5. Olitsky SE, Hug D, Smith LP. Disorders of vision. In: Kliegman RM, Behrman RE, Jenson HB, Stanton BF, editors. Nelson textbook of pediatrics, 18th ed. Philadelphia, PA: Elsevier Saunders; 2007. pp. 2573–76.
6. Appelboom TM. A history of vision screening. J Sch Health. 1985;55:138–41.
7. Hartmann EE, Dobson V, Hanline L, Marsh-Tootle W, Quinn GE, Ruttum MS. Preschool vision screening: summary of a task force report. Pediatrics. 2000;106:1105–16.
8. Warburg M. Visual impairment in adult people with moderate, severe, and profound intellectual disability. Acta Ophthalmol Scand. 2001;79:450–54.
9. Gilbert C, Foster A, Negrel D, Thylefors B. Childhood blindness: a new form for recording causes of visual loss in children. Bull World Health Org. 1993;71:485–89.
10. Resnikoff S, Pascolini D, Mariotti SP, Pokharel GP. Global magnitude of visual impairment caused by uncorrected refractive errors in 2004. Bull World Health Org. 2008;86:63–70.
11. Gilbert C, Foster A. Childhood blindness in the context of vision 2020 – the right to sight. Bull World Health Org. 2001;79:227–32.
12. Hyvärinen L. Vision in children, normal and abnormal. Toronto: Canadian Deafblind and Rubella Association; 1988.
13. American Academy of Pediatrics Section on Ophthalmology. Red reflex examination in neonates, infants, and children. Pediatrics. 2008;122:1401–4.
14. Evenhuis HM, Nagtzaam L. IASSID International consensus statement: early identification of hearing and visual impairment in children and adults with intellectual disability. Manchester: IASSID Special Interest Research Group on Health Issues; 1998.
15. Centers for Disease Control and Prevention. Down syndrome prevalence at birth. United States, 1983–1990. MMWR. 1994;43:617–22.

16. Shin M, Besser LM, Kucik JE, Lu C, Siffel C, Correa A. Congenital anomaly multistate prevalence and survival collaborative. Prevalence of Down syndrome among children and adolescents in 10 regions of the United States. Pediatrics. 2009;124:1565–71.
17. Akinci A, Oner O, Bozkurt OH, Guven A, Degerliyurt A, Munir K. Refractive errors and strabismus in children with Down syndrome: a controlled study. J Pediatr Ophthalmol Strabismus. 2009;46:83–86.
18. Stephen E, Dickson J, Kindley AD, Scott CC, Charleton PM. Surveillance of vision and ocular disorders in children with Down syndrome. Dev Med Child Neurol. 2007;49:513–15.
19. Merrick J, Koslowe K. Refractive errors and visual anomalies in Down syndrome. Down Syndr Res Pract. 2001;6:131–33.
20. De Cunha RP, Moreira JB. Ocular findings in Down's syndrome. Am J Ophthalmol. 1996;122:236–44.
21. Wong V, Ho D. Ocular abnormalities in Down syndrome: an analysis of 140 Chinese children. Pediatr Neurol. 1997;16:311–14.
22. Roizen NJ, Mets MB, Blondis T. Ophthalmic disorders in children with Down syndrome. Dev Med Child Neurol. 1994;36:594–600.
23. Kheptal V, Donahue SP. Cortical visual impairment: etiology, associated findings, and prognosis in a tertiary care setting. J AAPOS. 2007;11:235–39.
24. Edmond JC, Foroozan R. Cortical visual impairment in children. Curr Opin Ophthalmol. 2006;17:509–12.
25. Watson T, Orel-Bixler D, Haegerstrom-Portnoy G. VEP vernier, VEP grating, and behavioral grating acuity in patients with cortical visual impairment. Optom Vis Sci. 2009;86:774–80.
26. Watson T, Orel-Bixler D, Haegerstrom-Portnoy G. Longitudinal quantitative assessment of vision function in children with cortical visual impairment. Optom Vis Sci. 2007;84:471–80.
27. Holmes JM, Kraker RT, Beck RW, et al. A randomized trial of prescribed patching regimens for treatment of severe amblyopia in children. Ophthalmology. 2003;110:2075–87.
28. Repka MX, Beck RW, Holmes JM, et al. A randomized trial of patching regimens for treatment of moderate amblyopia in children. Arch Ophthalmol. 2003;121:603–11.
29. Mills MD. The eye in childhood. Am Fam Physician. 1999;60:907–18.

Chapter 19
Impact of Neurodevelopmental Disorders on Hearing in Children and Adolescents

Bharti Katbamna and Teresa Crumpton

Abstract Recent advances in maternal–fetal medicine and neonatology have led to unprecedented increase in the survival of severely preterm babies and babies with severe neurodevelopmental disabilities. These babies typically present with multiple neurosensory impairments and pose a significant challenge to neurodiagnosis and intervention. This review will describe some common neurodevelopmental disorders that impact the auditory system and present case studies to highlight the current technologies available to diagnose and treat the hearing problems.

Introduction

Since the earliest recommendations of the Joint Committee on Infant Hearing (JCIH) in 1971 [1], there has been a dramatic shift in the identification of babies considered to be at risk for hearing impairment, in that the list of specific criteria used to assess risk for hearing loss has been replaced with performance of hearing screening with the automated auditory-evoked brain stem response technique on site on every baby prior to discharge from the hospital [2]. Known as the universal newborn hearing screening program (UNHS), this program has already shown great promise for successful early identification and intervention of hearing loss. Data accumulated over the last 20 years clearly indicate that children identified and treated appropriately for hearing impairment before 6 months of age catch up with their normal hearing peers by 5 years of age and demonstrate essentially normal speech, language, and hearing development [3–5]. When multiple neurosensory systems are involved, however, the success of habilitating pediatric patients is highly dependent on multidisciplinary intervention. Moreover, due to overlapping and associative problems, habilitation in one area often produces changes in

B. Katbamna (✉)
Department of Speech Pathology and Audiology, Western Michigan University, Kalamazoo, MI 49008-5355, USA
e-mail: bharti.katbamna@wmich.edu

D.R. Patel et al. (eds.), *Neurodevelopmental Disabilities*,
DOI 10.1007/978-94-007-0627-9_19, © Springer Science+Business Media B.V. 2011

other areas; for example, multisensory (auditory–visual–proprioceptive) integration therapy may augment auditory cognition along with visual cognition and improve communicative skills of patients with neurodevelopmental disorders, and improvement in communicative skills may in turn help visual cognition. Thus, intervention in such cases may be most successful with multidisciplinary involvement. This review will highlight typical problems associated with the peripheral and/or central auditory nervous system involvement in the following common neurodevelopmental pathologies: auditory neuropathy spectrum disorder (ANSD), symptomatic congenital cytomegalovirus (CMV), and Down syndrome (DS).

Auditory Neuropathy Spectrum Disorder (ANSD)

ANSD is a new term for auditory neuropathy/dys-synchrony used to describe patients with normal cochlear outer hair cell function, but deficient neural conduction within the auditory pathway [6]. Cochlear outer hair cell function is typically gauged by measuring the acoustic (cochlear echoes or otoacoustic emissions; OAEs) or electrical (cochlear microphonics; CMs) responses from the cochlea to sound stimulation, whereas neural conduction is best assessed by measuring auditory-evoked brain stem responses (ABRs) to sound stimulation. Thus, patients with normal OAEs, at least initially, and/or CMs, but aberrant or absent ABRs may be diagnosed with ANSD. The hearing profile of ANSD patients may range from normal hearing sensitivity to a profound sensorineural hearing loss. Moreover, hearing loss may fluctuate over time and may be accompanied with poor speech listening abilities, especially in the presence of noise [7]. In some cases, fluctuating hearing loss may be precipitated by increase in body temperature (one case report linked it to a novel mutation of the otoferlin gene [8]), whereas in others no apparent causal relationship has been established [9, 10].

Other clinical manifestations include lack of suppression of OAEs with masking sounds presented either ipsilaterally or contralaterally, absent acoustic reflexes and elicitable eighth cranial nerve compound action potentials and ABRs to electrical (but not acoustical) stimulation. In normal subjects OAEs are suppressed by simultaneous presentation of masking sounds either in the same (ipsilateral) or in the opposite (contralateral) ear due to the inhibitory influences from the descending olivo-cochlear fibers that terminate on the outer hair cells. Patients with ANSD may show lack of OAE suppression due to the involvement of the efferent auditory pathway.

Likewise, ANSD patients show no acoustic reflexes; acoustic reflexes are mediated via the ascending eighth (auditory–vestibular) cranial nerve, to the central auditory pons and seventh (facial) motor nucleus of both sides, and a descending branch of the facial nerve which terminates on the stapedius muscle on each side. Thus, a moderately loud sound stimulus produces contraction of the stapedius muscle and allows assessment of the integrity of the eighth and seventh cranial nerves, as well as the intermediate regions of the arc. Lack of acoustic reflexes in ANSD patients is consistent with the eighth cranial nerve and/or seventh cranial nerve dysfunction.

Dysfunction of eighth cranial nerve in ANSD also comes from clinical observations of the inability of the eighth cranial nerve fibers to fire synchronously to auditory stimulus. Such a timing deficit would be expected to abolish both eighth cranial nerve compound action potentials and ABRs to sound stimulation. However, the eighth cranial nerve fibers retain the ability to respond to electrical stimulation yielding normal electrical compound action potentials as well as ABRs, indicating that ANSD cases may in fact be good candidates for and may benefit from cochlear implantation. In some instances though, the eighth cranial nerve is reduced or absent, so that both hearing aids and cochlear implants may not be good options.

Epidemiology

Prevalence estimates vary depending on patient populations examined by various studies. Prevalence rates have been shown to range from approximately 1 [11] to 10% in schools for the deaf [12–14] and approximately 10% in newborns [15] to 40% in neonatal intensive care unit (NICU) graduates diagnosed with hearing impairment [16].

Such prevalence numbers suggest a possible association of ANSD with a variety of risk factors for hearing loss and genetic factors. In fact, literature clearly supports the association between the presence of some perinatal diseases and neurological disorders and ANSD. Among the most common risk factors for hearing loss for which infants are admitted to the NICU include prematurity, hypoxia, and hyperbilirubinemia; and approximately 50% of all early-onset ANSD cases reportedly are associated with these perinatal conditions [17–19]. Likewise, family history may be a strong predictor of ANSD [17, 18] and hereditary disorders, specifically Charcot–Marie–Tooth syndrome, Friedreich's ataxia, Refsum's disease, hereditary motor–sensory neuropathies, and demyelinating diseases have been shown to be associated with ANSD [17, 18, 20, 21]. Some of these neurological disorders, like Charcot–Marie–Tooth syndrome and Friedreich's ataxia, account for later onset ANSD. Other genetic risk factors associated with ANSD include Waardenburg syndrome and neurometabolic and mitochondrial diseases [17, 22–24]. There is also evidence of ANSD in immune disorders like Guillain–Barre syndrome [24], infectious processes like meningitis [17], inflammatory neuropathies, cerebral palsy, severe developmental delays, and hydrocephaly [17, 24–25].

Diagnosis and Treatment

Epidemiology and etiology described above suggest multiple anatomic sites and pathological mechanisms for ANSD including dysfunction of inner hair cells, the nerves traversing the primary auditory pathway, the connecting synapses, and the auditory brain stem [16, 26, 27]. Thus, diagnosis should be based on assessment of these entities, the ultimate goal of assessment being the ability to differentially diagnose cochlear, eighth cranial nerve, and central auditory nervous system function both electrophysiologically and behaviorally using time-dependent and time-independent responses. Moreover, since clinical presentations of ANSD are highly idiosyncratic and may be transient or reversible over time, audiologic monitoring with ongoing assessments every 3 months or more frequently over the first 2 years of life or until the hearing profile is well defined should be considered. The diagnostic battery may include:

1. measurement of OAEs and CMs to assess the status of the outer hair cells of the cochlea and cochlear summating potential (SP) to assess the contribution of inner hair cells (both CMs and SP are stimulus-related cochlear receptor potentials, but whereas CMs are locked to the stimulus polarity, the periodic waveform inverting with the inversion of stimulus polarity from rarefaction to condensation phase, SP is locked to the stimulus time envelope, so that it is seen as a DC baseline shift within the same recording); note that OAEs are extremely low-level sounds produced by the outer hair cells of the cochlea in response to moderately loud sound stimuli and travel back from the cochlea (reverse transduction) via the middle ear to the outer ear; thus, middle ear and/or outer ear problems may preclude OAE assessment, so that high-frequency tympanometry may need to be performed before OAE measurements, to rule out outer and/or middle ear pathology, as well as to help interpret OAE test outcomes;

2. ABRs to assess the status of the eighth cranial nerve using both rarefaction and condensation polarity click stimuli to ensure that the responses are in fact coming from the eighth cranial nerve, rather than the cochlea (cochlear responses measured are primarily CMs and as mentioned above CMs lock to the polarity of the stimulus and invert when polarity is inverted, whereas ABR morphology is unaffected by stimulus polarity); moreover, the rapid onset/offset features of click stimuli mimic the transient onset/offset time characteristics of the eighth cranial nerve neurons (time dependent), so that responses to click stimuli provide a gauge of the ability of the neurons to fire synchronously;

3. auditory steady-state response (ASSR) is a newer electrophysiological procedure designed to test the auditory system with pure tone-like stimuli (time independent); pure tone stimuli used for ASSR are amplitude or frequency modulated (AM or FM) and the assumption is that the auditory neurons detect AM or FM modulation and therefore are responding to the carrier pure tones. Thus, this procedure provides a method of assessing the hearing ability with stimuli that are steady state rather than transient in nature, allowing hearing assessment of pathological cases like ANSD patients, in whom ABRs are not elicitable due to the neural timing deficit;

4. behavioral hearing test using both pure tones and speech stimuli to assess the perceptual aspects of hearing and to define the contour and degree of hearing loss.

In concert with the ongoing monitoring of the hearing status in ANSD, a variety of treatment options should be considered including fitting of assistive listening devices and/or mild gain amplification and ultimately cochlear implantation. Children diagnosed with hearing loss, but who are otherwise cognitively unimpaired may benefit the most from cochlear implantation. Other non-audiologic evaluation and treatment options include neurodevelopmental assessment to evaluate neurological and developmental status and need for medical management, genetic counseling to assess link to family history, speech reading and cued speech to supplement auditory information and enhance communication skills, sign language when auditory options are limited, speech and language evaluation and therapy to help facilitate speech and language development, family and psychological counseling and/or parent support groups to help better understand the limitations and/or successes with communication and other cognitive skills [28]. Case 1 described below demonstrates the complexity of diagnosing and managing infants from the NICU with ANSD.

Case Study 1

Case 1 was born after a 25-week gestation (birth weight of 961 g) and admitted to the NICU with admitting diagnoses of extreme prematurity, respiratory distress syndrome, and sepsis. She was treated for these and other multiple complications during the next 4 months of her stay at the hospital NICU and discharged at 2 months post-conceptional age. A hearing screening test performed with the automatic ABR technique prior to discharge from the hospital showed suspect results bilaterally. A comprehensive audiologic evaluation performed over the next month (2–3 months post-conceptional age) showed normal middle ear systems bilaterally as evaluated by 1,000 Hz probe tone tympanometry (see Fig. 19.1a) and cochlear hearing loss exceeding at least 30 dB in the 2–8 kHz range, since DPOAE results showed no repeatable responses in this frequency region in both ears (see Fig. 19.1b). ABR tests conducted with broad band click stimuli at 90 dB showed sinusoidal activity in the early part of the time window in both ears (see Fig. 19.1c). Moreover, phase reversal of the click stimuli from rarefaction (–) to condensation (+) produced phase inversion of the sinusoidal activity (see Fig. 19.1c) indicating that the responses were CMs emanating from the cochlea, rather than ABRs originating from the auditory brain stem. Since this pattern of responses is the hallmark of ANSD, the clinical impression was ANSD with at least a mild sensorineural hearing loss in the 2–8 kHz range in both ears.

Behavioral sound field testing conducted at 4–5 months of age showed responses to narrow band noise stimuli at moderate intensity levels in the low frequencies, but not in the high frequencies (see Fig. 19.1d) and tympanometry ruled out middle ear pathology (not shown), indicating a moderate sensorineural hearing loss in the low frequencies sloping to a severe to profound degree in the high frequencies in at least one ear. Note that sound field testing is conducted in a sound-treated room, where the sound is directed to one of the many loudspeakers placed typically at right angles to the patient directly in front and/or behind the patient. Thus, sound field testing provides estimates of hearing in the best ear, without reference to the

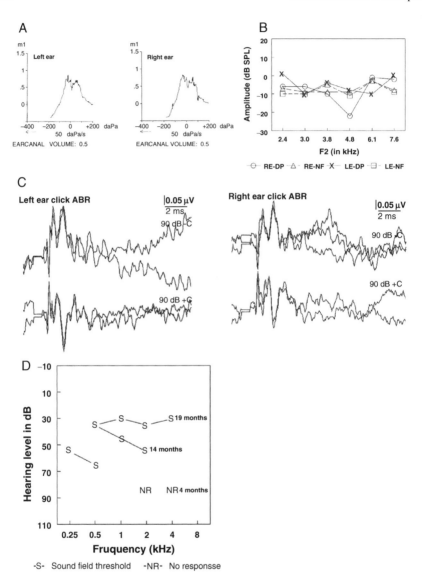

Fig. 19.1 Audiologic profile of case 1 diagnosed with ANSD showing **a** normal middle ear systems bilaterally on 1 kHz tympanometry; **b** no DPOAEs in the 2–8 kHz range in both ears (the noise floor [NF] levels are interweaving with the distortion product [DP] levels across the entire frequency range for right [RE] and left ears [LE]) indicating a cochlear hearing loss exceeding at least 30 dB levels; **c** sinusoidal activity in the early part of the time window that reverses with the phase reversal of the click stimuli (–C and +C), indicating that the responses are CMs rather than ABRs, a finding that is characteristic of ANSD; and **d** moderate to moderately severe hearing loss in the low frequencies, with essentially no measurable hearing at high frequencies in sound field testing at 4 months, but significant improvement at 14 months, shifting her hearing loss to the mild to moderate range, and further to borderline normal hearing following cochlear implantation in the right ear at 19 months of age

best ear. Based on the sound field assessment of hearing in this case, an otologic evaluation and a trial period with bilateral mild–moderate gain digital hearing aids were recommended, along with FM listening devices in the intervening period. The child's parents were keen on pursuing a trial with cued speech and in light of the fact that the child was responsive to her parents' voices and was beginning to engage in vocalizations and vocal play, fitting of FM listening devices was postponed. FM devices typically consist of a microphone-receiver system, where the signals from the microphone worn by the speaker are transmitted via a wireless high-frequency modulation (216–217 MHz dedicated radio frequency and hence, the name FM system) to a receiver worn by the listener. FM systems improve the signal-to-noise ratio substantially and alleviate listening difficulties, especially in unfavorable listening environments, like conversation with background noise or multiple speakers.

At 5–6 months of age the child was fitted with a hearing aid and in spite of auditory-verbal and cued speech communication therapy, private speech therapy, special education services from the local school district for speech-language stimulation, auditory receptive language development continued to be below par for her age during the next several months. The parents could not delineate if the hearing aid provided any true or objective benefit and the patient was referred to a cochlear implant program for an initial consultation. During the next several months, the child's hearing improved significantly; at 14 months of age she reported to the clinic with pressure equalization tubes bilaterally for middle ear infections she suffered during previous months and despite middle ear problems showed speech awareness thresholds at 30 dB and hearing levels in the mild to moderate range in sound field testing (see Fig. 19.1d).

During her entire first and second year, the child also received multidisciplinary evaluations and was diagnosed with cerebral palsy. She continued to receive speech–language–hearing intervention, along with occupational and physical therapy for her multiple physical disabilities. At 19 months of age she received a cochlear implant in her right ear and a hearing evaluation after activation of the implant showed borderline normal hearing in sound field testing (see Fig. 19.1d). A speech–language evaluation 1 year after activation of the implant showed language comprehension and expression at 15–18 months indicating that her performance age exceeded her hearing age. At this time, the father, an avid skier, also nudged her interest in skiing. He designed a walker with a ski and taught her to use the skis skillfully; this exercise has not only helped her physical and psychological disabilities immensely, but has spurred her speech–language development. At 4 years of age, the child's communication shows significant progression and her hearing evaluation shows near-normal hearing both with and without the cochlear implant. Such changes in hearing are consistent with the ANSD profile, so that decisions to implant may be quite challenging. However, since the first 6 months of life are critical for speech–language–hearing development, it may often be beneficial to err toward implantation for development of the best communication skills. The child is now 7 years of age and is in a classroom that is integrated with the public school system and continues to receive special education services. Her speech–language skills continue to reflect that her performance is ahead of her hearing age, even though she is lagging behind her peers due to multiple impairments.

Congenital Symptomatic Cytomegalovirus (CMV)

Congenital CMV is the most common viral, non-genetic cause of sensorineural hearing loss in the United States and approximately 1% of all newborns (~40,000/year) in the United States are infected with CMV [29]. Of these infected babies, approximately 10% are symptomatic at birth and majority of symptomatic babies (~90%) show significant neurologic sequelae, including hearing loss, mental retardation, microcephaly, seizures, and paresis/paralysis [29–33]. A recent survey of studies, conducted in Canada, Europe, and the United States that followed children with congenital CMV longitudinally for the sensorineural hearing loss, indicates that 22–65% of children with symptomatic infection show sensorineural hearing loss, as compared to 6–23% of those with asymptomatic infection [34]. Moreover, the onset of hearing loss varies, so that some children show hearing loss at birth, whereas others experience hearing loss later during the first few years of life, and regardless of the onset of hearing loss, there is no clear pathognomonic audiometric configuration associated with CMV, the hearing loss differing in severity and unilateral versus bilateral presentation, as well as possible progression and fluctuation over years [34].

The progressive and fluctuating nature of hearing loss suggests a chronic infection within the inner ear system or the auditory central nervous system (CNS). Studies in children with both symptomatic and asymptomatic CMV indicate that viral load, as measured in the urine or peripheral blood, is significantly correlated with development of hearing loss at birth and up to 6 months of follow-up [35, 36]. Moreover, children with progressive hearing loss continue to excrete virus in the urine for over 4 years, suggesting that progression of hearing loss may be related to ongoing replication of the virus and/or high viral load in congenitally infected children [37].

Postmortem analysis of infant inner ear in CMV-infected cases supports the above notion of CMV-induced chronic labyrinthitis. A number of studies have shown evidence of structural damage to the endolymphatic system, particularly the saccule and utricle, with lesser involvement of the cochlea post-CMV infection [38, 39]. Histological evidence of cytomegalic inclusion bodies in epithelial cells of the saccule, utricle, semicircular canals, Reissner's membrane, and stria vascularis [38–40] and hydrops of the saccule, utricle, and scala media, as well as degenerative changes in the stria vascularis, has also been documented [38, 39, 41]. Presence of viral DNA in the perilymph further consolidates the above findings and suggests that the virus may enter the endolymphatic system from the perilymphatic system via the stria vascularis [42, 43].

Epidemiology

Human CMV is a large DNA virus that belongs to the Herpesviridae family and like other herpes viruses (herpes simplex, varicella, Epstein–Barr) CMV remains dormant in the host for extended periods of time, with periodic reactivation [44].

Although 1% of newborns are infected with CMV in utero, 40% of children acquire it within the first few years of life [45]; pregnant mothers with primary infection pose the greatest risk for transplacental transmission of the virus accounting for a third of the fetal CMV infections [45] and one half of these in utero infections lead to symptomatic CMV [46]. Furthermore, the timing of the maternal infection is critical in determining the risk to the fetus; although pregnant mothers with nonprimary (previous) infections who are seropositive are less likely to transmit the virus to the fetus, they are more likely to get reinfected with a different strain of CMV thereby increasing not only the risk for transplacental transmission but also the likelihood of longer term neurological sequelae in infected babies [46, 47]. Postnatally, young children, symptomatic and asymptomatic, may shed virus at mucosal surfaces for a protracted period of time and they may serve as reservoirs for the virus, transmitting it to other children and pregnant women at mucosal surfaces via urine, saliva, or other bodily fluids [37, 48]. A basic hygiene practice like washing hands periodically has been shown to greatly reduce the infection rate in pregnant mothers [49]. The other major route of infection in young women is through sexual activity and blood transfusions, so that appropriate education of young women may help limit CMV infections [50].

Contribution of CMV to Risk Factors for Hearing Loss and Childhood Hearing Loss

A study by Rivera et al. [51] that examined demographic data, clinical and laboratory findings to determine if certain factors predicted hearing loss in symptomatic CMV cases, showed that none of the major factors including race, insurance status, hepatosplenomegaly, jaundice, microcephaly, seizures, thrombocytopenia, and referral status predicted hearing loss. The only two factors that were independently associated with hearing loss in symptomatic CMV children were intrauterine growth retardation and petechial rash exhibited by these patients [51]. Likewise, in asymptomatic cases, Fowler [52] showed that only low birth weight and prematurity predicted increased risk for sensorineural hearing loss, and these factors were associated with increased titers of urinary CMV and peripheral blood virus burden suggesting that increased viral burden may be predictive of increased risk for hearing loss in asymptomatic patients [52].

A number of studies in the 1980s also examined the relative contribution of congenital CMV to sensorineural hearing loss and reported very low rates of association between congenital CMV and hearing loss [34]. However, when nested polymerase chain reaction (PCR) on dried blood spots was used to identify CMV-positive children, sensorineural hearing loss of more than 40 dB was correlated with congenital CMV in 24.7% of children [53]. When a subgroup of children who showed greater than 70 dB sensorineural hearing loss was examined, the CMV-positive rate increased to 42.7% [53]. These findings indicate that CMV may account for a significant portion of childhood hearing loss, but that it continues to be overlooked as a prominent cause of childhood hearing loss due to the characteristics of the infection. Even the UNHS program designed to catch congenital hearing loss often cannot identify CMV-related hearing loss, due to the delayed onset of loss [34].

Diagnosis and Treatment

Since it is hard to predict which children with congenital CMV will develop hearing loss, if it is not already apparent at birth, and whether the hearing loss will progress further, many studies have examined and advocated screening for CMV first and in view of a positive test follow-up with serial monitoring of the hearing status and/or intervention of the hearing loss throughout childhood [34]. It is now quite clear that a positive viral load is highly correlated with development of hearing loss, regardless of whether the CMV symptoms are silent or not [35, 36]. Such a screening paradigm would not only facilitate early identification of hearing loss, but provide the opportunity to fit the children with hearing aids and/or cochlear implants, so as to facilitate normal speech–language learning and acquisition. Audiological evaluation at birth is typically based on assessing the integrity of (1) the outer/middle ear systems by tympanometry, (2) the cochlea via electrocochleography (CMs and summating potentials) and OAE assessments, (3) the auditory brain stem pathway by ABRs, and (4) finally, assessment of perceptual abilities for pure tone and speech stimuli via behavioral audiometry.

Although initial hearing aid selection is based on the first impression of the degree and configuration of hearing loss, the hearing aids should be adjustable to accommodate progressive deterioration in hearing loss. Thus, digital, programmable hearing aids may better accommodate the changing hearing profile of CMV-infected populations, since these hearing aids lend themselves to frequent reprogramming. Cochlear implantation may be an option if a profound hearing loss is identified at birth or subsequently during early childhood. There is clear evidence that children with CMV benefit from cochlear implants if they are not otherwise cognitively impaired due to severe CNS involvement. A study that compared benefits of cochlear implants in children diagnosed with connexin 26 deafness, that is not accompanied by any CNS sequelae, and in children with CMV who may have greater likelihood for CNS complications showed that both groups benefitted significantly from implants, although the CMV group lagged in language development compared to the connexin 26 deafness group [54]. Case 2 described below provides an audiological profile of a typical symptomatic CMV child whose hearing history was tracked over 2 years and who has benefitted significantly from the use of cochlear implants.

Antiviral Drugs and Hearing Impairment

A number of currently licensed drugs for CMV therapy work by blocking the viral DNA polymerase with different pharmacological actions. Although there is limited information on the utility of antiviral drug therapy in alleviating neuropathogenesis in CMV-infected infants, ganciclovir has been shown to be effective for short-term management of sensorineural hearing loss in infants in a recent phase III randomized double-blind study [55]. In this study, babies with congenital symptomatic CMV received intravenous ganciclovir for 6 weeks. The endpoint was improved ABRs between baseline and 6-month follow-up, as compared to normal ABRs at both time points in a control (no treatment) group. Of the 100 patients that were enrolled in the study, 42 patients received both baseline and 6-month follow-up ABRs. Twenty-one of the 25 patients who received ganciclovir showed improved hearing or normal hearing at both time points, compared to 10 of 17 of the control subjects. None of the 25 subjects who received ganciclovir showed worsening of hearing between baseline and 6 months, compared to 7 of 17 control subjects. Moreover, only 5 of the 24 subjects receiving ganciclovir therapy showed worsening of hearing at >1 year follow-up, compared to 13 of 19 control patients. Unfortunately, two-thirds of treated babies showed significant neutropenia during therapy. Thus, antiviral therapy requires careful consideration and monitoring, but may be protective against CMV-induced neurodevelopmental damage, especially to the auditory nervous system.

Case Study 2

Case 2 was a full-term baby, born at 40 weeks gestational age with an unremarkable birthing history. The mother reported an uncomplicated and unremarkable pregnancy and no history of drug or alcohol use. She also denied any family history of hearing loss on either the maternal or the paternal side. The baby, however, was diagnosed with neonatal jaundice and was admitted to the NICU for significantly elevated bilirubin levels. He received blood transfusion for hyperbilirubinemia and a screening test for CMV conducted during his stay at the NICU was positive. A hearing screening test performed prior to his discharge from the NICU showed referrals on both ears. A comprehensive audiologic evaluation performed at 3 weeks of age showed normal middle ears bilaterally, as evidenced by normal 1,000 Hz probe tone tympanograms (see Fig. 19.2a) and cochlear dysfunction as shown by lack of any repeatable responses in the 2–8 kHz range in both ears (see Fig. 19.2b). ABRs performed with broadband click stimuli (see Fig. 19.2c), as well as 500 and 1,000 Hz tone burst stimuli (see Fig. 19.2d, e), showed no responses at the maximum limits of the equipment. These findings together indicate a diagnosis of severe to profound sensorineural hearing loss in both ears. Behavioral audiometry showed hearing at the limits of the audiometer in the 0.25–2 kHz range with no measurable hearing at 4 and 8 kHz in the right ear and essentially no measurable hearing across the 1–8 kHz range in the left ear, confirming the diagnosis of bilateral profound sensorineural hearing loss (see Fig. 19.2f). The child was scheduled for hearing aid selection and fitting during the next month and received bilateral high gain digital hearing aids at 2 months of age. He was enrolled in early intervention program through the intermediate school district and also received auditory training at the university clinic.

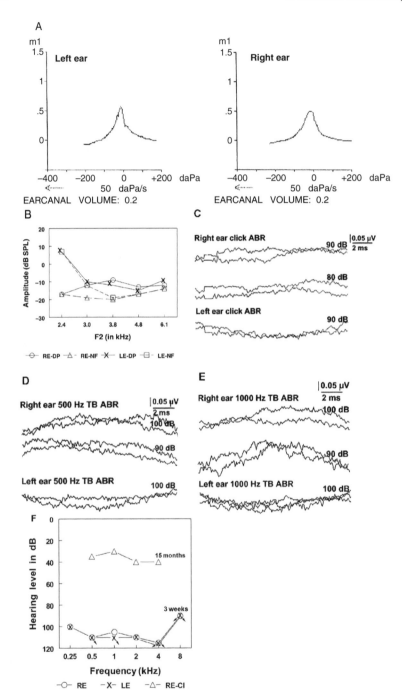

Fig. 19.2 (continued)

Over the next 12 months, he was evaluated on an ongoing basis and showed no functional benefit from amplification and at 14 months of age was fitted with a cochlear implant in the right ear. The implant was activated a month later and speech awareness was measured near normal levels (20 dB). He continued to receive speech–language–hearing intervention services and 1 year after activation both hearing and auditory skill assessments showed remarkable progress. His sound field audiogram showed a shift in hearing thresholds down to 30–40 dB levels, consistent with mild hearing loss (see Fig. 19.2f), whereas his auditory skills were scored near the top on a performance scale gauging vocal behavior, alerting responses to sounds, and deriving meaning from sound with the implant, using the Infant-Toddler Meaningful Auditory Integration Scale (IT-MAIS) developed by Zimmerman-Phillips et al. [56]. These outcomes suggest significant progress in responding to sound in his everyday environment.

During the next several months, however, he was evaluated by a team of multidisciplinary professionals, since he showed poor muscle tone and poor motor development. He was diagnosed with multiple cognitive and motor impairments, and although he did not present with chorioretinitis, he demonstrated visual problems. A cranial CT scan showed multiple areas of white matter abnormalities that corroborated the identified developmental impairments. He is currently receiving occupational therapy, physical therapy, services from a vision specialist, as well as a teacher of the hearing impaired for the recognized developmental impairments and continues to show slow improvement in all areas.

Trisomy 21 or Down Syndrome (DS)

Trisomy 21 or Down syndrome (DS) results from a chromosomal abnormality where somatic cells exhibit an extra chromosome in the 21–22 group; although majority (95%) of Down syndrome cases occur due to non-familial trisomy 21, approximately 3–4% of the phenotypes have been shown to result from unbalanced translocation between chromosomes 21 and 14 and the remaining 1–2% have

---

Fig. 19.2 Audiologic manifestations associated with a typical symptomatic CMV patient with essentially no measurable hearing at birth demonstrated by case 2 showing: **a** normal tympanograms and thus, no middle ear pathology bilaterally; **b** absent DPOAEs (distortion product [DP] levels overlapping noise floor [NF] levels for right [RE] and left ears [LE]); **c** no ABR responses to click stimuli indicating a profound sensorineural hearing loss in at least 2–4 kHz range bilaterally; **d** and **e** no ABR responses to low-frequency tone bursts at the limits of the intensity range indicating a profound sensorineural hearing loss in the 0.5–1 kHz range in both ears; and **f** behavioral audiometry outcomes corroborating the objective DPOAE and ABR test results of profound sensorineural hearing loss across 0.25–8 kHz range in both ears (RE: right ear; LE: left ear; *arrows* indicate no response), but remarkable augmentation in hearing with cochlear implantation in the right ear, hearing ability being measured just below the cutoff for normal hearing sensitivity in sound field testing 1-month post-implantation (RE-CI)

been attributed to mosaicism (presence of two cell lines, one normal, and one trisomy 21), the latter group showing less severe manifestations than the previous two phenotypes [57].

In spite of phenotypic differences, all DS cases show some common physical features including hypotonia, small brachycephalic head, epicanthic folds, flat nasal bridge, upward slanting palpebral fissures, small mouth, small ears, short stature, excessive skin at the nape of the neck, single transverse palmar crease, and a wide space between the first and second toe [57, 58]. DS is also one of the most common causes of developmental and intellectual disabilities. Mental impairment may range from mild (intelligent quotient: IQ of 50–70) to moderate levels (IQ: 35–50) and may be severe (IQ: 20–35) in a few individuals, although IQ does not typically predict social quotients, i.e., DS children tend to do better socially than predicted by their IQ levels [58]. Other associated common problems like congenital heart defects (50%), hearing loss (38–78%), ophthalmological disorders (60%), obstructive sleep apnea (50–75%), and less frequently celiac disease, hypothyroidism, arthritis, diabetes mellitus, leukemia, and seizures, often need medical attention immediately after birth, placing children with DS at a developmental disadvantage, particularly in speech, language, and hearing areas [57–59].

Ear Abnormalities and Hearing Loss

Morphological abnormalities of the external ear in children with DS include small, malformed, low set pinnae and/or narrow external auditory meatus and canals [60]. Stenotic ear canals and opening often result in cerumen accumulation that, in turn, may interfere with the diagnosis of middle ear pathology [60, 61]. Middle ear anomalies include various malformations of the ossicles including fixation of the stapes and deformity of the stapes superstructure (head, neck, and crura), residual mesenchymal tissue, poorly developed or pneumatized mastoid air cells, and large dehiscence of the facial canal [62–64]. Mid-face hypoplasia often produces a mal- or dysfunctional tensor veli palatini muscle of the palate, precluding adequate Eustachian tube opening and consequently, middle ear ventilation, placing children with DS at a high risk for chronic otitis media and cholesteatoma [62–64]; narrow, small, or collapsed Eustachian tube or lumen, in addition, may contribute to the risk for middle ear infections [65]. Inner ear abnormalities include a shortened cochlea, modiolus, cochlear nerve canal, internal auditory canal, reduced numbers of spiral ganglion cells, and a number of malformations of the vestibular system, the most common anomaly being absence or reduction of the lateral semicircular canal to a small bony island [63, 64].

Morphological abnormalities of the ear clearly suggest that children with DS may exhibit a hearing profile that may vary from normal hearing to profound sensorineural hearing loss, although conductive hearing loss appears to be most prevalent due to the presence of one or more structural anomalies of the middle ear. Balkany in 1979 [62] reported an incidence of hearing loss in a series of 107 DS cases to be 64%, of which 83% showed conductive hearing loss and 60% of those conductive losses could be accounted for by middle ear effusion and tympanic membrane perforation, whereas the remaining 23% were confirmed operatively with middle ear malformations; a small percentage (17%) showed permanent sensorineural hearing loss that may likewise be attributable to inner ear anomalies. These statistics have not changed over the years and have been confirmed recently by both cross-sectional and longitudinal studies [58, 61]. However, studies have also shown that the incidence of conductive hearing loss in children with DS may be significantly reduced with early, consistent, and aggressive otologic/audiologic evaluation and management [61]. In a 5-year longitudinal study, Shott et al. [61] showed that young children with DS (age at initial participation <2 years) who received otologic and audiologic evaluations every 6 months, as well as follow-up treatment with pressure equalization tubes to combat repeated bouts of infections (over half receiving multiple sets of tubes), also maintained near-normal hearing sensitivity over the span of the study. Thus, aggressive monitoring and treatment reduced the incidence of varying degrees of hearing loss from 81% down to 2%, where 98% demonstrated essentially normal hearing sensitivity and the remaining 2% showed mild hearing loss.

Epidemiology

Data from the most recent population-based birth defects surveillance programs analyzed by the Center for Disease Control and Prevention (CDC) indicate a DS prevalence rate of 9.2 per 10,000 live-born infants during the 1983–1990 period [66]. An update based on cross-sectional analysis of live-born infants with DS during the 1979–2003 period further indicates that the prevalence rate increased by 31%, from approximately 9 to 12 per 10,000 [67]. Moreover, the number of DS infants born to older mothers (>35 years) increased almost five times (38.6 per 10,000) compared to DS infants born to younger mothers (7.8 per 10,000; 67). Prevalence estimates beyond infancy in the 0- to 19-year age range for the year 2002 also showed an overall increase in prevalence, placing it at 1 per 1,000 children and adolescents [67]. These numbers suggest that improved early intervention and medical management of congenital heart defects and other conditions seen in DS have greatly improved the quality of life for individuals with DS, and as a consequence, increased life expectancy of individuals with DS [67].

Diagnosis and Treatment

The American Academy of Pediatrics recommends that infants with DS receive audiologic evaluation using objective test measures including ABR and OAE assessment by 3 months of age. Parental counseling to alert them regarding the high prevalence rates of middle ear problems in DS infants and need for monitoring middle ear and hearing status, so as to promote early identification and intervention, should also be part of the health-care supervision and guidance procedures. Thus, after initial objective assessment, behavioral testing should be conducted every 6 months until ear-specific hearing threshold information is available, followed by annual evaluations to monitor any changes in hearing [58, 61].

Age-appropriate hearing test batteries to diagnose hearing loss recommended by the American Speech–Language–Hearing Association for all infants that do not pass the initial hearing screening test performed prior to discharge from the hospital are also applicable to DS cases [68]. Thus, comprehensive audiologic testing for infants with DS:

1. from birth to 3 months of age (corrected for developmental delay) should include ABR, OAE, and high-frequency tympanometry. Middle ear pathology commonly seen in infants with DS may be misdiagnosed if high-frequency tympanometry is not utilized (see exemplary tympanometry recordings described below for case 3). Moreover, the ABR test protocol should differentiate between conductive, sensory, and neural types of hearing loss, and since DS cases are considered to be high risk for ANSD, neurodiagnostic assessments to rule out ANSD should be conducted. Typical ABR protocols include all the procedures described above in the diagnosis section of ANSD. If ANSD is ruled out, frequency-specific tone burst ABRs (presented via both air conduction and bone conduction pathways) may provide initial estimates of hearing thresholds;
2. for babies and toddlers with a developmental age of 6 months or greater, behavioral testing should be attempted. Visual reinforcement audiometry may be used to obtain behavioral thresholds in a sound field setting, and like the name suggests, animated toys may be used to reinforce a head turn toward sounds presented via a loudspeaker in a sound-treated room. Conditioned play audiometry may be more appropriate for children over 36 months of age. Often multiple sessions may be required to complete an audiogram with ear-specific threshold information. Due to the high prevalence of narrow ear canals, cerumen accumulation may occur frequently, adding another 10–30 dB of conductive component to the existing hearing loss; thus, otoscopy and tympanometry should be attempted at each testing session. Tympanometry can provide information on the integrity of the middle ear system that may not otherwise be obtained through otoscopy alone [60].

As mentioned above, aggressive management of otitis media under the supervision of an otolaryngologist ensures maintenance of normal hearing levels in children with DS [58, 61]. Although a pediatric office may be able to manage recurrent otitis media, supervision and care by an otolaryngologist may be necessary due to the need for microscopic ear examination, cerumen removal every 3 months until appropriate growth of the ear canal (typically 2–3 years of age) occurs, repeated insertion of pressure equalization tubes, and treatment of upper respiratory airway problems due to Eustachian tube malfunction and/or poor oral intake [59, 61]. The two case studies described below demonstrate how rigorous follow-up and intervention of middle ear infections helps ward off not only conductive hearing loss, but also upper respiratory problems and other extensive otologic/audiologic management (case 3) otherwise necessary for remediating complications associated with poorly managed recurrent middle ear infections (see case 4).

Permanent hearing loss, regardless of the origin of hearing loss (conductive, mixed, or sensorineural), identified in children with DS may be treated with traditional hearing aids, bone anchored hearing aid (BAHA) devices, or cochlear implants. Digital (programmable) hearing aids may be most effective in improving speech audibility of children with mild to moderate degrees of hearing loss. On the other hand, recurrent middle ear drainage and/or significant stenosis of the external auditory canal presented by many DS cases may preclude the use of traditional hearing aids. In such cases, bone conduction hearing aids or an osseointegrated titanium implant (BAHA system) may be appropriate. The BAHA device amplifies sound by conducting sound through bone, bypassing the middle ear, and directly stimulating the functioning cochlea. A small titanium fixture is anchored to the skull and after a short period the fixture osseointegrates with the bone of the skull (as alluded to by the name of the device). The sound processor is attached to the head via an abutment that may be connected or removed easily. An alternative BAHA sound processor mounted on a headband called the 'softband' may be a better option for children younger than 7 years of age. A recent study of children with DS who were fitted with the BAHA device showed improvement in the quality of life and satisfaction levels for not only the patients, but also the caregivers [69].

A limited number of DS children with severe to profound hearing loss have also been treated with cochlear implants. Special considerations for cochlear implantation in children with DS include frequent episodes of otitis media, temporal bone abnormalities including shorter cochlea and Mondini malformations, dehiscence of the facial canal, and absent cochlear nerve [64, 70]. Although DS children with additional disabilities may achieve post-implant outcomes below those of children without additional disabilities, objective improvements in auditory awareness and language use with and without supplemental sign language have been reported [70].

Case Study 3

Case 3 was a preterm baby born after 35 weeks of gestation, with a birth weight of 2,100 g. She was admitted to the NICU with an admitting diagnosis of prematurity and after 3 weeks of NICU care was discharged from the hospital. Hearing screening performed just prior to discharge showed a 'pass' outcome in the right ear and a 'refer' result in the left ear. Her mother reported an unremarkable prenatal, perinatal, and postnatal history, with no known history of hearing loss in the immediate family; however, the baby was diagnosed with DS prior to discharge. A comprehensive hearing evaluation at 39 weeks post-conceptional age showed essentially normal hearing with possible immature middle ear systems bilaterally. Tympanometric measurements performed with 678 and 1,000 Hz probe tones showed either noncompliant or poorly defined tympanograms, even though the results were normal with a low-frequency 226 Hz probe tone (see Fig. 19.3a; only right ear tympanograms shown).

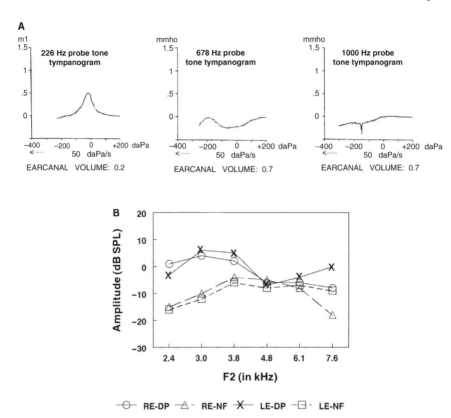

Fig. 19.3 DS cases 3 and 4 illustrating the outcomes of continual, aggressive identification and management of persistent middle ear pathology (**a–e**) and alternatively feeble monitoring of hearing loss and accompanying pathology, respectively (**f**); **a** tympanometric screening with 226 Hz probe tone, as opposed to 678 and 1,000 Hz probe tones, showing the sensitivity and utility of high-frequency probe tones in identifying middle ear pathology and immaturity that would have been otherwise completely missed by a low-frequency probe tone that displays normal findings at birth; **b** DPOAE results showing distortion product [DP] levels that are 5–15 dB greater than associated noise floor [NF] levels in the 2–4 kHz range in the right [RE] and left ears [LE], but no responses above 4 kHz in both ears; **c** ABRs to click stimuli displaying normal latency wave V from 80 dB down to 35 dB in the right ear and down to 40 dB in the left ear, with no reversal of waveforms when the polarity of the click stimuli is changed from negative (–C) to positive (+C) at 80 dB levels, in either ear; **d** pure tone audiometry results displaying air–bone gaps, defined as gaps in hearing as measured by air conduction (O for right ear: RE; X for left ear: LE) and bone conduction (<for right mastoid placement of the bone vibrator) due to conductive hearing loss of a mild degree in the 0.5–4 kHz range bilaterally; **e** borderline normal hearing in both right [RE] and left ears [LE]; and **f** pure tone audiometry results of case 4 showing significant air–bone gaps (air conduction thresholds illustrated as O for right ear: RE; X for left ear: LE; and bone conduction thresholds illustrated as open brackets '[' for right ear and close brackets ']' for left ear) indicative of maximum conductive hearing loss in both ears due to improperly managed middle ear pathology and consequent development of cholesteatomas in both ears

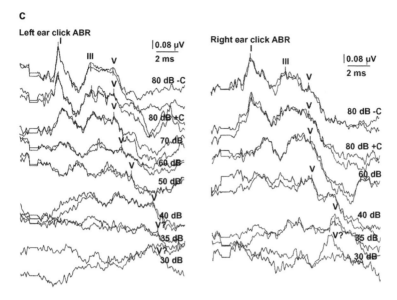

Fig. 19.3 (continued)

Note that high-frequency tympanometry during the first 6 months of life is replaced with low-frequency tympanometry after 6 months due to maturation of the middle ear; the middle ear resonant frequency of approximately 250 Hz at birth increases as age increases to approximately 1,200–1,500 Hz after 6 months. Thus, the probe tones must be swapped to prevent interaction of the probe tone frequency with the resonant frequency of the middle ear, necessitating the use of 1,000 Hz probe tone when the middle ear resonant frequency is 250 Hz and the use of 226 Hz probe tone after 6 months of life when the resonant frequency increases to 1,200–1,500 Hz.

DPOAE measurements showed robust responses in the 2–4 kHz range, but absent responses above 4 kHz in both ears (see Fig. 19.3b). ABR assessments performed at moderate to high intensity levels with broadband, negative-, and positive-polarity click stimuli showed waves I, III, and V with normal absolute latencies and normal interpeak intervals I–III, III–V, and I–V, with no significant interear differences. Furthermore, latency–intensity functions with click stimuli showed wave V down to 35 dB in the right ear and 40 dB in the left ear, the latencies at all intensity levels, except at 35 dB, being consistent with age-appropriate norms in either ear (see Fig. 19.3c). Thus, whereas high-frequency tympanometry results suggested immature middle ear systems, DPOAE, and click-evoked ABRs together indicated at least a mild hearing loss at and/or above 4 kHz in both ears; however, the contribution of aberrant middle ear systems to the DPOAE and/or ABR test outcomes could not be delineated. Thus, the mild hearing loss could have had both conductive and sensorineural components, but preservation of ABR morphology on phase reversal of click stimuli ruled out ANSD. In light of the diagnosis of DS and the

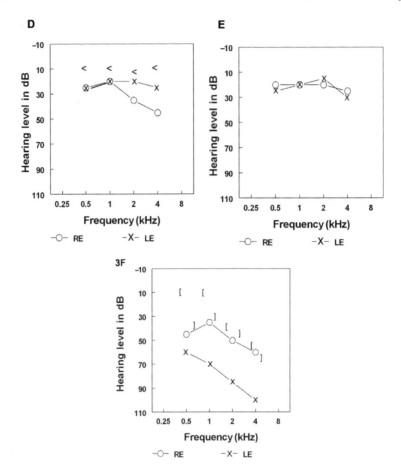

Fig. 19.3 (continued)

accompanying audiologic findings, otologic evaluation and follow-up, as well as a repeat comprehensive hearing evaluation in 2–3 months, were recommended.

The patient returned 3 years later due to the diagnosis of heart problems, that needed immediate attention and intervention; however, the patient received rigorous otologic intervention during the entire intervening period. Tympanometry performed with low-frequency probe tone showed flat tympanograms bilaterally, but middle ear infections could not be ruled out due to excessive cerumen accumulation in both ear canals (not shown). Pure tone audiometry showed mild to moderate hearing loss (see Fig. 19.3d) and in light of the flat tympanograms the patient was referred back to the otologist. Subsequent monitoring of hearing every 3–6 months, with repeated referrals to the otologist over the next 4 years, ensured preservation of hearing in the borderline normal to mild hearing loss range (see Fig. 19.3e). At 7 years of age, the child continues to demonstrate essentially normal hearing, but her communication skills are lagging slightly due to developmental delays imposed by DS.

Case Study 4

Case 4 was similar to case 3 in that the patient showed comparable findings on initial audiologic evaluation. However, due to limited access to otologic/audiologic management plans and/or neglect in seeking such care, recurrent middle ear infections led to progressive changes in the middle ear. The patient received three sets of pressure equalization tubes and underwent tonsillectomy before 4 years of age and then reportedly had a hiatus in appropriate care and/or received infrequent monitoring during the next 7 years. At age 11 years he presented with not only a moderate mixed hearing loss (both conductive and sensorineural components together) in the left ear and a sloping severe to profound mixed loss in the right ear (see Fig. 19.3f), but also bilateral cholesteatomas. Due to the deeper extension of the cholesteatoma in the right middle ear space, tympanomastoidectomy in the right ear along with facial nerve monitoring was recommended. The patient's parents were also advised about the need for repeated surgeries to clean the ear and reconstruct hearing. The patient is currently undergoing a second stage cleaning and repair. After appropriate healing, he will be fitted with BAHA or digital hearing aids depending on the severity and configuration of hearing loss in the right ear. Management of the left ear will proceed in a similar manner with surgical cleaning and repair, followed by audiologic assessment/intervention.

Conclusions

Neurodevelopmental disorders may impact the auditory system along the entire length of the auditory pathway. Thus, the integrity of each part of the auditory pathway including the outer/middle ear, inner ear, eighth cranial nerve, auditory brain stem, and overall perceptual ability must be assessed with appropriate technology, followed by otologic and/or audiologic intervention and management to ensure successful acquisition of speech and language and to abate developmental delays. Concurrent multidisciplinary evaluations and interventions should also be considered so as to reduce the effects of multiple disabilities, as well as capture the most critical period for speech–language and hearing development.

References

1. Committee on fetus and newborn. Joint statement on neonatal screening for hearing impairment. Pediatrics. 1971;47(6):1085.
2. American academy of pediatrics task force on newborn and infant hearing. Newborn and infant hearing loss: detection and intervention. Pediatrics. 1999;103:527–29.
3. Yoshinaga-Itano C, Sedey AL, Coulter DK, Mehl AL. Language of early- and later-identified children with hearing loss. Pediatrics. 1998;102(5):1161–71.
4. Downs MP, Yoshinaga-Itano C. The efficacy of early identification and intervention for children with hearing impairment. Pediatr Clin North Am. 1999;46(1):79–87.
5. Yoshinaga-Itano C. Early intervention after universal neonatal hearing screening: impact on outcomes. Ment Retard Dev Disabil Res Rev. 2003;9(4):252–66.

6. Guidelines development conference on the identification and management of infants with auditory neuropathy, International Newborn Hearing Screening Conference, Como, Italy, June 19-21, 2008.

7. Rance G, Barker EJ, Sarant JZ, Ching TY. Receptive language and speech production in children with auditory neuropathy/dys-synchrony type hearing loss. Ear Hear. 2007;25: 34–46.

8. Marlin S, Feldmann D, Nyugen Y, Rouillon I, Loundon N, Jonard L, Bonnet C, Couderc R, Garabedian EN, Petit C, Denoyelle F. Temperature-sensitive auditory neuropathy associated with an otoferlin mutation: deafening fever! Biochem Biophys Res Commun. 2010;394(3):737–42.

9. Berlin CI, Hood LJ, Goforth-Barter L, Bordelon J. Auditory neuropathy: three time courses after early identification. ARO abstracts. 1999;22:169.

10. Starr A, Sininger Y, Winter M, Derebery MJ, Oba S, Michalewski HJ. Transient deafness due to temperature-sensitive auditory neuropathy. Ear Hear. 1998;19(3):169–79.

11. Foerst A, Beutner D, Lang-Roth R, Huttenbrink KB, von Wedel H, Walger M. Prevalence of auditory neuropathy/synpatopathy in a population of children with profound hearing loss. Int J Pediatr Otorhinolaryngol. 2006;70(8):1415–22.

12. Berlin CI, Hood LJ, Morlet T, Den Z, Goforth L. The search for auditory neuropathy patients and connexin 26 patients in schools for the deaf. ARO abstracts. 2000;23:23.

13. Lee JSM, McPherson B, Yuen KCP, Wong LLN. Screening for auditory neuropathy in a school for hearing impaired children. Int J Pediatr Otorhinolaryngol. 2001;61:39–46.

14. Cheng X, Li L, Brashears S, Morlet T, Ng SS, Berlin C, Hood L, Keats B. Connexin 26 variants and auditory neuropathy/dys-synchrony among children in school for the deaf. Am J Med Genet. 2005;139(1):13–18.

15. Sininger YS. Identification of auditory neuropathy in infants and children. Sem Hear. 2002;23:193–200.

16. Rea PA, Gibson WPR. Evidence for surviving outer hair cell function in congenitally deaf ears. Laryngoscope. 2003;113:230–34.

17. Rance G, Beer DE, Cone-Wesson B, Shepherd RK, Dowell RC, King AM, Rickards FW, Clark GM. Clinical findings for a group of infants and young children with auditory neuropathy. Ear Hear. 1999;20(3):238–52.

18. Sininger YS, Oba S. Patients with auditory neuropathy: who are they and what can they hear? In: Sininger Y, Starr A, editors. Auditory neuropathy: new perspectives in hearing disorders, San Diego: Singular-Thomson Learning; 2001. pp. 15–36.

19. Madden C, Rutter M, Hilbert L, Greinwald JH, Choo DI. Clinical and audiological features in auditory neuropathy. Arch Otolaryngol Head Neck Surg. 2002;128(9):1026–30.

20. Starr A, Picton TW, Sininger Y, Hood LJ, Berlin CI. Auditory neuropathy. Brain. 1996;119 3:741–53.

21. Oysu C, Aslan I, Basaran B, Baserer N. The site of hearing loss in Refsum's disease. Int J Pediatr Otolrhinolaryngol. 2001;16:129–34.

22. Jutras B, Russell LJ, Hurteau AM, Chapdelaine M. Auditory neuropathy in siblings with Waardenburg's syndrome. Int J Pediatr Otorhinolaryngol. 2003;67(10):1133–42.

23. Corley VM, Crabbe LS. Auditory neuropathy and a mitochondrial disorder in a child: case study. J Am Acad Audiol. 1999;11:484–88.

24. Deltenre P, Mansbach AL, Bozet C, Clercx A, Hecox KE. Auditory neuropathy: a report on three cases with early onsets and major neonatal illnesses. Electroencephalogr Clin Neurophysiol. 1997;104(1):17–22.

25. Teagle HFB, Roush PA, Woodard JS, Hatch DR, Zdanski CJ, Buss E, Buchman CA. Cochlear implantation in children with auditory neuropathy spectrum disorder. Ear Hear. 2010;31(3):325–35.

26. Starr A, Isaacson B, Michaelewski H, Zeng F, Kong Y, Beale P, et al. A dominantly inherited progressive deafness affecting distal auditory nerve and hair cells. J Assoc Res Otolaryngol. 2004;5:411–26.

27. Starr A, Picton TW, Kim R. Pathophysiology of auditory neuropathy. In: Sininger Y, Starr A, editors. Auditory neuropathy: new perspectives in hearing disorders. San Diego: Singular-Thomson Learning; 2001. pp. 67–82.
28. Hall III JW. ECochG: clinical applications and populations; Auditory Neuropathy. In: Hall III JW, editor. New handbook of auditory evoked responses. Boston, MA: Pearson Education; 2007. pp. 138–53.
29. Demmler GJ. Summary of a workshop on surveillance for congenital cytomegalovirus disease. Rev Infect Dis. 1991;13:315–29.
30. Pass RF, Stagno S, Myers GJ. Outcome of symptomatic congenital cytomegalic infection: results of long term longitudinal follow-up. Pediatrics. 1980;66:758–62.
31. Ramsay ME, Miller R, Peckham CS. Outcome of confirmed symptomatic congenital cytomegalovirus infection. Arch Dis Child. 1991;66:1068–9.
32. Bopanna SB, Pass RF, Brit WJ, Stagno S, Alford A. Symptomatic congenital cytomegalovirus infection: neonatal morbidity and mortality. Pediatr Infect Dis J. 1992;11:93–99.
33. Noyola DE, Demmler GJ, Nelson CT, Griesser C, Wiliamson WD, Atkins JT, et al. Early predictors of neurodevelopmental outcome in symptomatic congenital cytomegalovirus infection. J Pediatr. 2001;138:325–31.
34. Fowler KB, Bopanna SB. Congenital cytomegalovirus (CMV) infection and hearing deficit. J Clin Virol. 2006;35:226–31.
35. Bradford RD, Cloud G, Lakeman AD, Bopanna S, Kimberlin DW, Jacobs R, et al. Detection of cytomegalovirus (CMV) DNA by polymerase chain reaction is associated with hearing loss in newborns with symptomatic congential CMV infection involving the central nervous system. J Infect Dis. 2005;191:227–33.
36. Bopanna SB, Fowler KB, Pass RF, Rivera LB, Bradford RD, Lakeman FD, Britt WJ. Congenital cytomegalovirus infection: association between virus burden in infancy and hearing loss. J Pediatr. 2005;146:817–23.
37. Noyola DE, Demmler GJ, Williamson WD, Greisser C, Sellers S, Llorente A, et al. Cytomegalovirus urinary excretion and long term outcome in children with congenital cytomegalovirus infection. Pediatr Infect Dis J. 2000;19:5050–10.
38. Myers EN, Stool S. Cytomegalic inclusion disease of the inner ear. Laryngoscope. 1968;78 11:1904–15.
39. Davis LE, Johnsson LG, Korufeld M. Cytomegalovirus labyrinthitis in an infant: morphological, virological and immunofluorescent studies. J Neuropathol Exp Neurol. 1981;40:9–19.
40. Bachor EH, Sudhoff R, Litschel R, Karmody CS. The pathology of the temporal bones of a child with acquired cytomegalovirus infection: studies by light microscopy, immunohistochemistry and polymerase chain reaction. J Pediatr Otorhinolaryngol. 2000;55: 215–24.
41. Rarey KE, Davis LE. Temporal bone histopathology 14 years after cytomegalic inclusion disease: a case study. Laryngoscope. 1993;103:904–9.
42. Sugiura S, Yoshikawa T, Nishiyama Y, Morishita Y, Sato E, Hattori T, Nakashima T. Detection of human cytomegalovirus DNA in perilymph of patients with sensorineural hearing loss using real-time PCR. J Med Virol. 2003;69:72–77.
43. Bauer PW, Parizi-Robinson M, Roland PS, Yegappan S. Cytomegalovirus in the perilymphatic fluid. Laryngoscope. 2005;115:223–25.
44. Nelson CT, Demmler GJ. Cytomegalovirus infection in the mother, fetus, and newborn infant. Clin Perinatol. 1997;24:151–60.
45. Kenneson A, Cannon MJ. Review and meta-analysis of the epidemiology of congenital cytomegalovirus (CMV) infection. Rev Med Virol. 2007;17:253–76.
46. Adler SP, Nigro G, Pereira L. Recent advances in the prevention and treatment of congenital cytomegalovirus infections. Semin Perinatol. 2007;31:10–18.
47. Bopanna SB, Rivera LB, Fowler KB, Mach M, Britt WJ. Intrauterine transmission of cytomegalovirus to infants of women with preconceptional immunity. N Engl J Med. 2001;344:1366–71.

48. McCluskey RR, Sandin R, Greene J. Detection of airborne cytomegalovirus in hospital rooms of immunocompromised patients. J Virol Methods. 1996;56:115–18.
49. Cannon MJ, Davis KF. Washing our hands of the congenital cytomegalovirus disease epidemic. BMC Public Health. 2005;5:70.
50. Staras SA, Flanders WD, Dollard SC, Pass RF, McGowan JE Jr, Cannon MJ. Influence of sexual activity on cytomegalovirus seroprevalence in the United States, 1988-1994. Sex Transm Dis. 2008;35:472–79.
51. Rivera LB, Bopanna SB, Fowler KB, Britt WJ, Stagno S, Pass RF. Predictors of hearing loss in children with symptomatic congenital cytomegalovirus infection. Pediatrics. 2000;110: 762–67.
52. Fowler K. Do perinatal factors predict hearing loss in children with asymptomatic congenital CMV infection? Am J Epidemiol. 2003;157:S84.
53. Barbi M, Binda S, Caroppo S, Ambrosetti U, Corbetta C, Sergi P. A wider role for congenital cytomegalovirus infection in sensorineural hearing loss. Pediatr Infect Dis J. 2003;22(1): 39–42.
54. Ciorba A, Bovo R, Trevisi P, Bianchini C, Arboretti R, Martini A. Rehabilitation and outcome of severe profound deafness in a group of 16 infants affected by congenital cytomegalovirus infection. Eur Arch Otorhinolaryngol. 2009;266:1539–46.
55. Kimberlin DW, Lin C-Y, Sanchez PJ, Demmler GJ, Dankner DW, Shelton M, et al. Effect of ganciclovir therapy on hearing in symptomatic congenital cytomegalovirus disease involving the central nervous system: a randomized, controlled trial. J Pediatr. 2003;143:16–25.
56. Zimmerman-Phillips S, Robbins AM, Osberger MJ. Assessing cochlear implant benefit in very young children. Ann Otol Rhinol Laryngol Suppl. 2000;109(12):42–3.
57. American Academy of Pediatrics Committee on Genetics. Health supervision for children with Down syndrome. Pediatrics. 2001;107:442–49.
58. Roizen N, Patterson D. Down's syndrome. Lancet. 2003;361(9365):1281–89.
59. Mitchell RB, Call E, Kelly J. Ear nose and throat disorders in children with Down syndrome. Laryngoscope. 2003;113(2):259–63.
60. Maurizi M, Ottaviani F, Paludetti G, Lungarotti S. Audiological findings in Down's children. Int J Pediatr Otorhinolaryngol. 1985;9(3):227–32.
61. Shott SR. Down syndrome: common otolaryngologic manifestations. Am J Med Genet C Semin Med Genet. 2006;142C(3):131–40.
62. Balkany TJ, Mischke RE, Downs MP, Jafek BW. Ossicular abnormalities in Down's syndrome. Otolaryngol Head Neck Surg. 1979;87(3):372–84.
63. Bilgin H, Kasemsuwan L, Schachern PA, Paparella MM, Le CT. Temporal bone studies of Down's syndrome. Arch Otolaryngol Head Neck Surg. 1996;122(3):271–75.
64. Blaser S, Propst EJ, Martin D, Feigenbaum A, James AL, Shannon P, Papsin BC. Inner ear dysplasia is common in children with Down syndrome (trisomy 21). Laryngoscope. 2006;116 12:2113–19.
65. Shibahara Y, Sando I. Congenital anomalies of the Eustachian tube in Down syndrome. Histopathologic case report. Ann Otol Rhinol Laryngol. 1989;98 (7) Pt 1:543–47.
66. Centers for Disease Control and Prevention. Down syndrome prevalence at birth – United States, 1983-1990. MMWR. 1994;43(33):617–22.
67. Shin M, Besser LM, Kucik JE, Lu C, Siffel C, Correa A; Congenital Anomaly Multistate Prevalence and Survival Collaborative. Prevalence of Down syndrome among children and adolescents in 10 regions of the United States. Pediatrics. 2009;124(6):1565–71.
68. American Speech-Language-Hearing Association. 2004. Guidelines for the audiologic assessment of children from birth to 5 years of age [Guidelines]. URL: www.asha.org/policy.
69. McDermott AL, Williams J, Kuo MJ, Reid AP, Proops DW. The role of bone anchored hearing aids in children with Down syndrome. Int J Pediatr Otorhinolaryngol. 2008;72(6):751–57.
70. Hans PS, England R, Prowse S, Young E, Sheehan PZ. UK and Ireland experience of cochlear implants in children with Down syndrome. Int J Pediatr Otorhinolaryngol. 2010;74(3): 260–64.

Chapter 20
Sexuality and Gynecological Care

Donald E. Greydanus and Hatim A. Omar

Abstract This chapter considers concepts of sexuality and gynecological care for children and adolescents with neurodevelopmental disabilities. Issues reviewed include normal human sexuality, sexuality education, sexual abuse, contraception, gynecological care, and sexual dysfunction. It is important for all children and youth including those with disabilities to have access to such important education and health care. All humans deserve optimum quality of life and those with disabilities should not be excluded from critical aspects of their own sexuality needs and management of gynecologic concerns or problems.

Introduction

Sex is a basic human need that arises in the subcortex and is controlled by the cerebral cortex in *Homo sapiens* [1]. The term sex is derived from the Latin word, sexus, that is rooted in the verb, secare – meaning to separate, cut, or divide. From an etymological perspective, sex refers to dividing plant and animal life (including human beings) into two separate groups, though the perplexities of human life complicate such a clear and pure separation because of such concepts as homosexuality, ambiguous genitalia, and transsexualism. Sexarche refers to the onset of coital behavior and sexarche initiates in most cultures of the world in the adolescent age group because of the inescapable influence of puberty. The role of the human brain in this regard is also important because of the impact of complex brain changes including the effect of key neurotransmitters such as dopamine, serotonin, and norepinephrine that are critical for normal sexual desire, sexual arousal, and orgasm in all human beings.

D.E. Greydanus (✉)
Department of Pediatrics and Human Development, Kalamazoo Center for Medical Studies, Michigan State University College of Human Medicine, Kalamazoo, MI 49008-1284, USA
e-mail: greydanus@kcms.msu.edu

D.R. Patel et al. (eds.), *Neurodevelopmental Disabilities*,
DOI 10.1007/978-94-007-0627-9_20, © Springer Science+Business Media B.V. 2011

Sexuality Education

Sexuality is complex process involving intricate interactions between one's biologic sex, sense of femaleness or maleness (i.e., core identity), and gender role behavior (sexual as well as non-sexual) [1]. Though parents and clinicians may assume that sexuality is not an important topic for discussion and education with children and youth with disabilities, research concludes that this is not the case [2–10]. Normal development for all children as well as youth and eventual acquisition of normal adulthood means that concepts of healthy sexuality must be learned and applied over a lifetime. This includes all children and youth, including those with neurodevelopmental disabilities such as mental retardation, autism, attention-deficit/hyperactivity disorder, cerebral palsy [11–16].

Parents and clinicians must understand that these children and youth remain at risk for adverse consequences of sexuality if not protected with key concepts of sexuality. Having a disability does not protect a child nor youth from sexual assault, unwanted adolescent pregnancy, or sexually transmitted diseases [1, 6, 17–20]. Some parents wish to closely protect their child or teen from harm and intentionally do not provide them with sexuality education. However, children do grow up and must learn to become adults caring for themselves as best as they can, often having sexual partners and becoming parents. Clinicians should not enable parents to ignore the emerging sexuality of their children. The role of the pediatric clinician is to help the child reach successful emancipation as an adult and not just get the child out of one's office in a timely manner.

Psychological Effects of Disability on Sexuality

Disability may complicate and even curtail the individual's attempt at acquiring a normal self-image in the inevitable journey from childhood to adulthood [1, 2, 11, 21–24]. These children or youth may experience rejection from peers for being different and may be subjected to being bullied or harassed. In attempts to prove normalcy, some may turn to sexual behavior. As puberty develops, youth become preoccupied with their changing bodies and are concerned with emerging body image issues that include comparisons with peers, worries about normalcy, and concepts of emerging sexuality with eventual sexual expression. Youth with disabilities have the added burden of dealing with real or perceived mental and/or physical abnormalities while seeking to develop a normal body image.

Concerns with abnormalities may lead to low self-esteem, poor body image, doubts about future self-sufficiency, doubts about the ability to reproduce and be a parent. This can lead to sexual experimentation in attempts to prove that one is normal and also because of the influence of peers and the media. Such experimentation may include masturbation, oral sex, vaginal sex, same-sex behavior. Media of the twenty-first century includes cable, movies, Internet social networks, and the print media which often teaches and stresses the belief that sexual behavior is

Table 20.1 Disorders associated with early/precocious puberty [1]

Cerebral palsy
Hydrocephalus
Obesity
Mental retardation
Williams syndrome
Meningomyelocele
Neurofibromatosis

important for all youth and that casual sex is the norm. The media teaches youth to have many sexual partners and not worry about such consequences as sexual abuse, rape, pregnancy, or diseases.

Some neurobehavioral conditions are associated with early or even precocious puberty (see Table 20.1) that can place this advanced adolescent in premature and unexpected sexual situations leading to abuse, unwanted pregnancy, and sexually transmitted diseases [1]. Sexual adequacy for adolescent females in contemporary society is often measured in terms of physical attractiveness. Concerns with unattractiveness due to perceived disabilities (i.e., low intelligence, Down syndrome appearance, physical limitations noted in cerebral palsy) may precipitate sexual behavior in attempts to prove normalcy without concern for negative consequences [1].

Low self-esteem may also result from the adverse effects of medication used to treat various conditions; thus, clinicians should carefully evaluate the effects of such drugs (as steroids, antipsychotics) on their young patients. Those individuals with neurodevelopmental disorders that are characterized by high levels of impulsivity (such as ADHD) may need continuous counseling regarding the consequences of high-risk behavior often seen with impulsive behavior.

Sexual Abuse

Unfortunately, sexual abuse is a common and devastating phenomenon in contemporary American society that affects children, youth, and adults. Those with disabilities, including mental retardation, are at increased risk for sexual assault [8, 15, 25–36]. Research notes 3 million cases of abuse in those with and without disabilities under 18 years of age, and these cases are categorized as sexual abuse (14%), physical abuse (26%), neglect (53%), and emotional abuse (5%) [1]. Studies note sexual abuse in 13% of females in the 8th and 10th grades versus 7% of males; sexual abuse reports rise to 27% in adult females and 16% in adult males [1]. The 2007 Youth Risk Surveillance Survey (YRBS) from the Centers for Disease and Prevention in Atlanta, Georgia, reported from their survey of high school students that nearly 10% (9.9%) of 15–19 year olds have been slapped, hit, or otherwise physically hurt by their boyfriends or girlfriends, and the prevalence rises as high as 15.7% [36]. Nearly 8% (7.8%) were forced to have sex in this YRBS study [36].

Table 20.2 Consequences of sexual assault [1, 31]

Psychosomatic disturbances (chronic headaches or abdominal pain)
Depression and other mental health disorders
Suicide attempts and completions
Pregnancy
Refractory seizure disorders
Runaway behavior
Juvenile delinquency and other youth violence
Juvenile prostitution
Severe parent–child/youth conflicts
School failure and dropout behavior
Sexually transmitted diseases
Chronic drug abuse
Chronic syncope
Eating disorders
Enuresis
Excessive masturbation
Sexual dysfunction
Sleep disturbances
Persistent hyperventilation syndrome

Unfortunately the risk for sexual assault rises in those with mental retardation and other disabilities [1, 31].

Rape is one of the fastest growing crimes of violence in America with most cases going unreported. As many as 70,000 cases of rape are reported in the United States each year, though the estimated annual number is over 500,000 [31]. In 2006 there were 272,350 victims of sexual assault (including rape and attempted rape) of all ages versus 191,670 in 2005; over 40% of rape victims are under 18 years of age and approximately one-sixth are under 12 years of age [33, 34]. Youth should be educated to this egregious example of violence including the growing tragedy of date rape and Internet predator abuse [33–37]. Clinicians should screen their patients for sexual assault including incest. Contemporary society is quite chaotic with high divorce rates, live-in-partners of parents, changing sex partners, and others. Potential consequences of sexual assault are noted in Table 20.2.

Clinician Counseling Concepts

Thus, clinicians should be prepared to provide education and counseling regarding sexuality issues for their children and adolescents with various disabilities [1, 15, 16, 31]. For example, discussions of masturbation can be directed to parents of young children, older children, and youth. The message is that masturbation is a normal aspect of human sexuality. Genital self-stimulation in children and youth with developmental disabilities may also result from diaper dermatitis in infancy, tight clothes, pinworm infection, phimosis, non-specific pruritus, and other medical issues. Youth should be warned about the classic paraphilic practice of sexual asphyxia syndrome (erotic asphyxiation, autoerotic asphyxia, breath control play) in adolescents and adults that involves masturbation with partial hanging in attempts to heighten orgasm; death from hanging (up to 1,000 per year in the United States) may result from this erotic paraphilia known at least since the 1600s.

Children and youth are naturally curious about sexuality issues and their questions can be addressed in a confidential, unprejudiced manner. Accurate, unbiased, balanced, and neutral sexuality information is important for all children and youth. Teach about the risks for sexual assault and evaluate for such a possibility in all children and youth including those with disabilities [6, 38–42]. Teach children and youth about appropriate and inappropriate genital/sexual touching; these vulnerable patients should understand self-protection skills. Information about prevention of sexual assault, pregnancy, and sexually transmitted diseases is important [15, 43–61]. Address issues regarding masturbation, menstruation, sexual behavior, reproduction, contraception, and other topics of interest and need to the pediatric patient [3, 31, 48, 49]. It is normal for some parents to avoid addressing these issues – the clinician should enter in as an important educator to these patients. Clinicians can address issues of social skills training (as for the child or youth with autism), possible lack of access to age-appropriate peers, lack of access to privacy, increased risk for bullying activity, and increased risk for sexual assault [31, 46, 51, 55].

Principles of Gynecological Care in Children and Adolescents with Neurodevelopmental Disabilities

Optimal gynecological care is recommended for all female children and adolescents, and this health-care maintenance should never be compromised because of lack of training or interest by the clinician nor because of the patient's degree of cognitive, mental, or physical disability [2, 10, 30, 31, 41, 52–60]. The gynecologic needs of all female pediatric patients are the same, though arriving at a correct diagnosis and providing optimal care may be more difficult or complicated because of various factors noted in those with neurodevelopmental disabilities (see Table 20.3) [30, 31, 41, 55–57].

It is vital for the clinician to obtain a complete gynecologic history, physical examination, and appropriate laboratory testing [58–60]. For example, collection of vaginal discharge for testing is with a cotton swab (calgiswab in prepubertal females) that is taken directly from the vagina or after normal saline irrigation [60]. It is not necessary to do endocervical sampling in the female child because the prepubertal vaginal lining is with columnar epithelium that allows for growth of *Neisseria gonorrhoeae* and *Chlamydia trachomatis*; thus, proper collection of the vaginal sampling will allow one to find these sexually transmitted organisms if present. Table 20.4 lists other tests that may be useful in evaluating gynecologic disorders in pediatric patients [58–60].

Communication with and education of the patient should always be in the appropriate developmental language. The parent or caregiver may be the main one to

Table 20.3 Factors complicating gynecologic care in females with neurodevelopmental disabilities [1, 31]

Cognitive disabilities with limitations in communication
Cognitive limits in gynecologic care noted in parents or clinicians
Refusal of patients to accept such care
Refusal of parents to allow such care
Refusal of clinicians to provide gynecologic care
Musculoskeletal complications: deformities, spasticity, contractures, autonomic dysreflexia, kyphoscoliosis, others
Coexistence of various neurological problems as epilepsy, tic disorders, others
Presence of decubitus ulcers leading to sitting position limits
Nutritional problems with complications of feeding tubes, gastroesophageal reflux

Table 20.4 Testing and specimen collection in pediatric gynecology [58–60]

Direct vaginal discharge collection in prepubertal females
Pap smear collection in post-pubertal females
Cervical testing in post-pubertal females for *N. gonorrhoeae* and *C. trachomatis*
Urine collection for *N. gonorrhoeae* and *C. trachomatis* using polymerase chain reaction (PCR) technology as an alternative to direct cervical sampling
Testing for *Shigella* in vaginal fluid of prepubertal females if indicated
Testing for Group A *Streptococcus* or other bacteria on vaginal fluid
pH of vaginal fluid
Wet mount with normal saline testing of vaginal fluid looking for clue cells trichomonads, others
Potassium hydroxide (KOH) testing of vaginal fluid looking for *Candida*
Anal swabs if indicated: brushing a cotton swab over the perianal region will stimulate an anal wink if present

communicate with if the patient is not able to deal with their issues due to physical, cognitive, or mental limitations. Depending on the age of the female patient and the specific circumstances, education can be given regarding the periodicity of gynecologic examinations, need for self-breast examinations (or exams by the caregiver if indicated), and options as needed regarding such issues as hygiene, menstruation, contraception [30].

In menstruating females, a careful menstrual history should not be forgotten by clinicians because the patient has a neurodevelopmental disability of varying severity [58]. The menstrual history includes age of menses, onset of menses (menarche), and a description of the menstrual flow (i.e., duration, frequency, presence of menstrual cramps) [58]. A menstrual calendar (recorded by the patient or, if necessary, by the caregiver) is very beneficial in identifying normal variations in adolescent menstrual patterns versus specific menstrual disorders, such as premenstrual syndrome, dysmenorrhea, or moodiness as well as agitation related to menstruation [57, 58]. Plotting behavior or mood changes can reveal unpleasant behaviors before the onset of a menstrual period. Physical and behavior changes that are identified need to be differentiated from a variety of urologic and gynecologic disorders [58].

Pediatric Gynecological Care

Complaints in the vulvovaginal area in female children are quite common and usually readily managed by the primary care clinician [31, 59, 60]. Asking the child about any concerns in this body system and a simple inspection of the external genitalia during general well-child evaluations are helpful to alert the child (and parents or guardians) that they can discuss the areas of pediatric gynecology and prepare the child if more detailed examinations are needed at some point. If this female has difficulty expressing herself, carefully search for clues to discomfort and disease. Such clues include a fever without clear reason or crying on urination with a foul-smelling urine that should evoke one to consider a diagnosis of urinary tract infection (UTI) [30, 31, 55]. Masturbation can lead to excessive vulvar irritation and inflammation while having a vaginal discharge with a history of frequent use of antibiotics may be an indication for *Candida albicans* vaginitis. If *Trichomonas vaginalis* is found on urinalysis, suspect sexual abuse.

Calming measures during the examination consist of such techniques as having the child gently placed in the mother's lap for the gynecologic examination and allow use of toys for the child. Various examining positions may be used including, as noted, having the young child sit in the mother's lap, lithotomy position (supine and feet in the stirrups), frog-leg, knee–chest position [60]. Sometimes sedation is necessary to conduct a proper examination, and the child should always be afforded a lack of excessive pain or discomfort. As part of preventive care measures, the patient and parent should be educated to the importance of the human papillomavirus vaccine for those 9–26 years of age in both females and males to prevent later HPV disorders including cervical cancer as an adult. Science predicts that untold thousands of females will be saved from cervical cancer death over the course of the twenty-first century because of the HPV vaccine and females with disabilities should not be excluded from such optimal, recommended, and well-researched preventive measures [31].

Vulvar Rash

Non-specific vulvovaginitis may develop often due to ineffectual hygiene, irritation from caustic agents (as bubble baths, synthetic undergarments), lack of estrogenization, and others [58–60]. Symptomatology may include redness of the vulva, vulvovaginal pain, discharge, and burning. Vulvovaginal cultures are negative, and management includes instruction in avoiding identified irritating agents, improving hygiene, and use of barrier creams. Oral antibiotics are useful if cultures are positive. If the child complains of pain with urination, consider a urinary tract infection (UTI) and obtain a urinalysis as well as urine culture. Anatomic defects (as urethral cyst, urethral prolapse, others) may cause leakage of urine with a secondary vulvar rash. Treat the UTI with appropriate antibiotics. Repeated infections should trigger further work-up for anatomic defects, and referral to a nephrologist or urologist is recommended along with appropriate imaging studies.

Vulvar erythema may also indicate diaper dermatitis in the infant, usually 9–12 months of age. In addition to the erythema, there may be skin erosion and a papular rash in the diaper area due to irritation from urine and stool; there may also be "satellite lesions" involving the skin folds due to *C. albicans* infection. Management includes hygiene with mild soap and warm water, use of petroleum jelly or zinc oxide creams, and possible use of low potency steroids. If *Candida* is a complication, brief use of antifungal cream or ointment will help. If an irritant rash occurs in the older girl, it may be due to an irritant causing contact dermatitis in the genital area with variable genital redness and maculopapular rash. Basic management includes removal of the irritating agent, use of a barrier cream, and possibly low potency steroid cream, as 1% hydrocortisone cream.

Vulvar erythema along with a painful rash and vaginal discharge points to a diagnosis of bacterial vulvovaginitis and may be due to a variety of bacteria, including *Streptococcus* (Groups A and B), *Escherichia coli, Shigella. Streptococcal vulvovaginitis* is quite common in girls and is due to autoinoculation from an ongoing pharyngeal infection or colonization; intense vulvar redness is characteristic of this streptococcal infection. The genital rash is red, maculopapular, and sometimes "sandpaper like." Management of bacterial vulvovaginitis includes appropriate topical and/or oral antibiotics.

Lichen sclerosus is a chronic disorder of unknown etiology that presents with vulvar skin thinning often in an "hourglass" pattern along with vulvar pruritus, excoriation, burning, bleeding, and secondary bacterial infection. The loss of vulvar architecture that results may be misdiagnosed as sexual abuse in the female child. Management includes use of topical steroids (as Clobetasol) tapered over several weeks. Barrier creams (as A&D ointment/magic barrier cream) is also used.

A vulvar rash may also be due to a drug-induced eruption which resolves with removal of the offending agent and sometimes use of steroid creams or even oral steroids for severe conditions. A scaly vulvar rash that is chronic may indicate psoriasis and may improve with steroid cream. Referral to a pediatric dermatologist or pediatric gynecologist is needed for severe and/or rapidly progressive conditions.

If the female child presents with several [often 2–6], painful vulvar/genital lesions that are raised and umbilicated, consider molluscum contagiosum that is caused by pox virus and due to either self-inoculation or sexual abuse. As with other confusing vulvar rashes, a biopsy can be helpful to make the correct diagnosis. Sometimes there is confusion between molluscum and warts from human papillomavirus infection. Molluscum management includes curettage, cryotherapy, and perhaps use of various medications in the immunocompromised child; these medications include imiquimod, cantharidin, cimetidine, ritonavir, and/or cidofovir. A pediatric dermatologist is recommended for resistant and/or extensive molluscum contagiosum infections [60].

Vaginal Discharge

Vaginal discharge in a prepubertal girl raises concerns of sexual abuse, and causative sexually transmitted diseases are considered in the differential diagnosis. Thus, a carefully history and early index of suspicion are important, since those with neurodevelopmental disabilities are at increased risk of abuse, as noted previously. The presence of a malodorous vaginal discharge should prompt the possibility of a vaginal foreign body, such as toilet paper, but virtually any object may be found – toys, beads, crayon, others. Vaginal bleeding may be seen as well.

A careful examination (sometimes under sedation) is necessary to find and remove the foreign body which may be accomplished in young girls via vaginal irrigation with normal saline placed by a pediatric feeding tube [60]. Antibiotics may be necessary if secondary bacterial infection is present and estrogen (Premarin) cream may be used in the vulvovaginal area in some cases. Toxic shock syndrome (TSS) may arise from a vaginal foreign body which requires treatment for shock as well as infection/sepsis in addition to removal of the foreign body. Other conditions may cause a malodorous discharge with local irritation and inflammation, such as a recto-vaginal fistula due to Crohn's disease or previous surgery. Surgical correction of the fistula is then needed. Vaginal discharge and perianal pruritus (pruritus ani) may also be seen in a young girl with pinworm vulvovaginitis due to infestation with *Enterobius vermicularis*. There is a fecal–oral transmission, and a scotch tape applied to the perianal area will help to identify this cause. A vaginal swab applied after shining a light on the area with subsequent microscopic examination will also identify the pinworm infestation. Management is with oral mebendazole (100 mg that is repeated in 7 days); treat family members as well and emphasize good hygiene with good hand washing to prevent repeat episodes.

Vaginal Bleeding

Vaginal bleeding may be an indication of sexual abuse in which there is genital/anal/perianal bruising and vaginal/rectal bleeding due to blunt penetrating trauma. Sometimes the damage is due to accidental trauma or injury from falls, for example. Sexual abuse and the suspicion of sexual abuse must be reported to local child protective agencies and/or local law enforcement. The child needs an immediate examination by a clinician trained in forensic evaluations with forensic material appropriately collected. Evaluation of potential or actual sexual abuse requires a team approach that involves a knowledgeable clinician, social worker, mental health counselor. The clinician should always remember that a number of conditions may be falsely confused with effects of sexual abuse – these include clitoral and/or labial hypertrophy, imperforate hymen, vaginal ridges/septum, ambiguous genitalia [60].

Another common condition that may be mistaken for sexual abuse is labial agglutination, a physiologic condition induced by the absence of estrogen in the prepubertal child. Management usually starts with "watchful waiting" and then application of topical estrogen therapy as twice daily use of conjugated estrogen (Premarin) cream for 2 weeks and then once a day for 1–2 weeks. Mechanical separation under local analgesia or anesthesia is used only as a last resort while surgical intervention is utilized if all else fails and/or for emergency urinary retention arises.

Vulvar hematoma may result from accidental straddle-type injures. A congenital vulvar hematoma may also been seen that is a collection of angioblastic mesenchyme. Though its finding may be alarming to the parents, it usually involutes between 2 and 10 years of age. Other vascular defects can be ruled out with imaging studies and approximately one in four requires medical or surgical management. Tight clothing may lead to this condition because of the impact of chronic trauma to thin, non-estrogenized vulvar tissue.

It should always be remembered that there are many causes for vaginal bleeding in a prepubertal girl that include vaginal infections (as Group A *Streptococcus*), lichen sclerosus, vaginal foreign body, precocious puberty, urethral prolapse, and genitourinary neoplasms (such as rhabdomyosarcoma and granulosa cell tumor of the ovary). Management of vaginal bleeding depends on the underlying etiology. For example, urethral prolapse causing vaginal bleeding is treated with conjugated estrogen (Premarin) cream. Treatment of some of these other causes has been reviewed previously.

Adolescent Gynecology

A thorough history and physical examination are necessary for the pubertal female as well. The exam should establish a sexually maturity rating or Tanner stage for the female that can be recorded and followed as she progresses from stage 1 to stage 5. Preventive health care for all adolescent females includes sexuality education as noted previously and encouragement of all recommended vaccines, including hepatitis B, hepatitis A, and human papillomavirus vaccines.

If she is not sexual active, a pelvic examination is usually not needed unless there is a history of sexual assault or the presence of specific gynecologic symptomatology [30, 31, 41]. A pelvic exam is also not immediately needed if she is not sexually active and yet requests contraception before sexarche or oral contraceptives are prescribed to treat menstrual disorders. A variety of techniques are noted in the literature to assist in a recommended pelvic exam in difficult patients such as those with contractures, cognitive limitations [31, 41, 55–61]. Such techniques include diverse adjustments in position (leg elevation without hip abduction, V-position, M-position, frog-leg position), careful use of the long, narrow Huffman–Graves speculum, or use of an exam without a speculum, one-finger bimanual exam, Q-tip Pap smear, or a rectoabdominal exam [1, 31, 41, 55]. As noted earlier, an examination under sedation may be needed as well as use of pelvic ultrasound, pelvic CT, or pelvic MRI.

Principles of periodic Papanicolaou (Pap) smears remain a controversial and ever-changing topic in adolescent gynecology, though current guidelines suggest such a procedure should start 3 years after onset of coitus (sexarche) or by age 21 if she is not sexually active [62]. The purpose of such exams is to screen for cervical cancer which is due to chronic HPV cervical infection and can cause death in adulthood. Conventional or liquid-based Pap smear techniques may be used. If the conventional Pap smear is selected by the clinician, a spatula and cytobrush or cervical broom is used and the specimen is smeared on a glass slide that is then fixed with a spray or liquid fixative [62].

Liquid-based smears utilize a cervical broom placing the collected cervical specimen in a liquid container. The liquid-based Pap smear can be beneficial in augmenting the collected specimen adequacy in situations where cervical visualization is difficult or impossible. Other advantages of the liquid-based method include having less extraneous matter on the smear, heightened sensitivity, and the potential for identifying sexually transmitted agents (such as the human papillomavirus [HPV], *N. gonorrhoeae*, and *C. trachomatis*) [63].

Any adolescent can be infected with various sexually transmitted disease (STD) agents whether involved in voluntary or involuntary sexual behavior. Vaginal discharge may be to such STD agents as *N. gonorrhoeae*, *C. trachomatis*, herpes simplex virus, *T. vaginalis*. Vaginal discharge in young adolescents may also be due to physiologic leukorrhea and confused with a STD. In physiologic leukorrhea there is a normal discharge that is due to estrogen stimulation occurring well before menarche (onset of menses) and varies from clear to white in color, mucoid to watery in consistency, and minimal to moderate in amount. Typically there is no odor or genital irritation, and the teenager or guardian may note yellowish staining of underwear that can be prevented by pretreating laundry with an enzyme-based bleach.

Vaginal discharge may also be due to bacterial vaginosis that is due to infection with anaerobic microbes, particularly *Gardnerella vaginalis*. It is not common in non-sexually active females and also not common in prepubertal females [60]. It may be noted in lesbians and females who use vaginal douching. Bacterial vaginosis is asymptomatic in some females, though most note malodorous vaginal discharge that is greyish with a "fishy" odor on KOH prep (positive whiff test). A wet mount of vaginal fluid reveals "clue" cells, and the pH of this fluid is over 4.5. In less common situations that are extensive or severe, there may be other problems such as dyspareunia or other pain (pelvic and/or abdominal). Standard treatment is with metronidazole (500 mg orally twice a day for 7 days) or gel (0.75%) – one full applicator (5 g) intravaginally once a day for 5 days.

Adolescent females may develop a number of genital conditions that may or may not be related to sexual behavior [52]. For example, the Epstein–Barr virus can be transmitted via intimate contact with a sex partner and lead to infectious mononucleosis. Hepatitis A and hepatitis B can be sexually transmitted and vaccination for both these viruses is recommended, as previously noted. Also as noted earlier, Group A *Streptococcus* may cause vaginal discharge and can be due to autoinoculation or sexual contact from a pharyngeal site. A forgotten, retained tampon (or other objects) can lead to foreign body vaginitis characterized by a very malodorous vaginal discharge; cognitively limited patients can vaginally insert a variety of objects, much like that noted with young children.

Clinicians may also find such conditions as tinea cruris, contact dermatitis, or molluscum contagiosum. Contact dermatitis can involve any part of the genitals and can be due to contact and sensitization from a variety of materials such as latex condoms or diaphragms, sexual lubricants, spermicides, deodorant soaps, bubble bath or bath salts, douches, underclothing dyes, patterned toilet tissue, "feminine hygiene" sprays or suppositories. Removal of the offending agent is needed along with sitz baths, topical compresses (Burrow's solution), and/or mild topical steroids.

Adolescents may be subjected to various infestations [52]. For example, intense vulvar pruritus (often worse at night) with excoriations can be found with the presence of the eggs ("nits") or active adult forms of Phthirius pubis that are evident on examination of pubic hair with a hand lens; these nits may also be found on perineum, axillary hair, or eyelashes. Crusted red papules may be seen at the sites of feeding. Pubic lice are acquired from sexual contact but may also be spread with fomites, such as bedding or clothes that are shared, such as with infected siblings and thus, involve children. Treatment is with 1% permethrin with second-line treatments such as use of lindane or pyrethrin; repeat the treatment in 7–10 days to kill lice hatched from the initial treatment. Petrolatum can be used to treat lice in eyelashes. Clothing and bedding should be thoroughly cleaned via laundering.

Another infestation that may occur is due to the mite, Sarcoptes scabiei, in which female mites burrow in the stratum corneum to deposit eggs leading to intense pruritus (worse at night) that can also result in various skin lesions, such as papules, vesicles, pustules, and burrows and linear or "S"-shaped tunnels may be seen on the hands (especially finger webs), wrists, axillae, belt line, and areolae. These lesions are also found on the penis and scrotum in males. The diagnosis is with microscopic examination of material scraped with a scalpel blade from non-excoriated lesions placed on a glass slide and covered with a cover slip, look for mites, eggs, or feces. Treat with 5% permethrin cream that is applied from the neck down for 8–14 h and repeated in 7–10 days to kill the mites that hatched from eggs after the initial treatment. Treat all members in the family and clean infested clothes and bedding; alternatively clothes and bedding can be stored in a plastic bag for 72 h.

Menstrual Disorders/Concerns

Any adolescent female may present with a variety of breast or menstrual disorders [52, 58]. Menstrual conditions can include amenorrhea (primary or secondary), dysmenorrhea, dysfunctional uterine bleeding (DUB), premenstrual tension syndrome [1, 2, 41, 56–58]. A recent study of adolescent females with Down syndrome, autism, and cerebral palsy noted a link between behavioral problems (as mood changes) and irregular menstrual bleeding, especially in those with autism [64]. Females with trisomy 21 have increased incidence for thyroid disorders that may lead to amenorrhea or dysfunction uterine bleeding. The presence of Turner syndrome should be considered in any adolescent female with short stature and amenorrhea because of premature ovarian failure. Youth with various neurodevelopmental disorders may be prescribed neuroleptic medication or anticonvulsants that may lead to drug-induced menstrual dysfunction [65].

In youth with severe cognitive limitations, education by the clinician may be confined to hygiene improvement and sex abuse prevention. Proper hygiene may be an issue for some patients and their guardians. The clinician may need to recommend various means to control problematic menstruation and related hygiene concerns; these recommendations may include behavioral modification training, use of non-steroidal anti-inflammatory drugs, prescription of hormonal treatment (i.e., Depo-Provera, combined oral contraceptives), or even gynecologic surgery (i.e., endometrial ablation or hysterectomy) [7, 15, 41, 56]. Perceived abnormalities may prompt the request for cosmetic surgery that may or may not be needed in attempts to prove one's self-esteem. Counseling can also help this vulnerable patient prevent unnecessary surgery, as noted with the recent trend for cosmetic surgery in those under 18 years of age, as breast augmentation and liposuction [66].

Contraception

Sexually active youth and those not having sex, but presenting with questions, should receive accurate and balanced information about contraception [1, 31, 49, 52]. In addition to pregnancy prevention, oral contraceptives can be presented as medication useful in treatment of a variety of conditions, including dysmenorrhea, dysfunctional uterine bleeding [52, 58]. As noted, the au courant media and social networking of the Internet are promoting a promiscuous society without fear of consequences from unprotected sex with multiple partners. Youth should be taught about STDs, effectiveness of condom use, and available contraceptive methods. Those who are sexually active should be screened for STDs and placed on acceptable contraception if requested by the teenager [2, 30, 49, 52, 55, 57, 61–65, 67–69]. Such instruction should also include accurate information about emergency contraception.

Methods such as the intravaginal ring and barrier contraception are often not the ideal choice for those with developmental disabilities unless this female possesses the physical and cognitive abilities to use the ring as directed or the barrier contraceptive with each act of coitus [49, 61–65, 67–69]. There may be concerns with estrogen-containing contraceptives because of risks for thromboembolic events or concerns with Depo-Provera because of risks for increased menstrual bleeding or loss of bone density.

Those with anorexia nervosa or if wheelchair bound may not be good candidates for prolonged Depo-Provera use [49, 68–71]. Nevertheless, the most popular contraceptive for adolescent females with developmental disabilities (such as cognitive limits) is often depo-medroxy-progesterone acetate (Depo-Provera), because of its high contraceptive efficacy for 3 months with each dose, its intramuscular administration, and its side effect of amenorrhea. As with all contraceptives and all medications, the risks of potential side effects must be balanced with the potential benefits of their use.

Thus, the clinician should provide careful, comprehensive counseling regarding contraception to these adolescent females. Concerns of fertility exist in the minds of adolescent and adult females with disabilities and should be addressed by the clinician in discussion with the patient or in actual testing as warranted by the specific situation [72]. Finally, the topic of sterilization for severely disabled youth remains a very controversial and complex topic in today's diverse society [54, 73–75].

Sexual Dysfunction

As the adolescent female progresses toward adulthood, issues of physical sexual expression and reproductive capacity become more important and, thus, sexuality education should be available from an informed, sensitive, and caring clinician who is not embarrassed with such topics. Discussion of sexuality can be complicated by cognitive dysfunction noted in various disabilities (see Table 20.5). Concerns of general society regarding the sexuality of adolescents including those with mental retardation and other disabilities have been present since *H. sapiens* emerged over 60,000 years ago. However, it is clear that healthy sexual functioning is an important part of healthy as well as joyful living, and a major cause of sexual dysfunction is lack of knowledge about normal sexuality.

A variety of sexual dysfunctions (see Table 20.5) are noted in adolescent and adult females including those with various disabilities. Sexual dysfunction may arise because of having certain disorders (i.e., cognitive limits, physical limits, mental disorders such as depression), medications used to treat various conditions, or complications that may arise, such as sexual abuse [76–78]. Prescribed medications that may induce sexual dysfunction include antidepressants (selective serotonin reuptake inhibitors [SSRIs] or selective norepinephrine reuptake inhibitors [SNRIs]), anticonvulsants (as valproic acid that leads to hyperprolactinemia and sexual dysfunction), and antipsychotics. Removal of the offending medications and replacement with those having less or absence adverse effect on sexual functioning are often helpful in this regard.

Sexual dysfunction that arises in adolescence may continue into adulthood when society becomes more accepting of sexual function in general. It is a general principle of medicine that pathophysiologic disorders (as diabetes mellitus, hypertension,

Table 20.5 Sexual dysfunctions in females

1. Lack of sexual desire
2. Inhibited sexual desire: hypoactive sexual desire disorder [HSDD]
3. Sexual pain disorder/dyspareunia
   (due to vaginitis, lichen sclerosus, imperforated hymen, pelvic inflammatory disease, congenital genital disorders, endometriosis, others)
4. Orgasmic dysfunction (anorgasmia)

Table 20.6 Disorders associated with intellectual disability

Autism
Cerebral palsy
Down syndrome
Fetal alcohol syndrome
Fragile X syndrome
Meningomelocele
Neurofibromatosis
Prader–Willi syndrome
Velocardiofacial syndrome
William syndrome
Others

obesity) should be identified and managed as soon as possible – such as during adolescence and before adulthood. The same principle applies to the development and correction of sexual dysfunction in adolescents. Failure to correct problems and disorders in adolescence typically leads to the worsening of these conditions in adulthood and with earlier complications or sequelae.

Youth with visible deformities may experience interference with sexual expression and need special counseling in this regard; these deformities include amputations, ostomies, paraplegia, or abnormal genitalia [1, 31]. Youth with colostomies can be anxious about the odor from the ostomy while those with arthritis may be in pain, or a youth with spinal cord lesions may have painful bed sores. Youth may be bullied by others especially if they appear different from peers because of having cognitive limitations, physical deformities, and/or mental disorders. Feelings of being inadequate and problems with sexual performance may arise in any youth or adult with regard to their sexual lives. However, perhaps the major discomfort is found in parents and society in general when considering the sexuality of their children with various disabilities (Table 20.6).

Conclusions

Adolescence brings complex challenges for parents, clinicians, society, and for the teenagers as well [79]. Consideration of healthy sexuality in adolescents including those with disabilities remains a controversial concept for contemporary society [80]. Adolescent females are involved in a wide variety of voluntary and forced sexual behavior, and the existence of neurodevelopmental disabilities does not negate these issues nor does it negate the importance of healthy sexuality functioning for these youth [85–88].

The 2002 National Survey of Family Growth reports that 47% of never-married female adolescents (aged 15–19 years) have been sexually active in contrast to 46% of the same age males [80]. The 2007 Centers for Disease Control and Prevention (CDC)'s Youth Risk Behavior Surveillance (YRBS) confirms such data noting that 47.8% of 15–19 year olds report being sexually experienced versus 46.2% in 1991

[36]. Indeed, sexuality is a ubiquitous and omnipresent part of human living and youth demand their share of this pervasive phenomenon.

Clinicians caring for youth need to be purveyors of sexuality education to youth and that includes provision of needed gynecological care to female adolescents with instruction in sexuality education that covers such controversial areas as masturbation, contraception, sexual dysfunction. Clinicians should learn basic principles of pediatric and adolescent gynecology for all female adolescents, including those with neurodevelopmental disabilities. Problems identified in childhood and adolescence can be corrected and lead to a healthier as well as happier adulthood. Health-care professionals should be educated to care for those with disabilities and focus on improving the quality of life for their patients [81–84]. Part of this effort must be focused on the sexuality and gynecologic needs of pediatric and adolescent females with neurodevelopmental disabilities.

References

1. Greydanus DE, Rimsza ME, Newhouse PA. Adolescent sexuality and disability. Adolesc Med Clin. 2002;13:223–47.
2. Shah P, Norlin C, Logsdon L, Samson-Fang L. Gynecological care for adolescents with disability: physician comfort, perceived barriers, and potential solutions. J Pediatric Adolesc Gynecol. 2005;18:101–4.
3. Neufeld JA, Klingbeil F, Bryen DN, et al. Adolescent sexuality and disability. Phys Med Rehabil Clin N Am. 2002;13:857–73.
4. Baxter P. Disability and sexuality. Dev Med Child Neurol. 2008;50:563.
5. Sawyer SM, Phelan PD, Bowes G. Reproductive health in young women with cystic fibrosis: knowledge, behaviour, and attitudes. J Adolesc Health. 1995;17:46–50.
6. Siddiqi SU, Van Dyke DC, Donohoue P, et al. Premature sexual development in individuals with neurodevelopmental disabilities. Dev Med Child Neuro. 1999;41:392–95.
7. Biggs WS. The family physician's challenge: guiding the adolescent with chronic illness to adulthood. Clin Fam Pract. 2000;2:1–11.
8. Cheng MM, Udry JR. Sexual behaviors of physically disabled adolescent in the United States. J Adolesc Health. 2002;31:48–58.
9. Suris JC, Resnick MD, Cassuto N, et al. Sexual behavior of adolescents with chronic disease and disability. J Adolesc Health. 1996;19:124–31.
10. Alexander B, Schrauben S. Outside the margins: youth who are different and their special health care needs. Prim Care Clin Office Pract. 2007;33:285–303.
11. Pratt HD, Greydanus DE. Intellectual disability (mental retardation) in children and adolescents. Prim Care Clin Office Pract. 2007;34:375–86.
12. Daily DK, Ardinger HH, Holmes GE. Identification and evaluation of mental retardation. Am Fam Phys. 2000;61:1059–67.
13. Tyler CV Jr., Bourguet C. Primary care of adults with mental retardation. J Fam Pract. 1997;44:487–94.
14. Murphy N, Young PC. Sexuality in children and adolescents with disabilities. Dev Med. 2005;47:640–4.
15. Murphy NA, Elias ER. Council on children with disabilities. Pediatrics. 2006;118:398–403.
16. American Academy of Pediatrics. Sexuality education of children and adolescents with developmental disabilities. Committee on children with disabilities. Pediatrics. 1996;97:275–8.
17. Freedman RI, Boyer NC. The power to choose: supports for families caring for individuals with developmental disabilities. Health Soc Work. 2000;25:59–68.

18. Rupp R, Rosenthal SL. Parental influences on adolescent sexual behaviors. Adoles Med State Art Rev. 2007;18:460–70.
19. Tannila A, Kokkonen J, Jarvelin MR. The long-term effects of children's early-onset disability on marital relationships. Dev Med Child Neuro. 1999;38:567–77.
20. Sulkes SB. Mental retardation in children and adolescents. In: Greydanus DE, Pratt HD, Patel DR, editors. Behavioral pediatrics. 2nd ed. New York, NY: iUniverse Publishing; 2006. pp. 66–83.
21. Goldson E. Behavioral issues in the care of children with special health care needs. In: Greydanus DE, Pratt HD, Patel DR, editors. Behavioral pediatrics. 2nd ed. New York, NY: iUniverse Publishing; 2006. pp. 182–205.
22. Birnkrant DJ, Hen J, Stern RC. The adolescent with cystic fibrosis. Adolesc Med. 1994;5: 249–58.
23. Rew L. Sexual health of adolescents with chronic health conditions. Adoles Med State Art Rev. 2007;18:519–29.
24. Greydanus DE, Fonseca H, Pratt HD. Childhood and adolescent sexuality. In: Greydanus DE, Pratt HD, Patel DR, editors. Behavioral pediatrics. 2nd ed. New York, NY: iUniverse Publishing; 2006. pp. 295–330.
25. Pratt HD, Greydanus DE. Violence: concepts of its impact on children and youth. Pediatr Clin North Am. 2003;50:963–1003.
26. Palusci VJ, McHugh MT. Abuse in the child and adolescent. In: Greydanus DE, Pratt HD, Patel DR, editors Behavioral pediatrics. 2nd ed. New York, NY: iUniverse Publishing; 2006. pp. 769–811.
27. Adams JA. Sexual abuse and the adolescent patient. In: Greydanus DE, Patel DR, Pratt HD, editors. Essentials of adolescent medicine. New York, NY: McGraw-Hill Medical Publications; 2006. pp. 333–40.
28. Broecker JD, Ross LS. Developmental delay, including Down syndrome. In: Hillard PJA, editor The 5-minute obstetrics and gynecology consult. Philadelphia, PA: Wolters Kluwer/Lippincott Williams Wilkins; 2008. pp. 90–91.
29. Gushurst CA, Palusci VJ. Medical evaluation of child sexual abuse. In: Greydanus DE, Patel DR, Reddy VN, Feinberg AN, Omar HA, editors. Handbook of clinical pediatrics: An update for the ambulatory pediatrician. Singapore: World Scientific; 2010. pp. 665–96.
30. Greydanus DE, Bhave S. Adolescents with mental retardation. Recent Adv Pediatr. 2006;17 14:174–92.
31. Omar HA, Greydanus DE, Tsitsika AK, Patel DR, Merrick J, editors Pediatric and adolescent sexuality and gynecology: principles for the primary care clinician. New York, NY: Nova Science; 2010.
32. Felitti VJ, Anda RF, Nordenberg D, et al. Relationship of childhood abuse and household dysfunction to many leading causes of death in adults: the adverse childhood experience (ACE) study. Am J Prev Med. 1998;14:245–7.
33. Victimization C, 2006. US Department of justice. Bureau of justice. Statistics, Washington DC. NCJ 219413 December, 2007. URL: www.ojp.usdoj.gov
34. Muran D. Sexual assault. In: Hillard PJA, editor The 5-minute obstetrics and gynecology consult. Philadelphia, PA: Wolters Kluwer/Lippincott Williams Wilkins; 2008. pp. 602–3.
35. MacKay AP, Duran C. Adolescent Health in the United States, 2007. Washington, DC: National Center for Health Statistics, Department of Health and Human Services Publications, 2008:1034.
36. Centers for Disease Control and Prevention Surveillance Summaries. MMWR 2008;57 (SS-4):1–136.
37. Alan Guttmacher Institute. Into a new world: young women's sexual and reproductive lives. New York, NY: Alan Guttmacher Institute; 1998.
38. Hibbard RA, Desch LW. Committee on child abuse and neglect and council on children with disabilities. Pediatrics. 2007;119 (5):1018–21.

39. Dupe SR, Anda RF, Felitti VJ, et al. Childhood abuse, household dysfunction, and the risk of attempted suicide throughout the life span. Findings from the Adverse childhood experience study. JAMA. 2001;286:3089–96.
40. Greydanus DE, Patel DR. The female athlete: before and beyond puberty. Pediatr Clin North Amer. 2002;50:222–40.
41. Quint EH. Gynecological health care for adolescents with developmental disabilities. Adolesc Med. 1999;10:221–9.
42. Sionean S, Clemente D, Wingoode GM, et al. Psychosocial and behavioural correlates of refusing unwanted sex among African-American adolescent females. J Adolesc Health. 2002;30:55–63.
43. Greydanus DE, Pratt HD, Dannison LL. Sexuality education programs for youth: current state of affairs and strategies for the future. J Sex Educ Ther. 1995;21 (4):238–54.
44. Ott MA, Santelli JS. Approaches to adolescent sexuality education. Adolesc Med State Art Rev. 2007;18:558–70.
45. Rome ES. Adolescent sexuality. In: Greydanus DE, Patel DR, Pratt HD, editors Essential adolescent medicine. New York, NY: McGraw-Hill Medical Publications; 2006. pp. 481–96.
46. Brown JD, Strasburger VC. From Calvin Klein to Paris Hilton and MySpace: adolescents, sex, and the media. Adol Med State Art Rev. 2007;18:484–507.
47. Greydanus DE, editor. Caring for your adolescent. 2nd ed. Elk Grove Village, IL: American Academy of Pediatrics; 2003.
48. Fonseca H, Greydanus DE. Sexuality in the child, teen, and young adult: Concepts for the clinician. Prim Care Clin Office Pract. 2007;34:275–92.
49. Greydanus DE, Rimsza ME, Matytsina L. Contraception for college students. Pediatr Clin North Am. 2005;52:135–61.
50. Pratt HD, Pratt MA, Sackett M. Youth survival: addressing the role of promoting the acquisition of the prosocial trial and other survival skills in youth. Prim Care Clin Office Pract. 2007;34:219–25.
51. Mitchell KJ, Finkelhor D, Wolak J. Risk factors for and impact of online sexual solicitation of youth. JAMA. 2001;285 3011–14:2001.
52. Greydanus DE, Patel DR, Patel HD, editors Essential adolescent medicine. New York, NY: McGraw-Hill Medical Publishing; 2006.
53. Greydanus DE, Strasburger VC. Adolescent medicine. Prim Care Clin Office Pract. 2006;33:269–612.
54. ACOG. Sterilization of women, including those with mental disabilities. In: Ethics in obstetrics and gynecology. The American college of obstetricians and gynecologists. 2nd ed. Washington, DC: ACOG; 2004. pp. 56–59.
55. Greydanus DE, Omar HA. Sexuality and disability. Pediatr Clin North Am. 2008;55 (6): 1315–35.
56. Owens K, Honebrink A. Gynecologic care of medically complicated adolescents. Pediatr Clin North Amer. 1999;46:631–42.
57. Greydanus DE, Omar H, Tsitsika A. Menstrual disorders in the adolescent female. Dis-a-Month. 2009;55:1–60.
58. Greydanus DE, Tsitsika A, Gains M. The gynecology system and the adolescent. In: Greydanus DE, Feinberg AN, Patel DR, Homnick DN, editors. Pediatric physical diagnosis. New York, NY: McGraw-Hill Medical Publishing; 2008. pp. 701–49.
59. Johnson J. The gynecology system and the child. In: Greydanus DE, Feinberg AN, Patel DR, Homnick DN, editors. Pediatric physical diagnosis. New York, NY: McGraw-Hill Medical Publishing; 2008. pp. 185–699.
60. Omar HA, Dekar A, Jackson W. Office gynecologic problems in prepubertal girls. In: Greydanus DE, Patel DR, Reddy VN, Feinberg AN, Omar HA, editors. Handbook of clinical pediatrics: an update for the ambulatory pediatrician. Singapore: World Scientific; 2010. pp. 665–98.
61. Omar H. Management of menstrual problems in adolescents with special health care needs. J Pediatr Adolesc Gynecol. 2003;16:51–56.

62. Geydanus DE, Omar HA, Patel DR. Cervical cancer screening in the adolescent female. Pediatr Rev. 2009;52:111.
63. Greydanus DE, Patel DR. Sexually transmitted diseases. In: Burg FD, Ingelfinger JA, Polin RA, Gershon AA, editors. Current pediatric therapy. 18th ed. Philadelphia, PA: Elsevier; 2006. pp. 326–9.
64. Burke LM, Kalpakjian CZ, Smith YR, Quint EH. Gynecologic issues of adolescents with Down syndrome, autism, and cerebral palsy. J Pediatr Adolesc Gynecol. 2010;23 1:11–15.
65. Greydanus DE, Calles JL Jr, Patel DR. Pediatric and adolescent psychopharmacology: a practical manual for pediatricians. Cambridge: Cambridge University Press, 2008:301.
66. Zuckerman D, Abraham A. Teenagers and cosmetic surgery: Focus on breast augmentation and liposuction. J Adoles Health. 2008;43:318–24.
67. Gittes EB, Strickland JL. Contraceptive choices for chronically ill adolescents. Adolesc Med. 2005;16:635–44.
68. Kaunitz AM. ACOG practice bulletin: the use of hormonal contraception in women with coexisting medical conditions. Internat J Gynaecol Obstet. 2001;75:93–106.
69. Greydanus DE, Matytsina L. Contraception in chronically ill adolescents. Int J Child Adolesc Health. 2010;3 (2):222–31.
70. Guijarro MJ, Valero G, Paule J, et al. Bone mass in young adults with Down syndrome. J Intellect Disabil Res. 2008;52 (Part 3):182–89.
71. Schrager S, Koss C, Ju AW. Prevalence of fractures in women with intellectual disabilities; a chart review. J Intellect Disabil Res. 2007;51 (Part 4):253–9.
72. Martin JR, Arici A. Fragile X and reproduction. Curr Opin Obstet Gynecol. 2008;29 (3): 216–20.
73. American Academy of Pediatrics, Committee on Bioethics. Sterilization of minors with developmental disabilities. Pediatrics. 1999;104:337–40.
74. Silber T, Batshaw JL. Ethical dilemmas in the treatment of children with disabilities. Pediatr Ann. 2004;33:752–61.
75. American College of Obstetricians and Gynecologists. Sterilization of women who are mentally handicapped. ACOG Committee Opinion 63. Washington, DC: ACOG; 1988.
76. Greydanus DE, Pratt HD, Baxter T. Sexual dysfunction and the primary care physician. Adolesc Med State Art Rev. 1996;7 (1):9–26.
77. Greydanus DE, Matytsina L. Sexual dysfunction in adolescent females. Curr Prob Obstet Gynecol. 2010;22:25–34.
78. Clayton AH, Hamilton DV. Female sexual dysfunction. Obstet Gynecol Clin North Am. 2009;36 (4):861–76.
79. Greydanus DE, Patel DR. Adolescent health. In: McDonagh JE, White JE, editors. Adolescent rheumatology. New York, NY: Informa Healthcare; 2008. pp. 291–310.
80. Abma JC, Martinez GM, Mosher WD, Dawson BS. Teenagers in the United States: sexual activity, contraceptive use, and childbearing: 2002. National Center for Health Statistics. Vital Health Stat. 2004;23 (24):1–2.
81. The Surgeon General. Call to action to improve the health and wellness of persons with disabilities. Accessed 2010 Jun 29. URL: http://www.surgeongeneral.gov/library/disabilities.
82. Kirschner KL, Curry RH. Educating health care professionals to care for patients with disabilities. JAMA. 2009;302 (12):1334–5.
83. Bononi BM, Sant'Anna MJC. Vasconcellos de Oliveira AC, et al. Sexuality and persons with Down syndrome. a study from Brazil. Int J Adolesc Med Health. 2009;21 (3):319–26.
84. Patel DR, Greydanus DE, Calles JL Jr, Pratt HD. Developmental disabilities across the lifespan. Dis Mon. 2010;56 (6):299–398.
85. Kellogg N. The evaluation of sexual abuse in children. Pediatrics. 2005;116:506–12.
86. Hegar A, editor. Evaluation of the sexually abused child. 2nd ed. New York: Oxford University Press; 2000.
87. Copeland-Linder N, Serwint JR. Posttraumatic stress disorder. Pediatr Rev. 2008;29:103–104.
88. Omar HA, Greydanus DE, Patel DR, Merrick J. Adolescence, chronic illness, and disability. Int J Disabil Hum Dev. 2008;7 (3):1–100.

Chapter 21
Dental Aspects

Ilan Feldberg and Joav Merrick

Abstract Oral hygiene and dental care is often neglected in persons with intellectual disability and good dental care can be difficult to acquire. Periodontal and dental diseases are common and can be a source of discomfort, fever, and challenging behaviors, especially because of communication difficulties. Hospitalization and treatment in general anesthesia may be necessary to provide adequate dental care, when outpatient care is impossible. Physicians should emphasize regular dental evaluations and consider mild sedation for outpatient dental visits. Evidence supports the need to develop strategies to increase patient acceptance for routine care, additional training for dentists to provide this care, and the development of more effective preventive strategies to minimize the need for this care. This chapter is based on the provision of dental service to people with intellectual disability in Israel during the past 30 years.

Introduction

In the past persons with intellectual disability (ID) were often neglected by the dental profession, because of different barriers, like insufficient knowledge and experience to treat this population, problems in the regular dental consultation if mixed population for dental visits, lack of collaboration with the patient, fear by the patient for treatment, lack of awareness by carers, and inadequate facilities and low compensation for treatment of patients that takes much longer to approach, assess, and treat [1, 2].

In general, people with intellectual disability have poorer oral health and oral hygiene than those without this condition. Data indicate that people who have intellectual disability have more untreated caries, higher prevalence of gingivitis, and

I. Feldberg (✉)
Health Services, Division for Mental Retardation, Ministry of Social Affairs, National Institute of Child Health and Human Development, IL-91012 Jerusalem, Israel
e-mail: feldberg5@walla.com

other periodontal diseases than the general population affecting their ability to chew, speak, and look attractive [3]. With increasing age and life expectancy this population will be in need of good dental care on a regular basis to prevent disease and increase their quality of life [4, 5].

A recent systematic review of 27 original studies [6] showed that people with ID have poorer oral hygiene, higher prevalence, and greater severity of periodontal disease. Caries rates were the same as or higher than the general population, but the rates of untreated caries were consistently higher. Two subgroups at especially high risk for oral health problems are people with Down syndrome and people unable to cooperate with routine dental care [6].

Our Experience in Israel

In Israel the Division for Mental Retardation (DMR) of the Ministry of Social Affairs and Social Services has the responsibility for the assessment, treatment, rehabilitation, and service for persons with ID. By the end of 2009 the total population in Israel was about 7.5 million and the DMR was in contact with about 30,000 persons of all ages with intellectual disability.

Residential care is provided to about 7,000 persons in 63 residential centers all over the country (see Tables 21.1 and 21.2) [7]; in about another 50 locations, residential care is provided to an additional 3,000 persons in hostels or in group homes in the community, whereas the remainder are served with day-care kindergarten, day-treatment centers, sheltered workshops, or integrated care in the community while living at home with their families. Dental services are provided free on a national basis by the DMR to all persons in residential care and optional to persons with ID living at home.

The first dental survey in Israel of the residential care population was conducted in 1971–1972 by the first medical director of the DMR together with the School of Dental Medicine at Tel Aviv University at three government residential care centers, including 573 residents with ID out of a total residential care population of 2,700 at that time period [8]. At this time period there were no dental clinics for this

Table 21.1 The population of persons with intellectual disability in 63 residential care centers in Israel in 2009

Age in years	Males	Females	Total	Percent
0–9	70	45	115	1.63
10–19	448	282	730	10.33
20–39	1,619	1,147	2,766	39.14
40–49	803	606	1,409	19.94
50–59	707	623	1,330	18.82
>60	330	387	717	10.14
Total	3,977	3,090	7,067	100.00
%	56.28	43.72	100.00	

Table 21.2 The level of intellectual disability (ID) in the population of persons with intellectual disability in residential care in Israel in 2009. Mild MR: IQ 55–70, moderate: IQ 35–54, severe: IQ 20–34, and profound: IQ < 20. Other: 79 persons, where the level of ID has not been determined at this moment

Age in years	Mild	Moderate	Severe	Profound	Other	Total	Percent
0–9	6	15	39	43	12	115	1.63
10–19	108	267	233	121	1	730	10.33
20–39	372	994	997	387	16	2,766	39.14
40–49	212	567	437	189	4	1,409	19.94
50–59	161	659	368	141	1	1,330	18.82
>60	84	400	160	63	10	717	10.14
Total	943	2,902	2,234	944	44	7,067	100,00
Percent	13.34	41.07	31.61	13.36	0.62	100.00	

population and the survey was conducted via a mobile dental clinic (a bus) with four dental chairs. The study showed that only 20% of the residents were able to fully cooperate with the dental procedure and treatment, while 84% of all residents were in need of treatment. About 50% of the residents needed pre-medication or general anesthesia in order to examine and treat them. Over 70% had suffered from caries in various degrees and 25% showed serious damage as indicated by seven and more decayed teeth per person. About 60% had lost one or more teeth and 17% more than seven teeth, whereas only 30% had fillings in one or more teeth. The total number of decayed teeth was 2,281 with a male to female ratio of 0.58:1.16% were caries free and the rest needed treatment with 45% showing severe or grave damage with more than seven affected teeth [8]. The first survey resulted in the establishment of dental clinics in residential care centers in Israel, with 15 clinics providing service to the whole population in residential care today and in recent years we have also opened up the service to people with ID living at home, persons with autism, and other severely disabled persons in residential care centers in Israel [9].

The second survey was conducted by the School of Dental Medicine at Tel Aviv University in 1993 [10] among 462 persons with ID in residential care with a randomly selected sample. A total of 362 were able to collaborate with the exam, and in the 2- to 11-year-old group decayed teeth was found at decayed, $D = 12.84$, no missing teeth, and only 1.89 filled teeth making a DMFT (decayed/missing/filled teeth) of 13.93. The 12- to 14-year-olds showed an active caries level of 12.15%, no missing teeth, filled teeth at 0.73%, and DMFT of 12.88. The 15- to 24-year-olds had caries level at 14.18% and DMFT of 17.96. The 25- to 34-year-olds showed a DMFT of 21.07 and the 35 years and older had an increased DMFT of 18.52.

The third large-scale survey in 1995 was conducted by the second medical director of the DMR together with the Hebrew University Hadassah School of Dental Medicine in Jerusalem [11] with a random sample of 387 persons in residential care. The sample was divided into four groups: (1) educable ($n = 70$), (2) trainable ($n = 92$), (3) behavioral problems ($n = 106$), and (4) severe physical handicap ($n = 119$). The total age-adjusted DMFT was 12.78 and differed significantly by behavioral group ($p < 0.001$); the MT was 10.70 for the educable group compared with 5.52 for the group with severe physical handicap. Total treatment needs included a participant mean of 3.32 for restorations and 0.61 for extractions. Residential care centers with a dental clinic had higher participant mean DMFT, DT, MT, and FT values ($p < 0.05$) compared with those institutions which had no clinics (16.04 vs. 9.74; 5.17 vs. 5.06; 9.45 vs. 4.16; 1.41 vs. 0.52, respectively). Age-adjusted Community Periodontal Index of Treatment Needs (CPITN) scores significantly differed by behavioral group; the group with ID and severe physical handicap had the highest CPITN 3 category mean score of 2.93 compared with $x = 1.89$ for the educable group; however, the educable group had the most sextants with no teeth ($x = 2.48$). Findings confirmed high dental morbidity and significant oral health differences by behavior group, age, and dental clinic status.

Community studies have been conducted, but usually with smaller number or specialized populations like Down syndrome [12, 13]. One general study [9] of aging and ID was conducted in Jerusalem area with persons aged 40 years and older living in community residence ($n = 65$) compared with those living with their families ($n = 43$). All 108 persons and caregivers were interviewed to ascertain health problems, sensory impairment, activity of daily living (ADL), cognitive skills, and leisure activities. Health problems had already developed by age 40 years. The most frequent were visual (33%), hearing impairments (20%), and dental problems (30%). The community residence group displayed more medical problems, whereas individuals living at home had more dental problems and this study resulted in residential care clinics opening up their service also for people with ID living at home [9].

The issue and problems we have observed in Israel are also found in other countries like the United States [14], the United Kingdom [15], and India [16].

What Have We Learned from Our Experience?

In the later half of the twentieth century, former President John F. Kennedy (1917–1963), who had a sister with ID, made the improvement of conditions for individuals with special needs a personal policy priority and in the 1970s, when acceptance of the de-institutionalization and normalization process that had started in Denmark and Sweden was widespread, many large institutions were closed and individuals were moved into community settings. This has not been the situation in Israel, where large institutions of the size seen in the United States never existed, as the average residential care center today in Israel consists of about 122 residents. We are therefore trying to make a policy, where dental service is provided by the residential care center (15 clinics today in Israel) to both residents and also persons with ID living in the community, because the general health and dental services in the community are not able to cope with this population and its special and complex needs.

We have by now established 15 dental clinics spread around Israel to meet the national need for this population. The clinics are located on the premises of residential care centers, usually in close connection with the general medical clinics with a waiting room area for groups of people from other centers or the community arriving for dental care after appointments. The clinics usually have two chairs in order for the dentist and the dental hygienist to work at the same time on several patients or in some cases two dentists working at the same time. The clinic is usually created in a friendly environment, but we are still working on improvements and have ideas to introduce the snoezelen concept in our clinics [17]. The clinics are accessible to and for patients in wheelchairs (see Fig. 21.1), equipped with lift (see Fig. 21.2) and papoose board (see Figs. 21.3 and 21.4) as standard equipment.

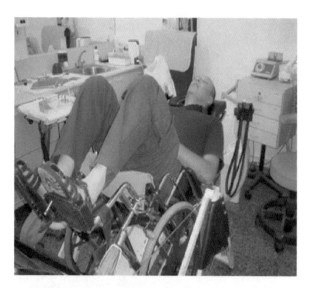

Fig. 21.1 Dental treatment for a patient in wheelchair

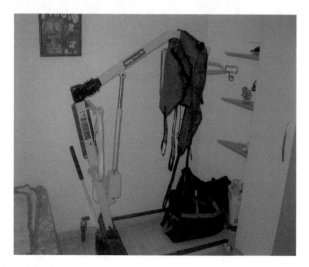

Fig. 21.2 Lift used for heavy immobile patients in order to prevent injuries to the dental clinic staff

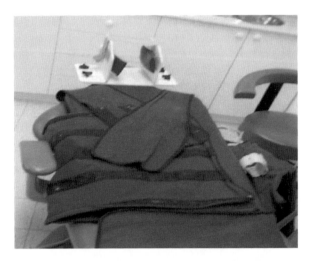

Fig. 21.3 Papoose board ready for the patient

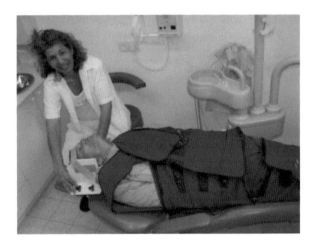

Fig. 21.4 Papoose board with patient

A papoose board (medical restraint device) is a device commonly used to immobilize a person for dental work, blood drawing, and minor medical procedures. The person is placed on a flat board and wide fabric straps are wrapped around the upper body, middle body, and legs. The restraints can be applied quickly to keep the person from struggling or resisting treatment and preventing self-damage and damage to the crew and the equipment. We feel that this procedure is preferable to sedation or general anesthesia (GA) and have now many years of positive experience with this procedure resulting in much less numbers of more risky and expensive GA. In recent years we have also introduced nitrous oxide or laughing gas in most of our clinics.

There are benefits of treatment under general anesthesia, like no problem of cooperation; multiple operations can be performed in one treatment, no experience of traumatic treatment for the patient, and convenience for the dental professional, who can work with the dental problems without interference under optimal conditions. General anesthesia on the other hand is not without risks, like mortality risk (3–6 cases per 100,000), morbidity risk, intubation and other complications, long durations between treatments which may cause a worsening deterioration, and loss of teeth and dental status. So we prefer to use the papoose board with as many patients as possible. In our last published annual survey of residential care centers [18] we found that out of 6,988 residents only 38 (0.54%) needed general anesthesia, which is a drastic decrease since our first annual survey in 1998 [19] when 266 out of 6,022 residents (4.42%) needed general anesthesia. This decrease is a result mainly of the introduction of papoose board, so we recommend it as standard equipment for all dental clinics working with this population.

A good, trained, experienced, constant, and dedicated staff is the success to a good treatment of this population, staff that will show respect and understand the patient. If the patient will see the same dentist, dental assistant, and dental hygienist again and again it will be a pleasure to come for the minimum of a yearly visit and mutual trust will be established.

On the first dental visit it is important to try and get a thorough history (both dental and medical) of the patient, assessment of caries risk, a review of dental development, an oral examination, treatment, and future prevention plan. Recording is important and we have implemented a national computerized recording system since 2002.

Behavioral technique of tell–show–do (TSD) is a familiarization technique in which the client is told what the operator is going to do in non-threatening terms. The operator then demonstrates or shows what he is going to do and then goes ahead and does it, but there are other issues involved:

- Voice control
- Desensitization
- Distraction
- Parental presence or absence
- Non-verbal communication
- Positive reinforcement

We have also encouraged frequent educational programs and training for the staff in order to communicate between the different teams and raise the educational level and provide a forum for discussion and supervision.

Dental Issues

Periodontal Disease

Genetics, medications, malocclusion, multiple disabilities, and poor oral hygiene combine to increase the risk of periodontal disease in people with intellectual disability. It is therefore important to encourage independence in daily oral hygiene. Ask patients to show you how they brush and follow up with specific recommendations on brushing methods or toothbrush adaptations. Involve your patients in hands-on demonstrations of brushing and flossing, because all people with teeth need brushing. Brushing followed by flossing is better if possible.

Some patients cannot brush and floss independently due to impaired physical coordination or cognitive skills. Talk to their caregivers about daily oral hygiene. Do not assume that all caregivers know the basics, but you should demonstrate proper brushing and flossing techniques. A power toothbrush or a floss holder can simplify oral care. Also, use your experiences with each patient to demonstrate sitting or standing positions for the caregiver. Emphasize that a consistent approach to oral hygiene is important and caregivers should try to use the same location, timing, and positioning.

Some patients benefit with the use of an antimicrobial agent such as chlorhexidine. Recommend an appropriate delivery method based on your patient's abilities. Rinsing, for example, may not work for a patient who has swallowing difficulties or one who cannot expectorate. If use of particular medications has led to gingival hyperplasia, emphasize the importance of daily oral hygiene and frequent professional cleanings.

Localized aggressive periodontitis, as found frequently in Down syndrome, is not dependent or connected to oral hygiene and can develop and cause teeth loss (mainly incisors and first molars) even in a perfect oral hygiene state.

Dental Caries

People with intellectual disability develop caries at the same rate as the general population. The prevalence of untreated dental caries, however, is higher among people with intellectual disability, particularly those living in non-institutional settings. Emphasize noncariogenic foods and beverages as snacks. Advice caregivers to avoid using sweets as incentives or rewards. Advice patients taking medicines that cause xerostomia to drink water often. Suggest sugar-free medicine if available and stress the importance of rinsing with water after dosing. We recommend preventive measures such as fluorides, sealants, and frequent visits to the dental clinic.

Malocclusion

The prevalence of malocclusion in people with intellectual disability is higher than that found in the general population, mainly with coexisting conditions and syndromes such as cerebral palsy, Apert syndrome, or Down syndrome. The ability of the patient or caregiver to maintain good daily oral hygiene is critical to the feasibility and success of treatment.

Missing Teeth, Delayed Eruption, and Enamel Hypoplasia

Missing teeth, delayed eruption, and enamel hypoplasia are more common in people with intellectual disability and coexisting conditions than in people with intellectual disability alone. Examine a child by his or her first birthday and regularly thereafter to help identify unusual tooth formation and patterns of eruption; 1–2 years late eruption is very common in Down syndrome. Consider using a panoramic radiograph to determine whether teeth are congenitally missing. Patients often find this technique less threatening than individual films. Take appropriate steps to reduce sensitivity and risk of caries in your patients with enamel hypoplasia. Fluoride application on tooth surfaces is very effective for caries prevention.

Oral Habits

Damaging oral habits are problems for some people with intellectual disability. Common habits include bruxism (grinding of teeth), mouth breathing, tongue thrusting, self-injurious behavior such as picking at the gingiva, biting the lips, and pica (eating objects and substances such as gravel, cigarette butts, or pens). If a mouth guard can be tolerated, prescribe one for patients who have problems with self-injurious behavior or bruxism.

Bruxism can come from many things ranging from anxiety to malocclusion of the teeth. It is important to determine whether the grinding is secondary to something else. If the cause of the bruxism is something bad for the person in other ways, such as chronic pain or anxiety, it is of course important to get to that problem first. If the grinding is caused by malocclusion of the teeth, a professional will have to determine if straightening or some other treatment is needed.

Injuries

Trauma or injury to the mouth from falls or accidents occurs in people with intellectual disability. Emphasize to caregivers that traumas require immediate professional attention and explain the procedures to follow if a permanent tooth is knocked out. Also, instruct caregivers to locate any missing pieces of a fractured tooth and explain that radiographs of the patient's chest may be necessary to determine whether any fragments have been aspirated.

Physical abuse often presents as oral trauma. Abuse is reported more frequently in people with developmental disabilities than in the general population.

Dental Care and Down Syndrome

Localized aggressive periodontitis is the most significant oral health problem in people with Down syndrome. Children experience rapid, destructive periodontal disease. Consequently, large numbers of them lose their permanent anterior and first molar teeth in their early teens. Contributing factors include poor oral hygiene, malocclusion, bruxism, conical-shaped tooth roots, and abnormal host response because of a compromised immune system. Some patients benefit the daily use of an antimicrobial agent such as chlorhexidine.

Children and young adults who have Down syndrome have fewer caries than people without this developmental disability. Several associated oral conditions may contribute to this fact: delayed eruption of primary and permanent teeth; missing permanent teeth; and small-sized teeth with wider spaces between them, which make it easier to remove plaque. Additionally, the diets of many children with Down syndrome are closely supervised to prevent obesity, which helps reduce consumption of cariogenic foods and beverages. By contrast, some adults with Down syndrome are at an increased risk of caries due to xerostomia and cariogenic food choices. Also, hypotonia and macroglossia contribute to chewing problems and inefficient natural cleansing action, which allow food to remain on the teeth after eating.

Several orofacial features are characteristic of people with Down syndrome. The midfacial region may be underdeveloped, affecting the appearance of the lips, tongue, and palate. The maxilla, the bridge of the nose, and the bones of the midface region are smaller than in the general population, creating a prognathic occlusal relationship. Mouth breathing may occur because of smaller nasal passages, and the tongue may protrude because of a smaller midface region. People with Down syndrome often have a strong gag reflex due to placement of the tongue, as well as anxiety associated with any oral stimulation. The palate, although normal sized, may appear highly vaulted and narrow. This deceiving appearance is due to the unusual thickness of the sides of the hard palate. This thickness restricts the amount of space the tongue can occupy in the mouth and affects the ability to speak and chew.

The lips may grow large and thick. Fissured lips may result from chronic mouth breathing. Additionally, hypotonia may cause the mouth to drop and the lower lip to protrude. Increased drooling, compounded by a chronically open mouth, contributes to angular cheilitis. The tongue and lips also develop cracks and fissures with age; this condition can contribute to halitosis.

Malocclusion is found in most people with Down syndrome, because of the delayed eruption of permanent teeth and the underdevelopment of the maxilla. A smaller maxilla contributes to an open bite, leading to poor positioning of teeth and increasing the likelihood of periodontal disease and dental caries. Orthodontic treatment should be carefully considered in people with Down syndrome.

Congenitally missing teeth occur more often in people with Down syndrome than in the general population. Third molars, laterals, and mandibular second bicuspids are the most common missing teeth.

Delayed eruption of teeth, often following an abnormal sequence, affects some children with Down syndrome. Primary teeth may not appear until age 2 years, with complete dentition delayed until age 4 or 5 years. Primary teeth are then retained in some children until they are 14 or 15 years. Irregularities in tooth formation, such as microdontia and malformed teeth, are also seen in people with Down syndrome.

Crowns tend to be smaller, and roots are often small and conical, which can lead to tooth loss from periodontal disease. Severe illness or prolonged fevers can lead to hypoplasia and hypocalcification.

Recommendations

We recommend a yearly routine visit to a dental clinic for all persons at all ages from the eruption of the first tooth. Even without teeth this regular visit is important to assure a healthy oral mucosa and fitting dentures if that is the case. Oral disease is often related to other medical problems and issues, so a close collaboration with the treating physician should exist.

The recent review by Anders and Davis [6] supported the need for further research in the following areas: development of strategies to increase patient acceptance of routine periodontal and restorative dental care, development of strategies to ensure that dentists and hygienists are prepared to provide this care, and development of effective preventive strategies to minimize the need for this care.

References

1. Waldman HB, Perlman SP, Swerdloff M. Children with mental retardation/developmental disabilities: do physicians ever consider needed dental care?. Ment Retard. 2001;39(1):53–56.
2. Waldman HB, Perlman SP. Why is providing dental care to people with mental retardation and other developmental disabilities such a low priority?. Public Health Rep. 2002;117(5):435–9.
3. Jurek GH, Reid WH. Oral health of institutionalized individuals with mental retardation. Am J Ment Retard. 1994;98(5):656–60.
4. Malmstrom H, Santos-Teachout R, Ren Y. Dentition and oral health. In: Prasher VP, Janicki MP, editors.. Physical health of adults with intellectual disabilities. Oxford: Blackwell; 2002. pp. 181–203.
5. Pearlman J, Sterling E. Dentistry. In: Rubin IL, Crocker AC, editors. Medical care for children and adults with developmental disabilities. Baltimore, MD: Paul H Brookes; 2006. pp. 435–49.
6. Anders PL, Davis EL. Oral health of patients with intellectual disabilities: a systematic review. Spec Care Dentist. 2010;30(3):110–17.
7. Merrick J. Survey of medical clinics, 2009. Jerusalem: Office of the Medical Director, Ministry of Social Affairs; 2010.
8. Sarnat H, Sterk VV, Amir E. The dental status of 572 institutionalized mentally retarded in Israel. Isr J Dental health. 1976;24(4):11–15.
9. Lifshitz H, Merrick J. Aging among persons with intellectual disability in Israel in relation to type of residence, age, and etiology. Res Dev Disabil. 2004;25(2):193–205.
10. Cohen S. Dental needs of the handicapped population living in institutions. Unpublished report, 1993.
11. Shapira J, Efrat J, Berkey D, Mann J. Dental health profile of a population with mental retardation in Israel. Spec Care Dentist. 1998;18(4):149–5.
12. Chaushu S, Yefenof EY, Becker A, Shapira J, Chaushu G. Parotid salivary immunoglobulins, recurrent respiratory tract infections and gingival health in institutionalized and non-institutionalized subject with Down syndrome. J Intellect Disabil Res. 2003;47(Pt 2):101–107.
13. Zigmond M, Stabholz A, Shapira J, Bachrach G, Chaushu G, Becker A, Yefenof E, Merrick J, Chaushu S. The outcome of a preventive dental care programme on the prevalence of localized

aggressive periodontitis in Down's syndrome individuals. J Intellect Disabil Res. 2006;50 (Pt 7):492–500.

14. Altabet S, Rogers K, Imes E, Boatman IM, Moncier J. Comprehensive approach towards improving oral hygiene at a state residential facility for people with mental retardation. Ment Retard. 2003;41(6):440–5.

15. Cumella S, Ransford N, Lyons J, Burnham H. Needs for oral care among people with intellectual disability not in contact with community dental services. J Intellect Disabil Res. 2000;44(1):45–52.

16. Jain M, Mathur A, Sawla L, Choudhary G, Kabra K, Duraiswamy P, Kulkarni S. Oral health status of mentally disabled subjects in India. J Oral Sci. 2009;51(3):333–40.

17. Merrick J, Cahana C, Lotan M, Kandel I, Carmeli E. Snoezelen or controlled multisensory stimulation. Treatment aspects from Israel. ScientificWorldJournal. 2004;4:307–14.

18. Merrick J, Kandel I, Lotan M, Aspler S, Fuchs BS, Morad M. National survey 2008 on medical services for persons with intellectual disability in residential care in Israel. Int J Disabil Hum Dev. 2010;9(1):59–63.

19. Merrick J. National survey 1998 on medical services for persons with intellectual disability in residential care in Israel. Int J Disabil Hum Dev. 2005;4(2):139–46.

Chapter 22
General Medical Care for Individuals with Developmental Disabilities

Joav Merrick and Mohammed Morad

Abstract In the past, most individuals with intellectual disability (ID) died at a young age due to their additional medical problems, congenital malformations, and infections, but today an increasing number of these children live into adulthood and we see the first generation of aging people with intellectual disability. This trend has resulted in not only pediatricians but also now adult physicians involved in the management of this population. Older people with ID have the same needs as other older people do, and they are subject to the same age-related impairments and illnesses. Moreover, because many disabled individuals live together with their families, the burden is double because the family members are also aging and, with time, will not be able to continue their caregiving. Medical needs from pediatric to adult care can be met by enrollment in universal health care or programs. Periodic health assessments and health care should be normalized and provided as an overall system of supports when needed or as assistance provided for the adequate self-directed use of general or specialty health services. Risk assessments and health reviews should be part of the individual's life plan and provided to detect diseases and conditions that could compromise longevity. This field of medicine also needs to evaluate the applicability of a new discipline of life span developmental medicine to lead in interdisciplinary care, health-care education, service delivery, and research for people with intellectual disability within an academic framework.

Introduction

The diagnosis of intellectual disability (ID), developmental disability, or mental retardation can sometimes be difficult due to various barriers, and some of these can also result in sub-optimal health care for this population in general. All in all

J. Merrick (✉)
National Institute of Child Health and Human Development, Health Services, Office of the Medical Director, Division for Mental Retardation, Ministry of Social Affairs and Social Services, POBox 1260, IL-91012 Jerusalem, Israel; Kentucky Children's Hospital, University of Kentucky, Lexington, KY, USA
e-mail: jmerrick@zahav.net.il

D.R. Patel et al. (eds.), *Neurodevelopmental Disabilities*,
DOI 10.1007/978-94-007-0627-9_22, © Springer Science+Business Media B.V. 2011

medical care to this population on a systematic level is a relatively new phenomenon dating back to the 1960s, when the US President John F Kennedy (1917–1963), who had a sister with intellectual disability, made improvement of conditions for individuals with special needs a personal policy priority and founded the National Institute of Child Health and Human Development and also developed the concept of university-affiliated facilities [1]. Optimal health care for children with chronic illness should [1]

- consider a holistic approach to the child (person) and his/her family;
- include a comprehensive assessment and evaluation taking into account the needs of the child and the family;
- encourage support for living at home as long as possible;
- support and encourage an environment that nurtures developmental progress;
- ensure access to comprehensive health, educational, and social care services;
- help the child and family to know and understand the work of the health-care system;
- find suitable resources;
- help to coordinate all agencies and entities involved in the care of the child and encourage smooth transition from pediatric to adolescent and adult care;
- support functional independence; and
- support the family unit, which often comes under extreme stress situations.

All in all it should be remembered that people with ID are entitled to the same health care that is available for the general population as a minimum, but it is know that people with ID [2]

- tend to have a higher level of morbidity and often multiple, complex, and chronic health problems;
- have higher prevalence of certain medical conditions (like, for example, epilepsy) and also life style-related health risks like obesity and on top also low physical activity and fitness;
- experience greater barriers to access health care (in surveys they are twice as likely to report unmet health-care needs [3]); and
- are less likely to participate in community preventive medicine programs that the general population are offered.

Different countries have developed various models for health care to the population of persons with intellectual disability. In the United Kingdom the Community Learning Disability Team [3] has been implemented, in the Netherlands the realization of a specialist physician for intellectual disability, while most other countries have relied on the mainstream health-care system to care for this population. A recent Cochrane meta-analysis [4] of organizing health-care services for persons with ID could not find any well-designed studies focusing on the issue of health service for persons with ID and physical problems, and very few studies concerned with mental health problems.

The health-care burden for a child born with intellectual disability is first of all on the child, then the family, and also society and the health-care system. The lifetime economic burden of a person with intellectual disability was estimated in 2003 in the United States at around 1 million dollars [5].

Infancy and Childhood

If the disability is diagnosed at an early stage, the health care will generally take place in a hospital setting and later often via a multidisciplinary child development center team. The focus from birth to 6 months of age will mainly be on medical issues (diagnosis, intervention, and early care and prevention of further damage) and support and help for the parents [1], but over time the medical (in this case usually pediatric care) issues and also parental assistance will diminish, while educational and residential programs take over in importance. In middle and late childhood, special education and social and recreational issues will have more significance for the individual and medical issues usually now be a small part of the life of the person [1]. It is important to stress that children with intellectual disability should receive the same standard health care as the general population and the same prevention and immunization program (unless contraindicated).

In this chapter we will not get into details around specific syndromes and their detailed health care, because there are resources available, like, for example, guidelines for health care in persons with Down syndrome at various stages of their lives [6–8]. An increasing number of children with syndromes, intellectual disability, and chronic illness are now living longer and entering adulthood, which presents now challenges for transition from pediatric to adult care [9].

Adolescence

The goals of the physician, family, and the adolescent to promote better outcomes are not always the same [10]. The adolescent is interested in the developmental task set out for adolescence (see Table 22.1) [11], whereas the physician and also the family are trying to achieve control (like, for example, blood glucose level in diabetes) and prevent or reduce further complications of the chronic illness.

Table 22.1 Developmental tasks of adolescence [11]

1. Autonomy or independence from parents and other adults
2. Increasing role of peer relationships
3. Developing a realistic body image
4. Self-identity formation that is realistic, positive, and stable
5. Sexual self-identity formation
6. Consolidation of a moral or value system (moral development)
7. Educational and vocational goal development

In order to provide better outcomes for adolescents with disability or chronic illness there will be a need to focus on [10] the following:

1. *Building the capacity of the adolescent*

   It is very important for the physician and health team responsible for health and treatment of adolescents with disability and chronic illness to understand the developmental tasks of adolescence (see Table 22.1) and the different coping mechanisms [12]: insightful acceptance (unusual in adolescents), denial (common strategy), regression (common), projection, displacement, acting out, compensation, or intellectualization. The adolescent can go through one or many of these and at different times, so it is important that the caregiver is aware and act accordingly with insight and wisdom.

2. *Building the capacity of the family*

   Parents often also go through psychological stages when confronted with diagnosis of a chronic illness and the worry about prognosis and survival [10] when diagnosis is in childhood or adolescence [13]. The health provider must be aware of the role of the family and not only guide the parents through this period but also provide them with information and a network to support them.

3. *Building the capacity in schools*

   On average adolescents in the 1988 NHIS [14] experienced 3.4 bed days and 4.4 school absence days related to their chronic condition in the year before the interview. It was also estimated that 23% of those with disabling chronic conditions were limited in their ability or unable to attend school on a long-term basis. The education system must take into account disabled adolescents and find ways to educate them even in case of hospitalization or having to stay home due to disease. Collaboration between the educational system, the health provider, and parents is essential.

4. *Building peer support programs*

   The peer group is very important for every adolescent and even more so for the one with chronic illness. Parents, school, and health provider must do their utmost to facilitate peer interaction and participation in programs.

5. *Building suitable community health care*

   It is important that the adolescent and his family will have access to a permanent health provider (a pediatrician, a specialist in adolescent medicine, or a family physician) that understands all the aspects of adolescence and the psychology involved and also the aspects of the specific disease or syndrome causing the chronic disability. This is important for continuity and optimal health care.

6. *Building suitable inpatient units*

   Adolescent medicine does not exist as a specialty in every country, every pediatric department, or medical center around the globe. Whatever the local situation it is important to build and arrange for suitable space and environment that can cater to the adolescent with chronic illness during hospitalization. This should include possibilities for educational and school programs also during hospitalizations.

7. *Building a model for transition to adult care*

With adolescence reaching adulthood also comes the responsibility for health care in the adult setting. Adolescents with disability often find this transition especially difficult [9, 10, 15, 16]. To facilitate this transition the physician in care can help by providing a comprehensive case summary and explain its contents with the adolescent, perform a physical exam with the adolescent as partner, facilitate support groups and networks, and continue care for a transition period or be available for both the adolescent and the new health provider.

More adolescents are found to have chronic illness, and some of these will be with lifelong disability. Several studies, especially in the United States with the National Health Interview Surveys (NHIS), have over time shown an increase in the prevalence of disability among adolescents, focused on issues concerned with insurance, and examined health utilization and school absence.

James M Perrin from Harvard Medical School in a review [17] reflected on the need for future research in the area of health service for adolescents with disabilities:

- In clinical and health service epidemiology there is a need for better description of the changing numbers of adolescents with disabilities and how their functioning has been affected
- Research on how to minimize the effects of disability on ability to engage in age-appropriate activities
- What makes a good transition to adult health care
- Research on social and structural determinants of new epidemics of chronic conditions and what determines if the condition with bring disability
- Research on what treatment and management that works and the cost benefits
- The role of the family and the role of primary and sub-specialty services
- Comprehensive studies of expenditures and utilization of services
- Research on appropriate measures of health status and quality of life

But often in daily clinical experience adolescents with a disability fall between systems and do not always receive optimal care, even though in this time period the medical needs are not demanding, since educational and social programs take precedence [1].

Adulthood and Aging

In the 1930s, the mean age at death for people with intellectual disability (ID) was about 19 years, in the 1970s about 59 years, in the 1990s increased to 66 years, and today close to general life expectancy, whereas for Down syndrome, the mean age at death was 9 years in the 1920s and 56 years today [18]. Such an increase in life span can be seen as the consequence of progress in medical technology and improved social awareness in the twentieth century. In the past, most individuals with intellectual disability died at a young age due to their additional medical problems, congenital malformations, and infections with the result that very few went through the aging process. This trend has resulted in not only pediatricians but also now adult physicians involved in the management of this population, and today we in fact really see the first generation of aging persons with ID, which is a challenge for service providers [9].

In the past decade it has been observed worldwide that there will be an increased number of persons over 65 years. This larger number of older people worldwide will require a better and more effective health and social service, because many will have chronic diseases in need of service and surveillance. This load will not only increase health, social, and long-term care expenses but also make public health interventions important in order to sustain good health and a good quality in life even in the face of chronic disease. It will also require a transition process from pediatric to adolescent care to adult care health providers, which so far have had little experience with adults with intellectual disability [19].

This increase in the number of older people in the general population is also reflected in the population of persons with intellectual disability (ID), and today the average life expectancy of older adults with ID is 66.1 years and growing [20, 21]. This population will present increasing challenges to the clinician, the social welfare, and to the public health system, characterized by increased rates of hearing and visual impairments, obesity, osteoporosis, dementia, and other chronic diseases with a need for more intensive medical surveillance and interventions [21].

In order to look more closely at aging in persons with intellectual disability we studied some 2,283 adults with intellectual disability aged 40 years and older in residential care centers in Israel in order to determine their health status [22]. Age was a significant factor in disease frequency, functional behavior, and age-related changes in organ system diseases. The frequency of all disease categories increased significantly with age, except for gastrointestinal, hematological, and infectious diseases. There were increases with age in both genders for cardiovascular disease, cancer, and sensory impairments. Cardiovascular disease was less prevalent than in the general population, suggesting that underdiagnosis of some diseases may be more common than expected in this population.

This study was a replication of an American large-scale population-based survey of health status and health services utilization among over 1,300 adults aged 40 years and older with ID living in small group, community-based residences in New York [23]. The main questions for both studies were whether the trends reported in previous studies could be confirmed in a large sample, whether these trends were comparable to data on older persons without ID, and what factors may place persons with ID at higher risk for declines in health and functional status as they age.

For this Israeli study [22] the response rate was 95%. The study population had a mean age of 49.8 years, indicating that the residents were generally younger, rather than older, adults. Most (88%) were under the age of 59 years. There were slightly more males (51%) than females (49%). The mean length of stay in current residence was 20.8 years (SD = 12.0) indicating a stable population. About 48% had severe or profound ID. Down syndrome was reported in 11% of the study population. Cerebral palsy (CP) as a coincident condition was reported for 14% of the adults. The mean BMI of the Israeli cohort was 25.7 with over one-third of the cohort (35%) classified as overweight with a BMI > 272.

Functional Behavior

About 25% of the cohort had impaired or limited vision. Impaired hearing was less prevalent as only 12% were reported to have impaired or no hearing. The prevalence of both visual and hearing impairments significantly increased with age ($p < 0.0001$). Inferred frailty, stemming from poor activities of daily living (ADL) skills and general functioning, was observed, but appeared within expected ranges of this population. In terms of impaired function, 17% were incapable of eating by themselves, 37% could not dress themselves, 28% could not toilet independently, and 55% were not capable of washing and bathing without assistance. In addition, 31% lacked complete bowel and bladder control (continence). The ability to independently toilet ($p = 0.035$), bathe ($p = 0.002$), and control continence ($p = 0.003$) all were significantly lower in older age groupings.

General Health and Health Services Utilization and Coordination

Irrespective of age group, over half of the cohort members were reported not engaging in any exercise. Very few adults experienced injuries. Nearly everyone saw a physician annually, and very few had been hospitalized or visited the emergency room in the last year. As would be expected, perception of health status declined and use of health services increased significantly with increasing age group.

In general, diseases occurred at about the same frequencies for males and females. However, age-related changes in most organ system diseases differed by gender. The prevalence of cardiovascular disease, cancer, as well as impairments of vision and hearing increased with age groupings for both genders. The only disease that did not significantly increase with age grouping in either females or males was hematologic disease. Psychiatric disorders decreased with age in both genders. Neurological disease decreased with age only in females, with most of the decrease occurring after age 70 years. The rate of neurological disease in this cohort was high (44% overall), but declined in older age groups, most likely reflecting early mortality among those adults, who were most impaired. Epilepsy and cerebral palsy were the two most frequent neurological conditions at 16 and 14%, respectively. The rate for cancer was generally low. The rate for adults with dementia was about 3%. Depression, anxiety disorders, and schizophrenia were found in less than 5% and bipolar disease in less than 1%. However, about 30% of the adults displayed some form of behavioral problems.

Cardiovascular Disease (CV) and Risk Factors

The apparently low frequency of CV disease in this study prompted further analysis of CV disease and risk factors. No specific CV diagnosis occurred at more than a rate of 13%. The frequency of hyperlipidemia and type II diabetes increased with age in the cohort. Body mass index (BMI) remained constant with increasing age group. This study population appeared to have lower frequencies of hyperlipidemia, hypertension, and diabetes than found in the general Israeli population.

A decrease in CV disease frequency with increasing cognitive severity was observed. The percentage of those adults with known CV disease risk factors like hyperlipidemia, BMI >27, type II diabetes, lack of weekly exercise, and hypertension decreased with more severe intellectual disability. Older people, those with high BMIs, those with diabetes, and those with hyperlipidemia, had greater frequencies of heart disease.

Health Needs of Adults with Intellectual Disability

With more persons with ID living longer comes an increase in age-related health problems seen in the general population, such as heart disease, cardiovascular disease, cancer, and visual and hearing impairments. Since many of the physicians and care staff involved with the health service of persons with ID came from the field of pediatrics, there will now be a need to take a long-term view and involve the fields of family medicine and geriatrics in the care. The physician working in family medicine in the community has very little training or experience working with ID, inspite of more people with ID living today in the community compared to residential care. We would like to share some of our experiences on health-related problems and needs of adult persons with intellectual disability relevant for family physicians or other allied professionals working with persons with ID both in residential care and in the community.

Mild and Moderate Intellectual Disability

The concerns will be the same as for the general aging population, but due to communication problems, lack of service, sometimes lack of interest, or commitment from the service providers, diagnosis or treatment can be ignored, overlooked, or delayed for this population [24]. This is unfortunate, because simple medical problems that could be solved will have adverse effects on the quality of life for the person with ID.

Cardiovascular disease was found to be less in persons with ID aged 65 years and older admitted to nursing homes than persons without ID (24.4 vs. 56.5%) [25], but there are very few studies on the prevalence of heart disease in this population [26]. A study from New York State [23] of 1,371 adult persons with ID living in the community showed that cardiovascular disease increased with increasing age and more likely among adults who were more functional and in adults with seizures and with the highest BMI.

The incidence of death from cancer in the United Kingdom for persons with intellectual disability has been lower than the general population (11.7–17.5 vs. 26%), but the incidence of cancer is now on the increase due to increased longevity [27, 28]. In New York State cancer increased significantly with age and was more likely to occur in females [23]. Gastrointestinal cancer was proportionally higher than the general population (48–58.5 vs. 25% of cancer deaths in the United Kingdom) [27, 28]. In a study of cancer and Down syndrome, a statistically significant excess of leukemia was found and in addition an excess of gastric cancer in institutionalized males observed [29].

Women with ID are much less likely to undergo cervical smear tests than the general population (19 vs. 77%) [30] and also less likely to have breast cancer examinations or receive mammography [31].

Visual and hearing impairments effect about half of the general population over 65 years and will also be seen in older persons with ID. Visual impairment was found seven times higher in adults with ID than the general population [32]. Cataract, glaucoma, macular degeneration, and diabetic retinopathy should be considered. Ocular and orbital abnormalities in persons with Down syndrome are numerous and reported with various occurrences: blepharitis (2–47%), keratoconus (5–8%), glaucoma (less than 1%), iris anomalies (38–90%), cataract (25–85%), retinal anomalies (0–38%), optic nerve anomalies (very few cases), strabismus (23–44%), amblyopia (10–26%), nystagmus (5–30%), and refractive errors (18–58%) [33]. Deafness is also common in this population [34], and impairment increases with increasing age [34]. Presbycusis (high-pitched tones become harder to hear) and hearing loss are also seen in this population as a result of impacted earwax [35].

Constipation is seen frequent with this population and can be a lifelong problem, which increases with age due to decline in mobility and less bowel motility or movement. Medication can also be a factor in constipation. Caretakers need to be aware of this problem, because of the dangers to accumulation and sometimes even intestinal perforation and death [36, 37].

In aging the bladder capacity and muscle tone will decrease and cause urinary incontinence, and in men enlargement of the prostate gland can also restrict urinary flow.

Dental problems in surveys of this population have identified poor oral hygiene, high prevalence of gingival disease, and untreated dental caries with dental care difficult to implement [38].

Health Concerns in Severe and Profound Intellectual Disability

Many persons with severe and profound ID will have associated medical problems and disease. In our review of mortality in this population in Israel [39] for the 1991–1997 period, 60% of the 450 cases were deaths before the age of 41 years and 68% in the severe–profound group. Cardiovascular reasons accounted for 35%, respiratory disease for 25%, and infectious diseases for 9% of the cases. The group with severe and profound ID, who survived into old age, will therefore have musculoskeletal problems, respiratory disease, and problems with swallowing; some will need gastrostomy and therefore demand a high service level.

Osteoporosis and increased fractures should be kept in mind in this population [40] due to immobility, nutrition, and lack of activity.

Health Concern in Down Syndrome

In the 1920s the life expectancy for persons with Down syndrome (DS) was only 9 years, but this has now increased to 56–60 years, which is still 20 years less than the general population [41].

Alzheimer disease (AD) was first described by Professor Alois Alzheimer, Germany, in 1906 [42], when he reported the case of Auguste D, a 51-year-old female patient he had followed at a Frankfurt hospital since 1901 up until her death on April 8, 1906. Even after her death he went on to study the neuropathological features of her illness. Shortly after her death he presented her case at the 37th Conference of German Psychiatrist in Tubingen on November 4, 1906, in which he described her symptoms:

- Progressive cognitive impairment
- Focal symptoms
- Hallucinations
- Delusions
- Psychosocial incompetence
- Neurobiological changes found at autopsy: plaques, neurofibrillary tangles, and artheriosclerotic changes

These symptoms are still the characteristics of AD today, which is the most common cause of dementia in Western countries. Clinically AD most often presents with a subtle onset of memory loss followed by a slowly progressive dementia that has a course of several years. The duration of AD can be 3–10 years from diagnosis to death, and this progress is more rapid in persons with DS, and usually seizures will present itself at the end stage. Epilepsy is seen in about 5% of persons with DS, but the combination of DS and AD will produce epileptic seizures in 85% of the cases.

Besides AD, persons with DS are prone to other medical problems when aging. A study from Holland [43] of 96 adults with DS from an institution investigated systematically over the period 1991–1995 with cytogenetic diagnosis mental functioning, dementia, ophthalmological and audiological assessments, and thyroid function. Seventy (73%) were older than 40 years and only 4.3% females. Three percent were with mild ID, 82% moderate and severe ID, and 15% profound ID; 19% had already dementia, but this number increased to 42% in persons above 50 years of age.

Epilepsia was present in 16.7% of all the persons, but in 50% of those with dementia. Vision problems were frequent with only 17% with normal vision and here again increase of problems with increase in age. In the 50–59-year age group 44.8% had moderate to severe vision loss. Seventy percent had moderate, severe, or very severe hearing loss, which was undiagnosed before systematic hearing tests were performed; 49% had thyroid dysfunction.

Besides from the above-observed health problems persons with DS have increased obesity, premature aging of the immune system resulting in various diseases, increased sleep apnea, and musculoskeletal problems [44].

Epilepsy and Cerebral Palsy

Persons with intellectual disability (ID), epilepsy, and seizures, who receive anti-epileptic drugs over long periods, will also be at an increased risk for premature mortality, increased risk of osteoporosis, and increased risks of falls.

A study of risk factors for injuries and falls [45] among 268 adults with ID from 18 nursing homes in Chicago revealed that 11% (30 cases) had reported injuries 12 months prior to the follow-up study. Over 50% of the injuries were caused by falls, and persons with a higher frequency of seizures, more destructive behavior, and usage of anti-psychotic drugs had the highest risk of injuries. Further analysis of the data revealed that persons over 70 years, ambulatory, and a higher frequency of seizures had the highest risk of injurious falls.

Studies of the effect of aging in persons with cerebral palsy (CP) are few, and studies with persons with both ID and CP are even less. Reason is that mobility would be decreased over the years and osteoporosis increased, increasing dependency on care over the years.

Older people with ID have the same needs as other older people do, and they are subject to the same age-related impairments and illnesses. Moreover, because many disabled individuals live together with their families, the burden is double because the family members are also aging and, with time, will not be able to continue their caregiving. As with older people in general, older people with intellectual disability also have the following needs:

- Social needs for people with intellectual disabilities should be met by making it possible for them to attend, use, and benefit from the social, recreational, and leisure resources and amenities that communities develop and operate for their elderly citizens.
- Housing needs can be met by supporting families when they are the primary carer or by providing financial resources for rentals or ownership of property. Housing can also be provided by brokering co-living arrangements with other people or by providing for small group homes or self-catered apartments.

- Medical needs can be met by enrollment in universal health care or programs. Periodic health assessments and health care should be normalized and provided as an overall system of supports when needed or as assistance provided for the adequate self-directed use of general or specialty health services. Risk assessments and health reviews should be part of the individual's life plan and provided to detect diseases and conditions that could compromise longevity.
- Activity or work is a normal part of life for everybody and should also be facilitated for this population, since we have seen that continued activation is preventative for old-age-associated depression and other emotional problems.
- Special care needs for age-associated conditions, such as Alzheimer's disease and related dementias, increasing fragility, or conditions or diseases compromising independent functioning, should be addressed with the focus on care in community or family settings. Institutionalization of persons with ID should not be based on old age alone.

Community Aspects

The number of persons with intellectual disability (ID) in general practice has been studied in Holland [46]. A general practice database with 62,000 patients had 318 persons (or 0.65%) with ID, which together with persons in residential care showed a total prevalence of 0.82%.

Barriers to treatment in general practice have been studied in Australia among 912 randomly selected general practitioners (GPs) [47], where communication difficulties with patients and other health professionals and problems in getting patient histories were the most significant barriers. Other difficulties were lack of training and experience, poor patient compliance, consultation time limitations, difficulties in problem determination, examination difficulties, poor continuity of care, and inadequate knowledge of services and resources, which resulted in the development of a practice guideline for primary health-care staff [2].

Researchers in Cardiff, Wales, have developed a health screening tool for persons with ID in general practice [48], which has also been used in general practice in New Zealand [49]. Here the introduction of an annual health screen resulted in medical findings of 72.6% of the 1,311 persons screened, which afterward required follow-up interventions.

A survey conducted through all US family practice residency directors [50] showed that 84% of the programs had provided residents with one or more experience about health-care needs of persons with ID and 60% had instructed residents in that area. Holland in the year 2000 established a chair in intellectual disability at the University of Rotterdam Department of Family Medicine and started a 3 year subspecialty in ID [51], where the first class of specialists in ID graduated in November 2003. In 2010 the second chair was established at the University Medical Center in Nijmegen.

Conclusions

We have seen an increase in the population of persons with intellectual disability surviving into adulthood and now also older age over recent years resulting in health problems emerging like in the general population, but sometimes at a much earlier stage, like Alzheimer disease in Down syndrome. There is therefore a need to provide more evidence-based practice standards to enhance health status, longevity, functional capability, and quality of life in this population [52] and transition from pediatric to adult care [9]. For the health professionals, there are also needs and efforts to be made in order to accomplish a transition from pediatric to adult care and expertize

- the acquisition of additional clinical and epidemiological knowledge regarding specific syndromes with linkages to basic science research in biomolecular genetics and metabolism;
- the development of adapted diagnostic and therapeutic methods for people who have difficulties with cooperation or communication;
- the development and evaluation of interdisciplinary interventions for complicated conditions (like sensory impairment, dysphagia, communication, and functional decline);
- the development of clinimetric measures in a number of areas (functional capability, quality of life, mental health, pain assessment, and clinical diagnosis) that are sensitive and specific, easy to administer, and applicable to persons with a wide range of mental and physical capabilities;
- the evaluation of clinical guidelines, including referral protocols, to support community-based primary care physicians, within specific health-care systems, to care for people with intellectual disabilities;
- the evaluation of the applicability of a new discipline of life span developmental medicine to lead in interdisciplinary care, health-care education, service delivery, and research for people with intellectual disability within an academic framework; and
- the development of the knowledge base regarding the health status and needs of people with intellectual disabilities living in less developed countries.

References

1. Rubin IL, Crocker A, editors. Medical care for children and adults with developmental disabilities. 2nd ed. Baltimore, MD: Paul H Brookes; 2006.
2. NSW. Department of Health. Health care in people with intellectual disability. Guidelines for general practitioners. North Sydney, NSW: DOH; 2006.
3. O'Hara J. Learning disabilities services: primary care or mental health trust? Psychiatr Bull. 2000;24:368–9.
4. Balogh R, Ouellette-Kuntz H, Bourne L, Lunsky Y, Colantonio A. Organising health care for persons with an intellectual disability. Cochrane Database Syst Rev. 2008;4:CD007492.

5. Centers for Disease Control and Prevention. Economic costs associated with mental retardation, cerebral palsy, hearing loss and vision impairment, United States 2003. MMWR. 2004;53:57–59.
6. Cohen WI, Nadel L, Madnick ME, editors. Down syndrome. Visions for the 21st century. New York, NY: Wiley-Liss; 2002:237–45.
7. Prasher VP, Janicki MP, editors. Physical health of adults with intellectual disabilities. Oxford: Blackwell; 2002.
8. Omar H, Greydanus DE, Patel DR, Merrick J, editors. Adolescence and chronic illness. A public health concern. New York, NY: Nova Science; 2010.
9. Bricker JT, Omar HA, Merrick J, editors. Adults with childhood illnesses: considerations for practice. Berlin: De Gruyter; in press.
10. Yeo M, Sawyer SM. Strategies to promote better outcomes in young people with chronic illnesses. Ann Acad Med Singapore. 2003;32:36–42.
11. Heaven P. Contemporary adolescence: a social psychological approach. Melbourne: Macmillan Education; 1994.
12. Coupey SM, Neinstein LS, Zeltzer LK. Chronic illness in the adolescent. In: Neinstein LS, editor. Adolescent health care. A practical guide. Philadelphia, PA: Lippincott Williams Wilkins; 2002. pp. 1511–36.
13. Kandel I, Merrick J. The birth of a child with disability. Coping by parents and siblings. ScientificWorldJournal. 2003;3(8):741–50.
14. Newacheck PW, McManus MA, Fox HB. Prevalence and impact of chronic illness among adolescents. Am J Dis Child. 1991;145(12):1367–73.
15. Blum RW. Introduction. Improving transition for adolescents with special health care needs from pediatric to adult centered care. Pediatrics. 2003;110(6Tt2):1301–3.
16. Merrick J, Kandel I. Adolescents with special needs and the transition from adolescent to adult health care. Int J Adolesc Med Health. 2003;15(20):103.
17. Perrin JM. Health services research for children with disabilities. Milbank Quart. 2002;80(2):303–24.
18. Janicki MP, Dalton AJ, Henderson CM, Davidson PW. Mortality and morbidity among older adults with intellectual disability: health services considerations. Disabil Rehabil. 1999;21:284–94.
19. Centers for Disease Control and Prevention (CDC). Trends in aging. United States and worldwide. MMWR. 2003;52(6):101–6.
20. Kandel I, Merrick E, Merrick J, Morad M. Increased aging in persons with intellectual disability in residential care centers in Israel 1999–2006. Med Sci Monit. 2009;15(4):PH13–PH16.
21. Fisher K, Kettl P. Aging with mental retardation: increasing population of older adults with MR require health interventions and prevention strategies. Geriatrics. 2005;60(4):26–29.
22. Merrick J, Davidson PW, Morad M, Janicki MP, Wexler O, Henderson CM. Older adults with intellectual disability in residential care centers in Israel: health status and service utilization. Am J Ment Retard. 2004;109(5):413–20.
23. Janicki MP, Davidson PW, Henderson CM, McCallion P, Taets JD, Force LT, et al. Health characteristics and health services utilization in older adults with intellectual disability living in community residences. J Intellect Disabil Res. 2002;46:287–98.
24. Kerr AM, McCulloch D, Oliver K, McLean B, Coleman E, Law T, Beaton P, Wallace S, Newell E, Eccles T, Prescott RJ. Medical need of people with intellectual disability require regular reassessment and provision of client- and carer-held reports. J Intellect Disabil Res. 2003;47:134–45.
25. Anderson DJ. Health issues. In: Sutton E et al., editors. Older adults with developmental disabilities. Baltimore, MD: Paul Brookes; 1993. pp. 29–48.
26. Merrick J, Morad M. Cardiovascular disease. In: O'Hara J, McCarthy J, Bouras N, editors. Intellectual disability and ill health. Cambridge: Cambridge University Press; 2010. pp. 73–7.
27. Cooke LB. Cancer and learning disability. J Intellect Disabil Res. 1997;41:312–16.

28. Duff M, Hoghton M, Scheepers M, Cooper M, Baddeley P. Helicobacter pylori: has the killer escaped from the institution? A possible cause of increased stomach cancer in a population with intellectual disability. J Intellect Disabil Res. 2001;45:219–25.
29. Boker LK, Merrick J. Cancer incidence in persons with Down syndrome in Israel. Down Syndr Res Pract. 2002;8(1):31–36.
30. Djuretic T, Laing-Morton T, Guy M, Gill M. Concerted effort is needed to ensure the women use preventive services. BMJ. 1999;318:536.
31. Davies N, Duff M. Breast cancer screening for older women with intellectual disability living in community group homes. J Intellect Disabil Res. 2001;45:253–7.
32. Warburg M. Visual impairment among people with developmental delay. J Intellect Disabil Res. 1994;38:423–32.
33. Merrick J, Koslowe K. Refractive errors and visual anomalies in Down syndrome. Down Syndr Res Pract. 2001;6(3):131–3.
34. Evenhuis HM. Medical aspects of ageing in a population with intellectual disability: II. Hearing impairment. J Intell Disabil Res. 1995;39:27–33.
35. Crandell CC, Roesser RJ. Incidence of excessive/impacted cerumen in individuals with mental retardation: a longitudinal investigation. Am J Ment Retard. 1993;97:568–74.
36. Bohmer CJM, Taminiau JAJM, Klinkenberg-Knol EC, Meuwissen SGM. The prevalence of constipation in institutionalized people with intellectual disability. J Intellect Disabil Res. 2001;45:212–18.
37. Morad M, Nelson NP, Merrick J, Davidson PW, Carmeli E. Prevalence and risk factors of constipation in adults with intellectual disability in residential care centers in Israel. Res Dev Disabil. 2007;28:580–6.
38. Walman HB, Perlman SP. Providing dental services for people with disabilities: why is it so difficult? Ment Retard. 2002;40(4):330–3.
39. Merrick J. Mortality for persons with intellectual disability in residential care in Israel 1991–97. J Intellect Dev Disabil. 2002;27(4):265–72.
40. Center J, Beange H, McElduff A. People with mental retardation have an increased prevalence of osteoporosis: a population study. Am J Ment Retard. 1998;103(1):19–28.
41. Merrick J. Aspects of Down syndrome. Int J Adolesc Med Health. 2000;12(1):5–17.
42. Alzheimer A. Uber einen eigenartigen schweren Erkrankungsprozess der Hirnrinde. Neurol. Centralblatt. 1906;23:1129–36. [German]
43. Van Buggenhout GJCM, Trommelen JCM, Schoenmaker A, De Baal C, Verbeek JJMC, Smeets DFCM, Ropers HH, Devriendt K, Hamel BCJ, Fryns JP. Down syndrome in a population of elderly mentally retarded patients: genetic-diagnostic survey and implications for medical care. Am J Med Genetics. 1999;85:376–84.
44. Merrick J, Ezra E, Josef B, Hendel D, Steinberg DM, Wientroub S. Musculoskeletal problems in Down syndrome. European Paediatric Orthopaedic Society Survey: The Israeli sample. J Pediatr Orthopaedics Part B. 2000;9:185–92.
45. Hsieh K, Heller T, Miller AB. Risk factors for injuries and falls among adults with developmental disabilities. J Intellect Disabil Res. 2001;45:76–82.
46. van Schrojenstein Lantman-de Valk HMJ, Metsemakers JFM, Soomers-Turlings MJMSJG, Haveman MJ, Crebolder HFJM. People with intellectual disability in general practice: case definition and case findings. J Intellect Disabil Res. 1997;41:373–9.
47. Lennox NG, Diggens JN, Ugoni AM. The general practice care of people with intellectual disability: barriers and solutions. J Intellect Disabil Res. 1997;41:380–90.
48. Jones RG, Kerr MP. A randomized control trial of an opportunistic health screening tool in primary care for people with intellectual disability. J Intellect Disabil Res. 1997;41:409–15.
49. Webb OJ, Rogers L. Health screening for people with intellectual disability: The New Zealand experience. J Intellect Disabil Res. 1999;43:497–503.
50. Tyler CV, Snyder CW, Zyzanski SJ. Caring for adults with mental retardation: survey of family practice residency program directors. Ment Retard. 1999;37(5):347–52.

51. Evenhuis HM, van Praag PH, Wiersema MI, Huisman S. Curriculum for the medical special-ist training for physicians for people with intellectual disability. Amsterdam: Dutch Society Physicians for People with Intellectual Disability (NVAZ); 1998.
52. Evenhuis HM, Henderson CM, Beange H, Lennox N, Chicoine B. Healthy ageing in people with intellectual disability. Physical health issues. Geneva: World Health Organization; 2000.

Chapter 23
Principles of Team Care for Children with Developmental Disabilities

Dilip R. Patel and Helen D. Pratt

Abstract Professionals who work with children and adolescents who have developmental disabilities will find themselves working with a number of other professionals on various "teams." These teams are typically composed of practitioners from more than one discipline working toward the single goal of providing comprehensive patient care. Research on medical and psychosocial teams confirms the overwhelming importance of clarity, commitment, and close positive exchanges among team members to promote successful teamwork. The effectiveness of teams is largely dependent on how the professionals work to accomplish meeting the needs of their patients. This chapter reviews multidisciplinary, interdisciplinary, and transdisciplinary approaches to delivering health care to children and adolescents who have developmental disabilities.

Introduction

Health-care delivery to children and adolescents who have developmental disabilities requires participation and sharing of expertise of multiple medical, social, and psychological disciplines. Multiple disciplinary approaches have been applied in education and training, service delivery, and research; however, our focus here is on service delivery to children with developmental disabilities [1]. Teamwork is promoted at all levels of health-care delivery with numerous purported benefits (see Table 23.1) of such approaches [1–8]. However, research-based evidence for effectiveness and utility of multiple discipline approaches is at best limited and equivocal. The effectiveness of team approach to delivering patient care varies widely depending on multiple factors. In this chapter we review the concepts of team processes and their application to delivering health care to children and adolescents who have developmental disabilities.

D.R. Patel (✉)
Department of Pediatrics and Human Development, Kalamazoo Center for Medical Studies, Michigan State University College of Human Medicine, Kalamazoo, MI 49008-1284, USA
e-mail: patel@kcms.msu.edu

D.R. Patel et al. (eds.), *Neurodevelopmental Disabilities*,
DOI 10.1007/978-94-007-0627-9_23, © Springer Science+Business Media B.V. 2011

Table 23.1 Purported benefits of multiple discipline approaches in health-care delivery

- Improves quality of care
- Reduces errors in health-care delivery
- Reduces duplication of services
- Provides cost-effective care
- Enhances efficiency of health-care delivery
- Addresses medical as well as psychosocial aspects of care
- Is more convenient for the patient and family or caregiver
- Increases patient and family or caregiver satisfaction
- Promotes development of innovative approaches and solutions to complex problems
- Meets the mandates of applicable laws
- Increases collaboration and networking among professionals
- Enhances individual professional development

Teams and Team Processes

Katzenbach and Smith defined a team as "a small group of people with complementary skills who are committed to a common purpose, performance goals, and approach for which they are mutually accountable" [9, 10]. Most teams in the setting of health-care delivery have 7–10 members, which lends itself to a more manageable group [11]. A team with a large number of members who are geographically more dispersed may have the potential for adversely affecting effective functioning of the team. The complementary skills considered essential of team members are interpersonal, functional, decision making, and problem solving [11].

Similar to a team, a work group is also comprised of a small group of people with a common goal [11, 12]. However, in a work group, each member functions individually and is accountable for the quality of his/her own performance. Unlike health-care delivery teams, a work group has a time-limited mandate to accomplish a specific goal. Work groups are formed on as-needed basis to address a particular issue that arises at a given time. According to Grigsby [12], a task force is a type of work group typically comprised of members who have specific expertise.

Professionals who work with children and adolescents who have developmental disabilities will find themselves working with a number of other professionals on various "teams." These teams are usually composed of practitioners from more than one discipline working toward a common goal of providing comprehensive patient care [1, 13–18]. The composition of team will vary depending on medical conditions that it is intended to provide services for. For example, a team that serves the health-care needs of children and adolescents who have multiple disabilities, predominantly of neuromotor nature, will typically include disciplines listed in Table 23.2. Coordinator of the team or the clinic plays critical role in the overall implementation and smooth operation of the entire program (see Table 23.3).

The effectiveness of teams is largely dependent on how the professionals work with each other to meet the needs of their patients. Depending on the setting, service delivery may occur in a shared place (a clinic) or separate places but is

Table 23.2 Members of multiple disability clinic team

Patient and his/her caregivers
Pediatrician
Orthopedic surgeon
Orthotist
Physical therapist
Occupational therapist
Physiatrist
Dentist
Dietician
Medical social worker
Clinical psychologist
Pharmacist
Nurse
Clinic coordinator
Neurologist
Speech pathologist
Audiologist

Table 23.3 Role of team coordinator in multiple disability clinic

- Schedule clinics, patient appointments, and appropriate staff to be present for the clinic
- Maintain and implement program/institutional policy and procedures
- Obtain appropriate medical information and past reports prior to patient visit
- Guide patient, family, caregivers, and staff through the clinic process
- Facilitate referral process
- Obtain, organize, and distribute the final written reports to appropriate practitioners and agencies
- Prepare and submit billing information to the billing/accounting department
- Make phone calls, send reminder letters to patients
- Work closely with the community and state agencies involved
- Assist patients/families enroll in special community and state special insurance programs
- Make sure appropriate interpreters for different languages are available
- Schedule and facilitate team meeting at the end of the clinic
- Work with nursing and institutional administrative staff to facilitate smooth operation of the clinic

coordinated. Team members are asked to conduct diagnostic assessment, deliver medical care, or evaluate functional needs of the patient (impact of illness or disorder on general health, vision, hearing, mobility, cognition, mental health, social function, and academic function). The patient's (or responsible caregiver's) ability to access and pay for health-care services is also assessed. Each team member puts forth his/her assessment data, with recommendations for interventions. Clinicians who provide therapy generally deliver treatment and report outcomes to the patient, to the patient's pertinent family members, and to the team. Members who evaluate functional impact are usually the members who served on the assessment team. Some teams have members who can provide all aspects of care and others have interchangeable members. Three types of teams, namely multidisciplinary, interdisciplinary, and transdisciplinary, are most frequently described in the literature [19–39]. These are reviewed in the sections that follow, with reference to their applicability to delivering health care to children and adolescents who have developmental disabilities.

Conceptualization of Multiple Discipline Teams

Discipline

In standard English language dictionaries, a discipline is variously defined as a branch of knowledge, instruction, learning, or education; or a field of study or activity [40].

Multiple Disciplinary

Choi and Pak [2] suggested that the term multiple disciplines (multiple disciplinary) should be used for a more general situation when the level or the nature of involvement and interaction of multiple disciplines in a team is not clearly delineated.

Unidisciplinary or Intradisciplinary

Satin refers to a unidisciplinary team as team that is comprised of two or more professionals in the same discipline with common skills, training, and language working together [41]. Tremendous expansion of knowledge base in different disciplines may necessitate professionals from the same discipline to share their individual expertise within the discipline with others in the same field to accomplish common goals. In that sense, unidisciplinary teams are also referred to as intradisciplinary teams.

Multidisciplinary

In a multidisciplinary team, each team member completes his/her training-specific assessment, intervention, and evaluation of the patient. Each team member draws on the skills and knowledge from different disciplines but functions within the boundaries of his/her discipline [2, 22]. The process is thus described as additive [2, 22]. Choi and Pak [2] gave $2 + 2 = 4$ as a mathematical example and a salad bowl as a food example to illustrate the concept of multidisciplinarity. Multidisciplinary teams were typically led by a physician who makes the final decision about the patient's care. In that sense it is hierarchical. The term multiprofessional team is used more widely in some European countries and Canada to describe multidisciplinary team.

Interdisciplinary

Members in an interdisciplinary team share the responsibility for making the ultimate decision about patient's care. The care plan is developed by the whole team, and it is the entire team's responsibility to follow through on it. The assessment and the care plan reflect the integration of expertise from individual disciplines. It is more of a group process. Each member of the team shares his/her expertise with others, and the team process is described as highly interactive. The process allows the team to "analyze, synthesize, and harmonize links between disciplines into a coordinated whole" [2, 23]. Choi and Pak [2] explained interdisciplinarity in terms of mathematical example as $2 + 2 = 5$ and in terms of food example, a melting pot.

However, truly interdisciplinary teams are probably few and far between, especially in a traditional medical facility. Interdisciplinary teams probably seem ideal to most members because they may not feel that their expertise is being undermined by one discipline. In some Children's Multiple Specialty Clinics the team is headed by a physician with a specialty in the disorder treated by that clinic. These teams typically coordinate their assessments and treatment. Sometimes the professionals who actually provide the care also participate in the assessment.

Transdisciplinary

Soskolne [30] defined transdisciplinary approaches to human health "as approaches that integrate the natural, social and health sciences in a humanistic context, and in so doing transcend each of their traditional boundaries." Members of a transdisciplinary team think beyond their individual disciplines and work toward formulating a novel solution or perspective to a given problem. Transdisciplinary approaches often lead to the development of entirely new fields of study or knowledge. Choi and Pak [2] viewed transdisciplinary approach as holistic and illustrated the concept with a mathematical example of $2 + 2 =$ yellow and a food example of a cake. In a transdisciplinary team, members share skills. There is an acceptance by the individual team member that another team member can do a better job in an area of his/her own expertise (role release) [2, 27]. Team members also acquire new skills and function beyond their discipline (role expansion) [2, 27]. Application of transdisciplinary team approach to delivering health care to children and adolescents who have developmental disabilities has not been reported.

Virtual or Electronic Teams

Widespread use of electronic communication has led to the development of virtual team processes [2, 11, 42–44]. The individual team members can be geographically dispersed but can work as a team in an interactive, integrated manner toward a common goal. Application and utility of such teamwork in the setting of health-care delivery to children and adolescents with developmental disabilities remains to be established.

Evolution and Comparative Characteristics of Teams

Teams may evolve naturally over time when a number of professionals from different disciplines are involved in delivering health care to the same patient and begin sharing information. These types of teams are much less common and take a long time to establish. More commonly, a team begins with a team leader who then carefully chooses members based on their expertise, discipline, and ability to work in a team setting. Choi and Pak published a comprehensive review of literature on multidisciplinarity, interdisciplinarity, and transdisciplinarity in health research, services, education, and policy [2, 5–10, 19–33, 40, 45, 46].

Developing Effective Teams

Research on multiple discipline teams confirms the overwhelming importance of clarity, commitment, and close, positive exchanges between team members to promoting successful teamwork [1, 13–18]. Several factors essential for developing and maintaining effective teams regardless have been described (see Table 23.4) [15, 46–51]. Teams that do not have clear goals, tasks, role delegation, or strong commitment to the team process will be ineffective. One set of researchers offers that the team leadership should not be discipline specific but should be dependent on the patient's presenting complaint as well as the ongoing management objectives. Strategies to enhance multiple disciplinary teamwork and barriers to effective team development are summarized in Table 23.5 [46].

Outcomes of Team Approaches in Health-Care Delivery

There is a paucity of published studies documenting the outcomes of multiple disciplinary team approaches in health care in general and in delivery of health care to children who have developmental disabilities in particular. Based on extensive reviews of literature, several authors found the evidence of effectiveness of multiple

Table 23.4 Essential factors for developing and maintaining effective teams

- Open and frequent communication between team members
- Clearly defined team philosophy
- A high degree of commitment to team process its members
- Autonomy for team members to function within the scope of their expertise
- Ability of team members to effectively cope with the issues related to service delivery to their patients (especially death and dying)
- Mutual respect and trust between team members and for the team process itself
- Effective coordination of work flow

Table 23.5 Strategies to enhance multiple disciplinary teamwork, summarized in an acronym TEAMWORK

	Strategy	Promoting the promoters	Barring the barriers	The 14 Cs of teamwork
T	Team	Good selection of team members Good team leaders Maturity and flexibility of team members	*Avoid* poor selection of the disciplines and team members *Avoid* poor process of team functioning	Coordination of efforts Conflict management
E	Enthusiasm	Personal commitment of team members	*Avoid* lack of proper measures to evaluate success of interdisciplinary work *Avoid* lack of guidelines for multiple authorship in research publications	Commitment
A	Accessibility	Physical proximity of team members The Internet and e-mail as a supporting platform	*Avoid* language problems	Cohesiveness (team sticks together) Collaboration
M	Motivation	Incentives	*Avoid* insufficient time for the project *Avoid* insufficient funding for the project	Contribution (feeling this is being made)
W	Workplace	Institutional support and changes in the workplace	*Avoid* institutional constraints	Corporate support
O	Objectives	A common goal and shared vision	*Avoid* discipline conflicts	Confronts problems directly
R	Role	Clarity and rotation of roles	*Avoid* team conflicts	Cooperation Consensus decision making Consistency
K	Kinship	Communication among team members Constructive comments among team members	*Avoid* lack of communication between disciplines *Avoid* unequal power among disciplines	Communication Caring Chemistry (personality, "good fit")

Adapted with permission from [47, table 1, p. E230].

disciplinary approaches to health-care delivery to be equivocal [52–61]. Authors note methodological flaws and difficulties in conducting such outcome studies including poor or no definition of types of teams, ill-defined or lack of theoretical concepts, variable populations served, different settings in which care is provided, variable organizational support and infrastructure, access to and availability of

Table 23.6 Assessment of need for multiple disciplinary process

• Assess if a single discipline approach is sufficient or not
• Identify reasons why a single discipline approach is considered to be insufficient
• Assess if the proposed disciplines are available
• Assess which disciplines and experts are available
• Assess potential role each discipline will play in the team
• Determine how the experts are expected to work (i.e., work together or to formulate a novel plan)
• Assess the availability of coordinators for the team operation
• Assess if an outcome evaluation process is in place
• Determine how outcome of success will be measured

Based on data from [4, pp. 434–6].

experts in different disciplines, and a wide range of health problems of varying severity served by the teams. There is no documented evidence of the effectiveness of application of the crew resource management model to reduce errors or improve quality in health-care delivery [11, 55].

The need for and effectiveness of team approaches to health-care delivery will vary depending on multiple factors including the specific problems being addressed, the ability of team members to work together, level of institutional and organizational support, fiscal viability of team approach, and access to and availability of needed disciplines. Such approaches have been reported to be more useful in delivery of care in the fields of rehabilitation, geriatrics, and psychiatry. Experience suggests that delivery of health care to children with developmental disabilities by an interdisciplinary team is highly desirable. It reduces unnecessary visits to emergency rooms and inpatient care, improves quality of care, fosters fruitful collaboration between disciplines, addresses complex psychosocial issues, and enhances patient and caregiver satisfaction about the care.

Not all medical conditions are necessarily best served by team approaches. A careful assessment should be undertaken before implementing an interdisciplinary team program for delivery of health care. Whitfield and Reid have proposed that several key questions must be asked before considering interdisciplinary population health research [4]. Their approach, although designed for application in research, can also be useful while considering implementation of an interdisciplinary team to deliver health care to children with developmental disabilities (see Table 23.6).

Conclusion

Application of multiple disciplinary approaches is widely promoted to deliver health-care services to children and adolescents with special health-care needs. Most widely described approaches are multidisciplinarity, interdisciplinarity, and transdisciplinarity. It is presumed and intuitive that such multiple disciplinary approaches will be cost-effective, improve quality of care, and reduce errors in delivery of health care. Many other benefits of such approaches are described. There is very little evidence that multiple discipline approaches to education, service delivery, and research are always necessary. Experience suggests that multidisciplinary and interdisciplinary approaches can be effective and beneficial in delivering health care to children and adolescents who have developmental disabilities; however, research must supplant experience and intuition, and is sorely needed and highly recommended.

Acknowledgment Adapted with permission from authors' previous work [62].

References

1. Pratt HD, Rickerts VI. Concepts of multidisciplinary versus interdisciplinary approaches to team work. Soc Adolesc Med Newsl. 2004;14(3):4, 7.
2. Choi BCK, Pak AWP. Multidisciplinarity, interdisciplinarity and transdisciplinarity in health research, services, education and policy: 1. Definitions, objectives and evidence of effectiveness. Clin Invest Med. 2006;29(6):351–64.
3. Heinemann GD, Zeiss AM. Team performance in health care: assessment and development. New York, NY: Plenum; 2002.
4. Whitfield K, Reid C. Assumptions, ambiguities, and possibilities in interdisciplinary population health research. Can J Public Health. 2004;95:434–43.
5. Schofield RF, Amodeo M. Interdisciplinary teams in health care and human services settings: are they effective? Health Soc Work. 1999;24:210–19.
6. McCallin A. Interdisciplinary practice. A matter of teamwork: an integrated literature review. J Clin Nurs. 2001;10:419–28.
7. Austin W, Park C, Goble E. From interdisciplinary to transdisciplinary research: a case study. Qual Health Res. 2008;18(4):557–64.
8. Kessel F, Rosenfild PL. Toward transdiciplinary research: historical contemporary perspectives. Am J Prev Med. 2008;35(2S):S225–34.
9. Katzenbach JR, Smith DK. The wisdom of teams. Boston, MA: Harvard Business School Press; 1993.
10. Katzenbach JR, Smith DK. The discipline of teams. Harv Bus Rev. 1993;71(2):111–20.
11. Parrish RAM, Oppenheimer S. The interdisciplinary team approach. In: Wolraich ML, Drotar DD, Dworkin PH, Perrin EC, editors. Developmental–behavioral pediatrics: evidence and practice. New York, NY: Elsevier Mosby; 2008. pp. 203–13.
12. Grigsby RK. Committee, task force, team: what's the difference? Why does it matter? Acad Physician Sci. 2008 Jan:4–5.
13. Brown KS, Folen RA. Psychologists as leaders of multidisciplinary chronic pain management teams: a model for health care delivery. Prof Psychol Res Pract. 2005;36(6):587–94.
14. Hall KL, Feng AX, Moser RP, Stokols D, Taylor BK. Moving the science of team science forward: collaboration and creativity. Am J Prev Med. 2008;35(2S):S243–49.
15. Jünger S, Pestinger M, Elsner F, Krumm N, Radbruch L. Criteria for successful multiprofessional cooperation in palliative care teams. Palliat Med. 2007;21(4):347–54.
16. Molinari E, Taverna A, Gasca G, Constantino AL. Collaborative team approach to asthma: a clinical study. Fam Syst Med. 1994;12(1):47–59.
17. Talen MR, Graham MC, Walbroehl G. Introducing multiprofessional team practice and community-based health care services into the curriculum: a challenge for health care educators. Fam Syst Med. 1994;12(4):353–60.
18. Whitmer K, Pruemer JM, Nahleh ZA, Jazieh AR. Symptom Management needs of oncology outpatients. J Palliat Med. 2006;9(3):628–30.

19. Poulton BC, West MA. Effective multidisciplinary teamwork in primary health care. J Adv Nurs. 1993;18:918–25.
20. Nolan M. Towards an ethos of interdisciplinary practice. BMJ. 1995;312:305–7.
21. Cole KD, Waite MS, Nichols LO. Organizational structure, team process, and future directions of interprofessional health care teams. Gerontol Geriatr Educ. 2003;24(2):35–49.
22. Natural Sciences and Engineering Research Council of Canada (NSERC). Guidelines for the preparation and review of applications in interdisciplinary research. Ottawa, ON: NSERC; 2004.
23. Canadian Institutes of Health Research (CIHR). Training program grant guide: strategic training initiative in health research. Ottawa, ON: CIHR; 2005.
24. Stokols D, Harvey R, Gress J, et al. In vivo studies of transdisciplinary scientific collaboration: lessons learned and implications for active living research. Am J Prev Med. 2005;28 (2 Suppl 2):202–13.
25. Nicholson D, Artz S, Armitage A, Fagan J. Working relationships and outcomes in multidisciplinary collaborative practice settings. Child Youth Care Forum. 2000;29:39–73.
26. Reilly C. Transdisciplinary approach: an atypical strategy for improving outcomes in rehabilitative and long-term acute care settings. Rehabil Nurs. 2001;26:216–20.
27. Kessler D. Transdisciplinary approach to pediatric undernutrition. Dev Behav News. 1999:8.
28. Stokols D, Misra S, Moser RP, Hall KL, Taylor BK. The ecology of team science: understanding contextual influences on transdisciplinary collaboration. Am J Prev Med. 2008;35(2S):S96–115.
29. Flinterman JF, Teclemariam-Mesbah R, Broerse JEW, et al. Transdisciplinary: the new challenge for biomedical research. Bull Sci. 2001;21:253–66.
30. Soskolne C. Transdisciplinary approaches for public health. Epidemiology. 2000;11:S122.
31. Benzecry SG, Leite HP, Oliveira FC, Santana E, Meneses JF, de Carvalho WB, Silva CM. Interdisciplinary approach improves nutritional status of children with heart disease. Nutrition. 2008;24(7–8):669–74.
32. Klein JT. Crossing boundaries: knowledge, disciplinarities, and interdisciplinarities. Charlottesville, VA: University of Virginia Press; 1996.
33. Lorimer W, Manion J. Team-based organizations: leading the essential transformation. PFCA Rev. 1996 Spring:15–19.
34. Mabry PL, Olster DH, Morgan GD, Abrams DB. Interdisciplinarity and systems science to improve population health: a view from the NIH Office of Behavioral and Social Sciences Research. Am J Prev Med. 2008;35(2S):S211–24.
35. Vyt A. Interprofessional and transdisciplinary teamwork in health care. Diabetes Metab Res Rev. 2008;24(Suppl 1):S106–9.
36. Institute of Medicine. Crossing the quality chasm: a new health system for the 21st Century. Washington, DC: National Academic Press; 2001.
37. Institute of Medicine. To err is human: building a safer health system. Washington, DC: National Academic Press; 2000.
38. Atwal A, Caldwell K. Do multidisciplinary integrated care pathways improve interprofessional collaboration? Scand J Caring Sci. 2002;16(4):360–67.
39. Choi BCK, Pak AWP. Multidisciplinarity, interdisciplinarity and transdisciplinarity in health research, services, education and policy: 3. Discipline, inter-discipline distance, and selection of discipline. Clin Invest Med. 2008;31(1):E41–48.
40. OneLook Dictionary Search. http://www.onelook.com/
41. Satin DG. A conceptual framework for working relationships among disciplines and the place of interdisciplinary education and practice: clarifying muddy waters. Gerontol Geriatr Educ. 1994;14(3):3–24.
42. Wiecha J, Pollard T. The interdisciplinary eHealth team: chronic care for the future. J Med Internet Res. 2004;6(3):e22.
43. Vroman K, Kovacich J. Computer-mediated interdisciplinary teams: theory and reality. J Interprof Care. 2002;16:159–70.

44. Furst S, Reeves M, Rosen B, et al. Managing the life of virtual teams. Acad Manage Exec. 2004;18(2):6–20.
45. Whitefield K, Reid C. Assumptions, ambiguities, and possibilities in interdisciplinary population health research. Can J Public Health. 2004;95:434–36.
46. Holistic Education Network. Transdisciplinary inquiry incorporating holistic principles. http://www.hent.org/transdisciplinary.htm (2008). Accessed 1 Sept 2008.
47. Choi BCK, Pak AWP. Multidisciplinarity, interdisciplinarity and transdisciplinarity in health research, services, education and policy: 2. Promotors, barriers, and strategies of enhancement. Clin Invest Med. 2007;30(6):E224–32.
48. Poulton BC, West MA. The determinants of effectiveness in primary health care teams. J Interprof Care. 1999;13:7–18.
49. Dukewits P, Gowan L. Creating successful collaborative teams. J Staff Dev. 1996;17(4):12–16.
50. Bronstein LR. A model for interdisciplinary collaboration. Soc Work. 2003;48(3):113–16.
51. American Academy of Family Physicians, American Academy of Pediatrics, American College of Physicians, American Osteopathic Association. Joint principles of the patient-centered medical home. http://www.medicalhomeinfo.org/ (2008). Accessed 1 Sept 2008.
52. Baker DP, Salas E, King H, et al. The role of teamwork in the professional education of physicians: current status and assessment recommendations. J Qual Patient Saf. 2005;31: 185–202.
53. Masse LC, Moser RP, Stokols D, et al. Measuring collaboration and transdisciplinary integration in team science. Am J Prev Med. 2008;35(2S):S151–60.
54. Orchard CA, Curran V, Kabene S. Creating a culture for interdisciplinary collaborative professional practice. Med Educ Online. 2005;10:11.
55. Pizzi L, Goldfarb NI, Nash DB. Crew resource management and its application in medicine. In making health care safer: a critical analysis of patient safety practices. Evidence Report/Technology Assessment: Number 43 (AHRQ Publication No. 01-E058). Rockville, MD: Search Results Agency for Healthcare Research and Quality; 2001. pp. 501–9.
56. Butterill D, O'Hanlon J, Book H. When the system is the problem, don't blame the patient: problems inherent in the interdisciplinary inpatient team. Can J Psychiatry. 1992;37:168–72.
57. Cashman SB, Reidy P, Cody K, et al. Developing and measuring progress toward collaborative, integrated, interdisciplinary health care teams. J Interprof Care. 2004;8:183–96.
58. Melzer SM, Richards GE, Covington MW. Reimbursement and costs of pediatric ambulatory diabetes care by using the resource-based relative value scale: is multidisciplinary care financially viable? Pediatr Diabetes. 2004;5:133–42.
59. Weaver TE. Enhancing multiple disciplinary teamwork. Nurs Outlook. 2008;56(3):108–14.
60. Schofield RF, Amodea M. Interdisciplinary teams in health care and human services settings: are they effective? Health Soc Work. 1999;24:210–19.
61. Jansen L. Collaborative and interdisciplinary health care teams: ready or not? J Prof Nurs. 2008;24(4):218–27.
62. Patel DR, Pratt HD, Patel ND. Team processes and team care for children with developmental disabilities. Pediatr Clin North Am. 2008;55(6):1375–90.

Chapter 24
Working with Families and Caregivers of Individuals with Developmental Disabilities

Helen D. Pratt

Abstract A physician's ability to provide quality care to their patients and their families is enhanced if he/she understands the impact of chronic disability on family (individually and collectively) function and development. Influencing factors include onset of the disability, intensity, severity, frequency, and complexity of interventions and resource availability. Chronic disability disrupts the lives of all members of the families. Early identification and intervention helps to mitigate the adverse impact (mental, physical, social, emotional, developmental) on function of chronic disabilities on the lives of family members.

Introduction

A physician's ability to provide quality care to their patients and their patients' parents and siblings is enhanced if he/she understands the impact of their patients' chronic disabilities (as identified in this book) on their family members (individually and collectively). Such knowledge can provide quality. Frequency of problems, intensity, severity, manifestation, impairments, and functional limitations are factors that affect the impact of chronic illness on family relationships. Early identification and intervention help to mitigate the adverse impact on function of chronic disabilities on the lives of the affected infant, child, adolescent, or young adult [1, 2]. This early effort can then be used to drive a range of treatment planning from medical treatment of the child to family planning for his/her parents to teaching family survival skills to parents and older siblings [3].

H.D. Pratt (✉)
Department of Pediatrics and Human Development, Kalamazoo Center for Medical Studies, Michigan State University College of Human Medicine, Kalamazoo, MI 49008-1284, USA
e-mail: pratt@kcms.msu.edu

Definitions

Developmental disabilities are a diverse group of severe chronic conditions that are due to mental and/or physical impairments. People with developmental disabilities have problems with major life activities such as language, mobility, learning, self-help, and independent living. Developmental disabilities begin anytime during development up to the age of 22 years and usually last throughout a person's lifetime (for example, autism spectrum disorders, cerebral palsy, hearing loss, intellectual disabilities, vision impairment, and birth defects) [4].

Manifestation of Disability

The personal and environmental impact of chronic disability on the individual, parents, siblings, or the family is dependent on several factors such as whether disabilities are overtly (publically, visually) or covertly (privately, not easily discernable to the public). Overt manifestations can exacerbate distress or garner public support or concern for the child and/or his parents. However, a sibling may be embarrassed at the visual display of the affected child's public displays of movement, vocalization, impulsive behaviors, unintelligible speech, or use of walking aide, or vocal displays of tics, etc. [5]. Private or covert disabilities may result in parents and siblings being questioned about the validity of their chronically disabled family member's behavior. Getting help for this child's disability may also be more difficult for parents [2].

Epidemiology

Most data found in researching epidemiology focused on the elderly, combination data for infants, children, and adults over 40 years of age. Those data were also disability specific and/or based on data from research by the Center for Disease Control in the Atlanta, GA, USA, area. Therefore the reader is referred to other chapters in this text that address specific disabilities [4].

Clinical Features

Chronic disabilities each disrupts the lives of all families and alters the typical developmental process (growth and maturation) of an infant, child, adolescent, and young adult. Although the physical effects may be disability specific, there are a few common affects on the (a) family dynamic, (b) parental intrapersonal relationship, (c) family interpersonal relationships with friends and extended family, (d) family member relationships with each other, and (e) sibling relationships with the affected child and with the parents [1, 2, 5]. Parental relationship dynamics requires them to expend extra efforts to meet the needs of the other children in the family and parents to care for their chronically disabled child, causes parental stress, increases the risk of the youth's development of another deficit in function. The connection between family health and parental health is widely accepted. Overburdened and distressed parents and parental interpersonal relationships negatively influence the parents' ability to meet the needs of their children, disabled or not.

Diagnosis

Diagnosis of chronic disability is addressed in disability-specific chapters included elsewhere in this book.

Impact of the Family's Environment

Immediate family and intimate environments are the primary influences in the lives of children prior to the age of 11 years. As the young adolescent's (ages 11–14 years) world expands from family focused to peer focused, the family's influence takes functions in the background. Youth in the middle adolescent stage of development perceive of how they are viewed by others and how they "fit" with peers as their primary influence. However, family always has a powerful influence and becomes more prominent as the individual matures. These factors (family, peers, and cultural environments) significantly influence that person's self-perception, attitudes about body (size, weight, and body fat), beauty, and their personal disability [2, 5].

Severe chronic disabilities increase the risk of mental or behavioral disabilities in the lives of the chronically disabled child and her family members. Families can provide a nurturing, supportive, protective environment where members are helped to grow and mature in a physically, mentally, and socially healthy manner. However, some families are not able to provide such an environment. Factors that impede healthy family environments have parents or children diagnosed with mental illness, have behavioral disorders, experience developmental disruptions, or the family dynamics are disrupted (divorce; death; birth of chronically ill child; or development of chronic illnesses, disabilities, or trauma). Chronic stress also impedes family function. Youth with developmental disabilities need protection and nurturance from parents, other family members, teachers, care providers, and peers to withstand these negative situations. Without this support they can develop profound sadness, distress, or even depression as a result [1, 6–8].

Parents usually lose access to support networks, experience isolation, anger, frustration, and loss of the dream of having a healthy "typically" developing child [1, 7, 9].

Physicians and parents need to be aware that the impact on family members and siblings in particular can range from mild to devastating. Family members of youth with chronic disabilities are at increased risk of developing psychological problems and behavioral problems [8]. Parents and siblings of youth who are technologically dependent may experience more severe distress. Fisher [10] offers that biomedical and technological advances have contributed to an increased survival of children with previous fatal diseases. These children are able to go home and live with their families. However, the intensity, duration, frequency, and complexity of their care create family environments that are no longer parent–child centered but now included parent–child-medical regimes–medical crises–medical and other intervention professionals. This creates stressed parents who are also overwhelmed, overworked, and under-rested. They experience a) increased loss of control of their lives, b) mixed with the uncertainty of outcomes with treatment, c) the end of hope for cures, d) the abundance of medical and medication regimes, e) fears of misdiagnoses, f) fear of death; lack understanding process and terminology, g) dealing with harsh reality of child's condition; h) face the harsh reality of their child's illness, i) changes in therapeutic regime, j) observe evidence of negative outcomes in other children with similar or the same disability; and k) fear that relinquishing some elements of control of their child could threaten their emotional equilibrium, causing parents anxiety [1, 9, 10].

Social Impact on Family

Parents of youth diagnosed with chronic disability may become socially isolated, not have entertaining space because of the major modifications to their homes to accommodate their child, experience a loss of privacy (conflicts and demonstrations of affection become public), and as a result the home loses its personal association with comfort security and privacy. Their daily lives become dominated by routine procedures relating to the care for their child with disabilities, especially with the technology-dependent child [1, 9].

Financial Impact

Accessing financial supports in the United States can cause parents and caregivers to experience difficulties coping with complex eligibility criteria and service restrictions associated with getting services and paying for them. Many families experience serious financial problems. Mothers often have to leave employment which reduces income, increased electricity, and long distance travel to receive specialized care. These issues also become a source of anxiety and stress [4].

Parent–Professional Relationships

Professionals need to remember that executive function is impaired under trauma and distressful times (focused attention, memory, and execution skills). Professionals can help by remaining calm, patient, and provide clearly written and bulleted information that is placed in a labeled binder (name of agency, provider, phone number, next scheduled visit, office hours, and emergency) or folder. When patients require special equipment, such tools become especially important [10]. Equipment should have written and visual instruction cards that are laminated and include a video with visual instructions for routine equipment care and for managing problems. Parents may demonstrate short patience, irritation, express feelings of being disrespected or treated like children by professionals who work with them. This is especially true for those professionals who must enter the patient's family home. It is vital for professionals to remember that the patient's parents or caregivers often have very little sleep, opportunities to distress, and/or lack adequate financial resources. There are often multiple urgent demands on their time, energy, and finances. Most intervention services are fragmented or duplicated and poorly coordinated in the absence of professional advocates who assume burden for the parents.

Parents need professionals to understand these issues and provide patient, supportive care and empathetic care delivery [10]. Parents want physicians and other professionals to view them as collaborators in their child's care. Case or nurse managers can provide crucial supports for parents of technology-dependent children. Most states provide such services through their community mental health programs including coordinating access to education, transportation, and respite care needs.

Professionals should serve as patient advocates and service providers. They should be trained in how to use enhanced communication techniques, team building, and developing healthy interpersonal relationships; this will minimize parental anxiety, feeling ignored, avoided, coerced, or disrespected by the professionals who are assigned to help them [9].

Assessment of Family Relationships

Assessing the impact of chronic disability on family function requires physicians and other professionals involved in the care of the identified patient to gather information about the patients' and parents' perception of multiple factors:

- What patients and parents believe about the prognosis of the disability.
- How much time, energy, and resources are required to care the chronically disabled child.
- How the parents and affected child see as the level of care required to maintain that child and what commitment the parents must make or invest.
- The financial cost of equipment, medical supplies, support personnel, hospital care, procedures, etc., required in caring for the chronically disabled child.
- The amount of resources left over for intra-parental relationships and sibling care.
- The numbers, frequency, and duration of evaluations and treatments (few months, a life time) required to treat the chronically disabled child.
- The numbers and types of professionals and support services required to care for the disabled child.

Treatment

Therapy should foster realistic beliefs and expectations of how families function and what children should and should not do. Psycho-education, cognitive restructuring, setting realistic expectations for children with developmental disabilities can teach parents key skills needed to improve their parenting effectiveness. Parents can learn techniques for strategic parenting; stress management; employing techniques such as meditation, relaxation techniques, and exercise for themselves and their children diagnosed with developmental disabilities. Such interventions help increase frustration tolerance and the ability to respond more calmly to difficult behavior. Parent training is an effective method to teach positive parenting and to teach parents how to control family stress [1, 2, 5].

Parents diagnosed with mental disorders will need extra support to help them parent their chronically ill child. Each of their children will need therapy to learn to develop healthy and effective detection and interpretation of social cues. These parents are at increased risk of raising children with emotional regulation problems during early and middle childhood and mood episodes during adolescence [11].

Every state in the United States provides education services for children who have developmental problems. These programs can start right after a baby is born and last until he/she turns 22 years. A list of resources for families of children with chronic disabilities can be found at the Center for Disease Control's web site entitled: National Dissemination Center for Children with Disabilities (NICHCY) [4].

Summary

A physician's ability to provide quality care to their patients and their patients' parents and siblings is enhanced if he/she understands the impact of their patients' chronic disabilities (as identified in this book) on their family members (individually and collectively). Chronic disabilities each disrupts the lives of all families and alters the typical developmental process (growth and maturation) of an infant, child, adolescent, and young adult. Early identification and intervention helps to mitigate the adverse impact on function of chronic disabilities on the lives of the affected infant, child, adolescent, or young adult. Parents can learn how to give attention to their child's special health care needs (mental, physical, social, emotional, developmental) and chronic conditions. Parents can learn techniques for strategic parenting; stress management; employing techniques such as meditation, relaxation techniques, and exercise for themselves and their children diagnosed with developmental disabilities.

References

1. Patel DR, Greydanus DE, Calles JL Jr, Pratt HD. Developmental disabilities across the lifespan. Dis Mon. 2010;56(6):299–398.
2. Pratt HD. Psychological issues in chronically ill adolescents. In: Omar HA, Greydanus DE, Patel DR, Merrick J, editors. Adolescence and chronic illness. A public health concern. New York, NY: Nova Science; 2009. pp. 151–63.
3. Council on Children with Disabilities. Section on Developmental Behavioral Pediatrics, Bright Futures Steering Committee, Medical Home Initiatives for Children with Special Needs Project Advisory Committee. Identifying Infants and Young Children with developmental disorders in the medical home: an algorithm for developmental surveillance and screening. Pediatrics. 2006;118(1):405–20.
4. Centers for Disease Control and Prevention. Developmental disabilities. http://www.cdc.gov/ncbddd/dd/resources.htm
5. Pratt HD. Neurodevelopmental issues in the assessment and treatment of deficits in attention, cognition, and learning during adolescence. Adolesc Med. 2002;13(3):579–98.
6. Pratt HD. Mental health aspects of chronic illness in adolescence. Int J Public Health. 2009;1(1):5–16.
7. Wirrell E, Cheung C, Spier S. How do teens view the physical and social impact of asthma compared to other chronic diseases? J Asthma. 2006;43:155–60.
8. Kyngäs H. Support network of adolescents with chronic disease: adolescents' perspective. Nurs Health Sci. 2004;6:287–93.
9. Kirk S. Families experiences of caring at home for a technology-dependent child: a review of the literature. Child Care Health Dev. 1998;24(2):101–14.
10. Fisher HR. The needs of parents with chronically sick children: a literature review. J Adv Nurs. 2001;36(4):600–7.
11. Muralidharan A, Yoo D, Ritschel LA, Simeonova DI, Craighead E. Development of emotion regulation in children of bipolar parents: putative contributions of socioemotional and familial risk factors. Clin Psychol Sci Pract. 2010;17(3):169–86.

Chapter 25
Allied Health Professionals and Intellectual Disability: Moving Toward Independence

Meir Lotan

Abstract Individuals with intellectual disability (ID) usually have to cope with an array of functional, mental, and physical challenges in addition to the primary diagnosis of ID. Despite the fact that this group of people represents about 2.5% of the world's population, they are still treated as a minority group. The vast versatility of syndromes, developmental challenges, and medical complexity results in infinite expressions of the ID diagnosis, although they are gathered under the same umbrella term. The management of individuals with ID necessitates treatment in a multitude of areas such as behavioral symptoms, early intervention, education, community-based support, medical challenges, activities of daily living, motor function, and old age, and the intervention approach recommended for this population would therefore be a teamwork model that integrates the knowledge of all allied health professionals into a holistic care management. The versatility of challenges of these clients makes working with them a complex and difficult task. They are one of the most multifaceted and demanding clients for the allied health professional, necessitating the initiation of a specific evaluation and the implementation of unique and creative therapeutic approach for each individual client. Alas, in most countries today there are no structured educational programs that prepare the allied health worker for such a challenge. This chapter will try and set some basic stepping stone into working with these individuals.

Introduction

"While we are among human being let us cultivate our humanity" [1].

Edouard Seguin (1812–1880) presented his innovative approach, which suggested that intensive sensory and motor intervention can help progress individuals with

M. Lotan (✉)
Department of Physical Therapy, Ariel University Center of Samaria, IL-40700 Ariel, Israel; Ariel and Israeli Rett Syndrome Association, National Evaluation Team, National Rett Syndrome Clinic, Chaim Sheba Medical Center, Ramat-Gan, Israel
e-mail: ml_pt_rs@netvision.net.il

D.R. Patel et al. (eds.), *Neurodevelopmental Disabilities*,
DOI 10.1007/978-94-007-0627-9_25, © Springer Science+Business Media B.V. 2011

intellectual disability (ID), more than 150 years ago [2]. Despite the work of Seguin and others, individuals with ID were defined as imbeciles, retarded, and uneducable, until not long ago. Despite the disbelief, intolerance, and reservations for this marginalized group, times are changing for our clients with ID, and with it the hope, that therapists working with individuals with ID can and should become the ones who carry the flags of change in our society.

This chapter will address therapists who work with individuals with ID and will therefore use point of reference for ways by which we can administer therapeutic means for this population. The chapter is based on existing literature as well as clinical experience working with individuals with ID at ages 0–80 and in all forms of facilities (day care, developmental, residential, and educational centers) for over 20 years.

Moral, Ethics, Empowerment, and Advocacy

Topics such as moral, ethics, empowerment, and advocacy have been presented by others in great depths, and this part of the chapter will merely present a hint of my perspective on these topics from the viewpoint of a clinician.

Valuable Individuals

Some have claimed that the intellectually "normal" human beings are morally more valuable than human beings with intellectual disabilities [3]. Such claims send a message that only the perfect is acceptable and the disabled may be discarded and thus brings us back to the practice of infanticide such as the one practiced in ancient *Carthage* [4]. I guess those suggesting such views may not have met many people with ID. Without any relation to their contribution this group of people is an important part of our society due to the direction they can make us take into becoming better humans. These individuals' uncorrupted souls can teach us much about patience for small changes, acceptance of ourselves and of other's imperfections, and attunement to minute human signal.

Pity Versus Compassion

I have many times heard the caregivers who work with individuals with ID say "Poor children, they are so weak, they should be resting and not working so hard" (especially when referring to physical therapy exercises). The concept of pitying this group of individuals could be harmful for them. Adopting this type of perspective may address them as sick and incapable and in need of nothing, but to be left alone. In view of this misfortunate standpoint people with ID have often been accepted as unhealthy by nature and therefore barred of health prevention, maintenance, or health promotion strategies [5]. As therapists it is our duty to change the way people look at individuals with ID, not with pity, but with compassion. In that manner they will be viewed as individuals with difficulties, but at the same time as individuals with goals, directions, and hope for improvement.

Physical Integration Versus Social Integration?

Integration is a well-known concept that has been pursued for many years [6, 7]; however, if one looks at different groups of people, one can actually see that they want to mingle among themselves rather than with others. People keep close to individuals of their own culture and religion, even people with the same disability (hearing impaired are a very good example). Why should people with ID be any different? Not only that, but the term integration is frequently distorted and skewed toward the physical aspect of integration rather than the social one. In many cases the integration is so extremely pursued that it becomes a target of its own with no regard to the wants and needs of the person with ID or to the consequences of this kind of integration. Merely placing individuals with ID in the middle of an urban society cannot be termed as integration [8]. Some evidence exists that mortality and morbidity are raised when moving from institutionalized settings to community settings [9, 10]. However, there are also correct ways of performing integration. In a project facilitated by a music therapist, children with ID were integrated into a regular school. Through a long process of activities, talks, and discussions with the children, the staff of both educational facilities, and the parents of both groups of children, personal, community, and social changes have been made in acceptance and overcoming diversity. This process was successful as the children without ID (who initially were afraid to interact with the children with ID) suggested having a mutual and collaborative summer camp together with the children with ID at the end of the first year. Initially this project was about to end after 1 year; however, the parents of the children without ID kept financing the project for two additional years [11, 12]. Changes such as these that implement slow and appropriate therapeutic processes and create acceptance to individuals with ID on an individual, community and social levels are blessed and should be pursued.

Research in Individuals with ID

There is a growing awareness of the importance of evidence-based medicine in guiding health-care delivery [13]. This implies for all clients, including individuals with ID. Yet, in a report released by the US federal government, Healthy People 2000, an expert panel wrote

> As with minority populations, the elements of this report that explicitly call for [health] improvements of people with disabilities are limited by the availability of data with which to set targets. One of the major challenges of the coming years is to improve our understanding of the needs of the full range of people with disabilities by improving the effectiveness of data systems [14, p. 40].

Due to the fact that studies on health promotion for people with disabilities are almost nonexistent [15], clinicians should pursue and conduct high-quality research projects and aspire to publish their intervention and experience so that others can benefit from successful interventions, while avoiding nonsuccessful ones. When performing research focused on persons with ID, ethical considerations are extremely important and should be carefully pursued, as many of these persons have difficulties in communication and in expressing their views [16].

Mediation of the Person with ID to Others

The same way we are determined to adjust the right amount of support to each of our clients with ID it is also our duty as advocacy massagers of integration to mediate our clients as human beings to others, who do not know them as we do, and see their only representation through their handicap and low intellectual capacity.

Keep an Eye on the Helpless and Give Them a Voice

The political weakness of the people with ID and their lack of voice may lead to their abuse by others [17]. The abusiveness and exploitation can take place by the hands of people "caring" for them, by relatives, neighborhood bullies, or the salesman who overcharge them. Nonintended abuse can also be presented by our misinterpretation of pain behavior. There have been reports about individuals with ID receiving less medication and delayed medical intervention due to their unique pain expression [18, 19]. Therefore the therapists, who work so closely with individuals with ID, should become their advocate, alert for any strange change in behavior [20], and seek the cause for such changes.

Therapeutic Intervention

When working with individuals with ID special care must be given to the special needs and characteristics of this population. It is given that the allied health personnel services are extremely intertwined with the daily experiences of this population; therefore, we carry a heavy responsibility for their health and well-being. Our training and the complex nature of this group of clients make it our responsibility to exercise our professional duties by always providing high-quality intervention. The intervention for this special group of clients should be performed under the following points:

- Turning disability into strength – In some occasions the child's disability can be utilized to his benefit by turning his limitations into a point of strength. For example, the individual with RS is forced to free her hands in order to perform

Fig. 25.1 Over turning
disability into resources

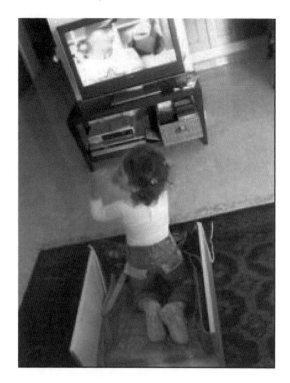

her stereotypical hand movement. On the other hand due to their multiple difficulties (changing muscle tone, apraxia, ataxia) most individuals with RS would
prefer to refrain from activity. Another point to consider would be that most of
these individuals are mesmerized by visual stimulus (an active TV or a computer
screen). Therefore, by placing the child with RS in a knee standing frame (see
Fig. 25.1) in front of a TV screen, we get her to actively and constantly change
position, as she stands on her knees to observe the program, but gets tired and
changes position to standing on all fours, but gets up again so she can do her
stereotypical movements, and so on.

- Attunement – When working with a speechless person we must always remember
  that even if people cannot speak, it does not mean that they have nothing to say.
  Due to the inability of the person with ID to alert us to his needs and wants in a
  conventional manner, we as therapists have to be ultra-attentive to nonverbal cues
  signaling pain, distress, complaints, or any other communicative message.
- Health promotion –For many years, the health care for individuals with ID
  has been directed at the primary prevention of disability rather than at prevention or reduction of secondary health conditions [21, 22]. Only in recent
  years has health promotion been given some attention in regard to individuals with disabilities [23]. Up-to-date intervention approaches should focus on
  reducing secondary health risks for those with ID by reducing or eliminating barriers that prevent them from participating in health-promoting activities. These

activities should include fitness programs, a well-balanced healthy diet, promotion of health behaviors [24].

- Empowerment – The word empowerment is constantly repeated when individuals with ID are concerned [25]. Yet, in relation to therapeutic interventions by allied health professions, health promotion for people with ID must become a major focus. Our aim as clinicians in the long run should be to prevent secondary health conditions by empowering people with disabilities to take control of their own health. This places more responsibility on individuals with ID as equals and able human beings and at the same time represents a more cost-effective, and certainly more humane, than watching people with disabilities decline in function from a lack of proper intervention. Allied health-care professionals should join in an effort to empower the lives of people with disabilities toward independence [24].

- Humanity – It is very easy to plunge into the challenging task of treating the "unfortunate" person with ID thereby missing the human being. As the child with ID grows, his environment and daily situation are added with more and more equipment, and the person might be lost inside the huge amounts of gadgets he uses: the crane, the splints, the corsets, the wheelchair, the bibs, the walker, and standing frame. During the sessions with the person with ID we should always relate to the person by talking or singing in order to create a human interaction.

- Interaction – Many research studies have suggested the importance of different therapeutic approaches and techniques for individuals with ID [26–29]; however, it is my strong belief (after more than 20 years of experience with this population) that it is not the therapeutic techniques and tools that you use, but rather the individual interaction you create as a therapist and a person with your client with ID. After you have established a strong human bond with the person with ID, the type of intervention you choose is sometimes less important and yet the sky could be your limit.

- Etiology-based intervention – Individuals with ID are often susceptible to different health conditions. Due to lack of a proper diagnosis/etiology, taking care of health-related issues of individuals with ID is often symptomatic; "if it's broken" we mend it, but intellectual disability is not a problem that needs fixing. What we actually treat is the health-related issues that correspond with a specific etiology. We take into consideration the congenital heart abnormalities of the person with Down syndrome [30], we manage the poor posture (due to laxity of ligaments) of the person with Fragile X [31], and we enhance communication of the person with Rett syndrome through assistive and augmentative communication (AAC) strategies [32]. Due to the fact that individuals with ID need more individualized, specialized, and structured intervention, differential diagnosis is extremely important for them as it holds substantial implications for prognosis and for the nature and intensity of the required intervention [33]. To allow proper intervention for all syndromes and conditions that incorporate the umbrella term intellectual disability we must invest time to enhance early diagnosis for our clients with ID. Only by knowing the specific diagnosis and thereby the specific health trajectory of our client, a proper "evidence-based" intervention program can be drawn and implemented.

- Uniqueness – Every person is unique and the person with ID is no exception, and therefore unique intervention is needed for each client. We cannot expect every person with ID to adapt to our way of work. Therefore, it is the responsibility of the therapist (after an in-depth evaluation) to adjust his intervention to the needs and characteristics of the client (i.e., the person with RS should receive a long adaptation period to the therapist and the therapy room, the person with visual impairments should be managed in a visually stimulating environment).

- Complexity – Many individuals with ID present an array of functional and medical difficulties. It is always very difficult to break through those barriers, and some people with ID will prefer to let go and withdraw into passivity. It is extremely frustrating for all working with this population due to the intense emotional input one conveys when in return the output can be scarce. The role of the therapist and caregiver is to find ways to overcome those barriers and unveil the person within the disability and the resources hidden behind the functional, emotional, or sensory difficulties.

- Communication – There are many needs for the person with ID, resulting in numerous persons who take care of those needs. In order for parents, therapist, and caregivers to enable the person with ID to make some progress, some form of coordination should take place among them. The transdisciplinary approach [34] has proven to be useful when working with individuals with disabilities and suggests a case manager who keeps the communication lines open among service providers, but even in simpler forms of therapeutic constellations, communication should always be pursued.

- Transparency – It is sometimes easier for the therapist to withdraw into the therapy room and "do his thing" without having any interruptions. I prefer working in the corridors and hallways. When doing so I am visible to the staff and they can see the person I am working with and what he can do. They can see that most of the things I do are not magical (I am also hoping they will be aspired to try and do similar interactions), but they can see the person who was just a minute ago a passive individual in a wheelchair, now walking, crawling, or even resisting to do any of the activities, but not passive any more.

- Love within boundaries – It is very easy to pity the young child with disabilities and to try and "help" him by doing the tasks for him. It is easier and faster for the caregivers to dress the child instead of letting him choose a shirt and struggle with it until it is on or to feed a child neatly instead of letting him self-feed, while making the table and floor around him looking like a battlefield. The conductive education (CE) concept suggests a psychosocial approach that combines intensive and demanding activities with an embracing support and respect for the person with ID and his limitations [35, 36], making the child a more active member in his society [37]. Nevertheless, we do not have to embrace a particular method in order to refrain from suggesting assistance that exceeds actual needs of the persons with a disability. The one thing that all individuals need is respect and love from the ones who care for them. Despite hard training and many complaints during the therapeutic session, one almost always get a big smile at the end if they sense that this hard endeavor is done with a loving caring attitude of the therapist.

- Therapeutic balance – The person with ID "needs" to take his medication, he "needs" to communicate, he "needs" to be fed correctly, he "needs" to be active ... and so on. Those immense needs must be balanced at many levels. It is natural for the parents of the young child with ID to try and reach his maximal potential by running from one therapeutic session to another (see paragraph on communication). Sometimes these intense therapeutic regimes might overburden the child, and it is the responsibility of the therapist to point it out to the parent/case manager. It might be that an overenthusiastic therapist may suggest a comprehensive, 24/7 intervention program, without taking into account the child's other needs. If the child's motor needs necessitates that he should sit unsupported on a stool, while his fine motor or nutritional needs necessitate that he is well supported during meal times, a compromise should be achieved to balance all those contradicting needs. It is our task as a therapeutic team to see that the person with ID is as active as possible with a complete and balanced program that covers all his therapeutic needs.

- Involvement – The human milieu surrounding the person with ID is extremely varied. Most of activities of daily living (ADL) are executed by individuals with basic training and knowledge regarding anatomy, physiology, and pathology of the people they are caring for. Can the caregiver understand the dangers of a hyperextended neck during eating and shaving? Does the parent know what hip dislocation is, and what could be its daily consequences if the child is poorly handled? The therapist's position and knowledge necessitate that he becomes involved in almost every aspect of his client with ID's life when intending to improve the quality of all management services provided to him/her.

- Mediation – It is well known that through the right intensity and quantity of mediation almost any person with ID can advance and function at some level. The therapists can adjust the right amount of support to each client in order to promote growth and enhance function.

- Transfer of therapeutic achievements outside the therapy room – The expectation that achievements from within the therapy session will extend into daily activities underpins all therapy practice. Positive experiences within the therapy impact upon the client with ID to achieve their full capacity outside the therapy room. Allied health professionals through collaborative consultation [38, 39] aimed at transferring information regarding each client's abilities to all those involved in the care of the client with ID. This information is later used to develop augmentative strategies for improvement that are adapted to the individual's needs and level of development [40]. Such augmentation may be in the form of muscle stretches and exercises from physiotherapists or adapted utensils and equipment from occupational therapists. Allied health assistants are sometimes employed to carry out some of the repetitive interventions that are considered helpful on a daily basis, but more commonly, teachers, caregivers, and parents should be engaged in the practice of these skills within daily situations.

- Motivation – Establishing a strong motivation factor is crucially important when aiming at a successful intervention with the person with ID.

A Case Story

YC is a 26-year-old man with a diagnosis of low-moderate ID, living in a residential facility. He is self-sufficient when it comes to eating and transitions, but needs some assistance in most of his ADL. His daycare center is about 100 yards from his dormitory. A few years back YC was showing severe medical problems, which manifested themselves especially in severe weakness, dizziness, and severe balance problems (which required intense help by a caregiver during ambulation and transitions). His condition was severe, and it seemed he was about to become wheelchair bound. To prevent him becoming a constant wheelchair user, the therapeutic team suggested an intervention program that would fit his daily routines, mainly including being taken to and from his daycare center by foot (instead of being wheeled in a wheelchair). The staff was unable to handle the program (half an hour daily) due to work load of daily duties and lack of cooperation by YC. Since his condition did not improve and the staff was unable to perform the program, the therapeutic team suggested assigning a volunteer who would implement the program and also take YC for daily walks in the afternoon (1.5 h daily). His cooperation remained low, and he was not showing any progress. Our OT decided to intervene, and she began taking YC for short walks (1 h weekly) starting with intense assistance and for very short distances. At the end of each walk she would call YC's mother on the phone (after coordinating it with her) and YC would tell his mother of his achievements. Within a few weeks he was independently doing all transitions and was walking independently for long durations of time. Today as a maintenance program, they still have their weekly trips around the residential center. YC walks unassisted for about 700 m a session in uneven terrain and gets to tell his mother of his endeavors.

This vignette suggests that a good motivating factor can achieve success with relatively little effort replacing hours of an unsuccessful intensive intervention. Therapeutic intervention confronts the person with ID at his weaknesses, and all of us need a very good reason to confront our weaknesses. The person with ID is no different. Due to low motivation [41] conventional programs that provide only remedial-type nature of intervention are not sufficiently motivating [42]. Thus, when seeking to activate individuals with ID, a broader perspective should be applied, taking into account the person's areas of interest [43]. The implementation of programs that incorporate motivational factors is highly recommended [41, 44] for this group of clients.

Anything can turn into a motivating factor if one can understand the person one interacts with. The suggestions below are just a partial list of possible motivational factors which have been found helpful in motivating individuals with ID to carry out crucial yet not always liked activities: a pep talk, a cup of coffee, a shiny journal, watching TV, listening to music, a program that meets the person character [41], usage of appropriate mediating environments [29, 45, 46], playing virtual reality games [47, 48], computer-based activities [49, 50], a toy (age appropriate), food items, talking to family members, outdoor activities [51], going to the mall or a coffee shop, a car ride, visiting a family member, creating an ornament to be hanged over the bed, new clothes, the use of animals [52], etc. The list is actually endless and can be fitted individually to almost everyone according to his specific needs and desires.

Therapeutic Needs

Persons with ID often have multiple and sometimes complicated medical problems [53]. In fact, a number of studies have documented substantially higher rates of both chronic and acute medical conditions in people with ID as compared to the general population [54]. Miniham et al. [55] reported that 99% of individuals with ID in a state institution had at least one chronic medical condition requiring regular follow-up (e.g., cardiac conditions, diabetes, ulcers, chronic otitis media, recurrent pneumonia, and progressive renal failure). Janicki et al. [56] found that 49% of people with ID admitted to hospitals had a visual impairment, 27% had a hearing impairment, and over 50% were obese. Likewise, Beange et al. [57] found that people with ID had increased cardiovascular risk factors and higher rates of medical consultations and hospital admissions than the general population, with 4.5 medical disorders per person on average.

The medical problems diagnosed in this population are diverse, ranging from limb contractures and scoliosis [58] to spasticity [59] and osteoporosis, particularly among non-weight-bearing patients [60]. Persons with ID often suffer from a host of behavioral and psychiatric problems as well [53]. These findings highlight the need for intense and specifically tailored therapeutic interventions for individuals with ID. However, as a minority group largely lacking empowerment and advocacy, they are constantly challenged by unmet health-care needs. Several investigations [57, 61] have suggested that the health mismanagement of this population has a severe impact on mortality [62], morbidity [56, 57], and quality of life [63].

Unmet Therapeutic Needs

Equivalent health care should be a minimum standard for every group of clients in all countries [64]. Yet despite existing evidence in the literature regarding the ill health of individuals with ID, this minority group still suffers from unethical figures of death and disability [65]. Since the global shift from institutional to community-based care, the primary health care of people with ID has been placed in the hands of general practitioners (GPs). However, studies which assessed the care of people with ID by community-based GPs have identified significant shortcomings [66, 67]. These studies suggested that people with intellectual disability suffer from an excessive number of unrecognized or poorly managed medical conditions. Moreover, many authors suggest that there is a lack of adequate health screening and preventative care in this population [68, 69].

In order to prevent complications associated with disability due to ID there is a need for a comprehensive and preventive therapeutic intervention. Such therapeutic agents should include physical therapy and hydrotherapy (to improve mobility and cardiovascular fitness, reduce spasticity, and prevent physical deformations), occupational therapy (to enhance function within activities of daily living and attend to sensory dysfunctions), speech therapy (to enhance communication skills and improve eating abilities), special education teachers (to gain computer access and enhance education and social skills), music therapy (for self-expression and emotional well-being) [70, 71]. It is suggested that health-care professionals should establish different evaluation forms specifically constructed and validated for individuals with ID. Moreover, the drive to establish and perform such evaluation forms should be demanded and initiated by health-care professional with interest in this group of clients [65]. Therefore, it is in the hands of therapists from all professions to enhance better care for our clients with ID establishing better and intensified evaluation and therapeutic interventions to answer their needs.

Holistic Evaluation

The concept that integrated teamwork can enhance the efficacy of services delivered to individuals with multiple disabilities is not new. This idea was first proposed by Whitehouse in 1951 [72]. Today, more than 50 years later, allied health professionals still find it difficult to be involved in integrated-type treatment, mostly due to the fact that each member of the educational/therapeutic staff was trained to work as an independent, therapeutic provider [72].

The variety of physical, cognitive, therapeutic, educational, and mental needs of clients with ID presents challenges to the allied health professionals responsible for their treatment. Accepting this point of view has led support services for pupils with special educational needs to change drastically during the past few decades. Today strong pressure is being exerted by support services to develop cooperative transdisciplinary teamwork. In many countries, such as Australia, England, the United States, France, and Holland, teamwork has become the guiding component for establishing the policies of education and welfare services. This in turn has led to comprehensive changes such as the development of cooperative assessment by a number of support services. In a broader sense, this process has also led to legislation obligating cooperation between different support services [73]. The rationale behind this policy is based on the fact that solving "complex problems" demands a wider scope of knowledge and more advanced capabilities usually not attainable by a single therapist [74, 75]. In actuality, this policy has brought about a process of change and a transition from treatment methods based on the medical model (such as the interdisciplinary and multidisciplinary approaches) to methods such as the transdisciplinary model better suited for the educational environment. The transdisciplinary model was first developed in 1976 by the United Cerebral Palsy Association's service for infants with cerebral palsy. After its assimilation this working model was recognized by health-related professions in fields of occupational therapy [76], physiotherapy [77], special education [78], nursing [79], and medicine [80].

This model was also recommended as a preferred approach for treating populations with multiple disabilities by care providers' organizations in the United States such as ASHA (American Speech–Language–Hearing Association), AOTA (American Occupational Therapy Association), APTA (American Physical Therapy Association), and TASH (The Association for persons with Severe Handicaps). Youngson et al. [81] described three types of transdisciplinary teams whose objectives encourage cooperation: application teams, discussion teams, and assessment teams.

The numerous and varied educational and therapeutic needs of individuals with ID, together with their relatively long life span [82, 83], demand a professional, transdisciplinary approach. Unfortunately, individuals with ID and their families do not always receive the best possible treatment [84]. Therefore, there seems to be a need to develop and improve appropriate management programs for this population. The model of the Israeli Rett syndrome evaluation group was developed with the intent of addressing the wide range of difficulties presented by this syndrome [85] and could be suggested as an appropriate model for individuals at all functional levels and all levels of IDD.

Intervention

It is important to emphasize that a child with ID has all the basic needs as any other child, that is, to be loved, talked to, and to be played with so that the child feels comfortable and emotionally secure. After establishing a safe base of support any child, with or without disabilities, will become secure in his ability to explore and learn the world around him [86].

An intervention program with this population should be the result of a well-performed evaluation, holistically employed by the child, his parents, caregivers, and therapists. The intervention program originating from such an evaluation should create a continuous network of human support around the individual with ID.

A growing body of research recommends that intensive, sustained treatment is important in improving the long-term outcome for people with ID [87]. Intervention planning should, on the one hand, be grounded in the present functional and medical reality but, on the other hand, should focus on the long-term vision/prognosis for the client's potential. Planning entails attention to evidence-based literature related to educational interventions, residential situations, and vocational programs [88, 89]. A well-functioning intervention program must also include appropriate involvement and collaboration with the client's family [90]. Intervention should be focused and individualized and must be broadly implemented to relate to the full range of impairments shown by the client [33]. Regardless of the individual's age, treatment planning should include provision for structured opportunities for learning and for generalization of what is learned. Individuals with ID require high-level general, medical, and allied health professional care which includes provision for routine preventive health measures and for the special needs of the multihandicapped person.

Usually many disciplines are involved in different aspects of the treatment of the clients with ID; therefore, it is important that one clinician be primarily involved with the parents to develop a plan of care for the child. This individual should also be responsible for service coordination and advocacy [87]. Clinicians should also help to coordinate services and work with parents to obtain appropriate educational programs, be an advocate for services such as respite care and support for the family, and provide consultation regarding prognosis of the disorder, therapeutic, medical, and pharmacology management [91].

According to Howlin [33] a successful intervention program with this population should include the following elements: a combination of behavioral, educational, and developmental approaches; a structured environmental therapeutic milieu; and social integration. I would add that a successful intervention should be intensive and tailored to each clients and family needs.

It is the belief of this author that individuals with ID can exceed many of their limitations if a comprehensive, individually tailored, and well-suited therapy program is implemented.

Intervention Across the Life Span

The age of people around the globe is gradually rising and so is the case with individuals with ID (see Fig. 25.2). Therefore the therapist working with this group of clients is bound to change the goals and direction of intervention as the child with ID grows to become an adult and a senior citizen with ID. Over their life span individuals with ID should receive changing therapeutic interventions from a young age

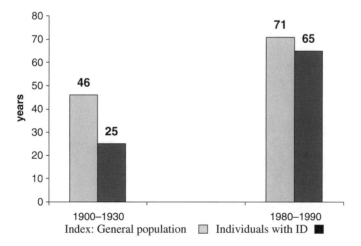

Fig. 25.2 Change in longevity for individuals with and without ID

to adulthood. And we should ask ourselves if such interventions live up to their designated goals: do they improve the state of the child at an early age? Do they have long-lasting effects? What should be changed when we set to manage the person with ID as he grows older? The next part of the chapter will discuss these questions.

Early Intervention

In the past, false assumptions as to the lack of potential and abilities of children with ID led to a denial of access to social, therapeutic, and educational opportunities that they needed. We now know that they can benefit from participating in therapeutic intervention and normal experiences [92]. According to Dineen [93] the components of a quality early intervention program are

- to begin as early as is possible,
- to include parents and families as full participants in the client's program, and
- to involve the multidisciplinary team in the assessment and planning of individual management.

Connolly and Russell [94] conducted an early interdisciplinary intervention program for this population and concluded that such a program was needed in order to help the participants in earlier attainment of many developmental tasks and enhanced functioning of the family unit. Based on reevaluating the results (three long-term follow-ups), it was found that achievements of the early intervention program for children with ID had long-lasting results [95] and participants in the early intervention program gained a foundation for subsequent learning and development [96].

One example of an attempt to evaluate specific motor training for children with ID was conducted in Sweden [97]. The intervention group consisted of 14 children and a control group of 6 children. The treatment began when the babies were 3 months old and lasted until they began to walk, focusing on increasing muscle tone, reducing incorrect patterns of movement, training typical movement patterns, and stimulating trunk rotation. The treated children performed better than the control children in four areas measured: gross motor, fine motor, kinesthetic perception, and tactile perception.

Since children with ID have been found to develop walking later than non-ID children [98], a special walking program has been implemented. The program involved seven infants with Down syndrome ranging in age from 8 to 11 months, who practiced daily on a treadmill and supervised by their parents. All infants responded by producing alternating steps [99]. Moreover, the experimental group learned to walk with help and to walk independently significantly faster than the control group. It was therefore suggested that treadmill training should be considered as an intervention approach for young children with Down syndrome [99]. The overall results provided evidence that with training and support, infants with Down syndrome can learn to walk earlier than they normally would [100]. Improvement in functional ability and fitness was reported for a group of children at a severe level of ID ranging in age from 5 to 10, after participation in daily treadmill program [101].

The long-term effects of such intervention programs were studied by Kolvin and associates [102], who conducted a long-term follow-up on 1,000 families receiving intervention for their child with special needs. The researchers claimed that the quality of physical and emotional care received by the child was the best outcome of intervention. They also claimed that quality care was able to overcome initial limitations and was found more important than lack of money, cognitive limitations, poor housing, or adverse life events reported by the participant's families.

Life span of individuals with ID has increased considerably within the last decades [103], and it is therefore important to continue intervention program throughout the life of the person with ID (and not only in their childhood), in order to maintain a healthy and active life and to become a healthy old individual with ID. With this in mind, the next part of the chapter will examine the efficacy of intervention programs that focus on adults with ID.

Intervention in Adults with ID

Heller et al. [104] found that a group of adults with ID, who participated in a fitness and health education program for 12 weeks (three practice days per week), changed their attitudes toward exercise and showed more positive expected outcomes, fewer cognitive-emotional barriers, and improved life satisfaction. These findings were very promising, since they suggested that implementing an appropriate educational physical program would enhance the participation of individuals with ID in such programs during adolescent and adulthood.

A group of adults with ID performed a jog/walk program [105]. The results suggested that adults with ID were able to improve their aerobic capacity when performing a systematic and well-designed aerobic training program.

Two treadmill training programs that lasted between 12 weeks and 6 months were held for young (mean age = 24.5 years) and aged adults (mean age = 63 years) with ID [106, 107]. Both programs showed significant improvement in muscle strength and dynamic balance. Carmeli et al. [108] implemented a treadmill walking program for adults with ID and arterial occlusive disease. Some of the participants showed significant improvements in walking speed, distance, and duration. Pain levels were reduced in those suffering from intermittent claudication. Blood hemodynamic parameters also showed significant improvements. This program demonstrated that besides improvements of the functional capacities, medical benefits can also be achieved by a low-intensity treadmill walking program of adults with ID. A 16-week long aerobic rowing ergometric training regime in adults with ID improved exercise endurance and work capacity of the participants [109]. An annual low-intensity treadmill intervention program, performed two times weekly, for adults with ID at a mean age of 42 years, presented significant improvements in fitness and reduced infirmary visitations in comparison to a matched control group, suggesting an improved well-being concept by the participants [110].

The accumulating evidence suggests that various physical activity programs for individuals with ID can positively and significantly improve numerous ill-health characteristics associated with primary and secondary health-related issues of this group of clients. It is also evident that such programs can be implemented cost-effectively with different age groups. In order for such programs to bare positive, long-lasting results, they need to be implemented for long durations and with high intensity. The next paragraphs will examine two main routes of intervention: direct and indirect care.

Direct Care

Many individuals with ID are extremely debilitated and handicapped by the vast array of neurological, orthopedic, and functional limitations posed by ID. Since the aim of the therapist is to improve the client's quality of life by overcoming or reducing these limitations, an individually tailored intervention program should be implemented.

It is important to state that individual intervention is not perceived as the ultimate intervention method but merely one basic step to support integration and independence of the individual. The individual intervention is the foundation upon which progress is based, especially for individuals with ID, or as Abraham Maslow (1908–1970) said, the individual therapy *may be conceived as a miniature ideal society of two* [111].

The direct care or hands-on intervention may start in the therapy room, but must simultaneously develop in the classroom, the residential environment of the person, and among his peer group and community. At the first encounters, the individual with ID might present difficulties typical of all newcomers. Such times have been reported as periods of anxiety both for the individual and for the parents [112].

It is recommended that initial contact between the client with ID and the therapist be conducted in a familiar, quiet place, with a caregiver/family member with whom the client is familiar and trusts. In such a favorable environment, bonding between the individual with ID and the therapist will create the necessary milieu for future functional advancement. Achieving rapport during the few first encounters is not always easy, and even after the establishment of such a connection, the advancement of the intervention with the individual with ID might sometimes be slow and demanding, requiring much patience by the therapist.

The connection between client and therapist is sometimes influenced by the emotions of the therapist working with the individual with ID. Therefore, in new and unfamiliar situations or when the therapist is tired, depressed, or nervous, results are seldom achieved [113]. If the therapist is attentive to him/herself and to the individual with ID, therapeutic results are much more easily gained. A deeper acquaintance with the person with ID, with his/her daily program and physical and human environment, will enable improved communication and meaningful attachment and, therefore, is highly recommended. Such bonding will enable the therapist to better decipher the client's signs and his understanding, and compliance with client will improve. As a result, the communicative "output" of the individual with ID might improve, helping in overcoming barriers in education and personal contact [112, 114, 115].

Despite the fact that it is probably a well-known feature to any therapist/educator, the author would like to reiterate that "individual intervention" does not mean that every therapist is totally devoted to his private therapeutic agenda and completely oblivious to other team members. Any therapist/educator working with an individual with ID must maintain professional relationships with their client's parents and other allied health professionals involved in his curriculum. It is advised that all team members (working according to a multi/transdisciplinary approach) join together and decide on combined goals for the client with ID, grouping their efforts and knowledge to advance the treatment of the individual with ID according to the collectively decided intervention plan. In some cases, parents will seek additional treatments for their child, and it is important that providers of such services coordinate their work with that of the educational facility [87].

Intervention goals are built in accordance with each client's abilities and needs and are led by the combined intention to achieve the highest functional level and the best quality of life attainable. Lewis and Wilson, when referring to individuals with Rett syndrome, contributed the obvious, yet important, statement that individuals with ID are "complete human beings" [112]. Therefore, the intervention for the individual with ID should be holistic, integrating all aspects of treatment, leading to the achievement of maximal functional gains in several developmental fields [112]. All therapeutic interventions should thrive to enhance performance by the individual within daily activities (eating, drinking, communicating, standing, walking, communicating, and socializing).

Dosage

Individuals with ID experience a range of comorbid conditions including sensory impairment and seizures. They are subject to orthopedic and other functional complications due to their primary disorder, such as limitations of movement, scoliosis, joint instability, bowel and bladder dysfunction, dysarthria and dysphagia, and altered growth and nutrition. People with ID are often excluded from school and community-based activities, because of lack of accessibility of these programs. Community centers were found to have participation barriers such as lack of safety, inaccessible equipment, lack of resources, transportation and financial barriers, and lack of knowledge by facility personnel about accessible involvement for individuals with ID. The physical and psychological consequences of this situation present complex diagnostic and therapeutic challenges for the allied health professional [116] working with this population. These challenges draw extreme financial resources,

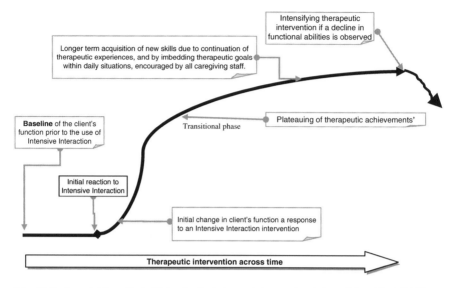

Fig. 25.3 A model for adjusted intensity in therapeutic interaction (adapted from Firth [119])

which grow with the continuation process of integration into community [117]. Due to such heavy economic budgets and the fact that our group of client is a minority speechless group, the therapeutic services they receive are always at a disadvantage in regard to their actual needs. In some cases, therapists tend to serve clients with ID with long-lasting ongoing intervention, yet there is growing awareness of the importance of evidence-based intervention in guiding health-care delivery to individuals with ID [13]. Allied health professionals have been exploring the possibility that long-term, ongoing work is not the most effective way to offer therapy services. The concept of titration (adjusting the dose of the intervention) is based on psycho-pharmaceutic concept. The concept is inquiring as to how much time and resources should be required in order to expect noticeable improvements. Hubble et al. [118] as well as others [119] charted the time trajectory of therapeutic benefit that has been repeatedly found effective. Their findings also suggested a plateau in outcomes after a given set of sessions. Intensive interaction is a model of communication with people, who have severe and profound disabilities suggested by Hewett and Nind [120]. This model can be similarly plotted to suggest a possible intervention model for other allied health professionals working with individuals with ID (see Fig. 25.3).

In accordance with this model it is suggested to apply therapy dosage (intensity) in the following manner:

1. An intense intervention is implemented until initial outcomes have been achieved.
2. The responsibility for maintaining outcomes is transferred to the person with ID and caregivers and implemented in daily routines.

3. Intervention is continued (less frequently). Intervention is not terminated, but a change in intensity is made to reflect an efficient and effective sustenance of outcomes.
4. Intervention is only intensified in response to diminished functional ability by the client, suggesting elevated therapeutic needs.

In the original findings by Firth [119] specific sets of intervention are presented. As individuals with ID represent a vast array of cognitive, sensory, and functional abilities I believe that the model should be accepted as a grand scheme and individually adapted to each of our clients.

Indirect Care and Counseling

Intervention with persons with ID is aimed at enhancement of abilities and compensation for difficulties and includes therapeutic intervention, adaptive techniques, environmental modifications, and assistive technologies [121]. The caregivers of the person with ID should not be limited to rely on health-related disciplines, such as physiotherapy, occupational therapy, music therapy, or others, and the therapeutic intervention should not be limited to what is administered in the treatment room or during individually applied sessions (also known as direct therapy). In order to attain a continuous effect, therapists and caregivers should work in cooperation with the families to construct a comprehensive intervention program that includes both the educational facility and the individual's residence. Kerr [122], when referring to individuals with RS, asserted that an activation program taught to caregivers was highly recommended throughout the life of the individual with ID, and she recommended that regular activity was essential for the long-lasting health of this population [122]. Moreover, support to the claim made by Kerr comes from several studies that have demonstrated the importance of family/caregiver involvement in exercising programs [123, 124].

It is therefore recommended that an exercise plan should be implemented by caregivers (as well as by the family and within the educational or residential facility of the person with ID) in order to construct a supportive network around the individual with ID. Such a day-by-day and hour-by-hour support will allow everyone involved in taking care of the client, to be aware of his\her needs and therefore support the supplementary management program.

The term "supplementary management program" implies continuous care for the individual by utilizing the time, intensity of appropriate handling, and suitable assistive devices. A supplementary management program will accompany and support the client's therapeutic regime throughout the day and across settings. Such a program can help him during the wearisome battles against the limitations that his specific disorder imposes. Since ID is constant and never relents, treatment management should continue through every available minute of everyday. This intense intervention could, however, wear out the caregivers. Therefore, such a program

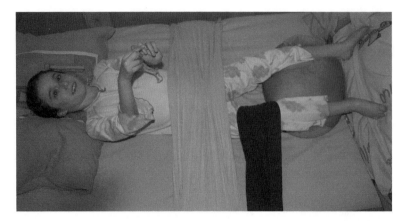

Fig. 25.4 A child using a bedside support against the development of windswept deformity

should be implemented wisely after adapting it to each individual's daily routines and the abilities and availability of the caregivers. We also recommend that such a program be supervised by an allied health team member acquainted with the child and aware of her/his specific needs. It is possible that intervention strategies might even be used during the resting hours of the individual with ID (see Fig. 25.4).

Figure 25.4 presents a child with a risk for developing windswept deformity prevented by nocturnal positioning, as well as utilizing her play and recreation time for introducing therapeutic elements without harming the joy of the user and the quality of her life. Figure 25.5 presents a child actively watching a TV program while practicing manual weight bearing.

Due to individual expression of ID and due to the ever-changing abilities and challenges of this group of clients, the caregiver should not limit him/herself to conventions that have already been tried. When there are no existing solutions, there is a need to use creativity, to explore some unusual thinking, and to experiment with new ideas. In the words of Yalom [125] taken from another professional context, but with the same spirit in mind, "*inspire yourself to create a new treatment for each client*" [125]. Anything that might get your client with ID to improve his disposition or performance is worth investigating.

When choosing the appropriate elements of a supplementary program, the following factors should be taken into consideration:

1. The client's physical profile (deformities, motor ability, and tendency toward pressure sores, weight of the person, muscle tone, and sensory sensitivity),
2. Environmental limitations (elevators, stairs, and available space in the house),
3. Behavioral needs (such as self-inflicted injuries, attention, and attention span),
4. Daily routine (the overall needs and routines of the family and caretaking staff), and
5. Future needs (change in function and change in medical condition).

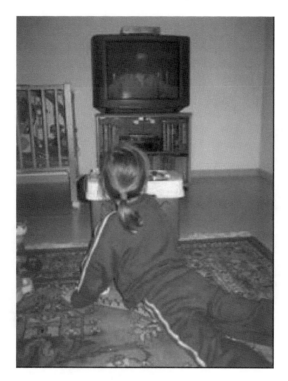

Fig. 25.5 A child kept active while watching a TV program

It is best to get the approval of the client's family physician to the program after screening the client's condition and accounting for the different aspects of the program.

It is recommended that all therapists working with the client will be involved in structuring the program in accordance to the child's needs and the caregivers' ability to comply. During each hour of the day and within every activity, the person with ID should always be driven to function toward his optimal/maximal level of functioning (as long as his safety and happiness are not compromised). For example, if the person is in need of a slight measure of assistance, support him only as much as he needs. By constantly doing so you will teach your clients to take responsibility over their body rather than becoming passive individuals relying on others.

When considering the duration of any activity, consult your child with ID. When the child is no longer in a good posture or when he starts complaining that it is time to change the intervention, change to another position within the intervention program, find better motivational agents (change to his favorite DVD), or reposition the child in a passive posture that has been found to comply with his therapeutic needs (see Fig. 25.6), as a resting position, before returning to another active posture or activity. The program should be flexible as it should adapt constantly to the changing state and medical conditions of the person with ID.

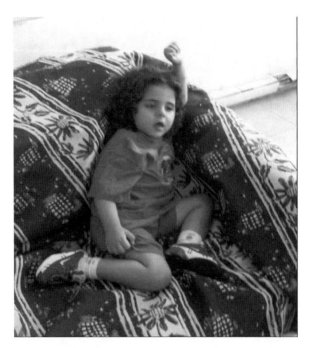

Fig. 25.6 Using a resting position that accommodates the anti-scoliosis regime (adapted from [124])

In Fig. 25.6 we can see a child resting between two active components of her daily program, in a passive position that elongates the left side of her trunk in correspondence with her anti-scoliosis regime.

Conclusions

Many barriers to the provision of health care for individuals with ID have been identified. Commonly mentioned barriers are communication difficulties between the health personnel and the patient, communication difficulties among health professionals, lack of ID-related knowledge, negative attitude presented by the medical staff toward individuals with ID, ethical issues and lack of appropriate procedures and guidelines for the therapeutic management of individuals with ID, difficulties with accessing the health-care system, short consultation times, special challenging behaviors expressed by individuals with ID, poor accessibility for health services, and the complexity of the medical condition of individuals with ID [126]. To overcome these barriers, a range of strategies has been recommended.

As Preventive Measures

- Provide more preventative health care [127].
- Present available and appropriate screening procedures by different health professionals [128].
- Establish better resources and specialist referral guidelines [55, 126].
- Educate toward better health promotion [129].
- Increase medical education and training in health-related professions [57, 126].
- Develop medical and allied health specialty in ID [126, 130].

In Regard to Ongoing Health Management

- Provide adequate time and reimbursement for consultations [131] and intervention.
- Ensure better communication strategies among other professionals or agencies [126, 132].
- Develop better information systems [61].
- Enable easier access to client's medical history [133].

When screening through the literature we can find that the last decades have presented with improved longevity for individuals with ID [134] which suggests an overall positive trend for this population (see Fig. 25.2).

Nevertheless, despite recent improvement and interest in care of individuals with ID, it is evident that health-related issues of this minority group are still being compromised in comparison to the general population. The source of this injustice is rooted in a complex set of barriers that can and should be overturned. Research into the quality of life, function, and intervention for individuals should be performed, clinical diagnosis for all with ID should be aimed at, educational programs for clinicians working with those individuals should be administered, multi-profession evaluation and intervention frameworks should be encouraged, and guidelines for assessment and intervention should be put forth and implemented for individuals presenting different etiologies.

References

1. Parmenter TR. Intellectual disabilities Quo Vadis? In: Albrecht GL, Seelman KD, Bury M, editors. Handbook of disability studies. London: Sage; 2001.
2. Talbot ME. Edouard Seguin. Am J Ment Defic. 1967;72(2):184–89.
3. Vehmas S. Discriminative assumptions of utilitarian bioethics regarding individuals with intellectual disabilities. Disabil Soc. 1999;14(1):37–52.
4. Williamson L. Infanticide: an anthropological analysis. In: Kohl M, editor. Infanticide and the value of life. New York, NY: Prometheus; 1978. pp. 61–75.

5. Tighe CA. Working at disability: a qualitative study of the meaning of health and disability for women with physical impairments. Disabil Soc. 2001;16:511–29.
6. Young L, Sigafoos J, Suttie J, Ashman A, Grevell P. Deinstitutionalisation of persons with intellectual disabilities: a review of Australian studies. J Intellect Dev Disabil. 1998;23(2):155–70.
7. Carnaby S. Reflections on social integration for people with intellectual disability: does interdependence have a role? J Intellect Dev Disabil. 1998;23(3):219–28.
8. Cummins RA, Lau ALD. Community integration or community exposure? A Review and discussion in relation to people with an intellectual disability. J Appl Res Intellect Disabil. 2003;16:145–57.
9. Strauss D, Shavelle R. Life expectancy of persons with chronic disabilities. J Insur Med. 1998;30:96–108.
10. Strauss DJ, Eyman RK, Grossman HJ. Predictors of mortality in children with severe mental retardation: the effect of placement. Am J Public Health. 1996;86:1422–29.
11. Elefant C. Must we really end? Community integration of children in Raanana, Israel. In: Stige B, Ansdell G, Elefant C, Pavlicevic M, editors. Where music helps. Community music therapy in action and reflection. Aldershot: Ashgate; 2010. pp. 65–73.
12. Elefant C. Musical inclusion, intergroup relations, community development. In: Stige B, Ansdell G, Elefant C, Pavlicevic M, editors. Where music helps. Community music therapy in action and reflection. Aldershot: Ashgate; 2010. pp. 75–90.
13. Lennox NG, Kerr MP. Primary health care and people with an intellectual disability: the evidence base. J Intellect Disabil Res. 1997;41(5):365–72.
14. Public Health Service. Healthy people 2000: national health promotion and disease prevention objectives. Washington, DC: US Department of Health and Human Services; 1991.
15. Patrick DL. Rethinking prevention for people with disabilities, part I: a conceptual model for promoting health. Am J Health Promot. 1997;11:257–60.
16. Brodin J, Renblad K. Ethical reflections in research on persons with intellectual disabilities. Tech Disabil. 2000;13:151–59.
17. Brown H, Thompson D. The ethics of research with men who have learning disabilities and abusive sexual behaviour: a minefield in a vacuum. Disabil Soc. 1997;12(5):695–708.
18. Stallard P, Williams L, Lenton S, Velleman R. Pain in cognitively impaired, non-communicating children. Arch Dis Child. 2001;85:460–62.
19. Gauthier JC, Finley GA, McGrath PJ. Children's self-report of postoperative pain intensity and treatment threshold: determining the adequacy of medication. Clin J Pain. 1998;14(2):116–20.
20. Von Tetzchner S, Jensen K. Interacting with people who have severe communication problems: ethical considerations. Int J Disabil Dev Educ. 1999;46(4):453–62.
21. Brandon J. Health promotion and wellness in rehabilitation services. J Rehabil. 1985;51: 54–58.
22. Stuifbergen AK, Becker HA. Predictors of health-promoting lifestyles in persons with disabilities. Res Nurs Health. 1994;17:3–13.
23. Renwick R, Friefield S. Quality of life and rehabilitation. In: Renwick R, Brown I, Nagler M, editors. Quality of life in health promotion and rehabilitation. Newbury Park, CA: Sage; 1996. pp. 26–36.
24. Rimmer JH. Health promotion for people with disabilities: the emerging paradigm shift from disability prevention to prevention of secondary conditions. Phys Ther. 1999;79(5):495–502.
25. Martin R. A real life-a real community: the empowerment and full participation of people with an intellectual disability in their community. J Intellect Dev Disabil. 2006;31(2): 125–27.
26. Ketelaar M, Vermeer A, Hart H't, Petegem-van Beek E, Helders PJM. Effects of a functional therapy program on motor abilities of children with cerebral palsy. Phys Ther. 2001;81(9):1534–45.

27. Lotan M. Alternative therapeutic intervention for individuals with Rett syndrome. ScientificWorldJournal. 2007;7:698–714.
28. Lotan M, Shapiro M. Management of young children with Rett syndrome in the multi-sensory environment. Brain Dev. 2005;27(Suppl 1):S88–94.
29. Lotan M, Hadar-Frumer M. Aquatic rehabilitation for individuals with Rett syndrome. Aquat Phys Ther. 2004;12(1):6–16.
30. Van Allen MI, Fung J, Jurenka SB. Health care concerns and guidelines for adults with Down syndrome. Am J Med Gen. 1999;89:100–10.
31. Sabaratnam M. Pathological and neuropathological findings in two males with fragile X syndrome. J Intellect Disabil Res. 2000;44:81–85.
32. Sigafoos J, Woodyatt G, Tucker M, Roberts-Pennell D, Pittendreigh N. Assessment of potential communication acts in three individuals with Rett syndrome. J Dev Phys Disabil. 1999;12(3):203–16.
33. Howlin P. Autism and intellectual disability: diagnostic and treatment issues. J R Soc Med. 2000;93:351–55.
34. Linder TW. Transdisciplinary play-based assessment (TPBA) A functional approach to working with young children. Revised ed. Baltimore, MD: Paul H Brookes; 1990.
35. Sutton A. Define to defend. Workshop given at the international conference celebrating 20 years of Tsad Kadima on: throughout life with cerebral palsy, partnership, environment and participation, Rishon LeZion, Israel, 2007.
36. Schenker R. Conductive education, history, definition, and basic concepts. Jerusalem: Tsad Kadima; 2007.
37. Hari M, Akosh K. Conductive education. London: Routledge; 1988.
38. Coufal KL. Collaborative consultation for speech-language pathologists. Top Lang Disord. 1993;14(1):1–14.
39. Rainforth B, York J, MacDonald C. Collaborative teams for students with severe disabilities: integrating therapy and educational services. Baltimore, MD: Paul H Brookes; 1991.
40. Lacey P, Ouvry C, editors. People with profound and multiple learning disabilities: a collaborative approach to meeting complex needs. London: David Fulton; 1998.
41. Lotan M. Quality physical intervention activity for persons with Down syndrome. ScientificWorldJournal. 2007;7:7–19.
42. Gignac MAM. Leisure time physical activity and well-being: learning from people living with arthritis. J Rheumatol. 2003;30(11):2299–301.
43. Temple VA. Barriers, enjoyment, and preference for physical activity among adults with intellectual disability. Int J Rehabil Res. 2007;30(4):281–87.
44. Rogers-Wallgren JL, French R, Ben-Ezra V. Use of reinforcement to increase independence in physical fitness performance of profoundly mentally retarded youth. Percept Mot Skills. 1992;75(3 Pt 1):975–82.
45. Lotan M, Gold C. Meta-Analysis of the effectiveness of individual intervention in the controlled multi-sensory environment (Snoezelen®) for individuals with intellectual disability. J Intellect Dev Disabil. 2009;34(3):207–15.
46. Lotan M. Management of Rett syndrome in the controlled multisensory (Snoezelen) environment. A review with three case stories. ScientificWorldJournal. 2006;6:791–807.
47. Lotan M, Yalon-Chamovitz S, Weiss PLT. Improving physical fitness of individuals with intellectual and developmental disability through a Virtual Reality Intervention Program. Res Dev Disabil. 2009;30:229–39.
48. Lotan M, Yalon-Chamovitz S, Weiss PLT. Virtual reality as means to improve physical fitness of individuals at a severe level of intellectual and developmental disability. Res Dev Disabil. 2010;31:869–74.
49. Hetzroni O, Rubin C. AAC instruction for children with Rett syndrome using assistive technology. Proceedings of the ISAAC, Dublin, Ireland, 1998. p. 361.
50. Hetzroni O, Schanin M. Computer as a tool in developing emerging literacy in children with developmental disabilities. Issues Spec Educ Rehabil J. 1998;13(1):15–21.

51. Greenaway R. A view into the future: the value of other ways of learning and development. In: Becker P, Schirp J, editors. Other ways of learning: the European Institute for Outdoor Adventure Education and Experiential Learning 1996–2006, Marburg, 2008. pp. 347–367.
52. Maciques Rodríguez E, Lotan M. Therapeutic horseback riding (hippotherapy) for individuals with Rett syndrome: a review with a case study. Int J Child Health Human Dev. 2008;1(1):39–53.
53. Prater CD, Zylstra RG. Medical care of adults with mental retardation. Fam Physician. 2006;73(12):2175–83.
54. Cooper SA. Clinical study of the effects of age on the physical health of adults with mental retardation. Am J Ment Retard. 1998;102:582–89.
55. Miniham PM, Dean DH, Lyons CM. Managing the care of patients with mental retardation: a survey of physicians. Ment Retard. 1993;31:239–46.
56. Janicki MP, Dalton AJ, Henderson CM, Davidson PW. Mortality and morbidity among older adults with intellectual disability: health services considerations. Disabil Rehabil. 1999;21:284–94.
57. Beange H, McElduff A, Baker W. Medical disorders of adults with mental retardation: a population study. Am J Ment Retard. 1995;99:595–604.
58. Lotan M, Ben-Zeev B. Rett syndrome. A review with emphasis on clinical characteristics and intervention. ScientificWorldJournal. 2006;6:1517–41.
59. Pfister AA, Roberts AG, Taylor HM, Noel-Spaudling S, Damian MM, Charles PD. Spasticity in adults living in a developmental center. Arch Phys Med Rehabil. 2003;84:1808–12.
60. Henderson RC, Lark RK, Gurka MJ, Worley G, Fung EB, Conaway M, Stallings VA, Stevenson RD. Bone density and metabolism in children and adolescents with moderate to severe cerebral palsy. Pediatrics. 2002;110(1 Pt 1):e5.
61. Kerr MP, Richards D, Glover G. Primary care for people with a learning disability: a group practice survey. J Appl Res Intellect Disabil. 1996;9:347–52.
62. Durvasula S, Beange H. Health inequalities in people with intellectual disability: strategies for improvement. Health Promot J. 2001 Aug;11:27–31.
63. Hensel E, Rose J, Stenfert Kroese B, Banks-Smith J. Subjective judgments of quality of life: a comparison study between people with intellectual disability and those without disability. J Intellect Disabil Res. 2002;45:95–107.
64. Lee SH, Smith L, d'Espaingnet E, Thompson N. Health differences for working age Australians. Canberra, ACT: Australian Institute of Health; 1987.
65. Beange H, Lennox N, Parmenter TR. Health targets for people with an intellectual disability. J Intellect Dev Disabil. 1999;24(4):283–97.
66. Beange H. The medical model revisited. Aust N Z J Dev Disabil. 1986;12:3–7.
67. Howells G. Are the medical needs of mentally handicapped adults being met? J R Coll Gen Pract. 1986;36:449–53.
68. Parmenter TR. An analysis of Australian mental health services for people with mental retardation. Aust N Z J Dev Disabil. 1988;14:9–13.
69. Barker M, Howells G. The medical needs of adults: primary care for people with a mental handicap. Occasional paper 47. Royal Coll Gen Pract, London, 1990.
70. Smith SW, Camfield C, Camfield P. Living with cerebral palsy and tube feeding: a population-based follow-up study. J Pediatr. 1999;135:307–10.
71. Ory A, Sansky Y, Keren G. The issue of life expectancy for patients with severe cerebral palsy. Forensic Med. 2002;27:50–64 [Hebrew].
72. Rainforth B, York J, York-Barr C. Collaborative teams for students with severe disabilities: integrating therapy and educational services. Baltimore, MD: Paul H Brookes; 1997.
73. Davis J, Rendell P, Sims D. The joint practitioner – a new concept in professional training. J Interprof Care. 1999;13(4):395–404.
74. Benierakis CE. The function of multidisciplinary team in child psychiatry – clinic and educational aspect. Can J Psychiatry. 1995;40:348–53.

75. Heinemann GD. Teams in health care setting. In: Heinemann GD, Zeiss AM, editors. Team performance in health care: assessment and development. New York, NY: Kluwer Academic/Plenum; 2002.

76. Dunn W. Models of occupational therapy service provision in the school system. Am J Occup Ther. 1988;42(11):718–23.

77. York J, Rainforth B, Giangreco MF. Transdisciplinary team work and integrated therapy: clarifying the misconceptions. Pediatr Phys Ther. 1990;2(2):73–79.

78. Campbell PH. The integrated programming team: an approach for coordinating professionals of various disciplines in programs for students with severe and multiple handicaps. J Assoc Pers Sev Handicaps. 1978;12(2):107–16.

79. Hutchinson DJ. The transdisciplinary approach. In: Curry JB, Peppe KK, editors. Interdisciplinary approach to human services. Baltimore, MD: University Park Press; 1987. pp. 65–74.

80. Bennet FC. The pediatrician and the interdisciplinary process. Except Child. 1982;48(4):306–14.

81. Youngson-Reilly S, Tobin M, Fielder A. Multidisciplinary teams and childhood visual impairment: a study of two teams. Child Care Health Dev. 1995;21(1):3–15.

82. Lotan M. The time is now – appropriate therapeutic intervention for individuals with Rett syndrome: a key not presentation at the annual conference of the Dutch Rett syndrome association, Utrecht, Holland, 2010 Sept 24th–26th.

83. Percy AK. International research review. Paper presented at the IRSA 12th annual conference, Boston MA, 1996 May 24–27, tape 622–15.

84. McDonnell S. Balancing family needs. A lecture presented at the annual Rett Syndrome Conference, Baltimore, MD, 2004.

85. Lotan M, Manor-Binyamini I, Elefant C, Wine J, Saraf E, Yoshei T. The Israeli Rett Syndrome Center. Evaluation according to the transdisciplinary play-based assessment. ScientificWorldJournal. 2006;6:1302–13.

86. Maslow A. Towards a psychology of being. 3rd ed. New York, NY: John Wiley; 1999.

87. Volkmar F, Cook EH Jr, Pomeroy J, Realmuto G, Tanguay P. Practice parameters for the assessment and treatment of children, adolescents, and adults with autism and other pervasive developmental disorders. J Am Acad Child Adolesc Psychiatry. 1999;38(12 Suppl):32S–54S.

88. Gerhardt PF, Holmes DL. Employment: options and issues for adolescents and adults with autism. In: Cohen DJ, Volkmar FR, editors. Handbook of autism and pervasive developmental disorders. 2nd ed. New York, NY: Wiley; 1997. pp. 650–64.

89. Harris SL, Handleman JS. Helping children with autism enter the mainstream. In: Cohen DJ, Volkmar FR, editors. Handbook of autism and pervasive developmental disorders. 2nd ed. New York, NY: Wiley; 1997. pp. 665–75.

90. Siegel B. Coping with the diagnosis of autism. In: Cohen DJ, Volkmar FR, editors. Handbook of autism and pervasive developmental disorders. 2nd ed. New York, NY: Wiley; 1997. pp. 745–66.

91. Marcus LM, Kunce LJ, Schopler E. Working with families. In: Cohen DJ, Volkmar FR, editors. Handbook of autism and pervasive developmental disorders. 2nd ed. New York, NY: Wiley; 1997. pp. 631–49.

92. Horgan M, Douglas F, editors. Children of the global village. Proceedings Conf Dublin Inst Technol, 2004 Apr 24th. http://omepireland.ie/downloads/Children%20of%20the%20Global%20Village.Proceedings%20of%20Conference%20held%20in%20DIT%20on%2024th%20April%202004.pdf. Extracted on July 2010.

93. Dineen M. Providing quality experiences for children with special needs. In: Horgan M, Douglas F, editors. Children of the global village. Proc Conf Dublin Inst Technol. 2004 Apr 24th.

94. Connolly B, Russell F. Interdisciplinary early intervention program. Phys Ther. 1976;56(2):155–58.

95. Connolly BH, Morgan SB, Russell FF, Fulliton WL. A longitudinal study of children with Down syndrome who experienced early intervention programming. Phys Ther. 1993;73(3):170–81.

96. Connolly BH, Morgan S, Russell FF. Evaluation of children with Down syndrome who participated in an early intervention program. Second follow-up study. Phys Ther. 1984;64(10):1515–19.

97. Bjornhage L, Lagerwall B, Ericsson-Sagsjo A, Waldenstrom E. Early motor training for children with Down syndrome. In: Chigier E, editor. Looking up at Down syndrome. London: Freund; 1990. pp. 163–71.

98. Kokubun M, Haishi K, Okuzumi H, Hosobuchi T. Factors affecting age of walking by children with mental retardation. Percept Mot Skills. 1995;80(2):547–52.

99. Ulrich BD, Ulrich DA, Collier DH, Cole EL. Developmental shifts in the ability of infants with Down syndrome to produce treadmill steps. Phys Ther. 1995;75(1):14–23.

100. Ulrich DA, Ulrich BD, Angulo-Kinzler RM, Yun J. Treadmill training of infants with Down syndrome: evidence-based developmental outcomes. Pediatrics. 2001;108(5):e84.

101. Lotan M, Isakov E, Kessel S, Merrick J. Physical fitness and functional ability of children with intellectual disability: effects of a short-term daily treadmill intervention. ScientificWorldJournal. 2004;4:449–57.

102. Kolvin I, Miller FJW, Scott DM, Gatzanis SRM, Fleeting M. Continuities of depravation. The Newcastle 1,000 family study. Aldershot: Avebury; 1990.

103. Patja K, Iivanainen M, Vesala H, Oksanen H, Ruoppila I. Life expectancy of people with intellectual disability: a 35-year follow-up study. J Intellect Disabil Res. 2000;44(5):591–99.

104. Heller T, Hsieh K, Rimmer JH. Attitudinal and psychosocial outcomes of a fitness and health education program on adults with down syndrome. Am J Ment Retard. 2004;109(2):175–85.

105. Tsimaras V, Giagazoglou P, Fotiadou E, Christoulas K, Angelopoulou N. Jog-walk training in cardiorespiratory fitness of adults with Down syndrome. Percept Mot Skills. 2003;96(3 Pt 2):1239–51.

106. Tsimaras VK, Fotiadou EG. Effect of training on the muscle strength and dynamic balance ability of adults with down syndrome. J Strength Cond Res. 2004;18(2):343–47.

107. Carmeli E, Kessel S, Coleman R, Ayalon M. Effects of a treadmill walking program on muscle strength and balance in elderly people with Down syndrome. J Gerontol A Biol Sci Med Sci. 2002;57(2):M106–10.

108. Carmeli E, Barchad S, Masharawi Y, Coleman R. Impact of a walking program in people with down syndrome. J Strength Cond Res. 2004;18(1):180–84.

109. Varela AM, Sardinha LB, Pitetti KH. Effects of an aerobic rowing training regimen in young adults with Down syndrome. Am J Ment Retard. 2001;106(2):135–44.

110. Lotan M, Burnstein S. Influence of a treadmill training program on adults with cognitive impairment. Annual Meet Israeli Physical Therapy Assoc. 2000 May.

111. Maslow A. Motivation and personality. 2nd ed. New York, NY: Harper Row; 1970.

112. Lewis JE, Wilson CD. Pathways to learning in Rett Syndrome. Teleford, Shropshire: Wozencroft Printers; 1996.

113. Rett A. Rett syndrome. An address at United Kingdom Rett Syndrome Association conference, Coleshill. 1985 Oct.

114. Woodyatt GC, Ozanne A. Communication abilities and a case of Rett Syndrome. J Intellect Disabil Res. 1992;36:83–92.

115. Woodyatt GC, Ozanne AE. A longitudinal study of cognitive skills and communication behaviours in children with Rett Syndrome. J Intellect Disabil Res. 1993;37(Pt 4):419–35.

116. Cooley WC. Providing a primary care medical home for children and youth with Cerebral palsy.(Clinical Report). Pediatrics. 2004;114:1106–13.

117. Thomas SB, Hawke C. Health-care services for children with disabilities: emerging standards and implications. J Spec Educ. 1999;32(4):226–37.

118. Hubble MA, Duncan BL, Miller SD. The heart and soul of change: what works in therapy. Washington, DC: American Psychological Association; 1999.

119. Firth G. A dual aspect process model of intensive interaction. Br J Learn Disabil. 2008;37:43–49.
120. Hewett D, Nind M, editors. Interaction in action: reflections on the use of Intensive Interaction. London: David Fulton; 1998.
121. Hoenig H. Assistive technology and mobility aids for the older patient with disability. Ann Long Term Care. 2004;12(9):12–13, 17–19.
122. Kerr AM. Understanding Rett disorder, A guide for professionals. An instruction DVD. Glasgow: University of Glasgow, Section of Psychological Medicine; 2006.
123. Heller T, Ying GS, Rimmer JH, Marks BA. Determinants of exercise in adults with cerebral palsy. Public Health Nurs. 2002;19(3):223–31.
124. Fox RA, Rosenberg R, Rotatori AF. Parent involvement in a treatment program for obese retarded adults. J Behav Ther Exp Psychiatry. 1985;16(1):45–48.
125. Yalom ID. The gift of therapy. Tel Avic: Kinneret; 2002 [Hebrew].
126. Godesh N, Menat H, Lotan M. Identifying limitations in health services for adults with ID in Israel. A final seminal work presented for the department of physical therapy. Ariel: Ariel University Center; 2010 [Hebrew].
127. Beange H, Bauman A. Caring for the developmentally disabled in the community. Aust Fam Physician. 1990;19:1558–63.
128. Wilson DN, Haire A. Health care screening for people with mental handicap living in the community. BMJ. 1990;301:1379–81.
129. Kerr MP, Richards D, Glover G. Primary care for people with a learning disability: a group practice survey. J Appl Res Intellect Disabil. 1997;9:347–52.
130. Crocker AC, Yankauer A. Basic issues. Ment Retard. 1987;25:227–32.
131. Beange HP. Caring for a vulnerable population. Med J Aust. 1996;164:159–60.
132. Lennox N, Chaplin R. The psychiatric care of people with intellectual disabilities: the perceptions of consultant psychiatrists in Victoria. Aust NZ J Psychol. 1996;30:774–80.
133. Burbidge M. Patient-held medical records for people with an intellectual disability. 10th World Congr Int Assoc Scientific Study Intellectual Disability, Helsinki, IASSID. 1996. p. 227.
134. Strauss D, Eyman RK. Mortality of people with mental retardation in California with and without Down's syndrome. Am J Ment Retard. 1996;100:543–653.

Chapter 26
Adoption

Gary Diamond and Yehuda Senecky

Abstract Adoption has become a socially accepted means by which a family grows, whether by choice, or where biological and psychosocial constraints prevent the process from occurring within the narrow context of the family's autonomous resources. The popularity of adoption is best reflected in its relation to live births, with the numbers in the Scandinavian countries and the USA approaching 1.1 and 3, respectively, per 100 live births. Falling fertility rates, as well as greater acceptance of children raised in more varied family settings, e.g., by single and older parents, single-gender couple living arrangements, have contributed to this trend. Many adopted children are considered to be "at risk" for both medical and developmental impairments, due to the adverse health status of the biological mother during the pregnancy, as well as their exposure to early environmental and emotional deprivation. To remedy these potential deficits, the adoptive family is encouraged to seek pre-adoption counseling and preparation, as well as access supportive services after the adoption in order to facilitate comprehensive medical screening and care, as well as optimize preventive and remedial efforts to minimize developmental and emotional–behavioral disabilities.

Introduction

Adoption refers to a process by which one assumes full and legal parenting rights of another individual, and in so doing, relieves the previous parent, whether biological or adoptive, of his moral and practical parental responsibilities. The practice of adoption is regulated by law and statutes, whether they be local, national, or

G. Diamond (✉)
Department of Pediatrics, Sackler School of Medicine, Tel Aviv University, Tel Aviv, Israel; Institute of Child Development and Neurology, Schneider Children's Medical Center of Israel, Clalit Health Services, 49202 Petah-Tiqva, Israel; Department of Pediatrics, Albert Einstein College of Medicine, Rose F Kennedy Center, Center for the Evaluation and Rehabilitation of Children, Bronx, NY, USA
e-mail: diamondg@clalit.org.il

D.R. Patel et al. (eds.), *Neurodevelopmental Disabilities*,
DOI 10.1007/978-94-007-0627-9_26, © Springer Science+Business Media B.V. 2011

inter-country. In the latter case, adoptions are regulated by the Convention on Protection of Children and Cooperation in Respect of Inter-country Adoption, formulated by the Hague Conference on Private International Law, implemented in 1995 and, since then, ratified by over 75 countries. International agreements and bilateral laws regulating inter-country adoption, such as the Hague Convention, require adherence to basic principles of fairness and morality, requiring the biological parent(s) to sign informed waivers of parental rights, to conduct the process of adoption outside the realm of the profit motive, and for countries to agree to safeguard the child's medical and psychological welfare, as well as his ethnic and cultural heritage [1].

Adoptions can take place either between family members or unrelated individuals. Indeed, the large numbers of adoptions occurring in the USA each year (approximately 127,000 for 2001) can in no small part (close to 50%) be attributed to other family members taking responsibility for a child suddenly bereft of a parent who has recently passed away [2]. Adoption differs from foster care, also sanctioned by law and regulations, in terms of its permanence and unequivocal nature regarding assuming the full range of responsibilities for the child. Foster care provides the springboard for close to 40% of the formal adoptions occurring in the USA each year [3].

Adoption is not synonymous with the term "orphan," since it is estimated that the number of true orphans, where the child is abandoned after the death of both parents, is actually quite small, estimated to constitute only 10% of the total [4]. The number of true orphans is relatively greater in sub-Saharan Africa, where large segments of the population have been decimated by the AIDS pandemic. Most of the children being adopted from abroad, most notably from Latin America, eastern Europe, and Asia, were born to single mothers, unable to care for them due to a combination of economic and social circumstances. In eastern Europe and the former Soviet Union, the majority of abandoned children were jettisoned by their families for economic reasons, with only 15% having been placed due to reasons of child abuse or neglect [5, 6].

Historical Perspective

Adoption has existed since the dawn of time. The Bible tells us, "Be your hand upon your trusted neighbor, whom you have adopted as your helper" (Psalms 80:18). "I, the Lord, adopted you unto myself," is found in the book of Isaiah 41:10. Moses, it will be remembered, was adopted by Pharaoh's daughter. Biblical parables typically stress the adoptee's ability to overcome great personal odds and to triumph as leaders of their people, this despite their inauspicious early beginnings.

Of the many kings and rulers of ancient Greece and Rome who were adopted, none is as famous as Oedipus, whose secret adoption lies at the heart of his own personal tragedy. The Koran (Sura 13) tells of the prophet Mohamed, who took for himself a son from among the slaves, yet who later rescinded the adoption for personal reasons. Napoleon enacted laws guaranteeing the legal rights of adopted children, thereby safeguarding their status in society, despite their origins being different from the milieu they eventually were raised in by their adoptive parents [7, 8].

Over the years adoption spread beyond the bounds of the immediate tribe or community and extended to raising children from different communities and ethnic backgrounds, as well as from different countries entirely. Despite its growing and widespread acceptance, adoption has never ceased to provoke controversy and public debate. With every passing generation, the debate flares anew, with changing and evolving issues, both morally and socially, coming to the fore.

Domestically, the most important development regarding the care of orphans prior to the World War II was the change in the perception of institutionalization in the eyes of the public and embodied in the position paper issued by the First White House Conference on the Care of Dependent Children in 1909. Within a 40-year period, beginning in 1923, the USA saw the percentage of orphaned children taken in by adoptive families jump from 2 to 33% [9].

With the arrival of tens of thousands of newly orphaned children, resulting from World War II, on American shores, adoption became an acceptable and widespread social norm. Surveys at the time reflected an overall "positive" attitude toward international adoption on the part of close to 90% of the American public, with close to 64% indicating a personal connection with either friends or family members who had adopted a child [10].

Far-reaching changes in social policy legislation, as well as an overall enrichment of vast segments of Western society, led to important changes in the patterns of adoption as well as considerably limiting the numbers of children who would be available for adoption at the local level. Social supports and disbursement of birth entitlements to young unmarried mothers in many Western countries removed the economic constraints on single mothers wishing to raise their babies by themselves, thereby thinning the ranks of infants abandoned to the care of the State. These developments led to profound changes in the demographic make up of children being offered for adoption. They were suddenly much older than they were previously at the time of adoption, and had been abandoned less for economic reasons, and more due to prevailing social stigma and psychological adjustment difficulties on the part of the biological family. Growing awareness on the part of adopting parents as to the emotional and behavioral fallout, resulting from environmental deprivation in congregate care settings for orphaned or abandoned children, led to parents wishing to seek adoptable infants as young as possible in more economically destitute countries where there remained a surplus of infants and young children available for adoption.

The growing demand for adoptable children from abroad was further fueled by two additional social and geopolitical developments: the increasing age at which mothers (as well as fathers, to a lesser extent) chose to bear children, with the attendant decrease in fertility rates in Western countries, as well as the fall of communism in Russia and eastern Europe in the late 1980s, thereupon releasing a torrent of babies and young children for adoption in the West. In 1970 the average maternal age at the time of their first parturition was 21.4 years, as opposed to 25 years in the year 2000. Today more than 20% of women choose to become pregnant after the age of 35 years, while their chances of actually becoming pregnant is 20% less than during their twenties. Miscarriage rates approach the 50% level during the fifth decade of a woman's life. Along with this, the social changes in east Asia and eastern Europe made a significant impact on Western, and specifically American, adoption statistics: by 2003 there had been a 334% increase in the number of successfully completed international adoptions to the USA, as opposed to abysmally low levels for 1992, only 11 years previously [11].

Epidemiology

Publications by the United Nations Children's Fund (UNICEF) and the United States Agency for International Development (USAID) from earlier in the decade placed estimates of the total pool of potential adoptees less than 15 years of age, having lost at least one parent, in African, Asian, and Latin American countries as being on the order of 108 million [12]. In the former Soviet Union there exist another estimated potential 100,000 adoptees. However, in the latter, the improved economic outlook, plus more progressive social legislation than is currently in place, promises to significantly alter future trends in adoption from that country.

Epidemiological analysis of figures for adoption to date generally spans the period between 1997 and 2007, the last year for which comprehensive data exist. International adoption figures generally date from April 1, 1998, when the Hague Convention regulations were widely ratified and placed in effect in most participating countries. General adoption figures place adoption from foster care (661,000, 37%) on an almost equal footing with adoption from private sources, outside of the foster care system (677,000, 38%). According to the Administration for Children and Families' analysis of data from the Adoption and Foster Care Reporting and Analysis System, most foster care adoptions (454,000, 69%) were carried out by an individual with experience in the foster care system, and in 23% of cases, by an actual family relative. Adoptions from foster care fared less well on physical and mental health-care measures compared with other groups, with 54% involving children with special health-care needs, which were significantly greater than for the general adoption figures of 39% and for the general population of children, with 14%. Most adoptive parents (85%) reported their children as being in "good health," even though close to 26% report having had to seek medical care for moderate to severe consequences of any one of 16 possible medical or psychological conditions during childhood or adolescence [13].

Adoptive children are more likely to have been diagnosed at one time with moderate to severe mental health symptoms, relative to the general pediatric population, with international adoptees faring better on the average by 50% than the general pool of adoptees (see Table 26.1).

International adoptions constitute approximately 25% of all adopted children, with a total of 444,000 being accounted for in the USA. Of these, 128,000 (29%) were considered to have special health-care needs. Children adopted internationally

Table 26.1 Social, behavioral, ADHD, and depression problems in general pediatric, adoptee, and international adoptee populations

Diagnosis	Social problems (>6 years, %)	Behavioral, conduct problems (>2 years, %)	ADHD (>6 years, %)	Depression (>2 years, %)
General	9	4	10	4
All adoptees	14	15	26	9
International adoptees	12	7	17	8

were more likely to have been adopted by married couples (82%), as opposed to 69% for the total pool of adoptees. In other countries, the percentage of inter-country adoptees by single parents are significantly greater [14].

Six out of 10 international adoptees in 2007 were from Asia (with the majority from China), with over 70% having been previously in congregate care. Congregate care, with its attendant psychosocial ramifications regarding the child's later physical and mental well-being, was most prevalent among international adoptees, with only 25% having resided with the birth family, compared with 59% who originated in foster care and 39% from private domestic adoptions. Nevertheless, these children's relatively good psychosocial adjustment attests to the importance of the age at the time of adoption, as well as to the efforts invested in treatment and prevention by inter-country adoptive parents, as well as significant challenges faced by children originating in the foster care system in the USA. The age at adoption tends to skew in favor of middle childhood, also reflecting the impact of foster care on the general adoption figures, with only 6% being adopted before the age of 2 years, with close to 30% coming from the 5- to 9-year-old age bracket. For international adoptees, the age of adoption is considerably younger, with 24% within the under 5-year-old age bracket, compared to 15% for that group out of the total population of adoptees.

The international adoption system has been marked by far-reaching changes in recent years, including cessation of adoptions from Romania in 2004, under pressure from the European Union, a freeze on adoptions from Guatemala in 2008, and application of more restrictive criteria by China in 2007. As a result, the number of adopted children from abroad has dropped, from a high of over 22,000 in 2004 to under 18,000 in 2008.

Of the entire pool of adopted children, over 71% had birth siblings, with the majority of whom contact was lost at the time of adoption, especially among international adoptees.

Most parents surveyed (87%) expressed satisfaction with the adoption. However, the significant numbers who did not belie the underlying problem of adoption disruption continue to plague adoptions in the USA [15].

Federal regulations, administered through the Department of Homeland Security and the Department of State, standardized the major steps in the process of international adoption, with formal entry through a state-licensed adoption agency or social worker, designated to perform a prerequisite home study. Depending on the state, and the regulations regarding eligibility for adoption by the provider country, restrictions on marital status, length and marriage, divorce, income, religion, health, and fertility status often apply [16–18]. According to provisions in the Child Citizen Act of 2001, the inter-country adopted child is granted US citizenship upon entry to the USA, provided that at least one adoptive parent is a US citizen, that he is less than 18 years of age, there is a full and final adoption completed, and he is admitted to the USA as an immigrant [19].

Medical and Developmental Concerns

Communicable diseases and congenital anomalies constitute two major areas of concern to parents adopting children, especially in those adoptions originating abroad. Serious systemic illness in the child is also uppermost in parents' minds prior to and immediately following the adoption. Adherence to recommendations regarding the validity of prior immunizations and scheduling "catch-up" vaccines is strongly urged of parents and treating primary care physicians with adopted children in their care [20, 21].

The American Academy of Pediatrics has set forth guidelines covering the medical issues of inter-country adoption and recommends testing for communicable diseases among the adopted children arriving from abroad: HIV-1 and HIV-2 (human immunodeficiency virus), hepatitis B and C, tuberculosis, syphilis, and parasitic enteropathogens. In addition, the appointed committee recommends further testing, to include complete blood count, serum lead levels, thyroid function tests, phenylketonuria, congenital malformations, inheritable metabolic diseases, and neuro-developmental testing and to include vision and hearing screening. Identification of a disease likely to endanger the child's life or of those in his immediate vicinity, such as AIDS (acquired immune deficiency syndrome, resulting from infection by HIV), requires special approval for entry into the country and is given under only the most unusual of circumstances [22].

Relying on prior testing is insufficient to meet the criteria set forth. Oftentimes prior testing had been conducted by local laboratories abroad without sufficient quality control supervision. Medical records had been shown to be inaccurate, if not downright falsified for a variety of reasons. Children had been brought to western countries in the past with a variety of ailments which potentially could have been prevented, if not actually treated, prior to their arrival [23–25].

Surveys conducted of the medical status of adopted children over the past decade indicated prevalence figures for children originating in eastern Europe of 15% for hepatitis B or C carriers, 4.8% had abnormal liver functions, 4.8% had strabismus or other visual impairments; 3.6% were affected by various degrees of hearing loss. Another 2.4% suffered from extreme failure to thrive (FTT), 3.6% from congenital cardiac malformations, and 3.6% from orthopedic anomalies. A total of 13% had neurologic dysfunction, including muscle weakness, hypotonicity, or movement disorders, and 5% were microcephalic, often associated with mental retardation or genetic syndromes affecting later behavior or cognitive development [14, 26, 27].

Where pre-adoption screening exists, a practice often inviting controversy over potential ethical dilemmas, close to 22% of adoptive families forwent the adoption because of fears related to abnormal medical or developmental findings, arising during the screening by consulting medical experts. Apparently the social norms and economic conditions prevailing in that country caused adopting families to be more circumspect, and thereby more vigilant regarding their abilities to cope with potentially disruptive medical and behavioral problems in the adopted child [14].

Emotional and Adjustment Difficulties in Adopted Children

Parental concerns regarding the ultimate welfare of their adopted child extend to their emotional and behavioral functioning as well. The longer the time passes after the adoption, the more these particular issues emerge as the overriding concern to parents, quickly eclipsing their original purely medically related worries.

The abnormal behaviors characteristic of adopted children in the period immediately following the adoption include autistic-like patterns, such as stereotyped movements of the head, such as nodding back and forth, actual head banging, and movements related to anxiety and fear [28]. In addition, there appears an increase in neuro-motor tone, similar to "freezing" or "stilling" posturing, a slowing of actual movements, similar to the way the body moves underwater, and a noticeable lack of facial expressions, especially of the mouth, accompanied by a paucity of sounds and words uttered under a variety of circumstances. Children are also more, or less, sensitive to feeling and touch and are especially maladroit at regulating their sensory functions. They find it difficult to adapt to new tastes as well as new textures of toys and food introduced into the oral cavity, avoid strong light and loud noises, especially those that are unfamiliar to them. This aversion often seems strange to parents who have visited them in the orphanage, often recalling the din of the constant chatter of children, caretakers shouting or admonishing the children, and the clanging of pots and pans from the kitchen or pantry. These problems of sensory regulation often affect the child's ability to adapt to the quiet of his new home, and even impact on his ability to retune his regulatory sleep patterns. As a result of the difficulties in regulating his sensory functioning, the child often undergoes serious disruptions in his emotional reactions, with angry and violent outbursts (or the converse – withdrawal and depression), fear of the dark, a resurgence of bed wetting, and soiling [29, 30].

The most profound long-term difficulties encountered include speech and language delays, at least until the end of the pre-school period, a tendency to suffer from distractibility and attention deficit disorder, with or without hyperactivity (ADHD), the ability to form viable and long-lasting friendships and social relationships, and the potential for mutuality in later intimate relationships. In many ways adopted children share many of the traits resembling individuals suffering from posttraumatic stress disorder (PTSD) [31].

Adopted children with physical growth retardation usually enter a "catch-up" phase after their adoption and usually by 4 years post-adoption, close any existing gap, relative to their native-born counterparts in Europe or North America. Nevertheless, the length of institutionalization at any early age plays a decisive role in this catch-up growth dynamic and for those children institutionalized from birth for longer than the usual maximal 2–2.5 years, the catch up is not always complete. The psychosocial deprivation at an early age in these cases leaves its indelible mark on their physical appearance as well, especially in terms of their ultimate growth parameters [27].

Many of the biological mothers who abandoned their children in different foreign countries, as well as indigent cases in Western countries, suffered from nutritional deprivation, as well as a myriad of intrauterine infections and substance abuse, including drugs, cigarettes and alcohol, with potential devastating effects on the developing fetus. Antenatal care is practically unheard of in these countries and the neonatal morbidity and mortality statistics reflect the heavy human price paid by those societies without the resources to invest in their future human resources. These antenatal risk factors are directly related to the high proportion of adopted children starting out in life both with outward signs of medical neglect, such as small head circumferences and stigmatized facial features, as in the fetal alcohol syndrome (FAS), as well as the less tangible behavioral and regulatory abnormalities in infant behavior, which often later evolve into problems of attention deficits, hyperactivity, emotional and behavioral difficulties, learning disabilities, or mental retardation [32].

A survey of immediate post-adoption developmental abnormalities in young adopted infants and children in the USA include gross motor delays (55%), fine motor impairments (49%), and speech and language delays (32–49%), as well as social and behavioral functioning and self-regulation (28%). These initial signs eventually evolve into the different aforementioned problem behaviors. The overwhelming quiet and lack of tactile and language stimulation, characteristic of long periods of time during their life in the orphanage and the absence of ongoing, reliable, and nurturing contact with the caretaker staff, leave an indelible mark on the young child's development [33].

Landmark studies of Romanian infants in Canada indicated the widespread presence of abnormal behaviors in the immediate post-adoption period: 33% had problems tolerating solid foods, 30% showed eating excessive amounts of food and hoarding behaviors, and 67% had stereotyped, repetitive autistic-like behaviors. Whereas most of these behaviors disappeared by the age of $4\frac{1}{2}$, many retained traces with more of a tendency to emotional outbursts, attention deficit disorder with hyperactivity (ADHD), and learning disabilities. The older the child was at the time of his adoption, the greater the tendency there was to retain these behaviors till later in life. Studies of adopted children who reached adolescence find higher than expected rates of depression, suicide attempts, and problems in building social relationships. The Romanian post-adoption studies in Canada also described "over friendly" maladaptive behavioral patterns of children toward strangers, especially at a younger age [34, 35].

Those adopted children who spent the initial first several months of their lives living with their biological mothers before being turned over to a local orphanage were found to be both at an advantage, having experienced in many cases a positive bonding experience with a nurturing mother, and also at a disadvantage, having undergone an especially traumatic rupture after the initial positive bonding experience during infancy [36].

Infant–Mother Attachment Theory

Early infant–maternal attachment constitutes the basis for healthy social and emotional development and has a determining influence on the individual's later development. Where attachment is a complete and healthy one, the infant learns to interact with his environment and develop a basic sense of trust with his primary caretaker.

John Bowlby developed his theory of attachment to describe the behavioral phenomena in infants and young children which he attributed to love, anxiety, abandonment, mourning, trauma, and depression at an early age. His descriptions were based on the premise that every child has a basic need to seek comfort and security from a dominant caretaker figure, usually his mother. This need is apparent from early infancy, persists for many years, and is especially obvious in novel situations, with a potential for danger and anxiety-provoking. The need for comfort, protection, and the development of trust, which permits the child to establish a firm emotional base from which he can continue to venture forth and explore a novel and potentially anxiety-producing world, evolves during the first 2 years of life. Those infants not having been able to develop this sense of trust, as is the case in many children abandoned from an early age, remain avoidant, suspicious, and insecure, possibly explaining many of the later behavioral problems witnessed in so many adopted children [37]. The abnormal behaviors described above, as well as additional observations by the medical teams visiting the orphanages first hand, include serious disturbances in and complete avoidance of normal oral and mouthing behaviors, used by infants to establish a bond of trust with the mother. Institutionalized infants in eastern Europe were noted to avoid placing any toys or objects in their mouths. Furthermore, abnormal social relationships with their young, 1- to 2-year-old peers were witnessed, including the establishment of a pecking order based on fear, retribution, violence, and censorship (Diamond et al., 2006, Pseudoneurological syndrome in institutionalized infants prior to bonding and adoption, "unpublished paper").

Intervention and Preventive Services

Developmental models of early attachment behaviors and their potential impact on later emotional and cognitive functioning reflect progress made in the understanding of the neuro-physiological mechanisms underlying early growth and development of the central nervous system in the infant and young child. Studies of imprinting and its associated neural plasticity stress the importance of early nurturing behavior and subsequent healthy emotional development. Attendant abnormal responses to stress, stereotyped behaviors, abnormal eating patterns and social dysfunction in primate studies were all expressions of maternal deprivation and a function of poorly developed dendritic arbors of neurons in the neocortex and the cerebellum [38–42]. Failure to develop healthy attachments during the first 2 years of life may prove maladaptive to both the cognitive and the emotional development of the child, where potential damage may have occurred to the developing neural circuits involved in emotional regulation and memory [43].

Just as in the case of children successfully raised by seemingly neglectful biological mothers, more often than not, a child raised in maladaptive foster or pre-adoptive congregate care experienced a "good enough" nurturing relationship with even a tangential caregiver, thus affording him the essential experience of positive early attachment [44].

By the same token that neural plasticity can augur poor long-term outcomes for neglected children, it can also signal the potential gains for early intervention, especially when children are adopted at a critical and younger age for compensatory "enriching and nurturing" mechanisms to be able to work [43, 45].

Adoptive parents need to be wary of premature placement of the young adopted child in congregate day care. They need to work hard at establishing new social and biological rhythms for themselves and their adopted child, including the eating habits, sleep cycles, and the mutually responsive patterns of oral and body language communication.

It is especially important to utilize counseling services by child care and developmental experts to guide these initial stages of adjustment and attachment building. Mundane issues, such as use of the pacifier, sleep and eating habits, television viewing, use of a car seat, toileting, abnormal behaviors and limit setting, all assume different proportions in the adopted child, given his previous life experiences, and require special sensitivity and expertise to guide the parents in smoothing over the "rough spots." Usual early childhood crises often assume epic proportions against the background of the momentous changes the adopted child has undergone. For the older adopted child, behavioral and social problems, learning difficulties and attention deficit, along with the issue of identity and questions about his previous life require professional advice and guidance, especially pertaining to the important step of opening a closed adoption file. In that case, counseling is vital when attempting to reestablish contact with the biological family of origin.

Long-term studies indicate developmental concerns by adoptive families in close to 67% of adopted children, with 8% showing early motor delays, 18% speech and language difficulties, and numerous cases of behavioral and learning problems [46].

Summary

Most domestic and inter-country adoptions are resounding success stories and parent satisfaction is impressive. Adoption presents great challenges to families and the opportunity to build new lives with great promise. For families who are unable to realize the dream of passing on their heritage and human gifts by utilizing their own innate biological and genetic potential, adoption offers a viable alternative. However, to do so requires much thought, planning, organization, resources, and professional guidance.

References

1. Hague Convention Proceedings, 1995.
2. National Council for Adoption, Adoption Fact Book, 2000.
3. US Child Welfare Information Gateway: trends in Foster Care and Adoption.
4. Convention on the rights of the child. UNICEF. http://www.unicef.org/crc/crc.htm
5. Johnson DE. Medical and developmental sequelae of early childhood institutionalization in international adoptees from Romania and the Russian Federation. In: Nelson C, editors. The effects of early adversity on neurobehavioral development. Mahwah, NJ: Lawrence Erlbaum; 2000. pp. 113–62.
6. Johnson DE. Adoption and the effect on children's development. Early Hum Dev. 2002;68: 39–44.
7. Diamond G, Arbel E. Adoption: Odyssey of a new parenthood. Tel Aviv: United Kibbutz Publishing/Workers' Library; 2009 [Hebrew].
8. Pollack D, Bleich M, Reid CJ Jr, et al. Classical religious perspectives of adoption law. Notre Dame Law Rev. 2004;79(2):693–753.
9. Barr B. Spare children, 1900–1945: Inmates of orphanages as subjects of research in medicine and in the social sciences in America. Dissertation. Stanford, CA: Stanford University; 1992.
10. National Adoption Attitudes Survey. Dave Thomas Foundation for Adoption. Evan B. Donaldson Adoption Institute. 2002 Jun.
11. Barad D. Age and female fertility. American Fertility Association. http://www.theafa.org/faqs/afa_ageandfemaleinfertility.html
12. UNAIDS/UNICEF/USAID. Children on the brink 2002: a joint report on orphan estimates and program strategies. 2002 July. http://www.unicef.org/publications/index_4378.html. Accessed 1 Mar 2005.
13. Vandivere S, Malm K, Radel L. Adoption USA (2007 National Survey of Adoptive Parents – US Department of Health and Human Services). http://aspe.hhs.gov/hsp/09/NSAP/chartbook/index.pdf
14. Diamond GW, Senecky Y, Schurr D, et al. Pre-placement screening in international adoption. Isr Med Assoc J. 2003;5(11):763–66.
15. US Department of Health and Human Services. Child Welfare information gateway. Adoption disruption and dissolution. Washington, DC: Department of Health and Human Services; 2004.
16. US Department of Homeland Security, US Citizenship and Immigration Services. Intercountry adoptions. http://uscis.gov/graphics/services/index2.htm
17. US State Department, Bureau of Consular Affairs. Overseas Citizens Services, Office of Children's Issues. International adoption. http://trave.state.gov/family/adoption/notices/notices_473.html
18. Johnson D. International adoption: what is fact, what is fiction, and what is the future? Pediatr Clin North Am. 2005;52:1221–46.
19. US Department of Homeland Security, US Citizenship and Immigration Services, Child Citizenship Act. Information for adoptive parents. 2001 Feb. http://uscis.gov/graphics/publicaffairs/backgrounds/cbground.htm
20. Saiman L, Aronson J, Zhou J, et al. Prevalence of infectious diseases among internationally adopted children. Pediatrics. 2001;108(3):608–12.
21. Centers for Disease Control and Prevention. General recommendations on immunization. MMWR. 2002;51(RR-2):1–35.

22. American Academy of Pediatrics. Medical evaluation of internationally adopted children for infectious diseases. In: Pickering LK, editor. 2000 Red book: report of the committee on Infectious Diseases. 25th ed. Elk Grove Village, IL: American Academy of Pediatrics; 2000. pp. 148–52.

23. Miller LC, Comfort K, Kelly N. Immunization status of internationally adopted children. Pediatrics. 2001;108:1050–1.

24. Staat MA, Daniels D. Immunization verification in internationally adopted children (abstract). Pediatr Res. 2001;49:468A.

25. Feikema SM, Klevens RM, Washington ML, et al. Extra immunization among US children. J Am Med Assoc. 2000;283:1311–17.

26. Johnson DE. Medical and developmental sequelae of early childhood institutionalization in international adoption from Romania and the Russian Federation. In: Nelson C, editor. The effects of early adoption on neurobehavioral development. Mahwah, NJ: Lawrence Erlbaum; 2000. pp. 113–62.

27. Mason P, Narad C, Jester T, et al. A survey of growth and development in the international adopted child. Pediatr Res. 2000;47:2009.

28. Rutter M, Andersen-Wood L, Beckett C, et al. Quasi-autistic patterns following severe early global deprivation. Book Suppl J Child Psychol Psychiatr. 1999;40:537–49.

29. Zeanah CH. Beyond insecurity: a reconceptualization of clinical disorders of attachment. J Consult Clin Psychol. 1996;64:42–52.

30. Zeanah CH, Boris N, Scheeringa M. Psychopathology in infancy. J Child Psychol Psychiatry Allied Discipl. 1997;38:81–99.

31. Scheeringa M, Zeanah CH, Peebles CD. Relational posttraumatic stress disorder: a new disorder? Paper 44th Ann Meet Am Acad Child Adolesc Psychiatr, Toronto, 1997.

32. Davies JK, Bledsoe JM. Prenatal alcohol and drug exposures in adoption. Pediatr Clin North Am. 2005;52:1369–93.

33. Weitzman C, Albers L. Long-term developmental, behavioral and attachment outcomes after international adoption. Pediatr Clin North Am. 2005;52:1395–419.

34. O'Connor TG, Marvin R, Rutter M, et al. Child-parent attachment following early institutional deprivation. Dev Psychopathol. 2003;15:19–38.

35. Ames E. The development of Romanian orphanage children adopted to Canada. Final report to the National Welfare Grants Program: Human Resources Development Canada. Burnaby, BC: Simon Fraser University; 1997.

36. Smyke A, Dumitrescu A, Zeanah C. Attachment disturbances in young children I. The continuum of caretaking causalty. J Am Acad Child Adolesc Psychiatry. 2002;41:972–82.

37. Bowlby J. The nature of the child's tie to his mother. Int J Psychoanal. 1958;39:350–73.

38. Harlow HF, Harlow MK. The affectional systems. In: Schrier AM, Harlow HF, Stollnitz F, editors. Behavior of non-human primates. Vol. 2. New York, NY: Academic Press; 1965. pp. 287–334.

39. Sackett GP. Prospects for research on schizophrenia. Neurophysiology. Isolation-rearing in primates. Neurosci Res Program Bull. 1972;10:388–92.

40. Bennett AJ, Lesch KP, Heils A, et al. Early experience and serotonin transporter gene variation interact to influence primate CNS function. Mol Psychiatry. 2002;7:118–22.

41. Struble RG, Riesen AH. Changes in cortical dendritic branching subsequent to partial social isolation in stumptailed monkeys. Dev Psychobiol. 1978;11:479–86.

42. Floeter MK, Greenough WT. Cerebellar plasticity: modification of Purkinje cell structure by differential rearing in monkeys. Science. 1979;206:227–29.

43. Hensch TK. Critical period regulation. Annu Rev Neurosci. 2004;27:549–79.

44. Winnicott DW. The ordinary devoted mother. In: Winnicott C, Shepherd R, Davis M, editors. Babies and their mothers. Reading, MA: Addison-Wesley; 1987. pp. 3–14.

45. Hannigan JH, Berman RF, Zajac CS. Environmental enrichment and the behavioral effects of prenatal exposure to alcohol in rats. Neurotoxicol Teratol. 1993;15:261–66.

46. Senecky Y, Diamond G, Zuckerman J, et al. Long term developmental, behavioral and health problems in children brought to Israel after international adoption. Paper, Nat Conf Child Dev Centers, Jerusalem, 2010.

Chapter 27
Palliative Care and End-of-Life Issues

Joav Merrick and Mohammed Morad

Abstract Today most children born with intellectual disability will enter adulthood. Some with the rarest syndromes or multiple associated disease will die in infancy or childhood, and here it is important that they will receive the same end-of-life service as the general population. Today, changing demographics that has resulted in a growing number of people with intellectual disability living into old age and suffering from the same diseases as the general aging population is creating a need for more organized palliative care for this population and to educate professionals to handle end-of-life issues with the persons with intellectual disability themselves dying, their families, and also care staff, who are not always prepared for these events.

Introduction

When a child is diagnosed with a serious condition, the life of the family changes due to the stress of the disease, travel and visits to treatment center(s), hospitalizations, economic burden, and uncertainty about prognosis and survival. Siblings are often forgotten during the medical treatments, because parental focus is on the sick child.

In palliative care, hope is an important part. Preserving hope and sometimes protecting the patient from disclosure of bad news are often playing parts, but it must be remembered that even very young children or children with a disability can understand the seriousness of a disease. Pediatric palliative care can therefore help the child to express emotions and cope through play, music, or other means or technologies.

J. Merrick (✉)
National Institute of Child Health and Human Development, Health Services, Office of the Medical Director, Division for Mental Retardation, Ministry of Social Affairs and Social Services, POBox 1260, IL-91012 Jerusalem, Israel; Kentucky Children's Hospital, University of Kentucky, Lexington, KY, USA
e-mail: jmerrick@zahav.net.il

D.R. Patel et al. (eds.), *Neurodevelopmental Disabilities*,
DOI 10.1007/978-94-007-0627-9_27, © Springer Science+Business Media B.V. 2011

In this time and age, children should basically live longer than their parents, but every year in any country around the world children die from congenital conditions, prematurity, heritable disorders, or acquired illness or trauma [1].

In this chapter we will discuss palliative care and end-of-life issues for children and adults with intellectual disability. Palliative care is defined as the active total care of patients whose disease is no longer responsive to current curative treatment [2], and the goal of care is to enhance quality of life in the face of an ultimately terminal condition. The treatment focus is on the relief of symptoms (like pain) and conditions (like loneliness) that cause distress and detract from enjoyment and quality of life. It should also ensure that bereaved families are able to remain functional and intact after the death of the child or person with intellectual disability.

Infants, Children, and Youth

Causes of death in children are usually different from the causes of death in adults, and therefore palliative care guidelines will be different for this age group. The American Academy of Pediatrics has developed guidelines [1] for palliative care in children that are general and not specific to intellectual disability, but we will convey the message from these guidelines in this chapter. The American Academy of Pediatrics recommended [1] the development and broad availability of pediatric palliative care services based on child-specific guidelines and standards with effective palliative care education of pediatric health-care professionals. The academy offers guidance on responding to requests for hastening death but does not support the practice of physician-assisted suicide or euthanasia for children [1].

In the service provided it is important to show respect and sensitivity for both the patients and the family. In consultation with the parents or guardian the plan of care should respect the wishes of the terminally ill (directly or via the wishes of the guardian) concerning testing, monitoring, and treatment. Although parents have the legal responsibility for medical care on behalf of their child, the concept of involvement of the child or person with intellectual disability is important. Even young children and people with intellectual disability may be able to express informed opinions about their medical care [3] and adolescents especially expect that they should have a say in what procedures they have to undergo. Professional staff (social work or psychology or psychiatry) should be able to discuss and understand at the level of comprehension and developmental stage the wish of the child or adolescent in question.

The provision of palliative care for children in a hospital, in hospice, or at home involves collaborations with many partners besides the child and family (remember not to forget the siblings), because of the physical, emotional, psychosocial, and spiritual/existential issues involved. This involves partnership with extended family, maybe the workplace of the parent(s), teachers and other kindergarten or school staff, various health professionals in the hospital and community setting, social worker, psychologist, religious involvement (rabbi, priest, or imam), and others in the environment of the specific family.

In addition to treat and reduce pain and other physical symptoms, physicians must provide access to therapies likely to improve the quality of life. Such therapies may include education, grief and family counseling, peer support, music therapy, child life intervention or spiritual support for both the patient and the siblings, and appropriate respite care to provide rest and renewed energy for the family [1].

The American Academy of Pediatrics [1] supports an integrated model of palliative care "in which the components of palliative care are offered at diagnosis and continued throughout the course of illness, whether the outcome ends in cure or death," since time of death is often difficult to predict. Dying with dignity and without pain or distress is the primary goal of the management.

Adulthood

Death in any family is a traumatic event that disturbs the regular course of life. The present population of persons with intellectual disability is most probably the first generation of aging people with intellectual disabilities ever living. The increase in their life expectancy makes the possibility of experiences with separation, death, and mourning a new reality for this population. Parents or sibling are passing away, and the person with intellectual disability continues to live [4].

In the past the majority of individuals with intellectual disability died at a young age and, therefore, never underwent the aging process. Compared to people without disabilities, the aging process creates many unique and complex tensions for aging individuals with intellectual disability, mainly as a result of often being dependent on others for daily support. In addition, they may demonstrate cognitive difficulties and deficient communicative skills. The situation may be worsened as a result of discriminatory social attitudes that impede and limit the access of aging individuals with intellectual disabilities to information and support. The increase in the life expectancy of people with intellectual disabilities is a "two-edged sword." These individuals enjoy the blessing of a long and healthy life; however, they also experience the pain and sorrow that often accompany the aging process. More people now have contact with separation, death, and mourning. Today, we witness an emerging phenomenon where traditional care providers, such as parents or siblings, are passing away, while their aging relatives with intellectual disabilities whom they supported are still living, sometimes with nobody left to care for them.

The issues of loss and bereavement are familiar ones to those who are involved with adults who have developmental disabilities. Unfortunately, there is little recognition of the impact of loss on this population. Usually with this group, the definition of loss tends to be a traditional one (i.e., death) rather than inclusive of the whole range of losses that an individual with developmental disabilities may experience. Individuals with intellectual and other developmental disabilities experience losses stemming from different sources. In addition to the "traditional" parting from a loved one who has passed away, they experience loss resulting from the replacement of a principal caregiver, from being arbitrarily transferred from one service or residential program to another and, similar to all aging individuals, from the loss of physical and cognitive functioning.

Even when there is recognition of the impact of losses on the individual, people who make up the person's support system may be unsure how to address losses. The loss of a significant relationship has an overpowering and often devastating effect on the lives of the individuals with intellectual disabilities, their families, and the services supporting them. In many cases, when the passing of a close relative of an individual with intellectual disabilities occurs, he is prevented from participating in the funeral. Often, the individual with disabilities is not told of the death for weeks or months after it has happened, or not told at all. Thus the basic rights of these individuals are seriously violated, and as professionals we should be profoundly disturbed by this phenomenon and search for appropriate solutions.

Harper and Wadsworth [5] stressed the tendency to see both intellectual disabilities and death as taboo subjects in Western society. For many, death is seen as "distant and unexplored territory." For most of our lives we live under the illusion that life is endless and that death is something that happens to others. For this reason, many families and professionals are unprepared to handle death and feel unqualified to deal with the task of breaking the tragic news to the person with intellectual disabilities. They may mistakenly believe that these individuals do not possess the capacity to understand the implications of death (that it is final, that it is not their fault), that they are unable to form or experience significant relationships, or that they are unable to feel sorrow or grief for the loved person who has died. Moreover, there are those who believe that it is better to divert the person's attention from the memory of the person who has passed away and thus help him to forget. Many erroneously feel that the person with intellectual disabilities has had a difficult and distressful life and should be protected from further pain and sorrow.

While the intentions of the family members and others may be noble, it is our opinion that this form of overprotectiveness is misplaced and indeed violates the basic human rights of the person involved. Many professionals claim that excluding the person with intellectual disabilities from the bereavement process is the cause of irreparable psychological harm and injury to his spiritual well-being. The lack of an appropriate opportunity to express his previous losses may trigger a delayed and exaggerated grief response in the person with intellectual disabilities who has not yet successfully completed an earlier grieving process.

It is of extreme importance that the person with intellectual disability is allowed to take part in ritual practices and customs when experiencing the death of a loved one. Jewish mourning rituals as we have discussed in an earlier paper [4], as a result of their practical and structured nature, are seemingly beneficial to bereft individuals with intellectual disabilities, assisting them in confronting their loss and grief and grasping the reality of death.

Causes of Death

In a study performed during 1991–1997 in all 53 residential care centers in Israel for persons with intellectual disability there were 450 cases of death [6]. Of those,

35% of deaths were due to circulatory and cardiac disease, 25% due to respiratory diseases, and only 6% due to cancer. Over the years there has been a slight increase in the number of cancer deaths due to the increased life expectancy of this population [7]. For the 1991–1999 period there were 43 cases or 7.2% of the total 600 cases of death, with brain and lung cancers the most frequent causes. For the 2000–2005 period there were 31 out of total 507 cases of death, with rectal cancer the most frequent cause. The calculated mortality rate for cancer in this population in 2005 was 59.3 per 100,000 [7].

The incidence of cancer in persons with intellectual disability (ID) is to some extent uncertain and often based on mortality studies. In several studies the cancer prevalence in this population has been reported lower than the general population with a variation of 4.6–17.4% compared to 20% in the general population [6]. Esophageal cancer in persons with severe/profound ID has been reported with a higher incidence, and death from gastrointestinal cancers has also been reported with a higher incidence in this population [8].

From Finland there have been several studies in this population [8, 9] related to the risk of neoplasms among people with intellectual disability. A total of 2,173 individuals with ID from a large, representative, nationwide population study conducted in Finland in 1962 were followed up for cancer incidence between 1967 and 1997. Standardized incidence ratios (SIRs) defined as ratios of observed to expected numbers of cancer cases were used, and expected rates were based on national incidence rates. The observed number of cancers in the cohort (173) was close to what was expected (SIR = 0.9, 95% confidence interval (95% CI) = 0.8–1.0). There was a significantly reduced risk of cancers of the prostate (SIR = 0.2, 95% CI = 0.0–0.5), urinary tract (SIR = 0.3, 95% CI = 0.1–0.7), and lung (SIR = 0.6, 95% CI = 0.4–1.0). The risk was increased in cancers of the gallbladder (SIR = 2.8, 95% CI = 1.1–5.8) and thyroid gland (SIR = 2.1, 95% CI = 1.0–4.8). The risks of lung and gallbladder cancers were the lowest and the highest, respectively, in those subjects with profound and severe ID, a group who also had significantly elevated SIRs for brain cancer (SIR = 3.46, 95% CI = 1.5–14.4) and testicular cancer (SIR = 9.9, 95% CI = 1.2–35.6). The incidence of cancer among people with ID was comparable with the general Finish population, despite their low prevalence of smoking and apparently decreased diagnostic screening activity. Nevertheless, a few types of cancer carry a higher risk in the population with ID, possibly because of conditions typical among this group, such as gallstones or esophageal reflux.

Palliative Care and End of Life

Before 1995 there were only four papers with the specific topic of death, dying, or end-of-life care in adults with intellectual disability [10], but a recent review from 2007 [11] found 45 journal papers, book chapters, and web-based articles with the primary focus on end-of-life care issues for this population. Almost half of these were from 2004 to 2005, so this shows a recent interest in this topic by professionals and researchers. Twenty-eight papers were from the United Kingdom, where this issue has been discussed and studied in more detail, 14 papers from the United States, and only 3 papers from other countries [11].

Death and dying are important but hidden issues in intellectual disability services, and there is limited literature around the personal experiences of death and dying from people with intellectual disabilities themselves [12].

In a recent small study drawn from four local authority areas in England and Wales [12] participants were recruited into one of four focus groups depending on the geographical area in which they lived. This study showed that when supporting and preparing adults with an ID in death and dying issues regardless of the environment (whether hospice or ID home) they were able to talk about their experiences of loss, death, and dying. Most people had stories to tell; professionals just need to take the time and opportunity to ask the right questions and facilitate such story-telling in a constructive and meaningful way.

From the same researchers [13] a small handy and instructive booklet has been produced for care staff and families to deal with this sensitive topic. They are not talking about a good death, but rather a good enough death. This booklet is geared toward people with intellectual disability living in a service or residential care setting, because most older people with intellectual disability will likely die in such a setting. There are good examples and advice on how to disclose the diagnosis, how to work with families and professionals, and palliative care, which should

- affirm life and regard dying as a normal process,
- not hasten or postpone death,
- provide relief from pain and other distressing symptoms,
- integrate social, psychological, and spiritual aspects of care according to the needs of the person and the family,
- offer a support system to help the person to live as actively as possible until death in his/her normal environment as long as possible, and
- offer a support system to help families, care staff, and other network cope during the final illness, burial, and help with their own bereavement after death.

Conclusions

Today most children born with intellectual disability will enter adulthood. Some with the rarest syndromes or multiple associated disease will die in infancy or childhood, and here it is important that they will receive the same end-of-life service as the general population in extreme cases like death at an early age.

Changing demographics that has today resulted in a growing number of people with intellectual disability living into old age and suffering from the same diseases as the general aging population will create a need for more organized palliative care and professionals who are able to handle end-of-life issues with the persons with intellectual disability themselves dying [14], their families, and also care staff, who are not always prepared for these events.

References

1. American Academy of Pediatrics. Palliative care for children. Pediatrics. 2000;106(2): 351–57.
2. World Health Organization. Cancer pain relief and palliative care. Geneva: WHO; 1990.
3. Tuffrey-Wijne I, Bernal J, Butler G, Hollins S, Using Nominal CL. Group technique to investigate the views of people with intellectual disabilities on need-of-life care provision. J Adv Nurs. 2007;58(1):80–89.
4. Kessel S, Merrick J. The benefits of Jewish mourning rituals for the grieving individual with intellectual disability. J Religion Disabil Health. 2001;5(2/3):147–56.
5. Harper DC, Wadsworth JS. Grief in adults with mental retardation: preliminary findings. Res Dev Disabil. 1993;14:313–30.
6. Merrick J. Mortality for persons with intellectual disability in residential care in Israel 1991–97. J Intellect Dev Disabil. 2002;27(4):265–72.
7. Merrick J, Merrick-Kenig E, Kandel I, Morad M. Residential care centers for persons with intellectual disability in Israel. Trends in cancer mortality during 1991–2005. Int J Disabil Hum Dev. 2008;7(4):447–50.
8. Patja K. Life expectancy and mortality in intellectual disability. Dissertation, Helsinki, 2001.
9. Patja K, Eero P, Iivanainen M. Cancer incidence among people with intellectual disability. J Intellect Disabil Res. 2001;45(Pt 4):300–7.
10. Tuffrey-Wijne I. The palliative care needs of people with intellectual disabilities: a literature review. Palliat Med. 2003;17:55–62.
11. Tuffrey-Wijne I, Hogg J, Curfs L. End-of-life and palliative care for people with intellectual disabilities who have cancer or other life-limiting illness: a review of the literature and available resources. J Appl Res Intellect Disabil. 2007;20:331–44.
12. Todd S, Read S. Thinking about death and what it means: the perspectives of people with intellectual disability. Int J Child Health Hum Dev. 2010;3(2), in press.
13. Blackman N, Todd S. Caring for people with learning disabilities who are dying. London: Worth; 2005.
14. Tuffrey-Wijne I, McEnhill L. Communication difficulties and intellectual disability in end-of-life care. Int J Palliat Nurs. 2008;14(4):189–94.

Chapter 28
Transition from Child-Oriented to Adult-Oriented Health Care

Dilip R. Patel and Donald E. Greydanus

Abstract The growing number of young adults with neurodevelopmental disabilities and chronic diseases necessitates a careful consideration of the issues involved in transition of these youth from a child-focused to an adult-oriented health-care system. Most adolescents accomplish the transition successfully as a natural process of growth and maturation in all spheres of life. Presence of chronic disease or disability, however, adds a significant dimension to the transition process and affects all areas of the adolescent's life – medical care, educational, vocational, daily living and activity, financial, and employment. The psychological and psychosocial impact of chronic illness or disability on the youth and family has been well documented. A brief overview of issues as they relate to transition of medical care of adolescents and young adults with chronic disease or disability from child-oriented to adult-oriented system of health care is presented here.

Introduction

Barbero, in a 1982 editorial entitled "Leaving the pediatrician for the internist," commented on the need for transfer of medical care for adolescents and young adults with chronic disease to the adult health-care system [1]. The 1984 "Youth with disability: The transitional years" conference and the 1989 Surgeon General Conference "Growing up and getting medical care: Youth with special health care needs" helped focus attention on the issues of transition [2, 3].

According to the Society for Adolescent Medicine, transition is the purposeful planned movement of adolescents and young adults with chronic conditions from child-centered to adult-centered care [4]. Transition services, as defined in the United States Individuals with Disabilities Act (IDEA) of 2004, are "a coordinated set of activities for a child with a disability that (A) is designed to be within a

D.R. Patel (✉)
Department of Pediatrics and Human Development, Kalamazoo Center for Medical Studies, Michigan State University College of Human Medicine, Kalamazoo, MI 49008-1284, USA
e-mail: patel@kcms.msu.edu

D.R. Patel et al. (eds.), *Neurodevelopmental Disabilities*,
DOI 10.1007/978-94-007-0627-9_28, © Springer Science+Business Media B.V. 2011

results-oriented process, that is focused on improving the academic and functional achievement of the child with a disability to facilitate the child's movement from school to post-school activities, including post secondary education, vocational education, integrated employment (including supported employment), continuing and adult education, adult services, independent living or community participation, (B) is based on the individual child's needs, taking into account the child's strengths, preferences and interests, and (C) includes instruction, related services, community experiences, the development of employment and other post-school adult living objectives, and, when appropriate, acquisition of daily living skills and functional vocational evaluation" [5].

The Consensus Statement on Health Care Transitions for Young Adults with Special Health Care Needs (supported by the American Academy of Pediatrics, American Academy of Family Physicians, American College of Physicians, and American Society of Internal Medicine) recommends to have a transition plan in place by the time the adolescent is 14 years old and to update this annually [6]. Some young adults may be ready to begin transition when they are 13 years old, whereas others may not be ready until they are 16 or 17 years old; thus, the transition plan must be individualized.

The Process of Transition

Transition is a process that takes place over time not as an event, such as transferring medical care from one physician to another [6–15]. Some authors have proposed that transition should begin on the day of diagnosis. The young adult and the family must be involved in the decision process, and health-care practitioners and parents should be prepared to let go. Parents report that not doing for their children what they can do for themselves is the most important component of transition planning throughout the child's growing years (Table 28.1).

Although some have argued for the pediatrician's continuing care for the young adult indefinitely, it is generally agreed that the medical needs of adults are best served in an adult-oriented health-care system by adult health providers [16–22].

Table 28.1 Main components of transition planning

Component	Description
Transfer of care	Care is transferred from child and adolescent health-care practitioners to adult medical practitioners
Access to care	Establish access to continuous and uninterrupted access to care
Skills acquisition	Acquisition by young adult of the knowledge and skills necessary to independently manage his/her medical treatment
School and workplace	Identification and advocating for needed accommodations in school or workplace for optimal functioning
Community resources	Identifying and accessing transition and adult community agencies and resources based on individual needs for services

Ideal care is age-appropriate and promotes independence and self-sufficiency as it shifts the decision making to the young adult. A well-planned transition helps assimilate a transition team, assesses transition readiness of the adolescent and the family, and facilitates the development of a team approach to medical care in the adult-oriented setting. The process of transition to adult-oriented care provides the adolescent with a hope for the future and helps enhance his/her sense of personal responsibility and control. Transition signals emancipation and prepares the adolescent and the young adult to become an independent health-care consumer. Adult patients in the pediatric setting may begin to feel uncomfortable, and this may adversely affect treatment adherence [23]. The transition process may facilitate treatment adherence and continuity of care. It provides an opportunity for an unbiased reassessment of the existing problems and possibly to uncover new problems [23].

The process of transition can be emotionally rewarding for the internist, and it may offer opportunities for professional fulfillment to the internist and collaboration and mutual learning for the pediatric and adult teams alike. The relatively protected and parent-oriented pediatric environment may reinforce dependence and continued parental responsibilities in providing for financial support, transportation, and other needs.

Modulating Factors

Transition is a complex process, and the interplay of many personal and systemic factors affects the process and its outcome either positively or negatively [3, 4, 7–9, 12, 24, 25].

The Adolescent and the Family

Over time the adolescent and pediatrician have come to know each other well and have developed a trusting relationship. In the protective pediatric environment, patients have become "accustomed to bargaining and partnership with their pediatrician." Moving into an adult-oriented system entails for the young adult a great degree of personal responsibility. The young adult now faces the challenges of establishing a new relationship with the new physician and meeting all the expectations of adulthood. Lack of appropriate support systems, severity of the chronic condition, delayed maturation and adaptation, inadequate coping style, and lack of personal motivation on the part of the youth all may interfere with the transition process. Family is the main support system. Parents may feel loss of control as their involvement gradually becomes mainly peripheral. Parents who have shared the many "ups and downs" together with the pediatric team may find it difficult to give up that support, and they may perceive the adult health system to be less involved and less sensitive to their needs. Parental inability to let go, emotional dependency, and need for control may hinder the process.

The Physician and the Medical Team

For the physician, readiness for transition on the part of the adolescent and the family may be difficult to assess. An adolescent's developmental and cognitive maturation, severity of the condition, availability of local resources, and strengths and weaknesses of the support systems all influence the readiness and timing of transition. Functional limitations tend to foster dependency in the youth with a chronic condition [22, 26, 27]. Variability in the capacity for transition makes it difficult to set rigid age criteria for transition of care. Timing of developmental tasks may occur earlier or later. Similarly, onset of puberty and progress of sexual maturation may also occur earlier or may be delayed [26]. An evaluation of biological and psychosocial maturity will help assess readiness for transition [22]. Hofmann and Gabriel [27] in their description of the adaptation process of youth with chronic illness noted that extending from late adolescence through young adulthood long-term adaptation focuses on patient's attainment of autonomy and optional emotional and functional adaptations to the condition.

The pediatrician is expected to extend care up to young adult years. Because of a strong emotional attachment with the patient and family, the pediatrician may show a great deal of apprehension about transfer of care and may unknowingly convey to the patient a sense of distrust for the competence and commitment of the adult health practitioner. A pediatrician may fail to recognize his/her own limitations and the youth's readiness for independent functioning. The pediatrician may become overprotective of the patient and may perceive the need for transition unnecessary. Losing a segment of his/her patients may be an economic consideration.

Adolescents with chronic conditions require a comprehensive team approach to management, and typical services have been rendered through specialized centers. There seems to be a lack of adequate training and experience for physicians and others outside such systems in managing these conditions. For the busy internist, the economic incentive in taking over care for young adults with chronic diseases may be none to minimal. In the pediatric setting, it has been well recognized that the most effective way of delivering services to youth with chronic conditions is an interdisciplinary team approach, but the adult-oriented system seems to have few similar models. Not uncommonly physicians who have long provided care to adults feel uncomfortable with this type of team approach.

The System of Health Care

With the current concerns over increasing costs of health care, financial issues continue to remain major barriers for youth with developmental disabilities to obtain appropriate services. Access to appropriate health care is limited for adolescents and young adults in general and for those with developmental disabilities in particular. Persons with developmental disabilities need comprehensive services requiring an interdisciplinary team and significant effort and time commitment. Availability of professional time may be limited because of inadequate reimbursement for the time and effort involved. Besides the lack of health insurance coverage and inadequate funding for transition programs, a lack of availability of comprehensive services is an important barrier to obtaining care. Adolescents and young adults with chronic conditions typically have many associated needs, such as special therapies, equipment, vocational training, and diets. Coordination of all the different services is crucial and requires knowledge of local resources. The adult system, not having had sufficient exposure, may need time and guidance to relate appropriate resources and coordinate the services.

Access to Adult Subspecialty Care

Most young people with developmental disabilities have at least one specialist to see if not more. This is a challenge because of difficulty in successfully engaging adult health-care physicians to help move these patients on to adult care. Several barriers to this have been identified. Pediatricians may have difficulty accepting that anyone else could take care of their patient as well as they can. Young adults and their parents or care givers who have known their pediatrician all of their lives are reluctant to move on. Because the underlying disorders are pediatric in nature, adult health-care physicians may not feel adequately prepared to manage them. On the other hand pediatricians may not feel adequately prepared to manage adult diabetes, heart disease, high blood pressure, and other adult onset illness.

Hospital Care

Where to hospitalize a young adult with developmental disabilities for inpatient care is another complicated issue. Young adults want to be on adult patient floors. They would like to be with peers. Nurses on the pediatric wards are generally not accustomed to adult-sized patients. The pediatric nurses also choose to take care of children and have a child-focused system of caring. From the adult nursing standpoint, they are not used to pediatric disorders such as cerebral palsy, Down syndrome, or autism. They are not used to having the parent being so involved in the patient's care. In the setting of a teaching institution medicine residents may not be adequately experienced in the care of young adults with developmental disabilities.

In the transition plan, the hospital of choice should be decided ahead of time. The care coordinator can help facilitate a visit to the hospital. Education for the nursing staff could be started by asking the nursing staff what their needs are and providing them with information and training. Care plans can be sent to the adult emergency department. During the first hospitalization and perhaps the second, the pediatrician could round with the adult medical team and answer questions about the pediatric condition or how the patient responds to being ill.

The Nature of Chronic Disease or Disability

The nature of specific developmental disability or chronic disease may also be a factor influencing the transition process. For example, generally for conditions for which an internist already has some knowledge and expertise (e.g., diabetes or end-stage renal disease), transition of care from pediatric to adult systems seems to occur as a natural process [28]. On the other hand, the internist may feel discomfort in taking over care for typically "pediatric" conditions (e.g., cystic fibrosis, congenital heart disease, or spina bifida).

Health-Care Transition Programs

Different approaches have been described, each with its own advantages and disadvantages [22]. The interdisciplinary team approach is a highly effective way for providing comprehensive services, although the availability of all needed team members may be limited outside a large institution. Provision and coordination of services by a primary care physician working concurrently with specialists without regard for the specific underlying condition represent the generic service model [22]. For certain chronic conditions, such as cystic fibrosis, hemophilia, and diabetes, services focused on the specific disorder have been developed. Transition takes place from the pediatric to the adult specialist. Although continuity of care for the specific condition is maintained, the primary care is usually missing. The family practice group working closely with specialists may provide continuity of care for the adolescent and young adult with chronic disease. The patient continues to see the same physician; however, care is modified according to the developmental stage and changing roles, and responsibilities are delineated for the adolescent and family [22].

The timing of transition to adult care depends on physical and psychological maturity of the patient and is largely influenced by the availability of local resources as well as the personalities and prejudices of the staff involved [19]. A general acceptance of the need for transition and commitment on the part of all involved greatly facilitates the process of transition. Key elements of successful transition programs include professional and institutional support, family support, decision making and consent, and professional sensitivity to psychosocial issues related to disability (Table 28.2).

As the adolescent matures into an adult, his/her needs change, and the support systems should accommodate to the biological and psychosocial maturation. It is generally accepted that the complex needs of the young adult with a chronic condition are best met by an interdisciplinary team approach to the care, with a well-coordinated effort of various professionals and community resources. The pediatrician should recognize his/her limitations and the need for transferring care of young adults to an adult health provider. The internist, on his/her part, should be comfortable with the team approach to care which takes into account the psychosocial maturation of the adolescent. Depending upon their cognitive abilities and psychosocial maturity, adolescents should be supported and encouraged to play an active role in their health care and independent decision making. A mature adolescent should be able to consent on his/her own accord for medical treatment in most

Table 28.2 Examples of possible barriers to successful transition

Level	Description
Individual	Reluctance of the adolescent or young adult to move into adult-oriented care
Family	Reluctance of the family to allow appropriate autonomy to the adolescent; reluctance of the family to allow adolescent to move into adult care
Systemic	Inadequate re-imbursement for practitioners for the time needed to plan and coordinate the transition services
Institutional	Lack of institutional support (time for planning, resources, personnel) for development of transition programs
Societal	Low expectations and social isolation of individuals with developmental disabilities – most significant factor
Practitioner	Difficulty identifying adult medical primary care and subspecialty providers who will take care of individuals with developmental disabilities

instances [22, 29, 30]. The family, the main support system for the adolescent, with appropriate professional guidance and support will adapt to the changing needs of the young adult and the challenges of the adolescent moving into adult health care.

The psychosocial issues associated with chronic conditions are relatively better recognized in the pediatric health-care setting. A transitional plan should facilitate the recognition of these in the adult care setting. Studies show that clinicians who discussed with their adolescent patients the ways in which the illness affected social interactions communicated more effectively than those who focused solely on signs and symptoms of physical disease [31]. Because of the very nature of the chronic condition, most medical care remains focused on the management of the chronic condition and its complications. Fortunately, most adolescents and young adults receive excellent subspecialty care; however, more often than not, the overall primary care, health supervision, and preventive care do not receive the needed attention. A transitional program should specifically help to ensure continuing primary care and coordination of primary care and specialty services.

Conclusions

Transition is a process and not an event, and it should allow gradual transfer of medical care from a child-centered to an adult-oriented system. The concept of transition is guided by the underlying philosophy that transition to adulthood and adult care will eventually occur. Because of advances in medical sciences, more children with traditional pediatric medical conditions now grow to become adults. To be consistent with the growth and maturation of these youngsters, the need for transition of medical care from pediatric to adult-oriented health-care systems is desirable. Funding for services and access to care remain major barriers to providing quality health care to youth with chronic conditions. A lack of research on the transition process makes it difficult to formulate recommendations.

The transfer of medical care from the pediatric to adult service may occur in different clinical settings. Because of the complex needs of the adolescents with chronic disease or disability, a variety of subspecialists are concurrently involved in providing medical care. Development of any specific approach is influenced by the availability of local resources. Research should help identify the characteristics of adolescents who most need a transition program, attributes of a successful program, and appropriate outcome measures. Research should help delineate and compare the different models for their effectiveness.

Acknowledgments This chapter is partly derived from author's previous works, Burdo-Hartman [32] and Patel [33].

References

1. Barbero GJ. Leaving the pediatrician for the internist. Ann Intern Med. 1982;96:673.
2. Blum RW, Leonard B, editors. Youth with disabilities: the transitional years. J Adolesc Health Care. 1985:6.
3. McGrab P, Millar H, editors. Surgeon General's Conference. Growing up and getting medical care: youth with special health care needs. Washington, DC: National Center for Networking Community-Based Services, Georgetown University Child Development Center; 1989.
4. Blum RW, Garell D, Hodgman CH, Jorissen TW, Okinow NA, Orr DP, Slap GB. Transition from child-centered to adult health-care systems for adolescents with chronic conditions: a position paper of the Society of Adolescent Medicine. J Adolesc Health. 1993;14:570–76.
5. United States Department of Education. Individuals with Disabilities Education Act: Part B. 2004 Section 602(34). http://idea.ed.gov/explore/search
6. Hirsch D, Kastner TA, Quint RD, Sandler AD. A consensus statement on health care transitions for young adults with special health care needs. Pediatrics. 2002;110(6):1304–5.
7. White PH. Transition to adulthood: adolescents with disabilities. In: Greydanus DE, Patel DR, Pratt HD, editors. Essential adolescent medicine. New York, NY: McGraw Hill Medical; 2006. pp. 51–78.
8. Betz CL. Facilitating the transition of adolescents with developmental disabilities: nursing practice issues and care. J Pediatr Nurs. 2007;22(2):103–15.
9. White P. Success on the road to adulthood: issues and hurdles for adolescents with disabilities. Pediatr Clin North Am. 1997;23(3):697–707.
10. Blomquist KB, Brown G, Peersen A, Presler EP. Transitioning to independence: challenges for young people with disabilities and their caregivers. Orthop Nurs. 1998;17(3):27–35.
11. Luther B. Age-specific activities that support successful transition to adulthood for children with disabilities. Orthop Nurs. 2001;20(1):23–29.
12. Kelly AM, Kratz B, Mary B, Rinehart PM. Implementing transitions for youth with complex chronic conditions using the medical home model. Pediatrics. 2002;110(6):1322–27.
13. Lotstein DS, McPherson M, Strickland B, Newacheck P. Transition planning for youth with special health care needs: results from the national survey of children with special health care needs. Pediatrics. 2005;115(6):1562–67.
14. Olson DG, Swigonski NL. Transition to adulthood: the role of the pediatrician. Pediatrics. 2004;113:e159–62.
15. Scal P. Transition for youth with chronic conditions: primary care physicians' approaches. Pediatrics. 2002;110(6):1315–21.
16. Kim H, Murphy N, Kim CT, et al. Pediatric rehabilitation: 5. Transitioning teens with disabilities into adulthood. PM R. 2010;2(3):S31–37.
17. Stewart D. Transition to adult services for young people with disabilities: current evidence to guide future research. Dev Med Child Neurol. 2009;51(Suppl 4):169–73.
18. Berkowitz S. Transitioning adolescents to adult care: putting theory into practice. Minn Med. 2009;92(3):42–44.

19. Cameron JS. The continued care of pediatric patients with renal disease into adult life. Am J Kidney Dis. 1985;6:91.
20. Peter NG, Forke CM, Ginsburg KR, Schwarz DF. Transition from pediatric to adult care: internists' perspective. Pediatrics. 2009;123(2):417–23.
21. Suris JC, Akre C, Rutishauser C. How adult specialists deal with the principles of a successful transition. J Adolesc Health. 2009;45(6):551–55.
22. US Department of Health and Human Services. Maternal and Child Health Bureau: moving on: transition from child-centered to adult health care for youth with disabilities. 44. Rockville, MD: US Department of Health and Human Services; 1992.
23. Slap GB. Youth in transition to adult health care. In: McAnarney ER, Kreipe RE, Orr DP, Comerci GD, editors. Textbook of adolescent medicine. Philadelphia, PA: WB Saunders; 1992.
24. Berg P. Youth in transition: developing appropriate services for adult survivors of pediatric disorders. Minneapolis, MN: National Center for Youth with Disabilities; 1988.
25. Bronheim S, Fiel S, Schidlow DB, et al. Crossings: a manual for transition of chronically ill youth to adult health care. Washington, DC: Georgetown University Child Development Center; 1988.
26. Blum RW. Chronic illness and disability in adolescence. J Adolesc Health Care. 1992;13:364.
27. Hofmann AD, Gabriel HP. Managing chronic illness in adolescence: a paradigm. In: Hofmann AD, Greydanus DE, editors. Adolescent medicine. Norwalk, CT: Appleton-Lange; 1989.
28. Resnick MD. Use of cutoff policies for adolescents in pediatric practice: report from the upper Midwest regional physician survey. Pediatrics. 1983;72:420.
29. Schidlow DV, Fiel SB. Life beyond pediatrics: transition of chronically ill adolescents from pediatric to adult health care systems. Med Clin North Am. 1990;74:132.
30. Hofmann AD. Legal issues in adolescent medicine. In: Hofmann AD, Greydanus DE, editors. Adolescent medicine. Norwalk, CT: Appleton-Lange; 1989.
31. Millstein SG, Alder NE, Irwin CE Jr. Conceptions of illness of young adolescents. Pediatrics. 1981;68:834.
32. Burdo-Hartman WB, Patel DR. Medical home and transition planning for children and youth with special health care needs. Pediatr Clin North Am. 2008;55(6):1287–98.
33. Patel DR, Rowlett JD, Greydanus DE. Youth with chronic conditions in transition to adult health care: an overview. Adolesc Med. 1994;5(3):543–51.

Chapter 29
Psychosocial Functioning in Youth with Chronic Illness

John A. Yozwiak, Regan E. Settles, and Rachel F. Steffens

Abstract A substantial number of children and adolescents experience chronic illness. Due to medical advances, many young patients survive into adulthood. A chronic illness has the potential to affect several facets of a young patient's life. The impact that chronic illness may have on various domains of psychosocial functioning will be reviewed. Youth with chronic illness and their families can experience a variety of consequences, but many adjust well and have favorable outcomes. However, factors associated with chronic illness and its treatment may influence the trajectory of development and functioning. The psychosocial treatment of youth with chronic illness will be covered. Issues pertaining to adherence to treatment regimens and means to enhance adherence will also be addressed. Recommendations for practice and future research will be offered.

Introduction

Approximately 15% of children in the United States have a chronic health condition [1, 2]. Chronic conditions faced by children and adolescents include cancer, cystic fibrosis, asthma, juvenile rheumatoid arthritis, diabetes, renal disease, heart disease, and hemophilia. Asthma is the most common chronic condition of youth in the United States, afflicting about 6 million children [1].

Children and adolescents with chronic illness face many potential challenges, such as demanding treatment regimens, treatment side effects, and in some cases the prospect of a foreshortened future. In addition to the physical sequela concomitant with many chronic conditions, young patients are confronted with the task of managing their emotional reactions to stressful events, adjusting to physical and

J.A. Yozwiak (✉)
Division of Adolescent Medicine, Department of Pediatrics, Kentucky Clinic, University of Kentucky College of Medicine, Lexington, KY 40536-0284, USA
e-mail: jayozw00@uky.edu

D.R. Patel et al. (eds.), *Neurodevelopmental Disabilities*,
DOI 10.1007/978-94-007-0627-9_29, © Springer Science+Business Media B.V. 2011

social limitations, and learning complex treatment regimens [3]. Youth with chronic illness face the additional challenge of handling issues pertaining to their illness and associated treatments while simultaneously attempting to complete developmental tasks, such as individuating from parental figures and identifying with a peer group. Adolescent patients must attempt to integrate their emerging personal identity with the reality of their medical condition and its associated effect on future educational and occupational opportunities [4]. The manner in which a chronic illness is managed by the patient, family, peers, and healthcare professionals can impact the course of development [5].

Due to advances in treatment, technology, and clinical care, young patients are surviving longer with illnesses and conditions that were once life threatening [3, 4, 6–8]. As a result of these advances, focus has now shifted from mortality risk factors to that of morbidity risk factors and the risk for further physical and psychosocial complications in adulthood. Since many youth with chronic illness are now surviving longer than they have in the past, it is critical that practitioners have a strong understanding of how chronic illness and its associated challenges affect various aspects of the lives of children as they progress through adolescence and into adulthood.

In this chapter, the impact on various domains of psychosocial functioning in children and adolescents with chronic illness will be reviewed. Psychosocial treatment, issues pertaining to treatment adherence, and considerations for practice and future research will also be addressed. Although young patients suffer from a wide range of medical conditions that have unique features, research suggests that the correlates of various chronic illnesses may be more universal. For instance, similarities exist among chronic illnesses with regard to chronicity, effects on a wide range of psychosocial variables, and the important role of treatment adherence [6]. Stein and Jessop [9] analyzed data from an institutional and a population-based study on the correlates of various illnesses and concluded that there may be more variability within illnesses than between them, and that diagnosis alone may not be an effective means of categorizing psychosocial variables. Based on these findings, a noncategorical approach to chronic illness will be taken throughout most of this chapter.

Psychosocial Functioning

Academic and Social Functioning

A chronic illness has the potential to impact academic functioning. Educational progression can be disrupted as a result of school absences to attend medical appointments or hospitalizations [10]. Chronic health conditions have been associated with placement in special education classes and grade retention [11], and children with chronic illness have higher rates of school absenteeism than their healthy peers [12]. Despite these risks, academic performance may not be destined to suffer [12]. However, frequent absences from school can reduce a young person's contact with classmates. Loss of social contact with peers can result in feelings of isolation, disturbance in the progression of social development, and problems with identity formation [5].

In addition to the social limitations resulting from missed school days, youth with chronic medical conditions may also face disruptions in their social functioning as a consequence of the physical aspects of chronic illness. For example, children who experience physical limitations tend to be less involved in social activities than youth without physical limitations. Likewise, children who experience pain associated with their illness tend to be less engaged in social activities than children who have no or occasional episodes of pain [13].

The effect of a chronic illness on social functioning may be especially acute for adolescents, as peer relationships take precedence at this stage of development. Social acceptance may be a concern if the medical condition is related to spending a great deal of time isolated from peers [14]. In addition, a chronic illness can enhance the perception that one is different from others, which may increase the distress experienced by an adolescent who is attempting to gain the acceptance of peers. This concern may be especially heightened if the adolescent's appearance is affected by the illness or treatment [15]. A chronic illness can also affect an adolescent's ability to achieve independence from family, develop a stable self-concept, formulate values, and plan for the future [14]. Parents may be hesitant to provide the adolescent with independence and autonomy because of concerns that their child will not be able to effectively manage the illness [15], which may further hinder interpersonal and social development.

Involvement in Risky Behaviors

Adolescents with chronic illness are more likely to be involved in risky behaviors than their healthy peers [16, 17]. Examples of risky behaviors include smoking cigarettes, illicit drug use, violent acts, disordered eating, and early sexual debut [17]. Factors underlying the increased involvement in these behaviors for adolescent patients have not been fully elucidated, but a number of potential risk pathways have been proposed. For instance, adolescents with chronic illness may engage in risky behaviors in order to gain the acceptance of their healthy peers by demonstrating normality; they may have difficulty obtaining access to prosocial peers and thus select risk-taking peers who may be more accepting of their chronic condition; they may be more prone to engage in risky behaviors due to a potentially shortened lifespan; or they may be drawn to risky behaviors as a mechanism to alleviate unpleasant emotions that are associated with their diagnosis and associated stressors [17]. Involvement in risky behaviors is especially pertinent to youth with chronic conditions because some of these behaviors may exacerbate symptoms of a chronic illness. For example, regular use of cigarettes can compromise the pulmonological functioning of patients with cystic fibrosis and patients with asthma. Therefore, it may be beneficial to include risk screening and preventive counseling as a component of treatment for adolescent patients.

Psychiatric Functioning

Youth with chronic illness may also be at greater risk for psychiatric difficulties than their healthy counterparts. The results from a survey of adolescents in Switzerland indicated that those who identified themselves as having a chronic condition were more likely to have attempted suicide in the previous 12 months than adolescents who did not identify themselves as chronically ill [16]. Population-based studies suggest that young patients are at greater risk for behavioral problems, emotional problems, and psychiatric disorder than their healthy peers [11, 18, 19]. Children with neurological disorders may be especially vulnerable to such problems [20]. The most common psychiatric conditions for children and adolescents across a range of chronic illnesses are adjustment disorders [3, 8, 21]. Adjustment disorders consist of disturbances in emotional and/or behavioral functioning which occur in response to an identifiable stressor [22]. Emotional and behavioral difficulties that are a byproduct of a chronic illness and its treatment may in turn influence the course of the illness, possibly impacting morbidity and mortality [21].

In addition to problems with adjustment, youth with chronic illness may be susceptible to symptoms of depression. Specifically, more adolescents with a chronic illness report symptoms of depression than their healthy peers, and adolescents who consider their condition to be moderate or severe report even higher levels of depressive symptoms than those who consider their disease severity to be only mild [23]. Additionally, adolescents with chronic illness have lower emotional well-being scores, report that they worry more about dying soon and about school or future work, and have poorer body image relative to their healthy counterparts [24].

A chronic illness in youth also has the potential to impact psychiatric functioning at later life stages. For instance, survivors of pediatric cancer may experience physical and psychological effects of their illness that first appear during the course of treatment and persist, whereas other effects may emerge after treatment completion [25]. Adolescent survivors of childhood cancer are more likely to engage in fewer social activities [26] and have more symptoms of depression and anxiety than their healthy peers [27]. Hobbie et al. [28] found that 20% of adult survivors of childhood cancer had a diagnosis of posttraumatic stress disorder at some point since the end of treatment. Clinical awareness of future psychiatric risk for patients after disease characteristics have ceased or after treatment completion may facilitate appropriate follow-up, monitoring, and referral provision.

Despite the aforementioned challenges and potential disruptions in psychosocial functioning that a chronic illness can pose, not all youth experience significant maladjustment. Barlow and Ellard [10] reviewed studies on the psychosocial well-being of children with chronic illness and concluded that these children were at a slightly elevated risk of psychosocial distress, but that only a minority experience distress that is clinically significant. Similarly, Lavigne and Faier-Routman conducted a meta-analysis on studies that examined children's adjustment to physical disorders and found that these children displayed an increased risk for adjustment problems, as well as internalizing and externalizing symptoms [29]. However, the degree of impairment varied by informant and by the methodology used in the studies. In a review of studies addressing depressive symptoms among children with chronic illness, Bennett reported [30] that these children were at a slightly elevated risk for symptoms of depression, but most did not meet the threshold criteria for clinical depression. The severity of the illness was not consistently associated with depressive symptoms. Moreover, Gledhill et al. [8] discovered from their review that most adult survivors of childhood chronic illness did not experience compromised psychiatric functioning when compared with healthy peers or the general population, but that the effects of a chronic illness may be different across individuals.

The impact of a chronic illness may be a function of the type and degree of physical impairment, the visibility of the illness, uncertainty about the course or nature of the disorder, irregular and unpredictable effects, high cost of treatment, pain, or other factors related to the illness and its treatment [14]. For example, among pediatric cancer survivors, behavioral and social difficulties have been associated with central nervous system tumors, leukemia, and neuroblastoma [27]. Additionally, poorer quality of life has been related to bone cancer, central nervous system cancer, at least two treatment series, and at least two organs with dysfunction at the end of treatment [31].

Non-illness factors may also impact the psychiatric functioning of young patients. For instance, in a sample of youth with asthma and a control group, a greater percentage of patients with asthma (16.3%) had at least one anxiety and/or mood disorder in the prior 12 months compared with those without asthma (8.6%) [32]. However, living in a single-parent household and more parent-reported externalizing behaviors, along with a more recent diagnosis of asthma and greater impairment in physical health, were also associated with a higher likelihood of psychiatric impairment. In addition, the variance in emotional well-being in adolescents with chronic illness has been shown to be accounted for more by body image, family connectedness, and concern about school and future work than by having a chronic medical condition [24].

Family Functioning

Pediatric chronic illness has the potential to impact the family system. Family members may be at risk for experiencing frustration, guilt, anger, depression, and anxiety [4]. For example, following a recent diagnosis of cancer in their children, many mothers and fathers experienced symptoms of acute distress, with some having acute stress disorder [33]. A number of parents also mourn the loss of their child's health [3].

Some parents encounter economic difficulties associated with reduced work attendance, decreased job mobility, and the costs related to treatment [3]. The social effects of having a child with a chronic illness may be particularly strong for the primary caregiver, as direct social contact and social activities may decrease [3]. Siblings may feel neglected and overshadowed [10] and may be at risk for experiencing behavioral problems [34]. Family maladjustment is of particular concern given that greater family conflict and maternal psychological distress have been shown to predict poor adjustment among children with chronic illness [35], and parental distress has been related to childhood distress [36].

Notwithstanding the risk for family difficulties, significant maladjustment and disruption in family functioning may not be inevitable for all families with a child or an adolescent with a chronic illness. The results of an epidemiological study revealed some indicators of parental psychosocial problems to be modestly elevated, such as maternal negative affect and rates of parental psychosocial treatment, but also showed that many families did not suffer a significant amount of dysfunction [37]. In some cases, the family can be a source of strength and resources [4]. A youth's illness might have a positive effect on family functioning, as families take on the challenge of caring for the young person and may experience greater cohesion [37]. Healthcare providers are cautioned against making assumptions that all families with a child or an adolescent with a chronic illness suffer from significant and clinically important family disruption and dysfunction. Instead, practitioners are encouraged to assess each family's individual strengths and weaknesses in the context of coping with the chronic illness [37].

Treatment Considerations

Healthcare providers are advised to be alert to common indicators of maladjustment and to respond rapidly with needed intervention [3]. Markers of psychological maladjustment include, but may not be limited to, medical symptoms that cannot be fully explained by organic factors, poor adherence to treatment recommendations, school refusal, and engagement in risky behaviors [5]. Comprehensive treatment includes not only a consideration of the biomedical aspects of the disease but also the developmental, psychological, and interpersonal effects of the illness and its treatment [4]. Treatment must focus on the individual and the family system, treat comorbid psychiatric conditions, and include education to the patient and the family about the illness and the treatment plan to enhance treatment adherence [5].

Psychosocial assessment of the various components of a young person's life throughout the course of the illness and treatment, along with the manner of coping that the young patient employs is imperative [3]. Comprehensive assessment can produce an accurate conceptualization of the patient's strengths and weaknesses, which in turn can inform treatment planning. An especially important treatment consideration is the functioning of the family system, upon which a burden might be placed secondary to the chronic illness [4, 6]. Healthcare providers are encouraged to monitor the impact of the illness on the social functioning of the caregivers [3]. The assessment of families should continue throughout the course of the patient's illness and treatment, as additional stressors may impact family members and alter their development and functioning.

Psychosocial interventions appear to hold promise for youth with chronic illness, which underscores the importance of their inclusion in the overall treatment plan when indicated. Beale reviewed the efficacy of psychosocial treatment for children and adolescents with a variety of chronic illnesses and tentatively concluded that such interventions are efficacious [38]. Illness type or intervention type did not moderate the effect sizes. Bauman et al. [39] reviewed 15 studies of psychosocial intervention programs for children with different chronic illnesses. The majority of the studies demonstrated evidence of efficacy. The domains of psychosocial functioning that were most affected were the psychiatric and behavioral domains.

Kibby et al. [40] reviewed the outcomes from 42 studies of psychological treatments for children and young adolescents with chronic medical conditions. Behavioral interventions were the most common form of treatment. These interventions consisted of behavior modification, cognitive-behavioral approaches, biofeedback, relaxation and imagery techniques, and distraction. The results support the general effectiveness of psychological interventions, and treatment gains were maintained for at least 12 months. In particular, behavioral interventions aimed at disease management and reducing the distress related to the medical condition and its treatment were effective. These interventions included increasing knowledge of the management of the illness, treatment of comorbid psychiatric conditions, and management of distress related to the treatment and medical procedures. Disease type, severity, and duration did not have an impact on the effectiveness of treatment [40].

Facilitating the use of active coping styles may also prevent disruptions in psychosocial functioning [13]. Active or direct coping skills, such as seeking social support, education, and involvement in decision making, are related to better adjustment than passive coping skills, such as avoidance [41]. Meijer et al. [42] examined the coping styles of adolescents with a variety of chronic illnesses. An active coping style appeared to be related to high social self-esteem, the use of adequate social skills, and reduced anxiety in social situations.

Educational support about the management of a chronic illness and its treatment can also enhance adjustment. For instance, children and adolescents with asthma who participated in an educational group about their illness and received instruction in stress management techniques demonstrated increased knowledge of their disease [43]. They also displayed a reduction in internalizing symptoms and improvements in completing daily household chores relative to participants who did not receive the intervention. Providing education and instruction to youth with other chronic conditions may also have a positive effect, particularly for patients who must adhere to a complex treatment regimen.

Additional group interventions targeting psychosocial adjustment have also been utilized in the overall management of youth with chronic illness. Although group interventions including emotional support groups, psychoeducational groups, and summer camps have been developed, empirical support for these groups is limited [44]. There is, however, strong support for adaptation/skill development groups that have the dual goals of enhancing psychosocial adaptation to the chronic condition and improving physical symptoms. These groups target areas such as family communication and functioning, social skills, problem-solving skills, symptom monitoring, and skills related to managing physical symptoms. Symptom reduction groups, which focus exclusively on changing behaviors to reduce or eliminate physical symptoms, are also well supported [44]. Social skills groups may be effective if part of the sequela of the medical condition includes physical restrictions or pain that limits social activities and social engagement [13]. A social skills group can provide instruction on prosocial behavior, conflict resolution, and empathy and perspective taking. Varni et al. [45] examined the impact of a social skills training program on the adjustment of children with cancer in a school context. Children who received training in social skills reported higher levels of perceived teacher and classmate social support nine months after treatment relative to pretreatment levels than children who participated in a school reintegration group. In addition, parents of the children in the social skills group reported a decrease in internalizing and externalizing problems and an increase in school competence in their children.

Incorporating knowledge of development in the treatment of youth with chronic illness is vital. For example, increasing the participation of young patients in their healthcare may promote their sense of autonomy and decision making, which in turn may enhance the perception that they are coping intentionally with their condition [5, 46]. Including adolescents in treatment considerations can augment their mastery and evolving sense of independence [4] and may foster a commitment to the treatment plan [47]. It may be productive to provide adolescents with an opportunity to discuss the illness in the absence of their parents in order to promote open communication [14], which may instill a sense of respect for their thoughts, concerns, and emotional reactions. Healthcare providers must strike a balance between encouraging autonomy and eliciting support needs with adolescent patients. Providers must encourage adolescents to appropriately rely on caregivers and practitioners to ensure adequate monitoring and treatment; however, they must avoid fostering the sick role and enabling excessive dependency that is developmentally asynchronous [21]. Practitioners are encouraged to highlight aspects of the young patient that are not related to the illness in order to promote growth in all areas of functioning [4]. A strength-based approach to treatment is recommended, which emphasizes the patient's unique strengths and assets not only for management of the chronic illness but also for healthy living and decision making [48]. The objective of a strength-based approach is not to resolve specific problems, but to promote patients who are "durably problem-resistant" [48].

Adherence to Treatment

Assessing adherence to the treatment regimen and treating suboptimal adherence are necessary components of the overall management of a chronic illness [3, 49]. Adherence to treatment in children may be more dependent on parental engagement, whereas adherence in adolescents is more contingent on the adolescent's involvement [5]. Suboptimal adherence may be more frequent during middle adolescence

[4], perhaps as a result of adolescents striving for autonomy from parents and other adults and a desire to be similar to their healthy peers. However, adherence may not simply be a function of age, as factors such as the treatment regimen and personal resources such as education and income also play a role [50].

Regular monitoring of adherence throughout the course of the illness can ensure optimal response to treatment. Healthcare providers are encouraged to routinely assess for adherence, be cognizant of the common barriers for nonadherence, and be capable of implementing interventions to surmount these barriers. Components of an assessment for adherence include an adherence history, the subjective experience of the illness and its treatment, family functioning, degree of social support, the impact of social and economic factors on the management of the illness, psychiatric functioning, and knowledge of medication names and dosages [47].

Barriers to treatment adherence are likely in many chronic illnesses, particularly illnesses that entail a complex treatment regimen and treatment with unpleasant side effects. Not only are aspects of the acute illness and treatment risks for nonadherence, but extended asymptomatic periods in adolescent patients are also a risk factor [47]. Abraham et al. [4] identified common reasons for nonadherence in a group of youth with HIV and their parents. Barriers to adherence included a fear of being different from others, a belief that the treatment is not helping because they feel better when not taking it, the perception that the price of lifestyle changes is greater than the benefit of the treatment, and a fear of physical changes as a result of the treatment. It is possible that some of these reasons for nonadherence exist among youth with other chronic illnesses. It is also important for practitioners to explore and address reasons for suboptimal adherence that may be specific and unique to the patient.

Adherence may be enhanced by the provision of clear and detailed information at a level that is commensurate with the cognitive abilities of the young patient [4, 46] and including the adolescent in treatment planning and decision making [47]. Practitioners are encouraged to be familiar with the developmental differences in a patient's ability to understand their medical condition and its treatment and tailor their style of communication accordingly (see Table 29.1 for a description of the stages of cognitive development and the progression of young patients' understanding of their illness). Additional means to improve treatment adherence include educational approaches, behavioral interventions (e.g., self-monitoring, goal setting), self-regulatory skills training [54], collaborative decision making with families [55], simplifying the medication regimen, and increasing the frequency of appointments [47]. Psychoeducational groups may also enhance adherence and change attitudes about medical service [44]. Across pediatric chronic illnesses, multi-component (i.e., multiple modalities, most commonly some variant of behavioral and educational treatment models) and behavioral interventions (e.g., problem solving, parent training) have produced marked effects on adherence behaviors [49]. Since intervention effects on adherence may diminish over time [49], regular and frequent monitoring is imperative.

Table 29.1 Illness understanding in children and adolescents [51]

Cognitive stage of development [52, 53]	Stage characteristics	Understanding of illness
Preoperational Age 2–7 years	• Mainly aware of immediately present experiences and able to understand only one aspect of a phenomenon at a time • Unable to differentiate between self and the external world • Utilize circular reasoning • Unable to generalize across situations	• Tendency to define illness only by being informed that they are ill or by being told about external signs of illness • Tendency to believe that they are sick because of a concrete action that they did or failed to do • May believe that they can recover from disease by adhering to strict rules or by the illness automatically "going away"
Concrete operational Age 7–11	• Understand more than one dimension of a situation • Become less egocentric and can use elementary logic to solve problems • Able to differentiate between self and others	• Define illness by a set of multiple, concrete symptoms • Tendency to believe that illnesses are primarily attributable to germs; thinking about germs tends to be magical and they may believe that recovery can occur by avoiding germs • Focus is on external causes; they may have a limited understanding of the role of the body in illness and healing • Tendency to be passive and do what they are told regarding care with the belief that following the physician's orders and taking medication are sufficient for healing
Formal operational Age 11 and up	• Able to transcend concrete here and now experiences and begin to think abstractly and hypothetically • Able to differentiate between self and others	• Able to understand illness in terms of internal structures and systems that can manifest in a variety of symptoms • Able to understand the role of their body in illness and recovery • Continued difficulty understanding prevention of illness

Conclusion

Although chronic illness has the potential to impact many domains of psychosocial functioning for children and adolescents, a myriad of potential outcomes for young patients may occur. Some evidence indicates that patients manifest disruptions in various areas of psychosocial functioning, whereas other data suggest that psychosocial impairment is minimal. The effects for parents with a child or an adolescent with a chronic illness seem to be similar to pediatric outcomes. Namely, parents may have an increased risk for adjustment problems but there is significant variability in psychosocial functioning and successful adjustment and adaptation are possible [56].

The results of treatment outcome studies appear promising and can inform practice. However, there remain some methodological limitations in current treatment literature. For instance, Bauman et al. [39] noted that some intervention studies did not provide a rationale for the use of specific measures and did not acknowledge that some measures had not been validated on children with health difficulties. Plante et al. [44] indicated that many studies did not measure hypothesis-specific outcomes. Additional limitations include a lack of standardized measures of illness or outcome, sample representativeness, control groups, and small sample sizes [5]. Moreover, there remains a lack of empirically sound intervention studies in certain areas of pediatric chronic illness. For example, Seitz et al. [57] highlighted the dearth of intervention research in adolescents with cancer.

Further research on the psychosocial functioning of youth with chronic illness is necessary. Research aimed at clarifying the correlates and risk factors for maladjustment, assessing various domains of psychosocial functioning, and delineating empirically sound interventions is needed. It is imperative to include measures that have been normed and validated on children and adolescents with chronic illness [39]. Some researchers have suggested that there may be greater variability within disease groups than between groups [12], which underscores the importance of within-group analyses [8]. Direct observations, structured interviews, and performance tests can provide additional information on psychosocial functioning and augment existing assessment approaches [56].

Given the variability in outcomes for young patients with chronic illness, a focus on the factors that promote resiliency, resistance to impairments in functioning, and factors related to positive growth continues to be important [10, 56]. Wallander and Varni [56] proposed a model of child adjustment to pediatric chronic physical disorders that included risk factors for adjustment problems (e.g., severity of the disease or disability, daily hassles, major life events), as well as resistance factors (e.g., temperament, problem-solving ability, cognitive appraisals, family environment, social support). Further exploration of the risk factors for maladjustment and the factors that promote resiliency can shed light on the variability in overall adjustment for youth with chronic illness.

Longitudinal designs are necessary to clarify the progression of adjustment to the different stages of a chronic illness [56]. Researchers who utilize this methodological approach can explore the changes and challenges faced by young patients as they attempt to cope with chronic illness in the context of the multiple developmental changes of childhood and adolescence. For instance, the relationship between changes in cognitive functioning and patients' understanding of their illness and adherence to treatment regimens can be more clearly elucidated. The late or long-term impact of chronic illness on a variety of areas of functioning well beyond the acute illness and treatment stage can also be examined. For example, survivors of cancer can experience physical and psychological effects after treatment has been completed [25–28], which highlights the importance of follow-up and longitudinal studies on the psychosocial functioning of patients with other medical conditions. In addition, longitudinal designs can be used to trace the effects of chronic illness on family members and overall family functioning across time [6].

Practitioners are encouraged to be familiar with the domains of psychosocial functioning that can be impacted by chronic illness [4], means to assess these domains, and empirically supported psychosocial interventions that can be employed when maladjustment is discovered. Multidisciplinary treatment teams are an ideal means of treating youth with chronic illness. Mental health professionals who specialize in assessing and treating the unique challenges faced by this population can be integral members of treatment teams. Thorough multidisciplinary assessment that begins at the time of diagnosis and is conducted throughout the course of the illness will enhance the identification of markers of maladjustment and foster the timely implementation of effective interventions.

Acknowledgments The authors are appreciative of the editorial assistance that was provided by Rebecca L Scotland, Ph.D.

References

1. Judson L. Global childhood chronic illness. Nurs Adm Q. 2004;28:60–66.
2. Stein RE, Silver EJ. Operationalizing a conceptually based noncategorical definition: a first look at US children with chronic conditions. Arch Pediatr Adolesc Med. 1999;153: 68–74.
3. LeBlanc LA, Goldsmith T, Patel DR. Behavioral aspects of chronic illness in children and adolescents. Pediatr Clin North Am. 2003;50:859–78.
4. Abraham A, Silber TJ, Lyon M. Psychosocial aspects of chronic illness in adolescence. Indian J Pediatr. 1999;66:447–53.
5. Geist R, Grdisa V, Otley A. Psychosocial issues in the child with chronic conditions. Best Pract Res Clin Gastroenterol. 2003;17:141–52.
6. McClellan CB, Cohen LL. Family functioning in children with chronic illness compared with healthy controls: a critical review. J Pediatr. 2007;150:221–23.
7. Merrick J, Carmeli E. A review on the prevalence of disabilities in children. Internet J Pediatr Neonatol. 2003;3:1.
8. Gledhill J, Rangel L, Garralda E. Surviving chronic physical illness: psychosocial outcome in adult life. Arch Dis Child. 2000;83:104–10.
9. Stein RE, Jessop DJ. What diagnosis does not tell: the case for a noncategorical approach to chronic illness in childhood. Soc Sci Med. 1989;29:769–78.
10. Barlow JH, Ellard DR. The psychosocial well-being of children with chronic disease, their parents and siblings: an overview of the research evidence base. Child Care Health Dev. 2006;32:19–31.

11. Gortmaker SL, Walker DK, Weitzman M, et al. Chronic conditions, socioeconomic risks, and behavioral problems in children and adolescents. Pediatrics. 1990;85:267–76.
12. Boekaerts M, Stress I. Roder, coping, and adjustment in children with a chronic disease: a review of the literature. Disabil Rehabil. 1999;21:311–37.
13. Meijer SA, Sinnema G, Bijstra JO, et al. Social functioning in children with a chronic illness. J Child Psychol Psychiatry. 2000;41:309–17.
14. Boice MM. Chronic illness in adolescence. Adolescence. 1998;33:927–39.
15. Huff MB, McClanahan KK, Omar HA. The effects of chronic illness upon mental health status of children and adolescents. Int J Disabil Hum Dev. 2008;7:273–78.
16. Miauton L, Narring F, Michaud PA. Chronic illness, life style and emotional health in adolescence: results of a cross-sectional survey on the health of 15–20-year-olds in Switzerland. Eur J Pediatr. 2003;162:682–89.
17. Suris JC, Michaud PA, Akre C, et al. Health risk behaviors in adolescents with chronic conditions. Pediatrics. 2008;122:e1113–18.
18. Cadman D, Boyle M, Szatmari P, et al. Chronic illness, disability, and mental and social well-being: findings of the Ontario Child Health Study. Pediatrics. 1987;79:805–13.
19. Hysing M, Elgen I, Gillberg C, et al. Chronic physical illness and mental health in children. Results from a large-scale population study. J Child Psychol Psychiatry. 2007;48:785–92.
20. Hysing M, Elgen I, Gillberg C, et al. Emotional and behavioural problems in subgroups of children with chronic illness: results from a large-scale population study. Child Care Health Dev. 2009;35:527–33.
21. Hatherill S. Psychiatric aspects of chronic disease in adolescence. CME. 2007;25:212–14.
22. American Psychiatric Association. Diagnostic and statistical manual of mental disorders. 4th ed. Washington, DC: American Psychiatric Association; 1994.
23. Key JD, Brown RT, Marsh LD, et al. Depressive symptoms in adolescents with a chronic illness. Child Health Care. 2001;30:283–92.
24. Wolman C, Resnick MD, Harris LJ, et al. Emotional well-being among adolescents with and without chronic conditions. J Adolesc Health. 1994;15:199–204.
25. Stein KD, Syrjala KL, Andrykowski MA. Physical and psychological long-term and late effects of cancer. Cancer. 2008;112:2577–92.
26. Pendley JS, Dahlquist LM, Dreyer Z. Body image and psychosocial adjustment in adolescent cancer survivors. J Pediatr Psychol. 1997;22:29–43.
27. Schultz KA, Ness KK, Whitton J, et al. Behavioral and social outcomes in adolescent survivors of childhood cancer: a report from the childhood cancer survivor study. J Clin Oncol. 2007;25:3649–56.
28. Hobbie WL, Stuber M, Meeske K, et al. Symptoms of posttraumatic stress in young adult survivors of childhood cancer. J Clin Oncol. 2000;18:4060–66.
29. Lavigne JV, Faier-Routman J. Psychological adjustment to pediatric physical disorders: a meta-analytic review. J Pediatr Psychol. 1992;17:133–57.
30. Bennett DS. Depression among children with chronic medical problems: a meta-analysis. J Pediatr Psychol. 1994;19:149–69.
31. Maunsell E, Pogany L, Barrera M, et al. Quality of life among long-term adolescent and adult survivors of childhood cancer. J Clin Oncol. 2006;24:2527–35.
32. Katon W, Lozano P, Russo J, et al. The prevalence of DSM-IV anxiety and depressive disorders in youth with asthma compared with controls. J Adolesc Health. 2007;41:455–63.
33. Patino-Fernandez AM, Pai AL, Alderfer M, et al. Acute stress in parents of children newly diagnosed with cancer. Pediatr Blood Cancer. 2008;50:289–92.
34. Tritt SG, Esses LM. Psychosocial adaptation of siblings of children with chronic medical illnesses. Am J Orthopsychiatry. 1988;58:211–20.
35. Drotar D. Relating parent and family functioning to the psychological adjustment of children with chronic health conditions: what have we learned? What do we need to know? J Pediatr Psychol. 1997;22:149–65.

36. Robinson KE, Gerhardt CA, Vannatta K, et al. Parent and family factors associated with child adjustment to pediatric cancer. J Pediatr Psychol. 2007;32:400–10.
37. Cadman D, Rosenbaum P, Boyle M, et al. Children with chronic illness: family and parent demographic characteristics and psychosocial adjustment. Pediatrics. 1991;87:884–89.
38. Beale IL. Scholarly literature review: efficacy of psychological interventions for pediatric chronic illnesses. J Pediatr Psychol. 2006;31:437–51.
39. Bauman LJ, Drotar D, Leventhal JM, et al. A review of psychosocial interventions for children with chronic health conditions. Pediatrics. 1997;100:244–51.
40. Kibby MY, Tyc VL, Mulhern RK. Effectiveness of psychological intervention for children and adolescents with chronic medical illness: a meta-analysis. Clin Psychol Rev. 1998;18:103–17.
41. Grey M, Cameron ME, Thurber FW. Coping and adaptation in children with diabetes. Nurs Res. 1991;40:144–49.
42. Meijer SA, Sinnema G, Bijstra JO, et al. Coping styles and locus of control as predictors for psychological adjustment of adolescents with a chronic illness. Soc Sci Med. 2002;54:1453–61.
43. Perrin JM, MacLean WE Jr, Gortmaker SL, et al. Improving the psychological status of children with asthma: a randomized controlled trial. J Dev Behav Pediatr. 1992;13:241–47.
44. Plante WA, Lobato D, Engel R. Review of group interventions for pediatric chronic conditions. J Pediatr Psychol. 2001;26:435–53.
45. Varni JW, Katz ER, Colegrove R Jr, et al. The impact of social skills training on the adjustment of children with newly diagnosed cancer. J Pediatr Psychol. 1993;18:751–67.
46. Schmidt S, Petersen C, Bullinger M. Coping with chronic disease from the perspective of children and adolescents – a conceptual framework and its implications for participation. Child Care Health Dev. 2003;29:63–75.
47. Smith BA, Shuchman M. Problem of nonadherence in chronically ill adolescents: strategies for assessment and intervention. Curr Opin Pediatr. 2005;17:613–18.
48. Chung RJ, Burke PJ, Goodman E. Firm foundations: strength-based approaches to adolescent chronic disease. Curr Opin Pediatr. 2010;22:389–97.
49. Kahana S, Drotar D, Frazier T. Meta-analysis of psychological interventions to promote adherence to treatment in pediatric chronic health conditions. J Pediatr Psychol. 2008;33:590–611.
50. DiMatteo MR. Variations in patients' adherence to medical recommendations: a quantitative review of 50 years of research. Med Care. 2004;42:200–9.
51. Perrin EC, Gerrity PS. There's a demon in your belly: children's understanding of illness. Pediatrics. 1981;67:841–49.
52. Piaget J, Innhelder B. The psychology of the child. New York, NY: Basic Books; 1969.
53. Wadsworth BJ. Piaget's theory of cognitive and affective development: foundations of constructivism. 5th ed. Boston, MA: Allyn Bacon; 2004.
54. Fielding D, Duff A. Compliance with treatment protocols: interventions for children with chronic illness. Arch Dis Child. 1999;80:196–200.
55. Drotar D, Crawford P, Bonner M. Collaborative decision-making and promoting treatment adherence in pediatric chronic illness. Patient Intell. 2010;2:1–7.
56. Wallander JL, Varni JW. Effects of pediatric chronic physical disorders on child and family adjustment. J Child Psychol Psychiatry. 1998;39:29–46.
57. Seitz DC, Besier T, Goldbeck L. Psychosocial interventions for adolescent cancer patients: a systematic review of the literature. Psychooncology. 2009;18:683–90.

Chapter 30
Parents and Siblings

Joav Merrick, Isack Kandel, and Mohammed Morad

Abstract This chapter looks at the effects on the family unit with the birth of a child with a disability. This event is always a crisis for the family, but with early and sensitive care and intervention for the involved child, the parents, and siblings much can be done to help the family. This support can help the family to adjust and become positively involved in the care and development of the child, even if that child is different and in need of special care. Siblings seem to have a positive role in the relationship and also concerning long-term support.

Introduction

With every child born the life of the whole family will change significantly and each of its members will have to adapt to the new situation. When the child is born with a disability, in addition to the regular adaptation the family must cope with stress, grief, disappointments, and challenges, which may lead to a serious crisis or even disruption of family life. Parents must coordinate assessments, evaluations, and various treatments maintaining contact with many professionals and numerous institutions or services. They find themselves faced with important decisions on behalf of the child, decisions on management of this new situation, and economic decisions that will affect the whole family.

Several researchers have found that children play a very important role in satisfying the needs of their parents [1, 2]. Children can be associated with materialism or competition and their parents' aspirations to achieve certain status or their desire to expand the family tree. Therefore it can be a terrible blow to the parents, when their child is unable to fulfill these wishes.

J. Merrick (✉)
National Institute of Child Health and Human Development, Health Services, Office of the Medical Director, Division for Mental Retardation, Ministry of Social Affairs and Social Services, POBox 1260, IL-91012 Jerusalem, Israel; Kentucky Children's Hospital, University of Kentucky, Lexington, KY, USA
e-mail: jmerrick@zahav.net.il

D.R. Patel et al. (eds.), *Neurodevelopmental Disabilities*,
DOI 10.1007/978-94-007-0627-9_30, © Springer Science+Business Media B.V. 2011

In general, one can observe several areas in which giving birth to a child is important for the parents. The child may be seen as the physical and psychological extension of his parents, possessing the hereditary combination of the characteristics of the latter. Where the child displays "good" characteristics, it is interpreted as a reflection of the positive side of his parents. Likewise, if his individual characteristics are negative or abnormal, they can be interpreted as a concealed or overt reflection of the characteristics of the parents. In many societies children are almost universally seen as an extension of their parents.

The child can also be seen as a means to satisfy the wishes of his parents, where their wishes and desires can come true. However, the child is not always able to fulfill and realize those wishes. The child may also be seen as a way for parents to achieve "immortality," by perpetuating their good name into the next generation.

The disability of the child also makes a difference. Researchers from Montreal [3] studied a group of children and their parents with Down syndrome, a group of children with congenital heart disease, a group with cleft lip and/or palate, and a control group without disability. Their study revealed that the parents of children with Down syndrome and those with congenital heart disease showed greater levels of parental stress and psychological distress in comparison to the other two groups. Mothers were found to report greater levels of stress and distress overall.

Later on in life the child himself/herself with a disability will have to cope with a variety of stress factors. Deutsch [4] described at least three categories: stress factors experienced by everyone (for example, a death of a relative), factors that are not at all stressful to the general population (for example, going to a store), and stress factors that are unique to persons with a disability (such as not being able to handle money). In order to cope and preserve his self-esteem the child with a disability may create a private world of his own and use various defense mechanisms to survive emotionally.

Parental Reaction to the Birth of a Child with Disability

The birth of a child with a disability can cause disappointment to his parents [1] and the reaction of the families seems to follow the five stages of Kubler-Ross grief elaboration theory (denial, anger, bargaining, depression, and acceptance) [5, 6]. This reaction is also similar to what we observe in parents with perinatal death or loss [7].

It should be emphasized that the functional crisis experienced by mothers and fathers of children with a disability may be accompanied by psychological stress, a feeling of loss, and low self-esteem. In addition, the fact that the child is unable to fulfill the expectations of the parents may also disappoint them. The birth of a child with a disability may result in a severe blow to the self-esteem of the parents, create disappointment, and result in the child becoming a social obstacle that will also cause feelings of shame and embarrassment.

Parent reactions to the diagnosis of the disability will not be identical. The intensiveness of reactions and their character depends on several dynamic factors, such as individuality, the character of social relations, feelings about the deviation, and the social status. In the literature [8], a wide range of reactions are mentioned, some considered more frequent than the others: anger, disappointment, shame, frustration, and grief. The coping process is not static, but a constantly changing cognitive and behavioral effort by the person to manage both external and internal stress factors and pressures.

Anger, disappointment, and shame [5–7]: these reactions result from the fact that the child is not the ideal child that the parent anticipated. The child is unable to fulfill the hopes and ambitions he/she was expected to. There are cases when parents unconsciously consider the child to be responsible for the crushing of their ambitions (as if he/she is "deliberately" disabled). However, since many parents consider it inappropriate to direct their negative feelings toward the children, anger may also be directed toward the parents themselves or toward others (for instance, the physician or other professionals for a variety of reasons, such as having made an incorrect diagnosis, insensitivity, offering false hope, or providing inadequate or ineffective treatment or services), with these feelings of jealousy and anger common in many families. The emotions may also be directed toward other families, who do not have to contend with such stress or those with disabled children who have higher functioning or improved to a greater extent. Sometimes, the opposite reaction can be observed, which is expressed in overprotecting the child. In other cases the parents see the disabled child as a symbol of their own personal failure. The feelings of a damaged self-esteem give rise to intensive feelings of inferiority and shame.

Frustration [9] over the fact that the child is not able to fulfill his parents' expectations can become even deeper as the slow development of the child makes him totally dependent on his parents, often especially his mother, seriously limiting her independence and freedom. In addition social and economic aspects of raising a child with disabilities may provoke additional anger and frustration. For example, difficulties in maintaining social communication, leisure activities, work projects, or economic plans. Frustration can belong to one of the two types: (a) frustration resulting from role organization factors, i.e., failure to organize a new role system, since the disabled child is not able to play the role he is expected to or (b) frustration resulting from the destruction of ambitions and wishes for a happy family life.

Often the initial diagnosis of the child's disability will produce a grief reaction in parents and other family members [3]. This may be the result of initial confusion and uncertainty. Grief and bereavement are normal reactions to the loss of an object (in this specific case the object is symbolic). By means of these feelings the human being temporarily retreats from involvement in the external world and allows his ego to focus on transferring the mental energy from the object on which it was concentrated to an alternative object. Transferring the energy is essential for successful conclusion of the bereavement process. However, this solution is not possible in case of the birth of a disabled child, since there is no final separation from the lost object, the child exists; thus, there is no opportunity to grieve over him without experiencing constant demands from his/her side. As a result of the demands, which are opposite to releasing oneself from the lost object and accepting the child, there is created a situation in which "chronic bereavement" is opposed to counterfeelings. Since this ambivalence cannot be accepted in the parents' consciousness, it is pushed aside and causes additional difficulties in finishing the lamentation process. Ambivalence toward the object is not a part of the usual bereavement, since the grief process itself is a temporary phenomenon.

Many parents also have little understanding of what the diagnosis of a given disease or syndrome entails and many will have various perceptions and speculations of the disease causing the disability. Parents should therefore be informed regarding the varied manifestations and aspects of the disability. Sometimes it is also very hard to predict the cause or development of the disability at an early age, which makes it even more difficult for the parents.

Grief is a complex reaction with the loss of the expected normal child and now the parents are faced with the necessity to develop new role of attachment to the abnormal child. Olshansky [10] described grief for a disabled child as a lifelong "chronic sorrow" that may accompany the parents all their life, regardless of whether the child lives at home or is in placement [11]. Although the intensity varies from one to another, it seems that all parents experience grief. Olshansky [10] argued that this type of grief should not be interpreted as a neurotic reaction, but rather it should be seen as a normal and natural reaction to the crisis. The crisis can take the following forms [1, 11]:

- The change crisis: this crisis takes place immediately after the diagnosis of the disability and is a most difficult experience. The parents are full of expectation for the birth of a normal child, and when they are informed about the disability, all their dreams are ruined, causing the traumatic reactions. This crisis is not a reaction to the handicap itself; rather, it is a reaction to the sudden change of reality.
- The ideological crisis: the change crisis is comparatively short; however, after the parents have digested the news, they are to confront with this experience everyday. This confrontation gives rise to strong emotional reactions, leading to an ideological crisis, which may last for a longer period of time. The parents are in a state of constant ambivalence. On the one hand they feel that they have to love and protect their child, but on the other hand social values cause them to feel discomfort, feelings of failure, and inability to accept the child as a "beloved" one. Such characteristic reactions as guilt, shame, overprotection, and grief appear at this stage.
- The reality crisis: this crisis is directly related to the objectively difficult conditions of bringing up a child with disability. The parents face numerous difficulties which influence their ability to manage the problem. The first difficulty is financial, since expenses grow considerably compared to their situation before or to that of other families. Many parents are disturbed by fears related to the influence the child has and will have on their lifestyle. Family members may stay in

seclusion at home and avoid spending their time in the way they used to, before the child was born. Many parents express concern regarding the coming of a time when they will not be able to take care of the child themselves.

The stages mentioned above are not necessarily pure, since there can be overlap, but in order to assist and support parents it is important to realize what stage of the crisis they are at.

The issue of gender differences in coping strategies has been studied by Sullivan [12] with 150 parents following the birth of a child with Down syndrome. Each parent was requested to answer a questionnaire (COPE inventory). It was found that females scored significantly higher than males in the areas of seeking instrumental and emotional support, in focusing on and venting emotions, and in suppression of competing activities. An additional study was carried out with 75 parents of young children, which displayed the same results. Although gender differences were found, no value may be ascribed to these different coping strategies.

Working through grief in the families of children with any disability is an ongoing process with periods of greater and lesser intensity to the grieving. This intensity may relate partly to developmental issues and events, such as birthdays or other rites of passage (e.g., Bar Mitzvahs, in Israel where all children are drafted to the Army, graduations, marriage of siblings), and may underscore how different the child is from his typical peers. Grief intensity may also relate to more personal, individual factors. Sometimes there is an alternation of hope and despair. Each new treatment or program for the child is often accompanied by an increase in optimism in the parents. If the new treatment or program is deemed unsuccessful, despair may follow, only to be replaced by hope once again, when a new plan is implemented.

Parental Guilt

Guilt is another common reaction to the diagnosis of a disability in a child. Sometimes that has been caused by the medical and professional community, who directly or inadvertently attributed a disease or condition in a child as parental failure [13], which later turned out to be based on a genetically disorder. The possible contribution of additional factors, such as environmental toxins, has also been discussed. Many parents wonder if they unwittingly did something to contribute to the disability in their child (such as exposure to x-rays, mercury from injections, or dental fillings).

An adult may experience guilt as a result of ideas and feelings, which are interpreted as forbidden or negative. The birth of a disabled child makes his parents feel disappointment, anger, and hostility toward the child. These feelings are interpreted as negative and can arouse guilt feelings and unconscious expectation that the child disappears. Guilty feelings are one of the most frequent reactions of the parents to the birth of a child with disability. There are parents, who feel rejection, disappointment, and anger, because their child is not the one they looked forward to. Since the parents cannot tolerate or suffer these negative feelings, they deny the feelings by directing the anger toward themselves – the feeling that this is a punishment for their past sins [11]. In other cases the guilt feeling is directed (as a result of negative feelings) toward other people, such as a spouse or a physician, or toward spiritual matters. We have often heard the following statements by parents with disabled children: "This happened as a punishment for me leaving the religion," "It is all my fault. Before I got married, I had been 'flirting about,' I made love before marriage and I always felt terrible about that, and now I have to pay for it."

Rosenzweig [14] has classified reactions to frustration by the following categories:

- Interpunitive reaction – a reaction of anger and guilt directed toward the "self." This reaction takes place when the super-ego does not allow realization of the aggressive feelings; rather, it turns them into guilt feelings and regret by means of keeping a distance and isolation.
- Extrapunitive reaction – a reaction of anger and hostility toward the external world, considering other people to be guilty. In this case as the super-ego is weak, it allows expressing the hostility feelings.
- Impunitive reaction – reactions of shame and guilt are slight, there is a compromise with the problem. This reaction is possible when the ego is strong and the self-esteem is positive. In pathological cases there is a process of keeping a distance, but in normal cases there is a process of sublimation.

Sometimes the guilt and shame are related to the inability of the parents to communicate with each other or with other family members [11]. We have seen over several years in Israel that parents leave their disabled children in the hospital. A nationwide study was conducted [15] in Israel during 1979–1983 and 1987–1991 to examine the factors affecting parental abandonment of infants with Down syndrome. The overall abandonment rate was 25%, where the major factors were the age of the mother, birth order, the health status of the child, and the study period. The trend to abandon these children has gradually been reduced over time.

Influence on Parental Married Life

The effects of the birth of a child with disabilities on the marriage of his or her parents have been studied by several researchers. An early study in 1964 conducted in Central California by Fowle at the University of the Pacific included a total population of 328 families with a child with severe intellectual disability aged 3–17 years. A selected experimental group of 35 families from a total group of 83 families who had hospitalized their child was matched with a control group of 35 families from a group of total 245 families who had not hospitalized their child. She could not find any significant difference in marital integration between the two groups, but there was a significant difference in the role tension of the siblings, especially in that of the oldest female sibling of the family [16].

A study of 142 families with a child born with spina bifida [17] (56 families with a surviving child) between 1964 and 1966 was examined in 1976. The divorce rate for families with a surviving child was found to be nine times higher than that for the local population and three times higher than that for the families, where the child with spina bifida had died. Marriages that followed a pre-nuptial conception were especially vulnerable with a separation/divorce rate of 50%. All divorced fathers and only one mother had remarried at follow-up. An additional study [18] also found the divorce rate 10 times higher in the families with a disabled child than in the general population.

The disability can cause damage to the married life of the parents in several different ways: it can create strong parental feelings, it can be a depressing symbol of a common failure, and it can change the family organization and create fertile ground for conflicts [19]. One frequent problem is the fact that burden for child care is not divided equally between the parents. In the common situation, the father is generally at work, while the mother cares for the child with the disability. The parents must organize a system of roles and a division of the burden of work in order to prevent the burning out of one partner [20]. In addition devotion of the mother to care of her child may make the father feel neglected, which sometimes can result in violence [21]. Sometimes the core of the conflict stems from the fact that each parent conceives the situation in a different way. One parent may relate to the child as a failed case, while the other as a capable or even a normal child. In addition there are parents, who are unable to live with what they see as shame or stigma [18].

It is therefore important that as soon as a child is born with a disability the parents should have the opportunity to talk and discuss the various issues with a competent professional, so that as many adverse reactions can be prevented. This way the family can be helped to adjust and become realistically involved with the care and development of the child [22].

Influence on Siblings

In the early study from California [16] in 1964 mentioned above, where two groups were compared (child with disability hospitalized versus child at home), the sibling role tension was also investigated. A total of 48 siblings in each group showed a significant difference with a higher sibling role tension in the group where the child with disability was kept at home. The study also showed that the oldest female sibling in families with a child with disability at home displayed more role tension.

A study was conducted with 327 siblings of disabled children compared with 248 siblings from a random sample of families in order to examine if the early family environment of siblings of disabled children had an influence on psychological functioning [23]. The results showed that younger male siblings, and especially those in close age-spacing relationship to the disabled child, scored higher on the psychological impairment than older male siblings. Contrary to these findings, the study showed that younger female siblings were psychologically better off than older female siblings and their age-spacing was not significantly related to psychological functioning.

A study from the United Kingdom with 183 children with intellectual disability (95 with Down syndrome) and their nearest in age sibling (with classroom control of the sibling) showed that behavior problems in the sibling were found most often where the child with intellectual disability had disturbed behavior and especially in the Down syndrome group [24]. The siblings in the non-Down group showed more reading problems and behavior disturbance in school than either the Down and the control group.

Results from a study at the University of Washington [25] of 110 children (8–15 years), half of whom had a disabled younger sibling, showed that distinct psychological predictors existed for the group with a disabled sibling with parental stress and some dimensions of the family social environment the most significant factors.

A 4-year follow-up study among orthodox Jewish families (82 families) in Illinois showed decrease in the negative impact of the child and increase in sibling and overall family adjustment. Parents cited religion as an important source of strength, while lack of time, behavior problems, and limited availability or use of professional assistance as continuing difficulties [26].

One study looked at the attitude of the sibling toward their brother or sister with a disability [27] and found that some of the very young siblings wanted to be similar and tried to imitate their sibling with a disability, especially if the sibling had physical disability. Before the age of 2 years children were able to recognize that their brother or sister were different and often imitated the parent's behavior toward the older child.

Researchers in Canada studied [28] unaffected siblings (137 in total) of children with pervasive developmental disorder (PDD) and Down syndrome with a control group over a 3-year period. A significantly greater number of adjustment problems were found in the siblings of PDD children and also caregivers of PDD reported the highest level of distress and depression, which persisted over the study period.

A Dutch study [29] looked at siblings of children with a physical disability (43 children) in order to investigate the sibling relationship, relationship with parents, and with others. The sibling reported difficulties with common activities and communication with the disabled sibling and expressed concern for the future and the health of their disabled sibling. Open communication and trust were the main characteristics in their relationship with parents, while having a sibling with a disability did not affect their relationship with friends.

In Israel we have seen several cases in residential care for persons with intellectual disability, where the parents kept it a secret in the family that they have a child with intellectual disability. The parents visited their child in the center, but their siblings knew nothing. When the parents died the siblings became guardian without knowing that they had a sibling with a disability. In the last 10 years we have therefore made major efforts to involve the whole family in visiting the disabled child in residential care and support siblings, who did not know of their brother or sister in care.

In a study [30] of Western Australian families with children with Rett (141 cases) and Down syndrome (186 cases), parents reported disadvances like time constraint, impaired socialization, financial and also physical burden in the care, lack of peer acceptance, and the dealing with strange behavior at social events. On the other hand they also reported that the siblings were very much aware, tolerant, and acceptant of disability and the sibling was compassionate, caring, and kind. The sibling was more mature for age, patient and supportive, and aware of their own health and abilities.

A recent review [31] of research between 1970 and 2008 concerned with adult siblings over 21 years of age concerning relationships, psychosocial outcomes, and involvement in future planning found a total of 23 studies. The studies showed that siblings overall had a positive relationship with their disabled sibling and they took supportive roles and participated in future planning. On the other hand there is a lack of research concerning intervention studies, a lack of perspective of people with disabilities for a mutual view at the relationship, and a lack of long-term research across lifespan to observe and understand how relationships and needs change over time.

Conclusions

This chapter looked at the effects on the family unit with the birth of a child with a disability. This event is always a crisis for the family, but with early and sensitive care and intervention for the involved child, the parents, and siblings much can be done to help the family. This support can help the family to adjust and become positively involved in the care and development of the child, even if that child is different and in need of special care. Siblings seem to have a positive role in the relationship and also concerning long-term support.

References

1. Wolfensberger W, Kurtz RA, editors. Management of the family of the mentally retarded. River Grove, IL: Follett Educational Corporation; 1969.
2. Blacher J, Meyers CE. A review of attachment formation and disorder of handicapped children. Am J Ment Defic. 1983;87(4):359–71.
3. Pelchat D, Ricard N, Bouchard JM, Perreault M, Saucier JF, Berthiaume M, Bisson J. Adaptation of parents in relation to their 6-month old infant's type of disability. Child Care Health Dev. 1999;25(5):377–97.
4. Stress DH. psychological defence mechanisms and the private world of the mentally retarded: applying psychotherapeutic concepts to rehabilitation. Psychiatr Aspects Ment Retard Rev. 1989;8:25–30.
5. Kubler-Ross E. On death and dying. New York, NY: Macmillan; 1969.
6. Calandra C, Finocchiaro G, Raciti L, Alberti A. Grief elaboration in families with handicapped member. Ann Ist Super Sanita. 1992;28(2):269–71.

7. Harmon RJ, Plummer NS, Frankel KA. Perinatal loss: parental grieving, family impact and intervention services. In: Osofsky JD, Fitzgerald HE, editors. Handbook of infant mental health. Vol. 4. New York, NY: Wiley; 2000. pp. 327–68.

8. Darling RB. Families against society: a study of reactions to children with birth effects. Beverly Hills, CA: Sage; 1979.

9. Waisbren SE. Parents's reactions after the birth of a developmentally disabled child. Am J Ment Defic. 1980;84(4):345–51.

10. Olshansky S. Chronic sorrow: a response to having a mentally defective child. Soc Casework. 1962;43:190–95.

11. Portowicz DJ, Rimmerman A. Parental reaction to the birth of a disabled child. Soc Welf. 1985;6(2–3):176–98 [Hebrew].

12. Sullivan A. Gender differences in coping strategies of parents of children with Down syndrome. Downs Syndr Res Pract. 2002;8(2):67–73.

13. Bettleheim B. The empty fortress: infantile autism and the birth of the self. New York, NY: Free Press; 1967.

14. The Rosenzweig Picture-Frustration (P-F) Study. Basic manual. St. Louis, MO: Rana House; 1978.

15. Sadetzki S, Chetrit A, Akstein E, Keinan L, Luxenburg O, Modan B. Relinquishment of infants with Down syndrome in Israel: trends by time. Am J Ment Retard. 2000;105(6): 480–85.

16. Fowle CM. The effect of the severely mentally retarded child on his family. Am J Ment Defic. 1968;73(3):468–73.

17. Tew BJ, Laurence KM, Payne H, Rawnsley K. Marital stability following the birth of a child with spina bifida. Br J Psychiatry. 1977;131:79–82.

18. McCormack M. A mentally handicapped child in the family: a guide for parents. London: Constable; 1978.

19. Featherstone H. A difference in the family: life with a disabled child. New York, NY: Basic Books; 1980.

20. Withers P, Bennett L. Myths and marital discord in a family with a child with profound physical and intellectual disabilities. Br J Learn Disabil. 2003;31(2):91–95.

21. Hutt ML, Gibby RG. The mentally retarded child: development, education and treatment. Boston, MA: Allyn Bacon; 1976.

22. Oates RK. Down's syndrome. Aust Fam Physician. 1984;13(1):50.

23. Breslau N. Siblings of disabled children: birth order and age-spacing effects. J Abnorm Child Psychol. 1982;10(1):85–96.

24. Gath A, Gumley D. Retarded children and their siblings. J Child Psychol Psychiatry. 1987;28(5):715–30.

25. Dyson L, Edgar E, Crnic K. Psychological predictors of adjustment by siblings of developmentally disabled children. Am J Ment Retard. 1989;94(3):292–302.

26. Leyser Y. Stress and adaptation in orthodox Jewish families with a disabled child. Am J Orthopsychiatry. 1994;64(3):376–85.

27. Hames A. Do younger siblings of learning-disabled children see them as similar or different? Child Care Health Dev. 1998;24(2):157–68.

28. Fisman S, Wolf L, Ellison D, Freeman T. A longitudinal study of siblings of children with chronic disabilities. Can J Psychiatry. 2000;45(4):369–75.

29. Pit-Ten Cate IM, Loots GM. Experiences of siblings of children with physical disabilities: an empirical investigation. Disabil Rehabil. 2000;22(9):399–408.

30. Mulroy S, Robertson L, Alberti K, Leonard H, Bower C. The impact of having a sibling with an intellectual disability: parental perspectives in two disorders. J Intellect Disabil Res. 2008;52(3):216–29.

31. Heller T, Arnold CK. Siblings of adults with developmental disabilities: psychosocial outcomes, relationships and future planning. J Policy Pract Intellect Disabil. 2010;7(1):16–25.

Chapter 31
Parenthood

Joav Merrick, Isack Kandel, and Mohammed Morad

Abstract Parenthood in persons with intellectual disability (ID) is an issue of concern for the family, guardians, and professionals as there are many sentiments and problems involved: financial, technical, medical, legal, and above all moral. People with intellectual, developmental, or other disabilities have feelings, want relationships, and some are able to have children also. The attitude of society has changed through time from the early eugenic concern with heredity and fertility, to a focus on the risk to the children due to parental neglect or abuse, to acceptance and a search for solutions to parental training and support. This change can be seen as a result of a shift from institutional care to community care and normalization. This chapter reviews available research, prevalence, service issues, and experience from around the world and relates to the situation in Israel. Jewish law has been very progressive regarding the possibility of marriage between persons with ID (in contrast to American law where historically this right has been denied, until recently). Recent research has shown that, in the case of such a union resulting in children, although they require some supervision, family, friends, and social welfare agencies have scrutinized these families so much that they are in constant fear of their child being taken away. There is little information on the number of such cases and an overall dearth of information on the effects on the children, although recent research has shown a varied picture of resilience and a close, warm relationship later on with the family and especially the mother.

Introduction

Parenthood in persons with intellectual disability (ID) is an issue of concern for the family, guardians, and professionals such as physicians, psychiatrists, psychologists,

J. Merrick (✉)
National Institute of Child Health and Human Development, Health Services, Office of the Medical Director, Division for Mental Retardation, Ministry of Social Affairs and Social Services, POBox 1260, IL-91012 Jerusalem, Israel; Kentucky Children's Hospital, University of Kentucky, Lexington, KY, USA
e-mail: jmerrick@zahav.net.il

D.R. Patel et al. (eds.), *Neurodevelopmental Disabilities*,
DOI 10.1007/978-94-007-0627-9_31, © Springer Science+Business Media B.V. 2011

counselors, social workers, child protection workers, clergy, officials in various institutions, or lawyers. The sentiments and problems involved (financial, technical, medical, legal, and above all moral) when persons with ID contemplate relationships, marriage, and parenthood make it a very difficult task for all involved.

People with intellectual, developmental, or other disabilities have feelings, want relationships, and are able to have children also. The attitude of society has changed through time from the early eugenic concern with heredity and fertility, to a focus on the risk to the children due to parental neglect or abuse, to acceptance and a search for solutions to parental training and support [1]. This change can be seen as a result of a shift from institutional care to community care and normalization [1].

Sexuality and Persons with Disability

Persons with physical, cognitive, or emotional disabilities should have a right to sexuality education, sexual healthcare, and sexual expression. Family, healthcare workers, and other caregivers should therefore receive training in understanding and supporting sexual development and behavior, comprehensive sexuality education, and related healthcare for individuals with disabilities. The policies and procedures of social agencies and healthcare delivery systems should ensure that services and benefits are provided to all persons without discrimination. Individuals with disabilities and their caregivers should have information and education about how to minimize the risk of sexual abuse and exploitation. People with physical or intellectual disabilities are mostly regarded as nonsexual by society, since sex is associated with youth and physical attractiveness and not with disability. If we accept that sexual expression is a natural and important part of human life, then the denial of sexuality for disabled persons would be to deny a basic right. There have been many barriers on sexuality over time to this population, both from workers who may be influenced by these views and from disabled people themselves in terms of gaining access to information and acceptance as sexual beings.

In relation to ID, society over time has taken the view that intellectually disabled people have no rights to pursue social and sexual relationships. There has been very little sex education for this population. Intellectually disabled people are sometimes regarded as sexually deviant, because they sometimes exhibit socially inappropriate sexual behavior. It is important for educators, particularly those involved in educational programs with disability workers or disabled people, to understand community attitudes toward disability and sexuality and the impact of these views on disabled people themselves.

Earlier Studies on Intellectual Disability and Parenthood

In her research into the marriage of persons with ID in the UK in the 1950s, Bass [2] observed that women who were sterilized succeeded more in their marriages. Due to this observation, she maintained that there should be a law to enforce the sterilization of women with ID (with their consent and that of the family), especially when there was genetic danger of giving birth to a retarded child.

In their follow-up of the marriage of one couple with ID, Bowden et al. [3] found that marital problems became worse with the birth of a child. A study of 130 persons with ID in Ireland in 1971 [4] found that only one-third of the couples were able to care for their children without outside help. Among the children of couples that did receive help, they did not find differences between these children concerning education in comparison with other children in the community and the children growing up in the home functioned better than those in institutions. They maintained that if a couple had children, but did not receive professional help, they would most likely fail. Mattinson [5], from the UK, examined 32 couples with ID living in residential care before their marriage. Children were born to 17 of these couples and 25% of all these children were placed in residential care due to their own ID.

Prevalence of Parenthood

Prevalence studies of parents with ID are hard to conduct, and information in this area is scarce. There are many reasons for this, some due to the fact that many parents are either not receiving service, some are not identified by the service system, and some are identified, but do not participate in any programs.

Some information can be found from the Arc's Department of Research [6] based on a study done by the Oregon Developmental Disabilities Council in 1989. The study identified 358 families in the state of Oregon with parents considered to have ID. Based on a 1990 Oregon population of 2,853,733, the number of parents with ID would equal 0.00013% of Oregon's general population. If these numbers reflect the general population of the USA, then 0.00013% of the US population of 249,632,692 in 1990 would equal 32,452 parents with ID, but that is probably a low estimate since many parents are not identified by the service system [6].

One national survey was conducted in Norway [7] in 1997 by sending a questionnaire out to all municipalities for the public health nurses. It showed that 23 persons with ID had given birth within the 12 months before the survey. A total of 126 children with parents with ID were identified, giving an incidence of 27 children per year and a prevalence of about 430 children under 16 years of age in this population of 3.4 million people.

The Concept of Marriage in Judaism

In the modern State of Israel, marriage is an act based on religious law or Halacha (religious Jewish law), and the rabbinate is the only established authority sanctioned to perform a marriage ceremony. In Judaism, marriage is the ideal human state of affairs and considered the basic institution established by G-d from the time of creation. In the Bible, it is clearly stated that the purposes of marriage are companionship and creation of the next generation with the following statement for companion: "It is not good that man should be alone, I will make him a help for him. . ... Therefore shall a man leave his father and his mother and shall cleave into his wife and they shall be one flesh" (Gen. 2:18, 24) and the other for creation: "Be fruitful and multiply and replenish the earth. . ..." (Gen. 1:28).

The marriage ceremony described in the Bible is referred to simply as "taking a wife" (Deut. 24:1), but from several cases (Jacob, Leah, and Rachel) it can be understood that there were socially defined rules and customs. In the Talmud (the oral law), the marriage ceremony has two parts. The first, kiddushin or erusin (betrothal), took place when the bridegroom gave any object of value (a ring, for example) to the bride and said in front of two witnesses: "With this ring you are consecrated to me according to the law of Moshe and Israel." The second stage took place at a later date (up to a year later) with the marriage proper or nisuin or the Chuppah effected after the bride was brought to the house of the groom and cohabited with him. Today in modern Israel, both the kiddushin and the Chuppah take place at the same event, usually in a wedding hall with the families from both sides and their friends. Different ethnic groups (like Sepharadim or Yemenite Jews) have variations with different traditions.

Legal Aspects of Jewish Marriage

According to the religious Jewish law, every man can marry following his "bar mitzvah" (ceremony at the age of 13 years) after which he is qualified and obligated to fulfill all the religious laws. From 0 to 13 years, he is called a minor (katan) without any legal status, but by 13 years he is called a gadol (an adult). A female is a minor until the age of 12 years, a "naarah" (an adolescent) until $12\frac{1}{2}$ years, and only afterward an adult. From 12 to $12\frac{1}{2}$ years, she will have to have the permission of her father to marry, but afterward she is considered an adult.

Child marriage as such in Jewish law is not a problem as long as the male is 13 years and the female $12\frac{1}{2}$ years old, but in modern Israel the law has been amended and a female cannot marry before the age of 17 years of age. A male who marries a female under 17 years of age will be punished by imprisonment, a fine, or both. However, district courts have jurisdiction to permit a marriage to a girl under 17 years when she has had a child or is pregnant by the male or if there are other special circumstances that permit the marriage, provided the girl is not under 16 years of age. Today this is very rare in Israel; however, with the immigration from Yemen or North Africa in the past, several cases took place.

The criterion for validity of a marriage is a minimal level of understanding (called daat kpeutot or the intellectual capacity of a 6-year-old normally developed child) and the comprehension of the act of marriage [8]. The status of a person with ID in Jewish law is complicated due to a lack of a definition in both the Bible and the Talmud [9]. The Halacha differentiates between people who have developed normally and those defined as deranged or deaf or shotah with a mental capacity disorder and thought process or behavioral process impaired [9]. The deranged can suffer from mental illness, melancholy, brain injury, or diseases of old age or any other reason, but the Halacha does not make a difference between them and does not categorize them according to etiology, but rather according to the level of functioning. Deafness was in the same category as deranged because communication was compromised.

Halacha recognizes situations in which a person functions at a level lower than "daat kpeutot," but is nevertheless capable of understanding the significance of the act of marriage. This possibility was described by Rabbi Raphael Lipman Halperin (the "Oneg YomTov," Poland, nineteenth century) and cited by Farbstein [10]:

> ... a man with a speech defect making his words extremely difficult to understand, and even people used to his company do not always understand his speech, and his mind is very weak, and does not even know how to count, he does not understand the meaning of divorce at all, and it never occurred to him to divorce, because never, since his birth, has he known that divorce exists in the world, and he does not even know anything about the Torah. And whatever he does, he does only because he has habitually seen others doing these things...

Entering into marriage for this person is valid, because we have seen that he can adopt acts that he regularly sees in his environment; this person has the legal status of one who is intelligent, because when something is explained, it makes sense to him.

In other words, the Rabbis took into account situations where people with ID may exhibit greater and lesser abilities in different areas of functioning, being very deficient in one domain while being able to understand complex actions in another. Therefore Rabbi Halperin maintained that if the person understood the meaning of being married, even if the person did not understand the ceremonial act of marriage, the act itself would be considered valid. This position has become Halacha or law.

Children

Once a Jewish man has passed "bar mitzvah," he is obliged to fulfill the command "be fruitful and multiply," but as mentioned above in modern society today, males wait a little longer in order to get married and multiply. In order to fulfill this commandment, both a male and a female child have to be born, so even after seven girls, the commandment has not been fulfilled.

So for a couple where one or both are persons with ID, there are no restrictions on having children according to Jewish law. Sterilization is another complicated matter, where Jewish law is against sterilization of men, it does not apply to women [11].

Interaction in Families with Intellectual Disability

One study conducted in Israel [12] was concerned with the lives of the families of four couples with ID. The findings were as follows:

- The effect of children on the life of the couple – This small case study [12] found that children had a negative effect on the functioning of the family. In families with one or more children, the level of positive interaction of the couple decreased, as opposed to families without children. In the families with children, there was less positive interaction on the part of the wife toward the husband and more negative responses from husband to wife when she approached him, as opposed to families without children. Interaction between parents and children was more negative in cases where there was positive interaction between the parents. Families without children exhibited a greater number of positive approaches from the wife toward the husband than in families with one child, in which the number of negative approaches and responses of husband and wife was higher. The fathers with ID could not care for their children properly and when the mothers tried to take care of their children and form positive relationships with them, then family functioning was significantly harmed. When the father with ID felt in competition with his child, he reacted with anger and acted negatively toward his wife. The wife with ID must on the one hand care for her children, but on the other she needed to maintain a normal relationship with her husband.
- The influence of several children on family life – In the families with fewer children, there were improved interactions between the couple. The number of children was related to three functions: parent relations, parent/children relations, and financial status. These functions become worse with more children. Parent relations and relations between parents and children were seen to be very clearly different between families with no children and a family with two children or more. No difference was found between families without children or with one child or more in relation to functions relating to finance, housekeeping, social life, community, and individual adaptation to the family.
- Concern for the children – There was a negative connection between concern for the children and between the two parents with ID. Deep concern for the children on the part of the mother resulted in a decrease in family function since the husband opted to stay away from the house as much as possible.
- Mental ability for parenthood – The ability of these couples to look after their children was low. They needed to depend on each other, in a childish manner, and draw much strength from each other. When a child was born to the family, they were unable to provide it with adult and responsible support that parents usually provide. The fathers, before very dependent on their wives, felt rejected and acted aggressively toward their children.
- Education worry – Education of the children (additional classes, contact with the teacher, buying books and other learning equipment) was considerably low. It was difficult for the parents to provide education and knowledge to their children, apart from the day-to-day worry of food and clothes. Parents expressed, more than once, their frustration concerning their inability to educate their children or guide their behavior and turned to the social workers and institutions to accept responsibility for the education of their children.
- Dependence on assistance from the environment and institutions – Assistance provided by the extended family created an important base for success of family

life. For families with a bad financial situation and fathers unemployed, assistance was generally provided by the wider family circle or by a support family in close contact with the couple. Sometimes, in extreme circumstances, the children were sent to residential care. This assistance from the wider family circle enabled the mother to be more available for her children. In providing assistance to the mother, the parents, brothers, or supporter decreased slightly the competition between the child and the husband. In this situation, the relations between the father and child increased significantly. The family could function better with the assistance of the extended family and various social institutions, but the extended family could not care for the children, who in most cases were cared for by strangers or referred to day care institutions. In the families where the child left the family for residential care, there came a certain amount of calm in the couple's relationship, so that the wife could devote herself to shaping her life and mutual relations with her husband and the husband could become more positive in his reactions and enjoy life again with his wife.

An obvious conclusion drawn from this small sample of four families in Israel pointed to the fact that individuals with ID can marry and live a harmonious and warm life together, but the aspect of children could add a significant factor of negative influence on the function of the family. This situation must therefore be seen as a challenge to social services to not only provide better support but also protect the children at the same time.

Discussion

In this chapter, we have discussed the attitude of Jewish law toward the marriage of persons with ID and found that there is no prevention of such a marriage. They may even have children within the framework of the law. Jewish law is more liberal than American law in this regard. The Mental Deficiency Act of 1913, as an example, made marriage illegal for persons with mental retardation everywhere in the USA [13]. This has changed and in the future we will see many more cases, even though data are scarce today. It has been estimated [13] that there are approximately 1.4 million parents with ID in the USA between the ages of 18 and 64 years with children under 18 years of age.

The main issue involved is the welfare of the children, both when we discuss children of parents with mental illness [14] or ID [15]. Data from the USA, the UK, and Australia [13] are beginning to demonstrate that parents with ID are

- overrepresented in childcare proceedings;
- less likely to have received support in their parenting;
- at greater risk to have their parental responsibility terminated on data that would never hold in a case of nondisabled parents;

- likely to have their competence as parents judged against stricter criteria or harsher standards than other parents;
- more likely to have their children removed and their parental rights terminated;
- disadvantaged in the child protection and court process by rules of evidence and procedure;
- less likely to receive support in correcting the conditions leading to termination.

And this even though we have little evidence that having parents with ID will have an adverse effect on the child. Researchers from the Sheffield Department of Sociological Studies [1] studied 30 people (16 men, 14 women), aged 16–42 years of age, who had grown up in a family with 1 parent (28 cases) with ID (usually the mother, 25 cases) with follow-up in-depth interviews. Of the 30 people, half themselves had learning difficulties, which was more than expected. None of these 30 people had had an easy childhood; 11 admitted to skipping school, 11 had been in trouble with the police (three served time in prison), 2 had attempted suicide, 11 were divorced, 16 had experienced some form of abuse, 7 presented or had overcome mental illness, and 8 suffered chronic illness. The overall findings showed that not all children were the victims of their situation and many demonstrated adaptability in coping with a life full of difficulties. There was not a direct correlation between parenting skills and child outcomes since outcome depended on more than just the parents, and it appeared that the support system had had a positive effect. These adults displayed a close relationship with their parents (especially their mother), which was the heart of their adult identity. A significant psychological aspect of couples with ID, and especially for the woman, is the need to bear a child. The woman regards a child as an emotional need, not a cognitive one; therefore, it is of more meaning than if it was a cognitive desire. For the couple, the pregnancy and birth symbolize a status of normal people; it is almost the only thing in which they can resemble normal people, thus here is a position in which they deal with an event having much decisive and existential meaning. This psychological appearance is also seen in the parents of the couple themselves. There exists an additional appearance of wishful thinking – that if their children with ID marry and bring children into the world, "then everything will be all right" and it will convey a sense of normality and approval that up until then did not exist.

Research workers and therapists working with the population of persons with ID refer to a sociopsychological appearance that they have confronted during their work with couples with ID called the "secondary gain." With marriage and childhood, all of a sudden they are interesting – with support and intervention from the community, the extended family, and social services.

In Jewish law, the "grow and multiply" command also relates to raising children and not just bringing them into the world. As for the phrase "raising children," opinions are divided, but the opinion that rules in the Jewish faith emphasizes the concern for the education of the children, not just their health and physical welfare. So in each case of a couple of persons with ID, the welfare services and providers must ask if the cognitive maturity of the couple enables them to raise their children correctly and understand their needs.

The following strategies may be useful to prevent the disadvantage and discrimination experienced by many parents with intellectual disability in the child protection and court process [16]:

- The development and implementation of a training module for child protection workers, lawyers, and judicial officers, based on up-to-date empirical research
- The development of video and accompanying plain text resources for parents with intellectual disability that explain the child protection process step by step and the rights of participants
- The development of a network of volunteers/advocates under the auspices of an independent third party to provide support to parents with intellectual disability during the child protection process
- Additional funding to support adequate legal representation of parents with intellectual disability, given that these parents require significantly more time both to be informed about the process and to provide their legal representatives with sound instruction
- A review of "expert" assessment practices and the development of guidelines which clearly specify the limitations of diagnostic–prognostic assessment and the need for functional assessment
- The development and maintenance of regional Internet web sites that provide listings of potential support services for parents with intellectual disability and their children.

It is important to relate to the each parent's individual abilities and their unique circumstances, since parents with intellectual disability are indeed suffering disadvantage and discrimination [16].

Conclusions

Jewish law has been very progressive regarding the possibility of marriage between persons with ID in contrast to American law, where this right historically had been denied because of the assumption that the children would be better off not being born or being cared for by others. In the case of such a union resulting in children, although they require some supervision, family, friends, and social welfare agencies have scrutinized these families so much they are in constant fear of their child being taken away. There is little information on the number of such cases and an overall dearth of information on the effects on the children, although one recent study from the UK has shown a varied picture of resilience and a close, warm relationship later on with the family and especially the mother.

References

1. Booth T, Booth W. Against all odds: growing up with parents who have learning difficulties. Ment Retard. 2000;38(1):1–14.
2. Bass MS. Marriage parenthood and prevention of pregnancy. Am J Ment Defic. 1963;68(3):318–33.
3. Bowden J, Spitz HH, Winters JJ Jr. Follow-up of one retarded couple's marriage. Ment Retard. 1971;9(6):42–3.
4. MacKay DN, Scally BG, Walby AL. Care of the mentally subnormal. Br J Psychiatry. 1971;119:341–47.
5. Mattinson J. Marriage and mental handicap. In: De La Cruz F, Laveck G, editors. Human sexuality and the mentally retarded. London: Butterworth; 1973. pp. 169–85.
6. Ingram D. Parents who have mental retardation. Fact Sheet. Silver Spring, MD: Arc; 1990.
7. Morch W-T, Skar J, Andersgard AB. Mentally retarded persons as parents: prevalence and the situation of their parents. Scand J Psychol. 1997;38:343–48.
8. Merrick J, Gabbay Y, Lifshitz H. Judaism and the person with intellectual disability. J Religion Disabil Health. 2001;5(2/3):49–63.
9. Lifshitz H, Merrick J. Jewish law and the definition of mental retardation: the status of people with intellectual disability within the Jewish Law in relation to the 1992 AAMR definition of mental retardation. J Religion Disabil Health. 2001;5(1):39–51.
10. Farbstein M. Legal principal and declarification of the daat concept and laws concerning the shotah. Jerusalem: Shaar Hamispat Institute; 1995 [Hebrew].
11. Jakobovits I. Jewish medical ethics. A comparative and historical study of the Jewish religious attitude to medicine and its practice. New York, NY: Bloch; 1959.
12. Levitan A. Interactions in families of mentally retarded people. Dissertation. Ramat Gan, IL: Bar-Ilan University; 1991 [Hebrew].
13. Randolph R. Information packet: parents with mental retardation and their parents. New York, NY: Hunter College School of Social Work; 2003.
14. Hetherington R, Baistow K, Katz I, Mesie J, Trowell J. The welfare of children with mentally ill parents. Learning from inter-country comparisons. Chichester: John Wiley; 2002.
15. Whitman B, Accardo P. When a parent is mentally retarded. Baltimore, MD: Paul H Brookes; 1990.
16. McConnell D, Llewellyn G. Stereotypes, parents with intellectual disability and child protection. J Soc Welf Fam Law. 2002;24(3):297–317.

Appendix A

About Michigan State University College of Human Medicine

The Department of Pediatrics and Human Development (PHD) at Michigan State University College of Human Medicine (MSUCHM) was developed in 1968 with the formation of the College of Human Medicine (CHM) at Michigan State University (MSU) in East Lansing, Michigan. It is a nationally recognized Department of PHD that involves four Michigan State University (MSU) campuses including East Lansing and Kalamazoo, Michigan. Michigan State University/Kalamazoo Center for Medical Studies (MSU/KCMS) is a nationally recognized university/community-based residency program with over 170 residents in over 12 disciplines including pediatrics that is located in Kalamazoo, Michigan, USA.

Mission and Service

The MSUCHM PHD has a unique balance between behavioral science, basic biological research, and clinical pediatrics. The department has a commitment to a comprehensive approach to the health and development of the child, adolescent, and the family. PHD has a unique blend of community-integrated medical training centers with a unified educational mission that serves medical students, pediatric residents, and four communities in Michigan, USA.

The mission is to "advance the healthy development and well-being of children and adolescents through innovative medical education, research, clinical care, and advocacy, emphasizing community-based partnerships." To this end, the department offers a broad range of clinical and laboratory services to the children and adolescents of Michigan. PHD draws on the talents of over 100 faculty members and over 500 volunteer teaching faculty members. The mission of the Kalamazoo, Michigan program (MSU/KCMS Pediatrics Program) is to train both medical students in their 3rd and 4th year as well as many residents in the field of pediatrics. MSU/KCMS Pediatrics is a fully accredited, 3-year program preparing physicians for board certification in pediatrics.

D.R. Patel et al. (eds.), *Neurodevelopmental Disabilities*,
DOI 10.1007/978-94-007-0627-9, © Springer Science+Business Media B.V. 2011

Values of MSU/KCMS include compassionate service, leadership training, commitment to lifelong learning, emphasis on teamwork, and commitment to excellence in health care. Trainees at MSU/KCMS become skilled at providing patient care that is compassionate, appropriate, and effective for the treatment of health problems and the promotion of health. They learn to demonstrate interpersonal and communication skills that result in the effective exchange of information and collaboration with patients, their families, and health professionals. They are taught to develop a commitment to carrying out professional responsibilities and an adherence to ethical principles throughout their training with a goal of these values becoming a lifelong habit that reveals professional compassion, integrity, and respect for others. Kalamazoo is the home of the Kalamazoo Promise, a truly unique program that guarantees college education for students who graduate from the Kalamazoo public schools.

Research Activities

MSU/KCMS has a variety of research projects in adolescent medicine, neurobehavioral pediatrics, adolescent gynecology, pediatric diabetes mellitus, asthma, cystic fibrosis, and pediatric oncology. MSU/KCMS Pediatrics is involved in a number of studies with the Children's Oncology Group in the United States.

MSU/KCMS Pediatrics has recently published a number of medical textbooks: *Essential Adolescent Medicine* (McGraw-Hill Medical Publishers), *The Pediatric Diagnostic Examination* (McGraw-Hill), *Pediatric and Adolescent Psychopharmacology* (Cambridge University Press), *Behavioral Pediatrics*, 2nd edition (iUniverse Publishers in New York and Lincoln, Nebraska), and *Pediatric Practice: Sports Medicine* (McGraw-Hill).

MSU/KCMS Pediatrics has edited a number of journal issues published by Elsevier Publishers covering pulmonology (*State of the Art Reviews: Adolescent Medicine – AM:STARS*), genetic disorders in adolescents (*AM:STARS*), neurologic/neurodevelopmental disorders (*AM:STARS*), behavioral pediatrics (*Pediatric Clinics of North America*), nephrologic disorders in adolescents (*AM:STARS*), college health (*Pediatric Clinics of North America*), adolescent medicine (*Primary Care: Clinics in Office Practice*), behavioral pediatrics in children and adolescents (*Primary Care: Clinics in Office Practice*), and developmental disabilities (*Pediatric Clinics of North America*). The department has also edited a journal issue on musculoskeletal disorders in children and adolescents for the American Academy of Pediatrics (*AM:STARS*).

The department has developed academic ties with a variety of international medical centers and organizations, including the Queen Elizabeth Hospital in Hong Kong, National Taiwan University Hospital (Taipei, Taiwan), Indian Academy of Pediatrics (New Delhi, India), and the University of Athens Children's Hospital (First and Second Departments of Paediatrics) in Athens, Greece.

Appendix B

About Division of Adolescent Medicine University of Kentucky

The division of adolescent medicine was founded in 1998 to provide state-of-the-art care for adolescent patients from all areas of the commonwealth of Kentucky, to serve as a statewide resource for education and training for local providers on adolescent issues, to study specific factors on the local level affecting youth in the state, to help teach medical students and residents, and to provide community service to help improve teen future in the commonwealth.

The division provides comprehensive, holistic team approach to adolescents, where teens receive all aspects of care from mental health to routine care from a team of professionals including physicians, mental health providers, social workers, nutritionists, and nursing staff. One unique program within the division is the Young Parent Program, where pregnant teens are cared for throughout pregnancy, then they and their babies are cared for together in the program.

The division is active in research with more than 10 peer-reviewed articles published each year as well as several books and special journal editions.

In the community, the program has founded several grass route programs to help prevent youth suicide, teen pregnancy, accidental death, and substance abuse among adolescents in Kentucky.

The division has provided more than 300 lectures, workshops, media events, and teaching for community providers, parents, teachers, and school counselors. It also provides advocacy work on behalf of teens with active work at the state legislative and executive government as well as local governments to help improve the lives of teens.

Collaborations

The division collaborates locally with school boards, youth service centers, state and local governments, other universities and child advocacy centers as well as with regional adolescent medicine programs.

It also collaborates internationally with the Institute for Child Health and Human Development in Israel, the Division of Adolescent Medicine at Santa Casa

University, Brazil, Quality of Life Research Center and Nordic School of Holistic Health, Copenhagen, Denmark, and the Department of Applied Social Sciences, Hong Kong Polytechnic University, Hong Kong.

The Vision

The vision of the Division of Adolescent Medicine is to improve the health and long-term well-being of Kentucky youth to grow into productive adults. We also envision global work to help positive youth development worldwide.

Target Areas of Interests

The interest areas of the division are all aspects of youth development and adolescent health with focus on prevention and community involvement in collaborations at the local, national, and global level with programs having the same goal.

Appendix C

About National Institute of Child Health and Human Development, Jerusalem, Israel

The National Institute of Child Health and Human Development (NICHD) in Israel was established in 1998 as a virtual institute under the auspices of the medical director, Ministry of Social Affairs and Social Services in order to function as the research arm for the Office of the Medical Director. In 1998 the National Council for Child Health and Pediatrics, Ministry of Health, and in 1999 the Director General and Deputy Director General of the Ministry of Health endorsed the establishment of the NICHD.

Mission

The mission of a National Institute for Child Health and Human Development in Israel is to provide an academic focal point for the scholarly interdisciplinary study of child life, health, public health, welfare, disability, rehabilitation, intellectual disability, and related aspects of human development. This mission includes research, teaching, clinical work, information, and public service activities in the field of child health and human development.

Service and Academic Activities

Over the years, many activities became focused in the south of Israel due to collaboration with various professionals at the Faculty of Health Sciences (FOHS) at the Ben Gurion University of the Negev (BGU). Since 2000 an affiliation with the Zusman Child Development Center at the Pediatric Division of Soroka University Medical Center has resulted in collaboration around the establishment of the Down Syndrome Clinic at that center. In 2002 a full course on "disability" was established at the Recanati School for Allied Professions in the Community, FOHS, BGU, and in 2005 collaboration was started with the Primary Care Unit of the faculty and disability became part of the master of public health course on "Children and Society." In the academic year 2005–2006 a one semester course on "Aging with Disability" was started as part of the master of science program in gerontology in our collaboration with the Center for Multidisciplinary Research in Aging.

Research Activities

The affiliated staff have over the years published work from projects and research activities in this national and international collaboration. In the year 2000 the *International Journal of Adolescent Medicine and Health*, in 2005 the *International Journal on Disability and Human Development* of Freund Publishing House (London and Tel Aviv), in the year 2003 the *TSW—Child Health and Human Development*, and in 2006 the *TSW—Holistic Health and Medicine of the Scientific World Journal* (New York and Kirkkonummi, Finland), all peer-reviewed international journals were affiliated with the National Institute of Child Health and Human Development. From 2008 also the *International Journal of Child Health and Human Development* (Nova Science, New York), the *International Journal of Child and Adolescent Health* (Nova Science), and the *Journal of Pain Management* (Nova Science) affiliated and from 2009 the *International Public Health Journal* (Nova Science) and *Journal of Alternative Medicine Research* (Nova Science).

National Collaborations

Nationally the NICHD works in collaboration with the Faculty of Health Sciences, Ben Gurion University of the Negev; Department of Physical Therapy, Sackler School of Medicine, Tel Aviv University; Autism Center, Assaf HaRofeh Medical Center; National Rett and PKU Centers at Chaim Sheba Medical Center, Tel HaShomer; Department of Physiotherapy, Haifa University; Department of Education, Bar Ilan University, Ramat Gan, Faculty of Social Sciences and Health Sciences; College of Judea and Samaria in Ariel and recently also collaborations has been established with the Division of Pediatrics at Hadassah, Center for Pediatric Chronic Illness, Har HaZofim in Jerusalem.

International Collaborations

Internationally with the Department of Disability and Human Development, College of Applied Health Sciences, University of Illinois at Chicago; Strong Center for Developmental Disabilities, Golisano Children's Hospital at Strong, University of Rochester School of Medicine and Dentistry, New York; Centre on Intellectual Disabilities, University of Albany, New York; Centre for Chronic Disease Prevention and Control, Health Canada, Ottawa; Chandler Medical Center and Children's Hospital, Kentucky Children's Hospital, Section of Adolescent Medicine, University of Kentucky, Lexington; Chronic Disease Prevention and Control Research Center, Baylor College of Medicine, Houston, Texas; Division of Neuroscience, Department of Psychiatry, Columbia University, New York; Institute for the Study of Disadvantage and Disability, Atlanta; Center for Autism and Related Disorders, Department Psychiatry, Children's Hospital Boston, Boston; Department of Paediatrics, Child Health and Adolescent Medicine, Children's Hospital at Westmead, Westmead, Australia; International Centre for the Study of Occupational and Mental Health, Düsseldorf, Germany; Centre for Advanced Studies in Nursing, Department of General Practice and Primary Care, University of Aberdeen, Aberdeen, United Kingdom; Quality of Life Research Center, Copenhagen, Denmark; Nordic School of Public Health, Gottenburg, Sweden; Scandinavian Institute of Quality of Working Life, Oslo, Norway; Centre for Quality of Life of the Hong Kong Institute of Asia-Pacific Studies and School of Social Work, Chinese University, Hong Kong.

Targets

Our focus is on research, international collaborations, clinical work, teaching and policy in health, disability and human development and to establish the NICHD as a permanent institute at one of the residential care centers for persons with intellectual disability in Israel in order to conduct model research and together with the four university schools of public health/medicine in Israel establish a national master and doctoral program in disability and human development at the institute to secure the next generation of professionals working in this often non-prestigious/low-status field of work.

Index